BSAVA Manual of Canine and Feline Rehabilitation, Supportive and Palliative Care:
Case Studies in Patient Management

Editors:
Samantha Lindley
BVSc MRCVS

Honorary Clinical Lecturer, Glasgow University Veterinary School
461 Bearsden Road, Bearsden, Glasgow G61 1QH, UK

and
Penny Watson
MA VetMD CertVR DSAM DipECVIM MRCVS

Queen's Veterinary School Hospital, University of Cambridge,
Madingley Road, Cambridge CB3 OES

Published by:

British Small Animal Veterinary Association
Woodrow House, 1 Telford Way, Waterwells
Business Park, Quedgeley, Gloucester GL2 2AB

A Company Limited by Guarantee in England.
Registered Company No. 2837793.
Registered as a Charity.

First published 2010
Reprinted 2018, 2021, 2023
Copyright © 2023 BSAVA

Illustrations 2.2 (parts), 5.7, 9.5a, 9.24, 10.2, 10.3, 11.1, 11.2 were drawn
by S.J. Elmhurst BA Hons (www.livingart.org.uk) and are printed with her
permission.

A catalogue record for this book is available from the British Library.

ISBN 978 1 905319 20 6

The publishers, editors and contributors cannot take responsibility for
information provided on dosages and methods of application of drugs
mentioned or referred to in this publication. Details of this kind must be
verified in each case by individual users from up to date literature published
by the manufacturers or suppliers of those drugs. Veterinary surgeons
are reminded that in each case they must follow all appropriate national
legislation and regulations (for example, in the United Kingdom, the
prescribing cascade) from time to time in force.

Printed in the UK by Severn Print, Gloucester GL2 5EU – a carbon neutral printer
Printed on ECF paper made from sustainable forests

18253PUBS23

Titles in the BSAVA Manuals series:

For further information on these and all BSAVA publications, please visit our website: **www.bsava.com**

Contents

Part 2: Rehabilitation, supportive and palliative care in practice: case studies

A variety of case scenarios in dogs and cats to illustrate the considerations to be made and the options available within a specific clinical setting. Information relating to the rehabilitation and palliation of each condition has been contributed to each case by the authors in the first part of this Manual.

Contributors

Rachel Casey BVMS PhD DipECVBM-CA Dip(AS)CABC CCAB ILTM MRCVS
RCVS and European Specialist in Veterinary Behavioural Medicine
Senior Lecturer in Companion Animal Behaviour and Welfare, School of Clinical Veterinary Science,
University of Bristol, Langford, Bristol BS40 5DU

Daniel L. Chan DVM MRCVS
The Royal Veterinary College, University of London, Hawkshead Lane, Hatfield, Herts AL9 7TA

Clive Elwood MA VetMB MSc PhD CertSAC DipACVIM DipECVIM-CA MRCVS
RCVS and European Specialist in Small Animal Medicine
Managing Director, Davies Veterinary Specialists, Manor Farm Business Park, Higham Gobion,
Hitchin, Herts SG5 3HR

Alex German BVSc PhD CertSAM DipECVIM-CA MRCVS
RCVS and European Specialist in Small Animal Medicine
Royal Canin Senior Lecturer in Small Animal Medicine, School of Veterinary Science,
University of Liverpool, Leahurst Campus, Chester High Road, Neston, Wirral CH64 7TE

Hilary A. Jackson BVM&S DVD DipACVD MRCVS
Dermatology Referral Services, Glasgow
Honorary Teacher at University of Glasgow Veterinary School

Melissa Java VMD DipACVECC
Center for Animal Referral and Emergency Services (CARES), 2010 Cabot Boulevard West,
Suite D, Langhorne, PA 19047, USA

Lesley King † MVB DipACVECC DipACVIM DipECVIM-CA
School of Veterinary Medicine, University of Pennsylvania, 3900 Delancey St, Philadelphia,
PA 19104, USA

Sorrel Langley-Hobbs MA BVetMed DSAS(O) DipECVS MRCVS
European Specialist in Small Animal Surgery
University Surgeon, Head of Small Animal Surgery, Department of Veterinary Medicine,
University of Cambridge, Madingley Road, Cambridge CB3 0ES

Karla Lee MA VetMB PhD CertSAS DipECVS MRCVS
European Specialist in Small Animal Surgery
Lecturer in Small Animal Surgery, The Royal Veterinary College, University of London,
Hawkshead Lane, Hatfield, Hertfordshire AL9 7TA

Samantha Lindley BVSc MRCVS
Honorary Clinical Lecturer, Glasgow University Veterinary School, 461 Bearsden Road,
Bearsden, Glasgow G61 1QH

Rachel Lumbis RVN BSc(Hons) PGCert(MedEd) CertSAN FHEA
Department of Veterinary Clinical Sciences, The Royal Veterinary College, University of London,
Hawkshead Lane, Hatfield, Herts, AL9 7TA

Natasha Olby VetMB PhD DipACVIM (Neurology) MRCVS
Department of Clinical Sciences, North Carolina State University, 4700 Hillsborough Street, Raleigh, NC 27606, USA

Gerry Polton MA VetMB MSc(Clin Onc) MRCVS
Head of Oncology, North Downs Specialist Referrals, Friesian Building 3&4, Brewer Street Dairy Business Park, Brewer Street, Bletchingley, Surrey RH1 4QP

Chris Seymour MA VetMB DVA DipECVAA MRCVS
Department of Veterinary Clinical Sciences, The Royal Veterinary College, University of London, Hawkshead Lane, Hatfield, Herts AL9 7TA

Brian J. Sharp MSc(VetPhys) BSc(Phys) BSc(Biol) PGCE PGDipHealthEd MCSP HPCReg ACPAT
Veterinary Physiotherapist, The Royal Veterinary College, University of London, Hawkshead Lane, Hatfield, Herts, AL9 7TA

Holly Smith RVN DipAVN(Surgical)
The Royal Veterinary College, University of London, Hawkshead Lane, Hatfield, Herts AL9 7TA

Peter Southerden BVSc MBA MRCVS
Eastcott Veterinary Hospital, 59 Bath Road, Swindon SN1 4AU

Polly Taylor MA VetMB PhD DVA DipECVAA MRCA MRCVS
European Veterinary Specialist in Anaesthesia
Independent Consultant in Veterinary Anaesthesia, Taylor Monroe Gravel Head Farm, Downham Common, Little Downham, Nr Ely, Cambs CB6 2TY

Penny Watson MA VetMD CertVR DSAM DipECVIM MRCVS
Bunning–Iams Senior Lecturer in Small Animal Medicine, Queen's Veterinary School Hospital, University of Cambridge, Madingley Road, Cambridge CB3 0ES

David L. Williams MA VetMB PhD CertVOphthal FRCVS
Associate Lecturer in Veterinary Ophthalmology, Queen's Veterinary School Hospital, University of Cambridge, Madingley Road, Cambridge CB3 0ES

Ruth Willis BVM&S DVC MRCVS, RCVS
RCVS Recognised Specialist in Cardiology
Holter Monitoring Service, 3 Kirkland Avenue, Blanefield, Glasgow G63 9BY

Foreword

Our abilities as veterinarians working in the first opinion or specialist setting are continually improving – we are increasingly better at diagnosing, treating and saving the pets entrusted to our care. However, to 'just fix' the obvious problem (say, cruciate rupture in a young dog) often results in sub-optimal outcome. At the other end of the spectrum, older patients often have perturbations of multiple systems and there is no 'easy fix'. In both these scenarios, health and function are optimized by a comprehensive approach to rehabilitation supportive and palliative care. Unique to the veterinary literature, this manual provides the practical knowledge to achieve this.

This *BSAVA Manual of Canine and Feline Rehabilitation, Supportive and Palliative Care* does an excellent job of explaining and showing how patient care can be optimized across these very different areas of pet health and wellness. The manual is truly unique – it brings together the principles of pain management, nutrition, physical therapies, rehabilitation and acupuncture and shows the readers how these can all be practically used to support the whole spectrum of veterinary patients. There is no other book that does this, and BSAVA is to be congratulated for supporting the development of this manual.

The international author list features well respected veterinarians and associated professionals, many at the top of their respective fields, all of whom bring their vast practical experience to this manual.

This is a manual that should be in every practice, and be read and referred to by every member of the practice team. It is not an overstatement to say it should form the basis of how patients are cared for, both within the practice and in the home environment.

Congratulations to Samantha Lindley and Penny Watson on having the vision to create this unique manual, and to BSAVA for supporting and driving its production.

B. Duncan X. Lascelles BSc BVSc PhD CVertVA DSAS(ST) DipECVS DipACVS MRCVS
North Carolina State University College of Veterinary Medicine
May 2010

Preface

Major advances in veterinary practice over the last 20–30 years, mirroring advances in human medicine, mean that we are now sufficiently skilled to have a growing population of companion animals undergoing previously uncontemplated surgical, medical, chemotherapeutic and radiotherapeutic treatments, and surviving what would, in the past, have been rapidly fatal conditions. These treatments are driven both by scientific advances and by owner demands. Owners have increasing expectations for intricate treatments, coupled with an increasing desire for increased quality *and* quantity of life for their pets.

All this is cause for celebration, but there are also causes for concern:

- After major spinal, soft tissue and orthopaedic surgery the need for rehabilitative medicine is great, but it is not a subject generally covered in the veterinary curriculum and the tendency is for it to be seen as less important than the procedures that indicate its use
- Chronic conditions such as musculoskeletal pain, chronic visceral disease and dermatological disease can cause prolonged suffering but can be frustrating to treat, leaving the veterinary team and the owners alike feeling helpless.

This manual is aimed at the whole veterinary team, drawing on all their skills to help patients achieve as full as possible function and quality of life after surgery, trauma or disease, and to manage chronic conditions effectively for the benefit of animal, owner and the practice team. The emphasis in this book is on evidence-based veterinary medicine. Of course, there remain large areas of veterinary medicine where evidence is poor and/or anecdotal; but there are also increasing numbers of studies being published that support the efficacy of nutritional, analgesic and physical therapies in the rehabilitation and palliation of our patients. With this in mind, this Manual focuses on supportive treatments with evidence of efficacy in human and, often, veterinary patients. Other, untested, more 'alternative', therapies have been left to other books.

While principles are outlined in the early chapters, the case-based scenarios form the core of this novel Manual. A unique integrated approach was used to generate these cases: one author was a 'mini-editor' for the chapter, defining the focus and important types of cases within their discipline, aiming to cover as broad a range of problems as possible. The expert authors in pain control, nutrition, behaviour, physical therapies and nursing then contributed to case templates, replicating an ideal 'team-based' approach to a case within the veterinary practice. For the editors, this book is the equivalent of stopping our colleagues in the corridor, or popping our heads around the office door, and asking them for their input on a particularly challenging case.

If you, as a member of the practice team, had easy access to experts in each field within palliative and rehabilitative care, you would be able to construct a complete plan of care for your patient, utilizing the skills within the practice and providing practical support for the owner. This book is your access to that expertise.

We have tried to provide cases that cover as many as possible of the issues raised in real life. This includes complications from patient temperament and body condition score, as well as concurrent disease. We hope that for most cases requiring rehabilitative and palliative care in the practice a similar example can be found here. Whilst it is expected that the practice team will have expertise and knowledge about the care of their patient, it is unlikely that they will have considered every aspect for every case. Therefore, as well as offering specific suggestions, each case will act as a checklist for the practice: when cases are very involved it is easy to miss out one of the approaches, such as considerations of fear and stress, or what the owner can do to stay more involved. Covering each aspect will give a truly integrated (i.e. 'holistic' in its true sense) approach to every patient.

Every day the veterinary practice team has to deal with some or all of the aspects covered within these pages. To some extent the broad concept of this book is something with which we are all familiar, but this is the first time that an attempt has been made to draw all the threads together.

This is a new venture for the BSAVA Manual series and has been a uniquely challenging book to edit. We would never have managed it without the patient help of all our authors and of the publications staff at Woodrow House, coping admirably with the multiple sections and repeated bouncing of cases between people. We would like to thank ALL the contributors and ALL those people who have provided photographs to help illustrate the case studies, as well as our colleagues who have helped us with ideas and suggestions. We have been really encouraged by everyone's enthusiasm and willingness to help. Last, but not least, we would like to thank our families for help with the photographs and for endless moral support.

We hope that you will find this book a constant source of practical information and help for your patients and all your team and dip in and out of it every day.

Enjoy it!

Samantha Lindley
Penny Watson
June 2010

Introduction

Samantha Lindley and Penny Watson

Supportive care in veterinary practice

The supportive patient care described in this Manual encompasses nursing, fluid and analgesic therapy, nutrition and physical therapies that are administered to the animal within the veterinary practice and at home, and which aid the patient's recovery and return to function. The case studies presented cover a wide variety of scenarios, from acute (often surgical) conditions that require careful support and rehabilitation, to chronic unresolving conditions where the quality and quantity of life of the patient can be considerably improved by careful palliation.

Rehabilitation

Rehabilitation is defined as a return to function. Although this definition appears clear, function will mean different things to different individuals.

For example, salvage surgery on a joint may return a dog to 'normal function' as a pet, but if the owner's aspirations were for an agility champion then the procedure and rehabilitation will be perceived by the owner to have failed. If the dog has a high drive for extensive running and exercise but cannot achieve this without a degree of discomfort and has to be restricted, then what is the value of rehabilitation? It could be argued that the owner had unrealistic expectations; it is vital to communicate with the owner about their expectations and expected outcomes at the outset. Results of force plate analysis (see Chapter 9) after different types of cruciate repair may be very informative to the veterinary surgeon, but what the owner wants to know is whether their pet will be able to return to his/her previous level of activity or exercise, whatever that may be. Also, for the dog, couldn't more to be done to limit his/her frustration?

For many patients, rehabilitation may be barely considered:

- A cat with a traumatic fracture is admitted, repaired and sent home. All being well, healing occurs and rehabilitation is achieved. Or is it? Is the cat using his/her repaired limb as well as he/she ought; if not, is this making the cat vulnerable to further injuries in the future? If the cat is not using the limb properly, is this because of continuing pain or reduced function, or both; and how can we tell?

- A dog with acute pancreatitis is treated with fluid therapy and analgesia while hospitalized, and sent home alive – to everyone's relief. But, is any consideration given to the short-, medium- and long-term dietary, analgesic and other needs of the dog when he/she is back at home, to stop him/her suffering from recurrent pancreatitis and significant postprandial pain?

The aims of rehabilitation are:

- To limit pain
- To return the animal to normal function where possible
- To reduce recovery times.

Rehabilitation requires patience and time. Realistic timelines need to be set, so that the practice and the owner can assess progress and identify when this is too slow or inadequate. Realistic outcome measures need to be set and there should, ideally, be input as appropriate from physical therapists, nurses and nutritionists, as well as veterinary surgeons and owners.

Palliation

The term 'palliative medicine' in the human field has become almost synonymous with cancer care, but true palliation is what most veterinary practices offer their patients most of the time. Palliative care aims to treat the clinical signs of a disease, without necessarily effecting a cure. It is therefore relevant for all chronic diseases, whether ultimately curable or not. For example, many dogs with chronic congestive heart failure and cats with chronic renal failure are treated palliatively for months to years, without any real expectation of a 'cure'. The dietary and therapeutic management of these animals can make a very real difference to their quality of life and also to their lifespan, such as in the well documented examples of extended life expectancy with dietary management of chronic renal disease in dogs and cats (see Chapter 5) or with the use of certain drugs in canine congestive heart failure. Likewise, chemotherapy and/or radiotherapy for many animals with malignant tumours can result in a significant period of remission, with return to normal or near-normal function, even if eventually the tumour recurs.

Perhaps the most common example of palliative care in veterinary medicine is the treatment of canine and feline osteoarthritis. As yet, there is no cure for osteoarthritis, but it can be managed well in many cases – to improve the patient's mobility and quality of life and, ultimately, to prolong the patient's life by avoiding euthanasia of an 'unacceptably crippled' animal. Management relies on accurately assessing the current problems of the patient, devising a plan to cover all essential aspects of palliation, and responding quickly to any changes in the animal's condition (e.g. an acute flare-up; see Chapter 3). Most veterinary surgeons do not think of this treatment as 'palliative care', but it is exactly this. Chronic skin conditions, as well as some chronic gastrointestinal, pancreatic and urinary tract diseases, are also managed with palliative care.

What rehabilitation and palliation mean to the patient

The main concern of all supportive care is clearly the welfare and quality of life of the patient. Minimizing pain, discomfort and stress, and optimizing return to function are the central aims.

Acute and chronic pain cause very similar physiological changes to those caused by acute and chronic stress. Diseases that cause pain and discomfort therefore not only have an immediate effect on the patient (feeling unwell) but also have potential long-term effects on the body as a whole. Itch, pain and disturbed urinary/gastrointestinal tract function may all disturb the quality of sleep. Reduction in sleep quality causes increases in anxiety, myalgia and emotional disturbances, which in turn impact on wellbeing and disease. Reducing acute and chronic pain, stress and conflict are key aims for our patients and are therefore considered first in Part 1 and and in individual cases in Part 2.

Chronic disease also impacts on the patient when the management restricts what he/she can do: play, exercise, eating, climbing up high to attain safety or comfort, and mental stimulation. If management can be improved and resources replaced, we are not only optimizing these factors for the patient but arguably and literally 'taking their mind off' the way the disease makes them feel (see Chapter 3).

What rehabilitation and palliation mean to the owner

The owner has a very important role to play in assisting with the rehabilitation and palliative care of their pet.

In the more short-term stages of recovery, when the animal is being treated in the practice, the owner has to understand, and be committed to, the treatment being undertaken – whether it is complex spinal or orthopaedic surgery, or intensive care of a dog with acute visceral disease. If the owner is not convinced that the animal is pain-free and stress-free, they may elect (understandably) for early euthanasia

rather than prolonged treatment. Financial considerations may also affect the amount of treatment to which they will agree.

In the longer term, the owner plays a central role in rehabilitation and palliation at home. The owner knows their pet best and so is most qualified to assess his/her progress and 'quality of life' (see below). In addition, the owner's help and commitment to physical and nutritional therapies is vital for their successful delivery.

Owners of patients with chronic disease often have more than their pet's problems to deal with. Any feelings of lack of control over the problem cause frustration, but often also drive them to seek answers elsewhere. Sometimes, searching for solutions from less orthodox sources brings these owners into conflict with the practice. Members of the practice team may feel that this represents a lack of trust in their professional skills or may become irritated at the alternative theories reported to them by the client. It is important to sympathize as much as possible with the position of the client and to keep an open mind about some of the therapies they want to discuss. Some therapies with implausible sounding mechanisms may achieve effects in other ways (see Chapter 8), so it is worth considering these before dismissing the intervention as 'rubbish' and risking offending and alienating the client. If the owner is seeking help from an alternative therapist, then communication between the veterinary surgeon and the therapist is also essential. The main rules of thumb to guide practice advice are:

- Is the 'alternative' therapy *safe* (not whether it is effective, since that information is generally not available)?
- Is the veterinary diagnosis being undermined or contradicted?

For example, it is clear that some Chinese and other herbal medicines will have potentially toxic effects in small animals (Ooms *et al.*, 2001; Ernst *et al.* 2006), so it is important to be aware as much as possible of all alternative dietary and other therapies the owner is accessing outside the practice. This information will only be readily divulged by an owner who trusts their veterinary surgeon, so building trust and effective communication with the client and avoiding a judgemental attitude is very important.

Owners often have strong views about feeding their animals and about dietary supplements. Giving tit-bits and the pet's feeding behaviour play a key role in the human–companion animal bond. However, as described in more detail in Chapter 6, obesity is very common in dogs and increasingly common in cats, and is a significant contributor to many chronic diseases. The veterinary surgeon or veterinary nurse will not be successful in persuading the owner to undertake an effective weight loss programme for their pet unless they communicate effectively and sympathetically in a non-judgemental way. If they do not, then the veterinary professionals will be perceived as interfering in the owner's bond with their animal in an unacceptable way.

Giving owners a sense of control over their patient's problem can be useful, if not imperative, in maintaining compliance and keeping them loyal to the practice approach. This includes consideration of what the owners can do themselves, but also how treatment protocols may affect the animals and their quality of life. Chapters 3 and 4 and the case examples in Part 2 of this Manual provide guidance and ideas about this area of management.

What palliation and rehabilitation mean to the veterinary practice

This book is aimed at the whole veterinary practice team. Most of the approaches discussed are relatively complex and potentially prolonged for the owner, patient and practice. Veterinary, nursing and reception staff need to be aware of the issues involved and that more can often be done to improve the animal's welfare and owner's sense of support from the practice. Good medicine, surgery and supportive care are good business: an integrated approach to these challenging cases will improve both client and practice satisfaction, rewarding work well done.

Chronic disease is difficult to deal with for patient, owner and practice. Chronic disease rarely lends itself to dramatic recoveries or miracle cures and is therefore, at the most basic level of human nature, potentially unrewarding as well as frustrating. Rewards are what keep people going, maintaining an interest in work and patients, and those rewards are usually far less tangible than monetary considerations. Evidence shows that events associated with strong emotions, such as a tremendously grateful and effusive client, enter our long-term memory as well as releasing mood-enhancing chemicals in our brains that drive us to look for more such experiences (Hamann *et al.*, 1999). Grey Mondays with ambivalent clients whose pets have a chronic disease that hasn't responded noticeably to treatment reinforce neither of these systems. Such cases then become associated with frustration and difficulty; it is all too easy to look for someone to blame for the lack of progress. Perhaps the owner is not complying as well as they ought; or perhaps the animal's illness is being used as an attention-seeking device.

Treatment and palliation of chronic diseases (such as osteoarthritis, cancer, feline lower urinary tract disease and chronic gastrointestinal diseases) require commitment from the owner and veterinary team, and constant communication and adaptation of diet and therapy as necessary. This is the stuff that day-to-day veterinary practice is made of: chronic, sometimes relapsing, sometimes refractory, diseases that can be frustrating to treat. However, those patients with chronic disease are the ones that keep returning to the practice and are on long-term medication and dietary modification. If palliation is achieved properly, sensitively and effectively for these patients, there are clear benefits for them, the owner and the practice. If palliation is not achieved, the owner may go elsewhere to seek better treatment (either another veterinary practice or 'alternative' therapies) or may, ultimately, seek euthanasia of their pet to alleviate his/her suffering, leaving both themselves and the veterinary practice team upset and frustrated. Euthanasia of a cat for recurrent, refractory inappropriate urination is not an uncommon occurrence – how much better to have been able to deal with the problem effectively to everyone's satisfaction.

Record keeping is an important, though often neglected, part of the process of client communication and supportive care of the patient, and is stressed at various points in this Manual. Keeping records of phone and verbal conversations and advice given to the owner, and keeping a kennel-side record of nutritional intake, defecation and urination, as well as treatments and fluid therapies, are essential parts of effective supportive care and communication.

Facilitating communication: an advocate for every patient?

One of the big challenges associated with complex and chronic conditions is ensuring that the owner can effectively communicate their worries and concerns to the practice and receive timely and individualized advice. By the very nature of these problems, information coming from the practice may be varied and delivered by different practice members at different times. Indeed, this Manual encourages all relevant members of the practice to be involved in using their own individual skills, but the danger for miscommunication here is obvious. One way to ensure effective communication and individual care is to appoint an *advocate* for each patient within the practice. This is the person to whom the owner can directly address their concerns and questions and who can then contact the relevant members of the team for their advice and input. The advocate may be the primary veterinary surgeon responsible for the case management, a veterinary nurse caring for the animal in the kennels, or another individual. If an owner is worried that their cat's homecare arrangements do not fit in with that individual's lifestyle, the advocate can approach the member of staff skilled in behavioural therapy to contact the owner and modify this. If the owner feels that they have somewhat fallen between two stools between the surgeon and the physician, the advocate can work to obtain a consensus between these two before passing on the advice to the owner. It is a responsible job but one that will be appreciated by owners, who often feel that there are so many different people dealing with their pet that they are not sure to whom they should be addressing their questions.

As far as the practice team approach is concerned, this role of advocate gives a special responsibility and sense of overall fulfillment, since every aspect of the patient's care is known to this person. In the busy day-to-day commitments of the veterinary practice, there will be one person flagging up the concerns and needs of each complex patient, rather than relying on the owner's personality to get things done. Not only will this be best for each patient's care, but will improve the sense of satisfaction and bonding with the practice.

The ethics of rehabilitation and palliative care

Just because we can do all this – should we?

Some of the techniques and cases described in this Manual may give rise to a certain amount of disquiet and debate amongst some practice members. There is much that can be achieved now in veterinary medicine; we are skilled at keeping patients alive and putting them back together after the ravages of trauma and disease. Owners themselves are often the means by which some of these efforts are curtailed, deciding that their pet's particular temperament is not suitable for prolonged therapy. Yet owners may feel guilty because the opportunity to prolong life is available but they are worried about the financial cost to themselves and the emotional (in the sense of suffering) cost to their pet.

Examples of chronic disease where such conflicts arise are chronic musculoskeletal and slowly degenerative spinal problems. Cats and dogs do not die of chronic muscular and joint pain, and it seems that they are now kept alive by our skills as physicians (providing optimum diets, avoiding inappropriate medications, identifying and treating life-threatening disease) to the point where the dramatic decision to end life (because of organ failure) is now often removed from the owner. Watching these animals become slightly more infirm, slightly more in pain and slightly less able to cope, month after month, becomes a source of very real anxiety to the owner, because they don't know when the situation will become unbearable for their pet and how they will be able to tell when it does. In reality, despite the concern of the owner, the final decision is often very obvious and much more so than they thought it would be, but that does not remove the preceding months of anxiety.

These concerns are not confined to owners of animals with chronic conditions. A dog with a serious medical disease, such as severe acute pancreatitis or neurological disease requiring brain or spinal cord surgery, may be kept alive in the intensive care unit with extensive monitoring and support, yet a limited chance of survival. This type of case often causes disquiet amongst the nursing staff as well as the owner. Questions such as 'Is it fair to do this?' or 'Isn't it time to euthanase this patient?' are often thought or voiced. The fundamental consideration in all cases must be the animal's quality of life (see below for discussion of assessment of quality of life) and welfare. The patient with acute pancreatitis can be nursed, provided pain is adequately controlled and that there is at least a realistic chance of recovery. While some members of the veterinary team have this expectation and knowledge, others may worry about the animal's quality of life and the likely outcome, and carry the belief that the case is 'hopeless'. Regular communication between members of the practice team is therefore important. Practice meetings should be arranged to discuss any critical or controversial inpatients, to allow all members of the practice to discuss and express their concerns, and for the team to reach a consensus about the way forward.

How do we decide between treatment and euthanasia?

As veterinary surgeons, we have the ability and responsibility to help owners make the choice between treatment or euthanasia for their pet. How do we approach this process? At the first level, this is a clinical decision based on the welfare of the animal: can the treatment we offer either realistically provide a return to function, or reduce suffering enough to justify continuing the animal's life? That decision will be based on the physical measures we take from our patients and clinical experience. Ultimately, our oath as veterinary surgeons is to promote the welfare of the animals under our care. The welfare of an animal in constant pain is poor; death is *not* a welfare problem (Webster, 1994).

Quality of life in the short, medium and long term has to be the most important consideration, over and above 'quantity' of life. Owners do not invariably appreciate this and, on occasion, can reflect their own feelings, needs and emotions on to their pet and struggle to keep an animal alive with an unacceptable quality of life. Some owners feel that taking the decision to euthanase their pet is the equivalent of murder. What right do they have to take that decision for anyone or 'play God' in this manner? As the veterinary practice involved we must remind them, and sometimes ourselves, that the ability to relieve suffering in this way is a privilege as well as a burden. Animals cannot 'look forward' beyond the pain they are experiencing now to a long and happy future: they live very much in the 'now' and it is our responsibility to make that 'now' as pain- and stress-free as possible. Chemotherapy protocols producing severe unpleasant short-term side effects in the expectation of a cure might be appropriate in consenting humans, but in small animals, less effective protocols with minimal side effects resulting in short-term remission and a return to normal function, but not a cure, might be preferable.

In contrast, an owner may request euthanasia at a time that appears 'premature' to the practice team. The owner must have the desire to continue; not only is cost a factor but the time involved in rehabilitating or caring for an infirm patient can be draining and may just be impossible in terms of the person's other commitments. The owner may be ill themselves, or have disabled relatives to look after, or be out at work all day and unable to nurse their pet. The emotional drain of interrupted nights' sleep and feeling responsible for their pet's condition will also have an impact in terms of the owner's own health and perspective on the problem. For those who appear to be making the decision prematurely, it must be remembered that there is more to the decision than a good prognosis for the patient. The prospect of prolonging the life of some dogs with lymphoma for significant periods of time is a reality, but the owner may have had bad experiences of chemotherapy themselves or may be unable or unwilling to cope emotionally with the knowledge that the lymphoma will recur at some time. Other owners may decline chemotherapy on the basis that their individual pet would not cope with the repeated trips to the veterinary clinic and frequent interventions, over and above any considerations of feeling unwell during the process. And this brings us to the crux of the matter – the individual.

What may be an unacceptable process to put one animal through may be perfectly 'worthwhile' apparently for another. If the patient enjoys interactions of any kind, likes close contact with his/her owner and being 'nursed', and is sociable, bright and outgoing, then the prospect of involved veterinary interventions may not be (if we could ask them) too daunting. An anxious animal, who does not cope well with routine trips to the clinic and may even display physical manifestations of such stressors, e.g colitis or cystitis, or one who is very sensitive to their owner's state of mind, or who has aggression problems that mean that either the practice or the owner have physical difficulty and risk in giving medication or nursing care, should be carefully considered before embarking on heroic surgery or procedures that may be technically impossible.

The individual owner, animal and owner–animal interactions needs to be assessed, and this is described in more detail in Chapter 4.

How do we assess quality of life?

There is no one set of physical parameters that, taken together, can add up to the magical score above which quality of life (QOL) is acceptable and below which euthanasia is wholly the right course. There is no way around considering each patient as an individual, with individual owners. Discussions of QOL in the veterinary literature often focus on minimizing pain (which is obviously important) but it is important to remember there is a lot more to QOL. Social relationships, mental stimulation, control over the environment, health, and freedom from hunger and thirst all contribute to QOL (McMillan, 2003).

QOL scores and questionnaires in human medicine have tended to be developed separately for different diseases and there has been a proliferation of papers in the veterinary literature over the last 10 years attempting to do the same thing. For example, QOL questionnaires have been developed for use in animals with osteoarthritis (Brown *et al.*, 2007), spinal disease (Budke *et al.*, 2008; Levine *et al.*, 2008), neoplasia (Mellanby *et al.*, 2003; Yazbeck and Fantoni, 2005) and cardiac disease (Freeman *et al.*, 2005; Oyama *et al.*, 2008). In human medicine, the patient themselves is usually the one who fills in the questionnaire. However, in some circumstances, this is not possible, such as with young children, the mentally ill or the very sick. In these cases, QOL is assessed by 'proxy informants' who know the patient well; these may be parents, spouses or other caregivers (Yazbeck and Fantoni, 2005). In veterinary medicine, QOL is ALWAYS assessed by proxy informants and these are usually the owners.

QOL questionnaires have generally been designed by the veterinary surgeon in charge of the study. Figure 1.1 shows examples of the types of question included in such questionnaires.

Questions about the PHYSICAL effects on the dog
• Does your dog still do what it likes? (playing, walking, etc. – this is also partly 'emotional')
• How often do you think your dog feels pain?
• Does your dog have an appetite?
• Does your dog get tired easily?
• How often does your dog vomit?
• Do your dog's intestines work properly?
• Can your dog still position him/herself to defecate and urinate?
• How does your dog sleep?

Questions about the EMOTIONAL effects on the dog
• How much attention is your dog giving to the family?
• How is your dog's mood?
• How many pleasures does your pet currently have in his/her life?
• How many pleasures did your pet have when he/she was feeling at his/her best?

Broad 'all-encompassing' questions
• How much do you think the disease is affecting your dog's quality of life?
• On a scale of 1 to 10, how willing would you be to take on the life your pet is now living?

1.1 Examples of questions included in quality of life questionnaires for dogs. Sources: McMillan (2003); Yazbeck and Fantoni (2005).

Brown *et al.* (2007) allowed more owner involvement by developing a questionnaire for use with dogs with osteoarthritis, using focus groups asking owners of affected dogs what should be included. However, as already stressed, each animal is an individual and it may therefore be unrealistic to expect one QOL questionnaire for a disease to apply to all cases equally. For example, a reduction in exercise would be expected to have a bigger impact on the QOL of a previously very active Border Collie than of a 'lapdog'. Enforced separation from the owner during treatment would have a much bigger impact on the emotional wellbeing of dogs predisposed to separation anxiety than of dogs apparently unconcerned by separation. Therefore, more recently, Budke *et al.* (2008) tried to develop an owner-perceived, weighted QOL questionnaire for use in dogs with spinal injury. Adapting a method used in human medicine, they asked owners to identify five 'key' areas of life or activities that they believed had the biggest influence on their dog's quality of life (Figure 1.2) and then to weight their relative importance. This individualized scoring scheme

Category	Examples
Mobility	Walking; running; jumping
Play or mental stimulation	Playing with toys; chasing salamanders
Health	Ability to urinate and defecate; willingness to eat and drink
Companionship	Affection; petting
Other [a]	'Leading a normal life'

1.2 Owners of dogs with spinal cord injury were asked to list the five areas of life that had most influence on their dog's quality of life (with no restraints). The responses could all be grouped into one of five domains (Budke *et al.*, 2008). [a] Not a very statisfactory domain – but only contained 1% of responses.

was then used to assess response to spinal surgery (Levine *et al.,* 2008). The change in owner-perceived score agreed with the change in neurological function score given by the veterinary surgeon, supporting the validity of the assessment.

It is clear therefore that assessment of the individual animal by the veterinary surgeon and owner is a key part of measuring 'quality of life'. This is as much a clinical consideration as interpretation of blood results or imaging, but it is difficult and rather emotive and time-consuming. It is not surprising that it is sometimes easier for veterinary surgeons to fall back on the comfortable technical question of 'Can we do this?' rather than adding '…and if we can, should we?' before undertaking complex surgical or medical treatments.

In reality, many practices and individual veterinary surgeons make these kinds of holistic decisions every day without formalizing them. This is because they know their clients and they know their patients. These veterinary surgeons and other practice members will have built up a pool of understanding of that client's and that patient's needs, temperament and financial limitations.

It is when that understanding does not exist, because the usual veterinary surgeon or patient advocate is away, or the patient and client are new to the practice or have had very little reason to attend the clinic except for routine checks, that the system can break down. In these circumstances, owners may feel that they have been 'bounced' into a decision with which they are not comfortable or have not been given the time to consider all the options and implications before opting for euthanasia.

Such decisions also put pressure on the practice. A decision to euthanase based on an owner's very good understanding of their pet and discussed with an individual veterinary surgeon may be anathema to other members of the practice, who feel that technically that patient had a good prognosis. In these circumstances, it is important that members of the practice can ask why, without it appearing to challenge clinical judgement, and that the veterinary surgeon involved can adequately articulate something that may feel as no more than an instinct based on clinical experience.

Ultimately, we should all be promoting quality of life above quantity of life: a longer life at the cost of poor QOL is, if anything, even less acceptable in veterinary medicine than in human medicine, as the veterinary patient is not able to consent to this choice. Most owners would chose QOL over quantity of life: one survey of owners of dogs with heart disease showed that most owners would trade time for QOL in their pet (Oyama *et al.,* 2008). The major challenge is how both veterinary surgeon and owner effectively assess QOL by proxy.

References and further reading

Brown DC, Boston RC, Coyne JC and Farrar JT (2007) Development and psychometric testing of an instrument designed to measure chronic pain in dogs with osteoarthritis. *American Journal of Veterinary Research* **68**, 631–637

Budke CM, Levine JM, Kerwin SC *et al.* (2008) Evaluation of a questionaire for obtaining owner-perceived, weighted quality-of-life assessments for dogs with spinal cord injuries. *Journal of the American Veterinary Medical Association* **233**, 925–930

Ernst E, Pittler MH and Wider B (2006) *The Desktop Guide to Complementary and Alternative Medicine.* Mosby Elsevier, Philadelphia

Freeman LM, Rush JE, Farabaugh AE and Must A (2005) Assessment of health-related quality of life in dogs with cardiac disease. *Journal of the American Veterinary Medical Association* **226**, 1864–1868

Hamann SB, Ely TD, Scott T *et al.* (1999) Amygdala activity related to enhanced memory for pleasant and aversive stimuli. *Nature Neuroscience* **2**, 289–293

Levine JM, Budke CM, Levine GJ *et al.* (2008) Owner-perceived, weighted quality-of-life assessments in dogs with spinal cord injuries. *Journal of the American Veterinary Medical Association* **233**, 931–935

McMillan FD (2003) Maximising quality of life in ill animals. *Journal of the American Animal Hospital Association* **39**, 227–235

Mellanby RJ, Herrtage ME and Dobson JM (2003) Owner's assessments of their dog's quality of life during palliative chemotherapy for lymphoma. *Journal of Small Animal Practice* **44**, 100–103

Ooms TG, Khan SA and Means C (2001) Suspected caffeine and ephedrine toxicosis resulting from ingestion of an herbal supplement containing guarana and ma huang in dogs: 47 cases (1997–1999). *Journal of the American Veterinary Medical Association* **218**, 225–229

Oyama MA, Rush JE, O'Sullivan ML *et al.* (2008) Perceptions and priorities of owners of dogs with heart disease regarding quality versus quantity of life for their pets. *Journal of the American Veterinary Medical Association* **233**, 104–108

Webster J (1994) *Animal Welfare: A Cool Eye towards Eden.* Blackwell, Oxford

Yazbeck KVB and Fantoni DT (2005) Validity of a health-related quality of life scale for dogs with signs of pain secondary to cancer. *Journal of the American Veterinary Medical Association* **226**, 1354–1358

2

Acute pain: assessment and management

Chris Seymour

Introduction

Effective treatment of pain is one of the veterinary surgeon's most important ethical responsibilities. To do this requires an appreciation of how painful certain procedures and conditions are likely to be, and the ability to recognize and quantify that pain. Pain scoring should be part of the routine ongoing assessment for each patient.

Pain has been defined by the International Association for the Study of Pain as '*an unpleasant sensory and emotional experience associated with actual or potential tissue damage, or described in terms of such damage*' (www.iasp-pain.org).

Because animals are unable to communicate verbally, Molony (1997) proposed that pain in animals be defined as '*an aversive sensory and emotional experience, representing an awareness by the animal of damage or threat to the integrity of its tissues. It changes the animal's physiology and behaviour to reduce or avoid the damage, to reduce the likelihood of recurrence and to promote recovery.*'

Physiological effects

• Neurohumoral alterations at site of injury [a]
• Alteration in synapses and nociceptive processing at the dorsal horn of the spinal cord [a]
• Neuroendocrine:
  o Increased catabolic hormones: cortisone, glucagon, growth hormone, catecholamines
  o Decreased anabolic hormones: insulin, testosterone
  o Increased plasminogen activator inhibitor (increased coagulation)
  o Sympathoadrenal via adrenal gland and lateral horns of spinal cord

Consequences
• CNS: distress, anxiety, depression, sleep disturbance • Cardiovascular: increased blood pressure, heart rate and vascular resistance, increased cardiac work • Respiratory: hypoventilation (respiratory acidosis), hyperventilation (respiratory alkalosis), inhibition of coughing • Gastrointestinal: ileus, nausea, vomiting • Genitourinary: urinary retention • Metabolic: see Neuroendocrine, above

2.1 Pathophysiological consequences of pain.
[a] Can lead to a state of persistent pain.
(Adapted from Farquhar-Smith, 2007)

As well as affecting behaviour, pain may also impair healing and cause long-term changes within the spinal cord and brain. Moreover, activation of the sympathetic and neuroendocrine systems by acute pain is harmful, and there is evidence that painful stressors, such as surgery, suppress immune function and may enhance tumour development (Page *et al.*, 2001). The pathophysiological implications of acute pain are summarized in Figure 2.1.

Relief of pain is thus necessary – not only from a moral and ethical standpoint, but also because it may have other undesirable consequences. **There can be absolutely no justification for using pain to limit an animal's activity after surgery or trauma or during treatment for painful medical conditions.** Considering that most small animal patients usually sleep if pain is properly managed, the misguided philosophy of keeping animals in pain to prevent movement is neither logical nor consistent with good practice. In addition, effective treatment of acute pain may help to limit central sensitization, with its associated hyperalgesia and

allodynia, and the development of chronic pain (see Chapter 3).

With advances in veterinary medicine and surgery, involving major interventions, the ability to recognize and treat acute pain has become even more important. Acute pain often has an obvious cause and is of relatively short duration (hours to days). The mechanisms of acute pain are now quite well defined and it can usually be successfully treated by targeting therapy, based on an understanding of the underlying pathophysiology. Combination treatment using analgesics with different modes of action (multimodal analgesia) now forms the basis of effective management. In contrast, chronic pain (see Chapter 3) is often unpredictable and the relationship with tissue damage is less clear.

Much work remains to be done to highlight which drugs and which combinations may be optimal for specific conditions. Only by further randomized, controlled, blinded clinical trials will this information become available.

Neurophysiology

A detailed description of the neurophysiology of pain is beyond the scope of this chapter, but excellent reviews are available (Julius and Basbaum, 2001; Muir and Woolf, 2001; Lemke, 2004).

Signalling processes

Several processes are involved in the perception of pain.

- **Transduction** involves the conversion of noxious stimuli into electrical signals by peripheral nociceptors.
- **Transmission** of these signals involves conduction along small myelinated (Aδ) fibres and unmyelinated C fibres to synapse with second-order neurons in the dorsal horn of the spinal cord (predominantly in laminae I, II and V).
- Two classes of dorsal horn neuron are involved:
  - o Nociceptive-specific neurons respond only to pain signals in Aδ and C fibres
  - o Wide dynamic range (WDR) neurons respond to both non-nociceptive impulses in Aβ fibres and nociceptive impulses in Aδ and C fibres.
- These second-order neurons then project to third-order neurons in the brain, which integrate spinal input and, finally, **project** to cortical areas, where painful stimuli are consciously perceived by the sensory cortex and parts of the limbic system.

These pathways, and the points at which analgesics exert their effects, are summarized in Figure 2.2.

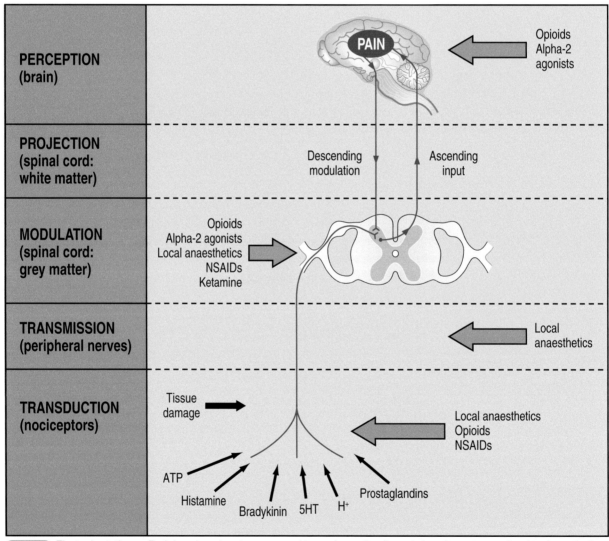

2.2 The pain pathway. Peripheral nociceptors respond to noxious stimuli, and signals are transmitted to the spinal cord via small myelinated (Aδ) and unmyelinated (C) nerve fibres. Impulses arriving at primary afferent nerve endings in the dorsal horn cause release of a number of neurotransmitters, including glutamate, substance P, calcitonin gene-related peptide (CGRP) and neurokinin, which activate second-order neurons. These neurons then transmit the signals to the brain, where the information is integrated and finally perceived as pain. Tissue damage causes release of pain-promoting substances from both surrounding tissue and the nerve endings themselves, leading to peripheral sensitization of nociceptors. Modulation of these pain signals occurs within the spinal cord (both inhibition and facilitation) and is under the influence of descending pathways from supraspinal sites. Pharmacological interventions that act at specific points of the pathway are indicated by orange arrows.

Mediators and modulation

In the periphery, tissue injury causes release of inflammatory mediators, such as hydrogen ions, bradykinin, histamine, 5-hydroxytryptamine, ATP, prostanoids and leucotrienes. All these sensitize nociceptors to both noxious and non-noxious stimuli (a phenomenon called **peripheral sensitization**). Impulses from peripheral nociceptors arriving at nerve terminals in the spinal cord release fast-acting neurotransmitters (e.g. glutamate) and slower-acting neuropeptides (e.g. substance P, calcitonin gene-related peptide (CGRP) and neurokinin), which then activate second-order neurons.

Nociceptive pathways are not 'hard wired'. Other sensory inputs (e.g. touch, temperature) and descending pathways from the brain (either inhibiting or facilitating transmission of noxious stimuli) can **modulate** activity in the dorsal horn. This is known as neuronal plasticity, and is vital to the development of the hypersensitive state that can follow acute pain.

Sustained stimulation of peripheral nociceptors can produce dramatic changes in the function and activity of the second-order neurons, a phenomenon called **central sensitization** (or 'wind-up'). The net result is that responsiveness of dorsal horn neurons, both to existing inputs and to previously sub-threshold inputs, is increased. This produces:

- Exaggerated responses to normal stimuli
- An increase in the size of the receptive field
- A reduced threshold for activation by non-nociceptive input (e.g. from mechanoreceptors).

The crucial event in this process appears to be activation of N-methyl-D-aspartate (NMDA) receptors by glutamate. With repetitive noxious input, this receptor is increasingly activated.

Modulation of pain signals in the dorsal horn is mediated by various neurotransmitters, including opioids, catecholamines (primarily acting at alpha-2 adrenoceptors), 5-hydroxytryptamine, gamma-amino-butyric acid (GABA) and glycine.

Assessment of acute pain

Pain can only be effectively managed when it is appreciated that it is present and at a level that warrants treatment. This is especially important in critically ill animals, where behavioural options for expression of pain may be limited. In animals, pain is what the observer says it is; because judgement of pain is subjective, animals can suffer if that judgement is incorrect (Robertson, 2008).

Unfortunately, there is no 'gold standard' for measuring pain in animals, so designing an analgesic plan for each individual can sometimes be very difficult. One approach is to give analgesics to any animal that has undergone surgery or trauma that would probably be painful in humans (Hellyer, 2002). However, some method of measuring the effectiveness of treatment is still needed with this approach, especially as some individuals undergoing the same surgical procedure or degree of trauma may experience or express their pain differently (Hellyer et al., 2007). The problem is how to link specific behaviours with pain and how to recognize them. In this respect, owner input is invaluable when deciding whether abnormal behaviour is linked to pain. Whatever system is used to measure pain, it should be part of an ongoing assessment of the animal's condition, along with temperature, pulse and respiration.

Pain scoring systems

A number of scoring systems have been used for assessing pain in animals (Figure 2.3). Any such system should be reliable, sensitive, quick and easy to perform in a busy practice, and have minimal variation between observers. Systems include the simple descriptive scale (SDS), the numerical rating scale (NRS) and the visual analogue scale (VAS). All these are relatively insensitive and also suffer from the disadvantage of being unidimensional, i.e. they measure only the *intensity* of pain and give no information on its *quality*. An interactive visual analogue scale (IVAS) is more sensitive because it involves interaction with the patient, although in some cases such interaction may be difficult (e.g. aggressive animals). Multidimensional pain scales also take the physiological and behavioural effects of pain into account and provide a fuller picture of the patient's pain experience.

Pain scale	Limitations
Visual analogue scale (VAS)	Significant inter-observer variability Sensitivity depends on observer training and experience Expresses summation of observer's interpretation of many different behaviours
Numerical rating scale (NRS)	Significant inter-observer variability Differences in pain severity between categories are undefined and inconsistent (uneven weighting) Expresses summation of observer's interpretation of many different behaviours
Simple descriptive scale (SDS)	Significant inter-observer variability Absence of selection criteria for behaviours assessed Low sensitivity Cannot identify small changes in the pain response In humans has been shown to artificially magnify the efficacy of analgesics
Composite scoring system	Time-consuming No selection criteria for the behaviours assessed Few validated tools in small animals
Multidimensional scoring system	Time-consuming No selection criteria for the behaviours assessed

2.3 Limitations of commonly used pain scoring systems. (Reproduced from *BSAVA Manual of Canine and Feline Anaesthesia and Analgesia, 2nd edn*).

Dogs

The Glasgow Composite Measure Pain Scale (CMPS) is a behaviour-based composite scale for assessing acute pain in dogs (Holton *et al.*, 2001). It consists of a questionnaire with a very detailed description of specific behaviours (both spontaneous and evoked), interactions with the patient and clinical observations. Each item assessed has a weighting assigned to it and the sum of the weights for these items gives the pain score for the animal. It is important to remember that this scale has been validated only in dogs experiencing acute pain, and is not suitable for use in cats. Similar scales, which consider both behaviour and physiological variables, have also been developed by the University of Melbourne and the University of Colorado.

More recently, a shorter version of the Glasgow CMPS has been developed (short-form composite measure pain score, CMPS-SF) for dogs in acute pain (Reid *et al.*, 2007). This is faster to perform in a busy practice setting and includes six behavioural categories (including mobility) with associated descriptive expressions ('items'). The items are placed in increasing order of pain intensity and numbered accordingly. The maximum score for the six categories is 24 (or 20 if mobility is impossible to assess). The total CMPS-SF score has been shown to be a useful indicator of analgesic requirement, and the recommended analgesic intervention level is 6/24 or 5/20. The form may be downloaded from www.gla.ac.uk/faculties/vet.

Cats

Assessment of acute pain in cats is currently more difficult because no validated multidimensional scoring systems exist, and signs of pain can be very subtle. Acute pain related to trauma may result in a depressed and immobile cat that tries to hide away from its surroundings and is unresponsive to stroking, or may result in aggression and extreme distress (see Chapter 4). Cats with abdominal pain often adopt a hunched posture, with a drooping head, elbows drawn caudally and stifles cranially, and tense abdominal muscles. Signs indicative of pain in cats are listed in Figure 2.4.

Based on these signs, a proposed scoring system for assessment of acute pain in cats is presented at the end of this chapter. This system depends on other factors apart from pain, such as the behaviour of the individual cat, which should also be taken into consideration when using it.

Management

Pain management strategies need to be tailored to each individual; the flowchart shown in Figure 2.5 can help this process.

Based on pathophysiological mechanisms, approaches to effective control of acute pain have been proposed to prevent both peripheral and central sensitization, and perhaps make development of chronic pain less likely. These include:

- **Pre-emptive analgesia**: treatment started before a painful procedure to reduce the consequences of nociceptive transmission. This has three goals:
  o Decrease acute pain after tissue injury
  o Prevent pain-related pathological modulation of the central nervous system ('pain memory')
  o Inhibit the persistence of pain and the development of chronic pain.

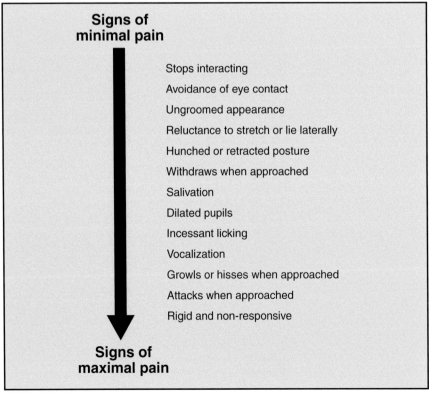

Signs of minimal pain

Stops interacting

Avoidance of eye contact

Ungroomed appearance

Reluctance to stretch or lie laterally

Hunched or retracted posture

Withdraws when approached

Salivation

Dilated pupils

Incessant licking

Vocalization

Growls or hisses when approached

Attacks when approached

Rigid and non-responsive

Signs of maximal pain

2.4 Signs indicative of pain in cats. (Reproduced from Cambridge *et al.*, 2000, *Journal of the American Veterinary Medical Association*, with the permission of AVMA).

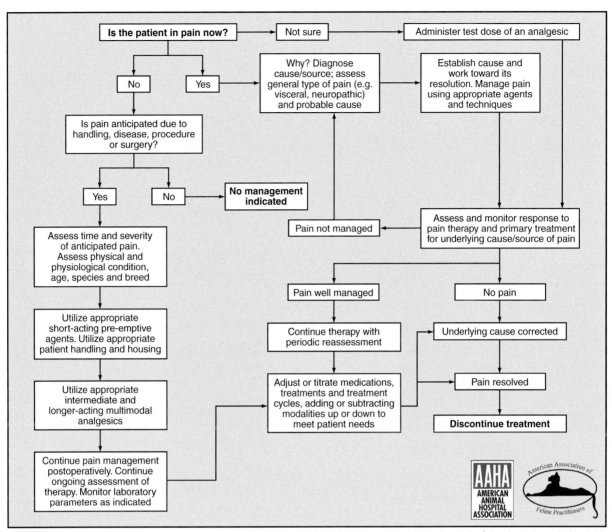

2.5 An approach to pain management in cats. (Adapted from Hellyer *et al.*, 2007, *Journal of the American Animal Hospital Association*, with permission of the American Animal Hospital Association. Copyright © 2007. To order this resource or obtain more information, go to www.aahanet.org).

Although there is some debate about the efficacy of pre-emptive analgesia (Dahl and Møiniche, 2004), it must still be recommended as best practice (Karas, 2009a). It may be that for pre-emptive analgesia to be truly effective, analgesia needs to be continued until wounds have healed.

- **Multimodal analgesia**: simultaneous use of more than one drug with different actions to produce optimal analgesia. Because drugs may have additive or synergistic effects, doses of individual types of drug can often be reduced.

Any plan requires a comprehensive understanding of the pharmacology of analgesic drugs. A detailed discussion is beyond the scope of this chapter but there are a number of excellent reviews (Robertson, 2005; Kerr, 2007; Lamont and Mathews, 2007). Figures 2.6 and 2.7 at the end of this section give doses, routes and comments on use for a number of drugs used in the management of acute pain in dogs and cats.

Opioids

Opioids still form the backbone of most analgesic plans.

- Opioids are often given intravenously during surgery or to those animals in severe pain, because bioavailability from intramuscular or subcutaneous injection is unpredictable if peripheral perfusion is poor, and repeated intramuscular injections are painful.
- Constant rate intravenous infusion is often used to avoid the peaks and troughs associated with intermittent administration (Lucas *et al.*, 2001).
- Administration via the epidural route (either as a single dose or repeatedly via an epidural catheter) is also a very useful technique and has been used successfully in many situations (Hansen, 2001).
- Transdermal delivery (fentanyl patch) is commonly used in dogs and cats, but there are still gaps in clinical knowledge about this route of administration: specific plasma concentrations required to obtain adequate analgesia in dogs and cats; variables that alter plasma concentrations; duration of effective plasma levels; and how chronic treatment and repeated placement of patches affect pharmacokinetics (Hofmeister and Egger, 2004).

Opioids activate peripheral, spinal and supraspinal opioid receptors. The commonest side effects are bradycardia, respiratory depression and urine rotention. In humans, opioids can sometimes increase rather than decrease sensitivity to noxious stimuli, and large doses of intraoperative opioids have also been shown to increase postoperative pain and morphine consumption. Also, prolonged use of opioids in human patients can be associated with a requirement for increasing doses and the development of abnormal pain (Koppert and Schmelz, 2007). Similar effects may occur in animals; therefore, when managing acute pain, consideration should be given to additional drugs that can decrease or prevent opioid-induced hyperalgesia (e.g. local anaesthetic agents, alpha-2 agonists, NMDA antagonists (ketamine) and non-steroidal anti-inflammatory drugs). This is another powerful argument for practising multimodal analgesia.

Local anaesthetics

This class of drug may be used by the traditional routes (perineural, epidural) but in recent years more interest has been shown in novel methods of delivery, such as intravenous, intra-wound and interpleural (Karas, 2009b).

In human medicine, lidocaine by constant rate infusion (CRI) has been shown to reduce postoperative pain and opioid consumption. The precise mode of action is unknown but probably includes both peripheral and central mechanisms, including blockade of voltage-gated sodium channels and inhibition of NMDA receptors. As lidocaine has been shown experimentally to reduce neuropathic and visceral pain, it may be of value in orthopaedic and neurological surgery, acute pancreatitis and trauma pain. Additional benefits are reported to be free-radical scavenging (helping to minimize reperfusion injury) and reduction of postoperative ileus (Cassutto and Gfeller, 2003; Cook and Blikslager, 2008). One study has demonstrated comparable levels of postoperative analgesia after intraocular surgery in dogs with either lidocaine or morphine (Smith *et al.*, 2001). Lidocaine is not recommended in cats because of concerns about cardiovascular depression, toxicity and lack of efficacy (Thomasy *et al.*, 2005; Pypendop *et al.*, 2006).

Interest has also been shown in longer-term application of local anaesthetics directly to the surgical wound via soaker catheters (Wolfe et al., 2006), to the brachial plexus (Moens and Caulkett, 2000) or into the interpleural space. Interpleural anaesthesia using a local anaesthetic may be of benefit in the management of post-thoracotomy pain (Stobie *et al.*, 1995) and cranial abdominal pain (Dravid and Paul, 2007) and warrants further investigation.

Ketamine

Given the crucial role of the NMDA receptor in central sensitization, ketamine (an NMDA receptor antagonist) would appear well suited for use in acute pain. Low, subanaesthetic doses are increasingly used in dogs and cats, as part of a balanced anaesthesia protocol (Slingsby and Waterman-Pearson, 2000) and/or postoperative analgesia (Wagner et al., 2002). However, there is little evidence that ketamine is analgesic in dogs when given alone. One other difficulty is that recommended doses are extrapolated directly from human medicine. Recent experimental evidence (Bergadano et al., 2009) suggests that doses higher than those currently used would be necessary to have an effect. There is also some clinical evidence that ketamine CRI during surgery does not reduce the requirement for postoperative opioid administration in dogs (Klöppel et al., 2009).

There is very little information on the role of ketamine as an analgesic in cats, although clinical experience suggests that it can be a useful adjunct when given by CRI. Indeed, ketamine may be of greater use in cats, given the concerns about lidocaine CRI in this species.

Further work is clearly necessary before firm recommendations can be made, and it is possible that higher doses may be associated with unacceptable side effects, such as dysphoria, which would make nursing more difficult.

Morphine + Lidocaine + Ketamine (MLK)

This 'cocktail' is favoured by some, but the evidence base for its use is rather sketchy and, as with all mixtures of drugs, it is impossible to change doses of one drug independently. Only one study has examined the use of MLK infusions in dogs (Muir *et al.*, 2003); this demonstrated that MLK reduced isoflurane minimum alveolar concentration (MAC) without adverse cardiovascular effects. However, the doses used may well be insufficient to control severe postoperative pain, and the author prefers the flexibility of using different analgesics by separate CRIs.

Alpha-2 agonists

Although alpha-2 agonists have potent analgesic properties, their use may be limited by the sedation and cardiovascular side effects that they produce. Traditionally, they have been used as part of preanaesthetic medication because of their sedative, analgesic and anaesthetic-sparing properties. They also have a synergistic action when used with opioids. Recent clinical research has investigated the use of dexmedetomidine by intravenous CRI for analgesia and as an anaesthetic adjunct. One study has shown that dexmedetomidine by CRI was as effective as morphine by CRI in providing postoperative analgesia to dogs undergoing invasive surgery (Valtolina *et al.*, 2009). Dexmedetomidine is unlikely to become a first-line analgesic drug but may be extremely useful as part of balanced multimodal analgesia.

Non-steroidal anti-inflammatory drugs

NSAIDs should be used with great care in seriously ill animals: their effects on renal function and the gastrointestinal tract are well known, and they may also interfere with platelet function. They should also be used with caution in animals with liver disease as they can cause hepatotoxicity.

In **dogs**, paracetamol may be a useful alternative to 'classical' NSAIDs and is available as a preparation for intravenous use. Tablets containing paracetamol in combination with codeine (Pardale-V) have market authorization in the UK for use in dogs. Paracetamol is probably underused where there are concerns about the side effects of 'classical' NSAIDs, and it may be a useful additional agent for neurological pain in dogs (Leece, 2007). Paracetamol should be avoided in liver disease because of its potential to cause hepatotoxicity.

> **WARNING**
> **Never give paracetamol to cats.**

Tramadol
Tramadol has both opioid and non-opioid mechanisms of action and has been used for management of acute perioperative pain in continental Europe, where a preparation for intravenous use is available (Mastrocinque and Fantoni, 2003). In the UK, only the oral form is available and it is finding increasing use in the management of moderate perioperative pain. Its main use, however, is for treatment of chronic pain (Murrell, 2009) (see Chapter 3).

Gabapentin
Gabapentin was originally introduced as an anticonvulsant, but has also been used to treat chronic pain in both humans and animals. Until recently, it was not thought to be useful for acute perioperative pain in humans. However, recent evidence from human medicine suggests that preoperative administration may be efficacious for postoperative analgesia and preventing chronic postsurgical pain. At the present time there is no evidence concerning its perioperative use in dogs or cats.

Drug	Route	Dose	Comments
Opioids			
Morphine [a]	i.m., i.v., s.c.	0.2–0.5 mg/kg q3–4h	Can cause histamine release intravenously; dilute and give slowly
	Epidural	0.1 mg/kg (diluted to 0.2 ml/kg with saline)	May be repeated every 18–24 hours by epidural catheter
	CRI	0.12–0.2 mg/kg/h	
Methadone [a]	i.m., slow i.v., s.c.	0.1–0.5 mg/kg q4h	Can cause bradycardia and apnoea when given intravenously
Pethidine (Meperidine)	i.m., s.c.	3–10 mg/kg q1–2h	**Do not give intravenously:** causes massive histamine release
Fentanyl [a]	i.v.	1–5 µg/kg q20–30min	Can cause bradycardia, apnoea
	CRI	Loading dose 1–2 µg/kg; follow with 0.05–0.15 µg/kg/min	
	Transdermal	4 µg/kg/h patch	May take 24 hours to reach effective plasma levels
Alfentanil [a]	i.v.	1–5 µg/kg	Short acting. Can cause bradycardia, apnoea
	CRI	Loading dose 1 µg/kg; follow with 1–2.5 µg/kg/min	
Remifentanil [a]	CRI	0.1–0.5 µg/kg/min	No loading dose required
Buprenorphine	i.m., i.v.	0.01–0.02 mg/kg q6–8h	May also be useful by oral transmucosal route if given at higher dose (0.12 mg/kg)
Butorphanol	i.m., i.v.	0.2–0.4 mg/kg q1.5–2h	
Local anaesthetics			
Lidocaine (authorized for infiltration and perineural use only)	Perineural	2–4 mg/kg	Duration 1–2h
	CRI	Loading dose 1–1.5 mg/kg; follow with CRI of 50 µg/kg/min	Use with caution in animals with liver disease
	IVRA (Bier's block)	2–4 mg/kg	
Bupivacaine [a]	Perineural	1–1.5 mg/kg	Duration 4–6h. **Do not give intravenously**
NMDA antagonists			
Ketamine	CRI	Loading dose 0.5 mg/kg; follow with CRI of 2–20 µg/kg/min (5 µg/kg/min common)	Maximum duration probably 24–36h. Higher doses can lead to dysphoria

2.6 Analgesics for management of acute pain in dogs. [a] Not authorized in the UK for use in dogs. IVRA = Intravenous regional anaesthesia. (continues)

Drug	Route	Dose	Comments
Alpha-2 agonists			
Medetomidine	i.m., i.v.	1–2 µg/kg	Can cause bradycardia Synergistic action with opioids
	CRI	1–2 µg/kg/h	No loading dose needed
Dexmedetomidine	i.m., i.v.	0.5–1 µg/kg	
	CRI	0.5–1 µg/kg/h	
NSAIDs			
Carprofen	s.c., i.v.	4 mg/kg	Injectable form authorized for single injection only Can be used perioperatively
	Oral	2–4 mg/kg (as single or two divided doses)	Postoperatively: authorized for use at 4 mg/kg/day for up to 5 days
Meloxicam	s.c.	0.2 mg/kg	Injectable form authorized for single injection only Can be used perioperatively
	Oral	0.2 mg/kg on day 1; then 0.1 mg/kg q24h	
Ketoprofen	i.m., s.c., i.v.	2 mg/kg	Maximum 3 days
	Oral	0.25 mg/kg q24h	Maximum 30 days
Firocoxib	Oral	5 mg/kg q24h	Authorized also for perioperative use at 5 mg/kg q24h for maximum 3 days, starting 2h before surgery
Tolfenamic acid	s.c., i.m.	4 mg/kg	Authorized for perioperative use. Subcutaneous injection can be repeated once
	Oral	4 mg/kg q24h	Maximum 3 days
Robenacoxib	s.c.	2 mg/kg	Authorized for perioperative use Single injection only
	Oral	1 mg/kg q24h	
Paracetamol (only oral form (combined with codeine) is authorized in dogs)	i.v.	10 mg/kg slow i.v. (over 20–30 mins)	May be useful for neurological pain
	Oral	10 mg/kg q12h	
Others			
Tramadol [a]	Oral	2–5 mg/kg q12h	More frequent administration (q6–8h) can be used if needed Avoid using with tricyclic antidepressants (e.g. clomipramine) and monoamine oxidase inhibitors (e.g. selegiline)
Gabapentin [a]	Oral	10 mg/kg	Precise dose for preoperative use unknown Use with caution in dogs with renal impairment and behavioural abnormalities

2.6 (continued) Analgesics for management of acute pain in dogs. [a] Not authorized in the UK for use in dogs. IVRA = Intravenous regional anaesthesia.

Drug	Route	Dose	Comments
Opioids			
Morphine [a]	i.m., i.v., s.c.	0.1–0.4 mg/kg q3–4h	May be less effective than in dogs due to lack of active metabolites
	Epidural	0.1 mg/kg (diluted to 0.2 ml/kg with saline)	
	CRI		Not recommended
Methadone [a]	i.m., slow i.v., s.c.	0.1–0.3 mg/kg q4h	
Pethidine (Meperidine)	i.m., s.c.	5–10 mg/kg q1–2h	**Do not give intravenously:** causes massive histamine release
Fentanyl [a]	i.v.	2–5 µg/kg q20–30min	Can cause bradycardia, apnoea
	CRI	Loading dose 1–2 µg/kg; follow with 0.05–0.15 µg/kg/min	
	Transdermal	25 µg/kg/h patch	May take 12h to reach effective plasma levels

2.7 Analgesics for management of acute pain in cats. [a] Not authorized in the UK for use in cats. (continues) ▶

Drug	Route	Dose	Comments
Opioids continued			
Alfentanil [a]	i.v.	1 µg/kg	Short-acting Can cause bradycardia, apnoea
	CRI	Loading dose 1 µg/kg; follow with 1 µg/kg/min	
Remifentanil [a]	CRI	0.1–0.5 µg/kg/min	No loading dose required
Buprenorphine	i.m., i.v., oral transmucosal	0.01–0.02 mg/kg q6–8h	
Butorphanol	i.m., i.v.	0.1–0.4 mg/kg q1.5–2h	
Local anaesthetics			
Lidocaine (authorized for infiltration and perineural use only)	Perineural	2–4 mg/kg	Duration 1–2h
	CRI		Not recommended
	IVRA (Bier's block)	3 mg/kg	
Bupivacaine [a]	Perineural	1–1.5 mg/kg	Duration 4–6h **Do not give intravenously**
NMDA antagonists			
Ketamine	i.v.	2 mg/kg	Maximum duration probably 24–36h Higher doses can lead to dysphoria
	CRI	2–10 µg/kg/min ?	No data on use of CRI in cats, but clinical experience suggests it may be effective
Alpha-2 agonists			
Medetomidine	i.m., i.v.	5–20 µg/kg	Can cause bradycardia Synergistic action with opioids
	CRI	1–2 µg/kg/h	No loading dose needed
Dexmedetomidine	i.m., i.v.	2.5–10 µg/kg	
	CRI	0.5–1 µg/kg/h	
NSAIDs			
Carprofen	s.c., i.v.	4 mg/kg	Single injection only Authorized for perioperative use
Meloxicam	s.c.	0.3 mg/kg	Single injection only Authorized for perioperative use
	Oral	0.1 mg/kg on day 1; then 0.05 mg/kg q24h	
Ketoprofen	s.c.	2 mg/kg	Maximum 3 days
	Oral	1 mg/kg q24h	Maximum 5 days
Tolfenamic acid	s.c.	4 mg/kg	Can be repeated once after 24h
	Oral	4 mg/kg q24h	Maximum 3 days
Robenacoxib	s.c.	2 mg/kg	Authorized for perioperative use Single injection only
	Oral	1 mg/kg q24h	Maximum 6 days
Others			
Tramadol [a]	Oral	2–4 mg/kg q12h	Avoid using with tricyclic antidepressants (e.g. clomipramine) and monoamine oxidase inhibitors (e.g. selegiline) Has been noted to cause seizures in cats at these doses
Gabapentin [a]	Oral	5–10 mg/kg	Few data available Use with caution in cats with renal impairment

2.7 (continued) Analgesics for management of acute pain in cats. [a] Not authorized in the UK for use in cats.

References and further reading

Bergadano A, Andersen OK, Arendt-Nielsen L *et al.* (2009) Plasma levels of a low-dose constant-rate-infusion of ketamine and its effect on single and repeated nociceptive stimuli in conscious dogs. *The Veterinary Journal* **182**, 252–260

Cambridge AJ, Tobias KM, Newberry RC and Sarkar D (2000) Subjective and objective measurements of postoperative pain in cats. *Journal of the American Veterinary Medical Association* **217**, 685–690

Cassutto BH and Gfeller RW (2003) Use of intravenous lidocaine to prevent reperfusion injury and subsequent multiple organ dysfunction syndrome. *Journal of Veterinary Emergency and Critical Care* **13**, 137–148

Cook VL and Blikslager AT (2008) Use of systemically administered lidocaine in horses with gastrointestinal disease. *Journal of the American Veterinary Medical Association* **232**, 1144–1148

Dravid RM and Paul RE (2007) Interpleural block. Part 1. *Anaesthesia* **62**, 1039–1049

Dahl JB and Møiniche S (2004) Pre-emptive analgesia. *British Medical Bulletin* **71**, 13–27

Farquhar-Smith WP (2007) Anatomy, physiology and pharmacology of pain. *Anaesthesia and Intensive Care Medicine* **9**, 3–7

Hansen BD (2001) Epidural catheter analgesia in dogs and cats: technique and review of 182 cases (1991–1999). *Journal of Veterinary Emergency and Critical Care* **11**, 95–103

Hellyer PW (2002) Treatment of pain in dogs and cats. *Journal of the American Animal Hospital Association* **221**, 212–215

Hellyer PW, Rodan I, Brunt J *et al.* (2007) AAHA/AAFP pain management guidelines for dogs and cats. *Journal of the American Animal Hospital Association* **43**, 235–248

Hofmeister EH and Egger CM (2004) Transdermal fentanyl patches in small animals. *Journal of the American Animal Hospital Association* **40**, 468–478

Holton L, Reid J, Scott E *et al.* (2001) Development of a behaviour-based scale to measure acute pain in dogs. *Veterinary Record* **148**, 525–531

Julius D and Basbaum AI (2001) Molecular mechanisms of nociception. *Nature* **413**, 203–210

Karas AZ (2009a) Pre-emptive analgesia: controversy over the evidence. *Proceedings, ECVAA Training Day, AVA Meeting, Helsinki, March 2009*, pp.20–22

Karas AZ (2009b) Somewhat less than local: efficacy and safety of intravenous and intra-wound infusion of local anaesthetics for postoperative analgesia. *Proceedings, ECVAA Training Day, AVA Meeting, Helsinki, March 2009*, pp.24–26

Kerr C (2007) Pain management I: systemic analgesics. In: *BSAVA Manual of Canine and Feline Anaesthesia and Analgesia 2nd edn*, ed. C Seymour and T Duke-Novakovski, pp.89–103. BSAVA Publications, Gloucester

Klöppel H, Adams VJ, Brearley JC *et al.* (2009) Opioid administration following spinal surgery in dogs receiving ketamine infusion compared to those not receiving ketamine: a retrospective study. *Proceedings, AVA Meeting, Helsinki, March 2009*, p.42 [Abstract]

Koppert W and Schmelz M (2007) The impact of opioid-induced hyperalgesia for postoperative pain. *Best Practice and Research in Clinical Anaesthesiology* **21**, 65–83

Lamont LA and Mathews KA (2007) Opioids, non-steroidal anti-inflammatories and analgesic adjuvants. In: *Lumb and Jones' Veterinary Anesthesia and Analgesia 4th edn*, ed. WJ Tranquilli *et al.*, pp.241–272. Blackwell Publishing, Ames, IA

Leece EA (2007) Neurological disease. In: *BSAVA Manual of Canine and Feline Anaesthesia and Analgesia 2nd edn*, ed. C Seymour and T Duke-Novakovski, pp.284–295. BSAVA Publications, Gloucester

Lemke KA (2004) Understanding the pathophysiology of perioperative pain. *Canadian Veterinary Journal* **45**, 405–413

Lucas AN, Firth A, Anderson GA *et al.* (2001) Comparison of the effects of morphine administered by constant-rate intravenous infusion or intermittent intramuscular injection in dogs. *Journal of the American Veterinary Medical Association* **218**, 884–891

Mahler SP and Reece JLM (2007) Electrical nerve stimulation to facilitate placement of an indwelling catheter for repeated brachial plexus block in a traumatized dog. *Veterinary Anaesthesia and Analgesia* **34**, 365–370

Mastrocinque S and Fantoni DT (2003) A comparison of preoperative tramadol and morphine for the control of early postoperative pain in canine ovariohysterectomy. *Veterinary Anaesthesia and Analgesia* **30**, 220–228

Moens NM and Caulkett NA (2000) The use of a catheter to provide brachial plexus block in dogs. *Canadian Veterinary Journal* **41**, 685–689

Molony V (1997) Comments on Anand and Craig, PAIN 67(1996) 3–6. *Pain* **70**, 293

Muir WW III, Wiese AJ and March PA (2003) Effects of morphine, lidocaine, ketamine and morphine-lidocaine-ketamine drug combination on minimum alveolar concentration in dogs anesthetized with isoflurane. *American Journal of Veterinary Research* **64**, 1155–1160

Muir WW III and Woolf CJ (2001) Mechanisms of pain and their therapeutic implications. *Journal of the American Veterinary Medical Association* **219**, 1346–1356

Murrell JC (2009) Tramadol. *UK Vet* **14**, 20–22

Page GG, Blakely WP and Ben-Eliyahu S (2001) Evidence that postoperative pain is a mediator of the tumor-promoting effects of surgery in rats. *Pain* **90**, 191–199

Price J and Nolan A (2007) The physiology and pathophysiology of pain. In: *BSAVA Manual of Canine and Feline Anaesthesia and Analgesia 2nd edn*, ed. C Seymour and T Duke-Novakovski, pp.79–88. BSAVA Publications, Gloucester

Pypendop BH, Ilkiw JE and Robertson SA (2006) Effects of intravenous administration of lidocaine on the thermal threshold of cats. *American Journal of Veterinary Research* **67**, 16–20

Reid J, Nolan AM, Hughes JML *et al.* (2007) Development of the short-form Glasgow Composite Measure Pain Scale (CMPS-SF) and derivation of an analgesic intervention score. *Animal Welfare* **16(S)**, 97–104

Robertson SA (2005) Assessment and management of acute pain in cats. *Journal of Veterinary Emergency and Critical Care* **15**, 261–272

Robertson SA (2008) Managing pain in feline patients. *Veterinary Clinics of North America: Small Animal Practice* **38**, 1267–1290

Slingsby LS and Waterman-Pearson AE (2000) The post-operative analgesic effects of ketamine after canine ovarohysterectomy – a comparison between pre- or post-operative administration. *Research in Veterinary Science* **69**, 147–152

Smith LJ, Shih A, Bentley E *et al.* (2001) Morphine or lidocaine infusion as a pre-emptive analgesic for intraocular surgery in dogs. *Veterinary Anaesthesia and Analgesia* **28**, 97–110

Stobie D, Caywood DD, Rozanski EA *et al.* (1995) Evaluation of pulmonary function and analgesia in dogs after intercostal thoracotomy and use of morphine administered intramuscularly or intrapleurally and bupivacaine administered intrapleurally. *American Journal of Veterinary Research* **56**, 1098–1109

Thomasy SM, Pypendop BH, Ilkiw JE *et al.* (2005) Pharmacokinetics of lidocaine and its active metabolite, monoethylglycinexylidide, after intravenous administration of lidocaine to awake and isoflurane-anesthetized cats. *American Journal of Veterinary Research* **66**, 1162–1166

Valtolina C, Robben JH, Uilenreef J *et al.* (2009) Clinical evaluation of the efficacy and safety of a constant rate infusion of dexmedetomidine for postoperative pain management in dogs. *Veterinary Anaesthesia and Analgesia* **36**, 369–383

Wagner AE, Walton JA, Hellyer PW *et al.* (2002) Use of low doses of ketamine administered by constant rate infusion as an adjunct for postoperative analgesia in dogs. *Journal of the American Veterinary Medical Association* **221**, 72–75

Wolfe TM, Bateman SW, Cole LK *et al.* (2006) Evaluation of a local anaesthetic delivery system for the postoperative analgesic management of canine total ear ablation – a randomized, controlled, double-blinded study. *Veterinary Anaesthesia and Analgesia* **33**, 328–339

▶ **Sample pain assessment form for cats**

Owner		Date				
Patient		Time				
General subjective impression	No pain Unbearable pain	↓	0 1 2 3	0 1 2 3	0 1 2 3	0 1 2 3
General behaviour	Choose between the following signs: • Altered respiratory pattern • Hunched posture • Unwilling to move, stiff • Excited, vocalizing, hides in far side of cage • Does not groom • Licking or looking at the wound • Urinating or defecating without moving • Anorexia		□ □ □ □ □ □ □ □	□ □ □ □ □ □ □ □	□ □ □ □ □ □ □ □	□ □ □ □ □ □ □ □
	None of the above is observed 1 of above is observed 2–4 of above are observed 5–8 of above are observed		0 1 2 3	0 1 2 3	0 1 2 3	0 1 2 3
Interactive behaviour	Bright, reactive to voice and stroking Tries to react Reacts slowly Does not react or shows aggressive behaviour		0 1 2 3	0 1 2 3	0 1 2 3	0 1 2 3
Increase of heart rate above baseline value	<10% 11–30% 31–50% >50% or impossible to assess	Baseline:	0 1 2 3	0 1 2 3	0 1 2 3	0 1 2 3
Reaction to wound palpation	No reaction (vocalization or movement) after 4 palpations Reaction (vocalization or movement) • During 4th palpation • During 2nd or 3rd palpation • During 1st palpation Impossible to assess		0 1 2 3 3	0 1 2 3 3	0 1 2 3 3	0 1 2 3 3
Intensity of reaction	No reaction Mild reaction Head turning or vocalization Tries to bite, aggressive or impossible to assess		0 1 2 3	0 1 2 3	0 1 2 3	0 1 2 3
TOTAL SCORE	1–5: mild pain 6–10: moderate pain 11–18: severe pain					
Treatment plan						

Pain assessment form for cats. (Reproduced, with permission, from Mahler and Reece, 2007)

3

Chronic pain

Samantha Lindley and Polly Taylor

Introduction

The management of chronic pain is an emerging discipline in veterinary medicine. It requires an understanding of chronic pain that is beyond that of 'acute pain that has lasted a long time'. This chapter will address some of the intellectual dilemmas of chronic pain and then set out a practical approach to assessing and treating chronic pain. There are no definitive 'best' approaches to chronic pain, and the reader is encouraged also to consult other sources (e.g. Mathews, 2008; Robertson, 2008). Chronic pain requires a multimodal approach to analgesia, and the involvement of the owner – to improve compliance and effectiveness, and to give them a sense of control over their pet's pain and the restrictions it may cause. The approach to chronic pain has the potential to involve the whole practice team in working towards the wellbeing of the patient.

Pain and suffering

The terms 'pain' and 'suffering' are usually used synonymously, but it is more accurate to recognize them as separate experiences. Pain is the sensory experience; suffering is the emotional experience that is often (but not always) associated with the sensation of pain. This is important, because not all pain inevitably leads to suffering, and some interventions relieve suffering without improving a subjective score of pain.

If an animal patient is in pain, it is generally considered that it should be given the benefit of the doubt that it is also suffering.

Definition of chronic pain

Chronic pain is not just acute pain that has lasted for a long time. It is defined in various ways but often as 'pain that persists beyond the time of healing', which is accurate but not all-inclusive, as it does not cover such condtions as arthritis that will never 'heal' but certainly have the potential to cause chronic pain. Pain that persists beyond a rather arbitrary time limit such as 6 months is also sometimes defined as 'chronic'.

It may be better to think of chronic pain as pain that is 'maladaptive', i.e. not useful, in a biological sense, to the sufferer. Acute pain, and all the fear and anxiety with which it is associated, is vital to help reduce damage to the body, where possible, and to trigger healing mechanisms. The sensation of pain is not just unwelcome for its own sake, but it also signals potential tissue damage that will limit function and, ultimately, survival. As Chapter 2 explains, however, this is not a reason to allow patients to suffer with acute pain. The veterinary team attempts to limit or remove the tissue damage causing the pain and thus to remove the body's need to 'recognize' that pain. Yet, from the understanding that feeling (and *suffering from*) pain is important for survival comes the sense that some owners have that *all* pain is useful and that we should not 'just be masking it', as if this removes its usefulness to the patient.

It is important to be very, very clear: chronic pain is not remotely useful to the patient.

- It causes a reduction in sleep and sleep quality, which causes more chronic pain.
- It causes alteration in posture, which puts strain on musculoskeletal structures, thereby causing more chronic pain.
- It alters mood and alters the very mechanisms by which the individual copes with pain, again leading to more chronic pain and more suffering.

Why, then, does chronic pain exist? It is there because the mechanisms that make it so trying to the sufferer are the same mechanisms behind the acute pain that keeps the body alive and functioning. Chronic pain is, in essence, a side effect of that lifesaver. It is tiresome, depressing and debilitating but, ultimately, no individual ever died of chronic pain (although some may have died because of it).

Chronic pain causes the same changes in the body as chronic stress (Figure 3.1) (Lamont *et al.,* 2000). This is a useful axiom to convince owners to use adequate pain relief for their pets. It should also be clear from Figure 3.1 that many patients who present as anxious, and who may be presented for behavioural problems such as separation anxiety or sound sensitivity, may in fact be suffering from pain, since trembling, panting, pacing and mood changes are also signs of pain. Sensations of anxiety and pain are inseparable if untreated.

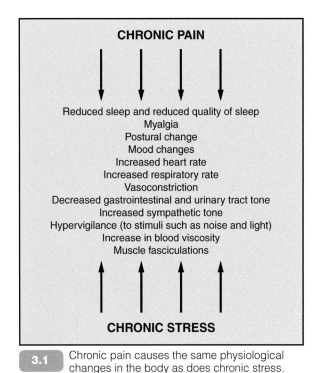

CHRONIC PAIN

Reduced sleep and reduced quality of sleep
Myalgia
Postural change
Mood changes
Increased heart rate
Increased respiratory rate
Vasoconstriction
Decreased gastrointestinal and urinary tract tone
Increased sympathetic tone
Hypervigilance (to stimuli such as noise and light)
Increase in blood viscosity
Muscle fasciculations

CHRONIC STRESS

3.1 Chronic pain causes the same physiological changes in the body as does chronic stress.

Chronic pain may involve either or both of the following:

- **Nociceptive pain** – arising from an intense, noxious stimulus
- **Neuropathic pain** – arising directly from a nerve or from abnormalities in central processing.

A summary of chronic pain is given in Figure 3.2.

- Chronic pain is maladaptive, i.e. of no biological use to the animal
- Chronic pain causes suffering
- Chronic pain is a stressor and gives rise to the same physiological changes as any other kind of chronic stress
- Chronic pain is different from acute pain, not merely because of its duration, but because the plasticity of the nervous system leads to changes in neurons and their receptive fields and the recruitment of nerves not normally associated with transmitting pain
- Chronic pain does not therefore present a consistent picture between individuals
- Chronic pain does not reflect the degree or even presence of pathology
- In some cases chronic pain 'becomes the disease'.

3.2 A summary of chronic pain.

Neurophysiology

The neurophysiology of pain is described in Chapter 2. The simple description of 'physiological' pain uses the 'transmission-of-a-message' picture; however, chronic pain is a different and more complex phenomenon.

In some senses, and according to the International Association for the Study of Pain, the use of the term 'pain pathways' is inaccurate for chronic pain (Merskey and Bogduk, 1994). Pain and suffering are perceived by the brain and therefore pain is 'whatever

the patient says (or in the case of animals and humans who cannot verbalize – thinks) it is'. This may be a better way to think of chronic pain than the classic Cartesian view of a sensation that is transmitted by the body and then 'recognized' by the brain. John Bonica, the father of the understanding of chronic pain in human medicine, described pain as a 'low fidelity signal' (Terman and Bonica, 2001). In other words: pain, or the peripheral stimulus we think of as 'pain', does not arrive as a discrete signal to the nervous system and get transmitted to the brain as a faithful representation of that signal. There is no genuine and reproducible 'representation', because pain is 'whatever the patient thinks it is' and what the patient thinks pain is depends on the resting state of their individual nervous system (including their emotional state), the intensity and duration of the stimulus, intercurrent disease, the amount of attention they pay to the stimulus (the 'cognitive component') and the amount of control they feel they have over the stimulus. A sudden competing stimulus such as a life-threatening event (e.g. a near-miss road traffic accident) or a potentially life-enhancing stimulus (e.g. the arrival of a mate) may reduce the perception of pain to almost negligible.

As an example, radiographically demonstrable osteoarthritic changes *do not correlate at all* with the pain experienced by the patient, regardless of species. This is partly because there may be other, radiographically invisible, sources of pain (soft tissue such as the synovium and muscle), but also because of this low fidelity phenomenon. Animals may run about apparently pain-free with severely radiographically affected joints or may be crippled when the radiographic changes are only minor.

Peripheral sensitization

Peripheral sensitization is mediated by chemical mediators such as the potent vasodilator calcitonin gene-related peptide (CGRP) and substance P, which are released after damage to tissue. By creating a sensitizing 'soup' and attracting more inflammatory mediators, these neurotransmitters lower the response threshold for Aδ and C fibres, thereby creating a zone of 'primary hyperalgesia' around the original site of the tissue damage. The animal therefore protects that area because it is more sensitive. This protection allows healing to take place (Lamont *et al.*, 2000).

Wind-up

'Wind-up' is physiological, i.e. a normal response to a pain stimulus for every individual. Every animal experiences wind-up when they experience pain. It occurs when the synaptic action potentials generated by the stimulated Aδ and C fibres cause an increased and extended potentiation in the neurons of the dorsal horn of the spinal cord. This effect is mediated by N-methyl-D-aspartate (NMDA) receptors. The result for the animal is that a few brief seconds of nociceptive input (such as a surgical incision) causes pain lasting several minutes. The understanding of this phenomenon, and the importance of preventing it, forms the basis of perioperative analgesia.

Central sensitization

Although used synonymously with wind-up in many texts, central sensitization is distinct when used to describe a pathological state. It can be thought of as wind-up that has not 'wound down'.

Central sensitization involves dynamic changes in dorsal horn neuron excitability: the receptive fields of the neurons are modified; nerves that do not normally respond to pain, such as Aβ fibres, are recruited; and areas of secondary hyperalgesia develop (i.e. sensitive areas beyond the original injury). Thus, pain, independent of the progress – or even presence – of pathology, is perceived as worse by the patient.

This plasticity of the nervous system, and the changes that occur in an individual, account for much that is confounding and frustrating for the clinician in the recognition and treatment of chronic pain. It means that the pain perceived becomes separated from the pathology. In the most extreme example, chronic pain *becomes the disease*. It cannot be predicted which individual patients will develop central sensitization, although it seems likely that inadequate treatment of acute and chronic pain is at least a risk factor. The phenomenon is not an inevitable consequence of chronic pain, but it is a serious one for the welfare of the patient (Sternbach,1981).

Central sensitization involves a disturbance or abnormality in the way that pain is processed and so it is also often included in any discussion of neuropathic pain.

Neuropathic pain

This describes:

- Pain arising as a result of direct damage to a nerve
- Pain due to abnormalities of central processing (see above)
- Pain involving descending inhibitory pathways.

The pain caused by direct damage to a nerve, such as nerve root irritation or a neuroma, is characterized in human patients by a sharp, burning, lancinating pain. This sensation has to be inferred from the behaviour of veterinary patients. Jumping, or starting as though stung, are relatively common descriptions, but the behaviour can be as subtle as turning to look at the affected area, progressing to suddenly jumping up and running away from their immediate location, through to panicking and trying to escape, or attacking the area of the body from which the pain appears to be coming. This last behaviour occurs in some cats with spinal pain, where the tail is often targeted. Dogs with neuropathic pain have been presented, anecdotally, with fearful behaviours such as trying to escape from the room or house.

Central sensitization in practice

When a patient develops central sensitization (sometimes known as 'chronic pain syndrome') the separation of pathology and the perception of pain is complete in terms of trying to make any sense about how the patient feels and what the clinician sees as the pathology. There may be no pathology to be found, or it may have resolved or been removed. The questions 'Why is this patient apparently feeling so bad?' and/or 'Why does this owner think their pet is in so much pain when there is nothing to find….' or, worse, '…when I've fixed it?' may be asked. These should be alarm signals for the possibility of central sensitization.

Other clues to this phenomenon may occur during clinical examination.

- **Allodynia** is the interpretation of a normally non-painful stimulus as pain.
- **Hyperalgesia** is an exaggerated response to a painful stimulus.

It is hard to be absolutely sure of the correlation between the presence of hyperalgesia and allodynia, and the way animal patients feel most of the time (i.e. when they are not being prodded). However, a correlation is seen in human patients and in the pain clinics of one of the authors: the presence of allodynia and hyperalgesia do appear to correlate with significant ongoing behavioural signs of suffering.

Pain modulation: descending inhibitory pathways

Descending inhibitory pathways from the brain (e.g. periaqueductal grey and thalamocortex) modulate pain and other sensory inputs and effectively 'damp' pain at every spinal segment. Without such pathways, or when they do not function normally, every microtrauma and minor nociceptive input is perceived as far worse than would be expected. This central modulation of input is mediated by the neurotransmitters serotonin (5-hydroxytryptamine), noradrenaline and endorphins, amongst others, acting at the dorsal horn of the spinal cord. Loss of these inhibitory controls contributes to chronic pain and the signs of central sensitization. Attempting to enhance or augment these effects forms the rationale behind the use of some medications often used in chronic pain problems, such as the tricyclic antidepressants (amitriptyline) and tramadol (Mathews, 2008; Roberston, 2008).

Figure 3.3 summarizes the concepts discussed above.

Acute pain	Both acute and chronic pain may be nociceptive or neuropathic in origin, or have a mixed picture: e.g. intense muscular pain secondary to nerve root irritation
Chronic pain	
Nociceptive pain	Caused by an intense, noxious stimulus threatening damage to tissue
Neuropathic pain	Directly involves nerves or an abnormality of central processing
Sympathetically mediated pain	An incompletely understood pain syndrome described in humans (complex regional pain syndrome) and characterized by cold, painful areas (often limbs) and abnormal reactions to peripheral inputs

3.3 Terminology of clinical pain. (continues) ▶

Peripheral sensitization	Primary peripheral afferent nociceptors are sensitized by inflammatory mediators and, as a result, the affected area is more painful than the surrounding uninjured area
Wind-up	An increased and extended potentiation in the neurons of the dorsal horn of the spinal cord, mediated by *N*-methyl-D-aspartate (NMDA) receptors. The result for the animal is that a few brief seconds of nociceptive input (such as a surgical incision) causes pain lasting several minutes
Central sensitization	An increase in the excitability of dorsal horn neurons and an increase in their receptive field, causing development of allodynia and/or hyperalgesia. The term is often used synonymously with 'wind-up' but it may be more useful to think of it as pathological whereas wind-up is physiological (normal)
Hyperalgesia	Exaggerated pain response to a normally painful stimulus
Allodynia	Where a normally non-painful stimulus, such as light touch, gives rise to pain

3.3 (continued) Terminology of clinical pain.

Assessment of pain and suffering

The sensory and emotional (affective) components of pain, whilst usually experienced almost simultaneously, are distinct (Figure 3.4).

There is no definitive answer to determining how much pain and suffering are present, but it is clear from the numerous pain assessment and quality of life scores (see Chapter 2) that change in an individual's behaviour is the key to assessing pain (Wiseman-Orr *et al.*, 2004, 2006; Freeman *et al.*, 2005).

It is important to have an idea about the degree of suffering because this will determine how robustly one should approach the analgesic regime. It would be possible to set up a few treatment protocols for chronic pain and apply these to every case, after taking into account any particular contraindications for

that individual, but this would inevitably result in the over-medication of many individuals and, possibly, the under-medication of a few. Such an approach does not take into account the variable nature of chronic pain, nor the resistance of many owners to medication unless the necessity for it is well explained. It would also be unsatisfying as a clinical approach and would not take into consideration the different influences of the components of pain.

Components of pain

One way of guiding the clinician (and suggesting which members of the team may be best recruited into helping a patient) is to look at the components that make up the pain experience in the individual being assessed. There are four main components to pain: sensory; emotional; motor; and cognitive.

- The **sensory** component (Figure 3.5a) is the sensation that is experienced and that is called 'pain' by humans. It carries only sensation, but no suffering. It is hard to separate the sensory from the emotional (suffering) component of pain, because humans tend to remember only pain that made them *suffer*, but the two components can be separated and this is the basis of treament with opiates. With opiate analgesia, human patients describe themselves as being 'apart' from the pain: they still have the sensation of pain but they do not care about it any more; sometimes they describe the sense of physical separation from the pain.
- The **emotional** component of pain is the suffering it causes (Figure 3.5b). In chronic pain the suffering component is significant and dealing with the suffering is of paramount importance, because if the patient does not *care* about the pain then that pain does not matter, unless it is going to cause dysfunction and disability. Assessing the degree of suffering in veterinary patients is difficult.
- The **motor** component of pain concerns the movements that the patient makes in order to limit (and sometimes to get attention and

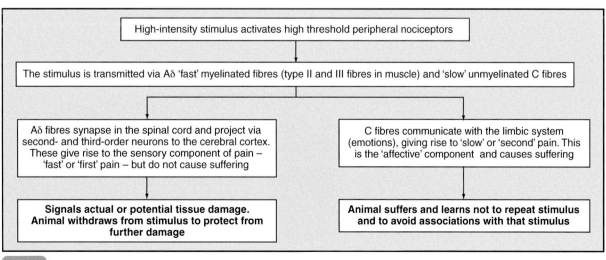

3.4 Pain and suffering.

High-intensity stimulus activates high threshold peripheral nociceptors

↓

The stimulus is transmitted via Aδ 'fast' myelinated fibres (type II and III fibres in muscle) and 'slow' unmyelinated C fibres

Aδ fibres synapse in the spinal cord and project via second- and third-order neurons to the cerebral cortex. These give rise to the sensory component of pain – 'fast' or 'first' pain – but do not cause suffering

C fibres communicate with the limbic system (emotions), giving rise to 'slow' or 'second' pain. This is the 'affective' component and causes suffering

Signals actual or potential tissue damage. Animal withdraws from stimulus to protect from further damage

Animal suffers and learns not to repeat stimulus and to avoid associations with that stimulus

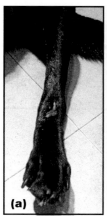
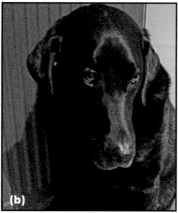
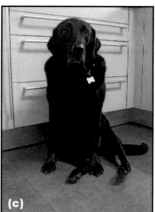

3.5 **(a)** The *sensory* components of this dog's pain are Achilles tendon rupture and surgical complications. **(b)** The *emotional* component of the pain is the way the dog feels about this sensation, in this case obvious from his expression. **(c)** The *motor* component is the predictable lifting of the injured leg whenever it feels painful.

sympathy for) its pain. Classically, this manifests as lifting a painful leg (Figure 3.5c) or the 'praying' stance characteristic of cranial abdominal pain, but reluctance to jump in the car or avoidance of specific behaviours that cause pain, such as being groomed or using a litter tray, are also examples.

- The **cognitive** component of pain is the way that the patient thinks about the pain. This is a major part of chronic pain in people: the more the patient thinks negatively about their pain and focuses on it, the worse the perception of the pain becomes. One of the main ways of helping chronic refractory pain in human patients is through cognitive behaviour therapy – teaching the patient to think differently about their pain. This approach is unfortunately not directly useful to animal patients, but by occupying them and enriching their environment, it should be possible to reduce or change this cognitive component.

Practical applications

Splitting pain into its component parts can help by determining the emphasis to be put on a particular part of the treatment plan.

The *sensory* component of osteosarcoma is usually the most significant element in the patient's pain because these tumours are usually very painful. Trying to make the patient feel happier by playing mentally stimulating games or stroking it will have a marginal effect if the sensory component of the problem is not dealt with, and this significant sensory component will be the primary influence on the *emotional* component, i.e. it is what makes the patient suffer most.

A patient with moderate osteoarthritis whose activities and resources are restricted because of its *disease* and not because of its *pain* (e.g. a Labrador on a weight-reduction diet, no longer allowed to play throw and fetch with its favourite toy) may be suffering more from frustration and hunger than from pain, but has more opportunity to perceive its pain because there are fewer competing influences, i.e. less to take its mind off its pain. In this case the *cognitive* input needs to be changed by devising mentally stimulating games, changing feeding regimes, and using touch and massage to make the patient feel good. In this case, the sensory component is not

the major influence on the suffering and this needs to be taken into account for the animal's welfare as a whole. The analgesic input for this patient will be very different from that of the osteosarcoma patient, but that does not mean that the pain management input is less overall, because of the additional measures that can be taken to stimulate the patient.

This approach can guide the clinician as to where to concentrate the skills of the practice:

- If the *cognitive* component is important, a veterinary nurse with skills and interest in behaviour therapy may well be able to help the owner devise ways in which to help the patient (see Chapter 4)
- A strong *sensory* component may need surgical removal (amputation for the osteosarcoma), aggressive medical intervention (fluids, analgesics, antibiotics) or surgical modification (joint replacement or arthrodesis).

Triangulation

This is the approach used in the pain clinic run by one of the authors (SL). It is unvalidated, but produces a distribution of outcomes that could be reasonably expected from chronic pain patients: a few patients who appear to be coping well and have their pain well managed; a few patients who are suffering so significantly that they either need urgent further investigation or a robust multimodal approach to pain relief; and the majority of patients, who vary in the degree of suffering from requiring relatively conservative additions to their analgesic regime to an extensive programme tackling all four components of pain.

John Webster (2005) described the difficulty of trying to be certain about areas of science such as welfare. As a sailor he used the analogy of taking one's bearings to be more confident about a yacht's position: taking one or two bearings could still leave a good deal of uncertainty, but taking three bearings reduces the 'triangle of uncertainty' about where one is. He used this analogy when assessing certain measures of welfare: there is not one single measure that makes one confident that an animal's welfare is good or bad, but taking a number of measurements increases one's confidence that the assessment is a reasonable one. Figure 3.6 illustrates the points of the triangle.

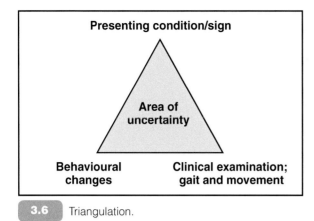

3.6 Triangulation.

Having realized that this was what was essentially being carried out at the pain clinic (SL), this system was adapted to look at chronic pain:

- The first point of the triangle, i.e. the presenting sign or condition, *may* be indicative of pain, but equally may be misleading
- Behavioural changes on their own may be suggestive of pain, but unless the animal's environment has been taken into account these could also be misleading
- The physical examination (which may include further tests and their interpretation), the third point of the triangle, may confirm or confound the combined information from the behavioural and presenting signs assessment.

If all three points of the triangle indicate pain and suffering, then the area of uncertainty about that suffering is reduced (Lindley, 2007).

Behavioural changes

Behavioural indications of pain in dogs and cats are listed in Figures 3.7 and 3.8.

Behaviours for which the animal has a high motivation are important to assess. If a dog has a high motivation to chase a ball, for example, then the fact that it continues to do this with enthusiasm does not rule out pain and suffering. However, if the same patient will *not* engage in this behaviour then it would indicate that its suffering is profound.

There are some patients for whom the owners describe no behavioural changes, yet their gait and physical examination strongly suggest very severe pain. These animals always appear to have had conditions that have been present for some time, often years, such as hip dysplasia; sadly, the conclusion must be that they have suffered pain for years so there are no behavioural changes to measure. The reason for the presentation is usually an acute flare-up in the condition or because postural strain has finally taken its toll on the rest of the musculoskeletal system. Confirmation of the hypothesis about pain having been present for longer than the owner thinks can be seen when the animal is finally given sufficient analgesia and its behaviour changes in a positive direction, beyond that which the owner expects.

Changes in:

- Exercise tolerance, including the patient's initial enthusiasm to exercise as well as how long they would exercise if given a free run
- Play: enthusiasm to play and initiation of play
- Spending time with the owner, e.g. are they more 'clingy' or more distant
- Greeting the owner when they arrive home or come downstairs in the morning
- Attitude to other dogs/people
- Sensitivity to noises
- Ability to be left alone
- Attitude to travelling in car
- Attitude to children
- Attitude to young or boisterous dogs
- Appetite
- Sleeping position
- General activity
- General demeanour

NB: Any of these may change with other changes in environment (e.g. the loss of a human owner or sibling pet, the arrival of a baby) and will depend upon the general sensitivity of the patient

Specific behaviours strongly suggestive of pain

- Jumping or starting behaviour
- Excessive licking of, or gnawing at, an area of the body (in the absence of dermatological disease)
- Panting and/or pacing for no obvious reason (i.e. ambient temperature is normal and the animal has no other reason for anxiety)
- Restless when trying to settle and sleep

3.7 Behavioural indications of pain in dogs.

Changes in:

- Climbing or jumping on to high areas
- Grooming/hygiene
- Activity
- Play and initiation of play
- Time spent with owners
- Demeanour and mood
- Use of scratch post
- Toileting habits

NB: Any of these may change with other changes in environment (e.g. the loss of a human owner or sibling pet, the arrival of a baby) and will depend upon the general sensitivity of the patient

Specific behaviours strongly suggestive of pain

- Jumping, starting or attacking areas of the body such as hindlimbs or tail (suggests hyperaesthesia)

3.8 Behavioural indications of pain in cats.

Examination for hyperalgesia and allodynia

This will be covered here in detail because it is not mentioned in many other texts, whereas general examination techniques for visceral pain are covered in texts and general veterinary teaching.

In both cats and dogs, palpation of tense or guarded muscles and joints is likely to be painful, even if there is no pre-existing pain. Anxiety in both the cat and dog will make the examination more suggestive of pain, since fear exacerbates pain. Yet pain exacerbates fear, so information as to whether the animal is usually anxious during examinations will be helpful. Ensuring the patient is as relaxed as possible is essential:

- There is no substitute for taking time
- Talk to the animal gently and engage the owners. If the owners have confidence in the clinician, many pets will relax because the owner is relaxed
- Owners usually know whether their dog is more relaxed when examined on the floor or on the table
- Food will relax some dogs; gentle petting and massage others
- Cats usually enjoy being rubbed around their chins and ears. Keeping one hand in gentle contact with them whilst examining is helpful
- Groomers that mimic a massaging action can be helpful in some animals. Touch is in itself powerful too, dropping blood pressure and releasing mood-enhancing neurotransmitters in animals that do not resent grooming or close human contact (Odendaal, 2002) (see Chapter 8).

Examination of the part of the patient that is suspected to be the source of pain should be reserved until last. Once pain has been caused, the examination is effectively over in terms of any further useful information to be gained. Sometimes this approach will reveal surprising information: the dog that presents with a forelimb lameness may be found to have much more significant pain in its back and possibly one or both hindlimbs; or an animal presenting with apparent back pain may be far more tender on palpation of its cranial abdomen or over its bladder.

Start with a *gentle* touch. The technique of examining muscles is not taught in veterinary (or medical) undergraduate training but is a skill worth acquiring. Pressing muscles hard just hurts, but graduating the touch from light to firm is the key to identifying changes in central perception.

- Allodynia is the perception of light touch as pain. Most commonly this manifests as a movement away (flinching) from light touch, or shuddering, or fasciculations of the muscle when the fingers are passed lightly over a given area.
  Fasciculations are not the same as trembling of the whole animal and should be distinguished from such. Sometimes an animal will move its head towards the area touched, as though a snap or bite is intended. Owners will often report that the animal resents or resists grooming or stroking in that same area.
- Hyperalgesia is the exaggerated response to a painful stimulus. It is arguably harder to be certain of hyperalgesia than of allodynia, unless an algometer is used to give a consistent pressure, but that is not practical in a normal examination nor for internal structures. With experience, an adverse response to a relatively firm pressure that would cause no overt resentment in a normal patient can be interpreted as hyperalgesia.

Once light and then relatively firmer touch and pressure on the skin, muscles, soft tissues and joints have been carried out and assessed, firmer pressure, joint palpation, range of movement, swelling, heat and visceral pain can be assessed in the usual way.

Gait and movement

Gait and movement are included in the third point of the triangle. Arguably, they could be considered as a separate item, but it is harder to be convinced about changes in this category when there is a pain source other than musculoskeletal. For musculoskeletal pain the gait of the animal should always be watched (using video if this gives a more genuine account, especially in cats), assessing walking, running, and going up and down stairs (dogs) or on and off high surfaces (cats). If time allows, it is helpful to watch the animal move about the consulting room freely: lying down, standing up, sitting, moving slowly. It may be that a dog presented for forelimb lameness demonstrates unequivocally that it has primary hindlimb and back pain by the way it tries to get up. Subtle shifts in weight bearing may also be noted. For animals whose pain source is not musculoskeletal, some characteristic motor patterns may be noted in a relaxed animal: e.g. pawing at the face; 'praying' or stretching; excessive yawning; jumping, starting or looking round suddenly; hunched posture; licking at the abdomen.

A pragmatic approach to the treatment of chronic pain in dogs and cats

The principles of approaching treatment of chronic pain are summarized in Figure 3.9.

1. Identify the presenting sign and/or condition

Identifying the presenting sign should be straightforward, but the sign will not necessarily, nor even commonly, equate to the diagnosis. The presenting sign is usually whatever the owner decides to bring to the attention of the veterinary surgeon; for example, the dog cannot jump in the car; the cat is urinating inappropriately. Sometimes this sign will accompany a pre-existing diagnosis, such as osteoarthritis or cystitis, but the two need not necessarily be related. In a pain clinic setting, the 'fact' of the condition may be presented, i.e. 'my dog/cat has osteoarthritis/cystitis and I need to know what this means and how it is affecting him/her'.

2. Identify and reconcile the owner's concerns and expectations

It is often obvious what the owner is concerned about but it is important to make sure that, whatever it may be, this is understood clearly at the beginning of the consultation. Some examples:

- The clinician may be concerned about the level of pain and suffering for the animal, whilst the owner is concerned about whether or not that animal may eventually be able to perform agility, or become a show animal, or get through the night without toileting on the floor

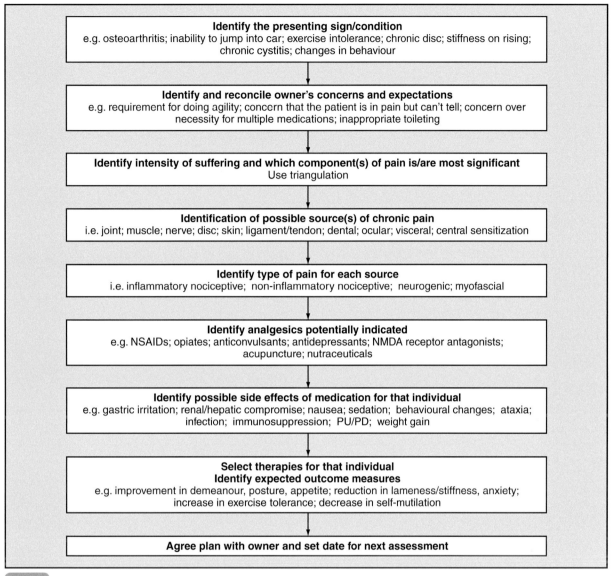

Identify the presenting sign/condition
e.g. osteoarthritis; inability to jump into car; exercise intolerance; chronic disc; stiffness on rising; chronic cystitis; changes in behaviour

Identify and reconcile owner's concerns and expectations
e.g. requirement for doing agility; concern that the patient is in pain but can't tell; concern over necessity for multiple medications; inappropriate toileting

Identify intensity of suffering and which component(s) of pain is/are most significant
Use triangulation

Identification of possible source(s) of chronic pain
i.e. joint; muscle; nerve; disc; skin; ligament/tendon; dental; ocular; visceral; central sensitization

Identify type of pain for each source
i.e. inflammatory nociceptive; non-inflammatory nociceptive; neurogenic; myofascial

Identify analgesics potentially indicated
e.g. NSAIDs; opiates; anticonvulsants; antidepressants; NMDA receptor antagonists; acupuncture; nutraceuticals

Identify possible side effects of medication for that individual
e.g. gastric irritation; renal/hepatic compromise; nausea; sedation; behavioural changes; ataxia; infection; immunosuppression; PU/PD; weight gain

Select therapies for that individual
Identify expected outcome measures
e.g. improvement in demeanour, posture, appetite; reduction in lameness/stiffness, anxiety; increase in exercise tolerance; decrease in self-mutilation

Agree plan with owner and set date for next assessment

3.9 An approach to the treatment of chronic pain.

- The clinician may be concerned about the existence of a lameness or the differential for frequent vomiting, whereas the owner may only be concerned about whether pain is present
- The surgical removal of a tumour may be of paramount importance to the clinician as part of the animal's treatment, but the owner may be desperately concerned about whether their pet will cope with the intervention as a whole
- Relief of pain and discomfort may be the aim of the clinician, but the owner's agenda may be to keep the patient off medication wherever possible.

Asking the question 'What concerns you most?' is therefore necessary to avoid unpleasant surprises and potential problems with communication or compliance later in the process.

3. Identify intensity of suffering and which component(s) of pain is/are most significant

This can be achieved by:

- Considering the components of pain involved
- Triangulation (see above).

There may be reasons other than pain for the presenting sign:

- At the simplest level, a cat may be withdrawn and 'grumpy' because the household has become very busy or redecoration has removed the cat's core territory and security
- A dog may not jump in the car because the car has been changed and is too high or awkward, or the dog may have received an electrostatic shock on a previous attempt
- The presenting condition need not necessarily be causing pain, even though it is a risk factor for the presence of pain, e.g. osteoarthritis may be present but may not currently be causing pain.

4. Identify possible sources of chronic pain

This will guide the clinician towards the analgesic(s) most likely to be of use in this patient.

Possible sources of pain include:

- Skin – some dermatological conditions are obviously painful. Intense pruritus may lead to self-mutilation and tissue damage; it has recently been suggested that itch is more akin to neuropathic pain, which may explain why it is so challenging to treat
- Muscle – includes myositis, muscle spasm and myofascial pain. Each of these responds to different approaches. Key points to remember are:
  - o In humans, the longer the duration of muscle pain and the more intense the pain, the more widespread is the referral pattern (Kellgren, 1938); albeit that referred pain can only be inferred from examination and the behaviour of veterinary patients, it may be assumed that this will also be the case in animals
  - o Muscle pain can be intense and debilitating
  - o Myofascial pain (see Chapter 11) which arises from myofascial trigger points (the 'knots' that can be easily found in the shoulder girdle muscles of most humans over 25 years of age) is apparently not well controlled by conventional analgesia. Trigger points can arise secondary to somatic and visceral pain, as well as from age degeneration, postural strain, nerve root irritation and blunt trauma (Gerwin, 1994; Simons *et al.*, 1999)
- Joints and associated structures – synovium, ligaments and tendons. Pain from these structures can be intense, but tends to be fairly localized
- Discogenic pain – there is still some controversy about the source of pain when a disc prolapses, although some is evidently caused by pressure on local nerve roots (radiculopathy) and some by a local inflammatory reaction mediated by neurotransmitters such as brain-derived neurotrophic factor (BDNF), glutamate and substance P (Onda *et al.*, 2003). Secondary muscle pain is common
- Neuropathic pain (see above) – assess for hyperalgesia and allodynia. These are challenging pains to treat, and can also be associated with secondary muscle pain as a mixed picture
- Dental pain – abscess, gingival disease. This kind of pain is apparently tolerated remarkably well by many patients, but owners often report dramatic behaviour changes after tooth removal, indicating that pain has caused more suffering than was supposed
- Visceral pain – gastrointestinal pain, pancreatic pain, bladder pain. Any human who has experienced visceral pain will testify that it is a uniquely debilitating pain, even more difficult to describe than other pains
- Ocular pain – potentially intense and localized.

5. Identify the type of pain for each source
Identifying, if possible, whether pain is nociceptive or neuropathic will guide the clinician as to the type of analgesia required.

6. Identify analgesics potentially indicated
Factors to consider:

- The severity of suffering
- The prescribing cascade
- Contraindications related to the patient and condition
- Side effects that would be particularly debilitating for this patient or of particular concern for this owner
- Cost (where it has been raised as a concern)
- Difficulties in drug administration (particularly pertinent for cats)
- Additional therapies: acupuncture; hydrotherapy; physiotherapy; touch; massage; heat or cold; mental stimulation; nutraceuticals.

Figure 3.10 shows how multimodal analgesic treatment, both pharmacological and non-pharmacological, may be used for a range of clinical situations.

Nociceptive pain (visceral, musculoskeletal, dental, dermatological) without central changes or significant suffering
• NSAIDs • Nutraceuticals; physio/hydrotherapy; pentosan polysulphate (no evidence for direct analgesia but appears to help in some cases) • Acupuncture
Where suffering is intense but NSAIDs contraindicated or not effective enough
• Tramadol [a] • Amantadine [a] • Paracetamol with codeine (not cats) • Cinchophen with prednisolone • Acupuncture • Gabapentin [a] • Amitriptyline [a] or imipramine [a]
Where signs or pathology indicate neuropathic pain (including disturbances in central processing)
• Gabapentin [a] • Amitriptyline [a] or imipramine [a] • Acupuncture • Tramadol [a] • Amantadine [a]

3.10 Multimodal analgesia for chronic pain. See Figure 3.11 (and product data sheets) for dose rates, contraindications and adverse reactions. [a] Not authorized in the UK for use in small animals.

Drug treatments
Analgesics and analgesic doses are described in many texts (including the *BSAVA Small Animal Formulary*) and by many different authors; since many of the medications used for chronic pain states in animals are not authorized for safety or efficacy in dogs and cats, the dose rates vary from text to text. Figure 3.11 lists the commonly used chronic pain medications with notes on their use and adverse effects in dogs and cats.

Non-pharmacological interventions
Non-pharmacological interventions for chronic pain include acupuncture, hydrotherapy and physio-therapy (see Chapters 9, 10 and 11). The main consideration for any device (or treatment) whose mechanism is unknown or unproven is that it should be *safe* (safety includes a consideration of delaying effective treatment; see Chapter 8), although the financial implication for owners may also be significant.

Drug and action	Doses/use in dogs	Doses/use in cats	Comments
NSAIDs (Anti-inflammatory and analgesic)	As per data sheets. 6 weeks may be required for wind-down of chronic pain	Meloxicam now authorized for cats in the UK. Dose as per data sheet	Meloxicam appears to be metabolized via oxidative pathways rather than by glucuronidation in the cat and is therefore better tolerated than other NSAIDs
Tramadol [a] (Partial opiate; reduces suffering)	2–5 mg/kg orally q12h or 2 mg/kg i.v. once; but doses of 2–10 mg/kg orally q8h quoted. Lower doses (1–2 mg/kg q12h) often appear to be effective	2–4 mg/kg orally q12h or 1–2 mg/kg s.c. once. Seizures reported in cats treated at these doses. Slower elimination time in cats, so keep dose and frequency low	Difficulty dosing smaller dogs and cats as smallest capsule 50 mg, but the compound is very stable so capsules can be split for smaller dose size. Side effects include vomiting, diarrhoea, sedation, dullness, dysphoria
Gabapentin [a] (Action not entirely understood; membrane stabilizer; enhances descending noradrenergic pathway)	3–10 mg/kg orally q8–12h	3–10 mg/kg orally q8–12h	Smallest capsule 100 mg. Side effects include vomiting, diarrhoea, polyuria/polydipsia, itching (at high doses), sedation. Signs of toxicity or sensitivity are ataxia, stumbling or tripping; reversible on withdrawal
Tricyclic antidepressants [a] (Enhance adrenergic transmission, i.e. augment descending inhibitory pathways)	Amitriptyline: 1–2 mg/kg orally q12h Imipramine: 0.5 mg/kg orally q8h	Amitriptyline: 0.5–1 mg/kg orally q24h Imipramine: 0.5–1 mg/kg orally q12–24h	Both A and I can be bitter and difficult to administer to cats. Antidepressant effects take up to 4 weeks: analgesic effects appear to be much faster (1–2 days) although this must depend on the source of pain and state of the nervous system. Competent renal and hepatic function are necessary for complete clearance and excretion. Cardiotoxic (dysrhythmogenic) in overdose. Do not use with tramadol (theoretical risk of serotonin syndrome). NB Clomipramine, although authorized for separation anxiety in dogs, not generally considered useful in pain because of greater serotonergic than noradrenergic effects
Paracetamol (acetaminophen) [a] (Analgesic and antipyretic; analgesic action reported to be enhanced when used with other analgesics in human medicine)	10 mg/kg orally q12h Paracetamol with codeine: Pardale V authorized as per data sheet, but dose as for paracetamol component	**Do not use in cats**	
Amantadine [a] (NMDA receptor antagonist)	Doses suggested range from 3–5 mg/kg orally q24h to 1–2 mg/kg orally q12h. Caution would suggest starting at lower dose rate once a day, i.e. 1–2 mg/kg q24h	1–4 mg/kg orally q24h, starting at the lowest dose and gradually increasing	GI signs have been seen in at least one canine patient; GI signs and CNS signs reported in humans
Buprenorphine [a] (Opioid: partial mu agonist, kappa antagonist)	Not practical for long-term use, although oral transmucosal route (0.12 mg/kg q6–8h) has been described in dogs	0.01–0.02 mg/kg by oral transmucosal route q6–8h (Figure 3.12)	Although more commonly used in transition period between acute and chronic pain, there is no reason not to use it more long term if tolerated by the patient and necessary for its wellbeing
Cinchophen plus prednisolone (NSAID plus steroid) (Prednoleucotropin)	25 mg/kg orally q12h	**Do not use in cats**	Occasionally, this combination will give pain relief where all other NSAIDs have been tried and failed

3.11 Commonly used analgesics in chronic and neuropathic pain. [a] Not authorized in the UK for use in animals. The dose rates for unauthorized medications are based on experience and practice. In patients with multiple pathologies or a tendency to adverse reactions or on multiple medications, starting at a lower dose rate may be sensible to help limit side effects.

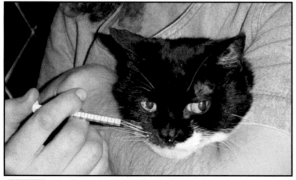

3.12 Oral transmucosal administration of buprenorphine.

Transcutaneous electrical nerve stimulation

TENS works in the same way as 'rubbing it better', i.e. via Aβ fibres in the skin and presynaptic inhibition in the dorsal horn of the spinal cord, mediated by gamma-aminobutyric acid (GABA) (Melzack and Wall, 1965; Wall and Sweet, 1965). TENS has been used since 1985 in the human field and is useful in a number of human medical acute and chronic conditions, such as angina pectoris, labour pain and acute orofacial pain (Thompson, 1998).

There are different types of TENS now available. The conventional type employs high-frequency, low-intensity stimulation and is the one with which most people are familiar. Pulsed TENS employs low-frequency/low-intensity stimulation and ALTENS (acupuncture-like TENS) uses low-frequency/high-intensity stimulation. These modifications were developed in an attempt to deal with different kinds of pain, both acute and chronic, suffered by patients.

The problems with using any form of TENS in non-human animals are: electrode placement needs to be quite precise (i.e. where the pain is); and, with conventional TENS, once the device is turned off, the pain returns quite quickly. Human patients tend to wear their device most of the day when they have chronic pain and to adjust the intensity of stimulus according to their pain level. Most of the high-quality evidence in animals is in models of experimental and acute pain inflammation, which makes it difficult to extrapolate to its use in chronic pain in animals. TENS is widely recognized as a useful pain-relieving technique in humans and it is natural for its use to be explored in the veterinary field, despite the potential problems cited. TENS is discussed more fully in Chapter 9.

Transcutaneous spinal electroanalgesia

TSE appears to work by sending an electrical stimulus via the skin to the spinal cord, thereby inhibiting onward transmission of pain, but the precise mechanism is unknown (MacDonald and Coates, 1995). There is usually no sensation experienced by the patient, but they often become very sleepy and relaxed. The commercially available devices only deal with chronic pain and will not mask acute pain, so they are safe to use at home (Figure 3.13) and give the owners a sense of control over their pet's pain. However, there is no evidence currently available for the use of TSE in the cat or dog, and the studies in humans to date have been negative or equivocal.

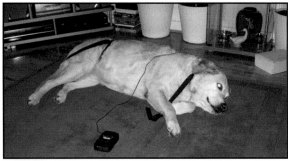

3.13 A relaxed patient undergoing transcutaneous spinal electroanalgesia.

Magnets

There are many magnetic products available for humans and pets that are promoted to relieve pain, but the scientific evidence appears to be scant. The most commonly suggested mechanism is via improved blood flow and tissue oxygenation but this does not appear to be supported.

7. Identify possible side effects for the individual

- For all medications, any individual may develop gastrointestinal signs. This may be a response to the medication or, in more unusual cases, to the capsule within which the medication is enclosed.

- NSAIDs should be avoided in renal and hepatic disease or in animals with, or predisposed to, gastrointestinal ulceration. Monitoring for renal side effects during long-term use or in high-risk patients is essential.

- Sedation: sometimes this is not noticed until the animal stops taking the medication, so it may not be obvious. It is possible that what the owner thinks is sedation is general dullness arising from nausea or disorientation, or relaxation as a result of reduction in pain. Either way, if the animal is not 'happier' than they were before they started the medication, at least a trial withdrawal should be considered. Some sedation may be short-lived, e.g. with the tricyclic antidepressants (TCAs), and wear off as the liver induces enzymes to metabolize the medication, so this should be accounted for before withdrawing the drug.

- Dysphoria (or euphoria): this can occur with any of the opiate drugs, and with tramadol if the patient is particularly sensitive to the opiate component of the drug. This may be acceptable when using the drug short term to deal with intense pain, but should not be accepted as a long-term side effect.

- Behavioural changes can occur with any of the centrally acting drugs; these changes may range from agitation to aggression.

- Gabapentin commonly causes dizziness in human patients; signs of specific toxicity in animals are stumbling or tripping up. This may be a genuine ataxia or may be due to dizziness. The dose should be reduced or the drug withdrawn.

- Weight gain may occur with chronic usage of TCAs and has been reported with gabapentin. This will impact on the prognosis of musculoskeletal disease if significant, but it usually tends not to be dramatic and is not generally a reason to withhold these drugs.

- TCAs and prednoleucotropin tend to depress T4, so this should be borne in mind if the patient is borderline hypothyroid or when interpreting blood samples.

- Anecdotally, there are few reports of long-term problems with most of these unauthorized products, though time and experience may temper these observations. Animals on TCAs should be monitored, since TCAs require competent renal and hepatic function to be cleared and are to be used with caution in cardiac dysrhythmias. Gabapentin is processed by the liver in the dog before being excreted, so its use in a patient with concurrent liver disease should be considered with relative caution (Mathews, 2008).

It is important, when describing possible side effects to the owner, that they are reassured that they are uncommon and that their pet will not have to 'put up' with them. They should be informed that if side effects occur, the drug dose will be reduced or the drug withdrawn. This sounds self-evident but many owners will assume that these are side effects that their pet will have to live with in order to have the 'right' medication, so it is worthwhile re-iterating that the main concern is for the animal's overall wellbeing.

8. Select therapies and identify potential outcome measures

For each therapy, the owner should have an idea of the outcome expected (Figure 3.14). It may be that they just expect their pet to be 'happier' and more interactive, or to sleep better, or to stop the excessive licking of a body area. If there is hyperalgesia and/or allodynia present, then these may need to be resolved before there is a major change in the movement or major presenting signs of the patient, but the owners will probably describe their pet as 'happier', possibly picking up a toy for the first time in a while, perhaps being more affectionate. These are important observations as they reflect a *decrease in suffering*.

Analgesia: veterinary treatment
• Medication
• Diet
• Nutraceuticals
• Acupuncture
• Transcutaneous spinal electroanalgesia
• Touch
• Physiotherapy
• Hydrotherapy

Techniques for the owner
• Touch, flat hand massage, stretching (muscles and joint mobilization)
• Optimizing core territory for a cat (see Case 14.1 for details)
• Manipulation of feeding: food balls, hide and seek, controlled delivery of food over an extended period requiring mental stimulation and play
• Play: appropriate play for the condition; mental stimulation instead of vigorous play
• Exercise: varied walks, avoidance of hard substrates, socialization if enjoyed; reduce pulling by non-pulling harnesses
• Comfort: watch the animal's choice and buy beds accordingly
• Heat: if the patient seeks heat, use warmed towels over painful areas
• Coolness: if the patient wants to lie on the cool grass or tiles, provide cooled towels for distraction
• Consider ease of movement around the house: non-slip rugs, lead support going up and downstairs if stairs must be tackled and the animal is hesitant

Potential desired outcomes
• Improvement in demeanour (i.e. reduction of suffering)
• Reduction in lameness
• Improved mobility (musculoskeletal)
• Reduction in palpable pain
• Improved range of movement (of joints)
• Reduction in signs such as yawning, stretching, lip licking, salivating, plant consumption
• Improvement of hunched appearance
• Improvement in appetite
• Improvement in toileting (resolution of diarrhoea, constipation, frequency of urination, stranguria, distress on straining)
• Reduced visceral signs
• Positive changes in behaviour – more interactive, more affectionate, more relaxed

3.14 Summary of chronic pain treatment and outcomes.

9. Agree plan with owner and agree date for next assessment

For the owner to comply with the plan it must be discussed and agreed upon. Similarly, a date at which the animal can be re-examined and any progress or problems assessed should be arranged.

Osteoarthritis

This is one of the most common chronically painful conditions in dogs and cats and is worth a special mention. The aim of treating arthritis is two-fold:

- To slow down the progress of the disease towards an end-stage joint
- To drive a chronic active state to a chronic silent state – where there is no pain – independent of any progression of disease.

The first aim is the hardest to achieve, but the second is equally important to the animal. A practical approach to ensuring that all the areas that can influence the disease are covered has been devised by Carmichael (2006) and involves a straightforward ABCDE approach.

- **A = analgesia,** including NSAIDs, tramadol, acupuncture.
- **B = bodyweight.** Weight loss significantly reduces the pain associated with osteoarthritis in dogs and, in some specific circumstances, can also reduce the progression of disease (see Chapter 6). Research is underway to determine what proportion of weight needs to be lost before a significant improvement is seen; this would be very helpful for owners to give them a target for which to aim. However, weight loss is not the only consideration: muscle atrophy may be severe and some arthritic patients are cachexic, so appropriate nutrition and exercise are needed to address this.
- **C = control** – of complications and of comfort, and to impart a sense of control to the owner.
  - o For owners to feel that they can be in control of their pet's pain is an important part of managing chronic pain.
  - o Complications include side effects of the medications, lack of owner compliance, and factors hindering the improvement of the patient (like bodyweight or the need to exercise vigorously to be contented).
  - o Comfort includes considerations of beds, ramps, surfaces walked on, avoiding pulling on the lead, and the use of heat or cold to provide easing and distraction from pain. For cats this means modifying their core territory so that they both feel better about their pain and can acquire all their resources despite pain and mobility restrictions (see Chapters 4 and 14).
  - o **C** also stands for **common sense**: to paraphrase Carmichael (personal communication), 'if the dog with hip arthritis can run about and the only thing it cannot do is get in the car, then the dog needs a ramp and not a hip replacement'.

- **D = disease modification.** This includes trying to slow the progress towards end-stage joints and resultant salvage surgery (joint replacement, femoral head excision, arthrodesis). Slowing the progress is difficult to achieve and to prove but it may be achieved: by the use of nutraceuticals (although the results of research on this are variable and controversial – see Chapter 7); by sensible, relatively non-concussive exercise; and by maintaining an optimum weight for the animal. Avoiding excessive weight gain in large-breed dogs during growth has been shown to be particularly effective in reducing the severity of developmental joint disease such as hip dysplasia.
- **E = exercise.** Osteoarthritis in the chronic active phase indicates the need for controlled, regular exercise. The amount and type should be judged by the animal's reponse: is it stiff after exercise or resting; does it slow down at a certain point on the walk; do particular signs occur after too much exercise? It is important to give the owner guidance about a specific amount of exercise (e.g. 'three 10-minute walks, on a lead, on flat ground, without pulling') and how to modify this depending on the response to treatment.

Hydrotherapy and physiotherapy may be included in all categories A–E.

Chronic pain clinics

The aims of a veterinary pain clinic are:

- To assess the current pain state of the patient
- To assess how much any restrictions caused by the disease or its management are affecting the patient's life (e.g. restriction of food, favourite play, exercise; see Chapter 4)
  - o Restriction of exercise often means that a dog is not meeting other dogs and people as much as previously and tends to be walked (on concrete) around the same, restricted area
  - o For cats, the inability to reach high places, difficulty in managing high-sided litter trays and the need to climb to reach their food may represent real stressors on top of the pain they are already experiencing
- To explore the possible causes of pain and, therefore, the best approach for that individual, whilst taking into account the owner's concerns and having time to allay them if possible
- To find ways of helping the owner to feel that they are in control. For human patients, having control over their chronic refractory pain is an important part of the treatment (Jensen *et al.*, 1991) but owners also seem to need to feel that they have some control over their pets' pain. If an owner has given the total pain medication for the day, but still feels that their pet is in pain, it is helpful if there are measures they can take to safely help that pain. These measures include: massage, relaxation therapy, play therapy, and the use of heat or coolness to distract or ease pain

- To use an integrated approach to pain: this will include orthodox medications and more 'advanced' medications, but also acupuncture where appropriate, hydrotherapy and physiotherapy where indicated, and environmental enrichment. In this way the aim is to deal with *all* the components of pain, not just the sensory components
- To identify realistic outcomes for the owner and provide support for them and their pet
- To provide a genuinely 'value added' service for the client. The advantage of an 'advocate for the patient' (see Chapter 1) within the practice, to whom the owner can turn when they are worried and who will bring those concerns to the notice of all practice personnel who have dealings with that patient, can be appreciated.

References and further reading

Carmichael S (2006) Putting theory into practice – best practice management for osteoarthritis. *European Journal of Companion Animal Practice* **16** (1), 27–31

Freeman LM, Rush JE, Farabaugh AE and Must A (2005) Assessment of health-related quality of life in dogs with cardiac disease. *Journal of the American Veterinary Medical Association* **226**, 1864–1868

Gerwin RD (1994) Neurobiology of the myofascial trigger point. *Ballière's Clinical Rheumatology* **8**(4), 747–762

Jensen MP, Turner JA and Romano JM (1991) Coping with chronic pain: a critical review of the literature. *Pain* **47**, 249–283

Kellgren JH (1938) Observations on referred pain arising from muscle. *Clinical Science* **3**, 175–190

Lamont LA, Tranquilli WJ and Grimm KA (2000) Physiology of pain. *Veterinary Clinics of North America: Small Animal Practice* **30**(4), 703–728

Lindley S (2007) Recognising pain in cats: a challenge for our times. *Proceedings of the Mosaic Symposium, Seville 2007*, pp.12–14.

MacDonald AJR and Coates TW (1995) The discovery of transcutaneous spinal electroanalgesia and its relief of chronic pain. *Physiotherapy* **81**, 653–661

Mathews KA (2008) Neuropathic pain in dogs and cats: if only they could tell us if it hurts. *Veterinary Clinics of North America: Small Animal Practice* **38**(6), 1365–1414

Melzack R and Wall PD (1965) Pain mechanisms: a new theory. *Science* **150**, 971–979

Merskey H and Bogduk N (1994) *Classification of Chronic Pain, 2nd edn.* IASP Press, Seattle

Odendaal J (2002) *Pets and our Mental Health: The Why, the What, and the How.* Vantage Press, New York

Onda A, Murata Y, Rydevik B *et al.* (2003) Immunoreactivity of brain-derived neurotrophic factor in rat dorsal root ganglion and spinal cord dorsal horn following exposure to herniated nucleus pulposus. *Neuroscience Letters* **352**, 49–52

Robertson SA (2008) Managing pain in feline patients. *Veterinary Clinics of North America: Small Animal Practice* **38**(6), 1268–1290

Simons DG, Travell JG and Simons PT (1999) *Travell and Simons' Myofascial Pain and Dysfunction: The Trigger Point Manual. Volume 1: Upper half of the Body.* Williams and Wilkins, Baltimore

Sternbach RA (1981) Chronic pain as a disease entity. *Triangle* **20**, 27–32

Terman GW and Bonica JJ (2001) Spinal mechanisms and their modulation. In: *Bonica's Management of Pain*, ed. JD Loeser, pp. 74–152. Lea and Febiger, Philadelphia

Thompson J W (1998) Trancutaneous electrical nerve stimulation (TENS). In: *Medical Acupuncture, A Western Scientific Approach*, ed. J Filshie and A White, pp. 177–192. Churchill Livingstone, Edinburgh

Wall PD and Sweet WH (1965) Temporary abolition of pain in man. *Science* **155**, 108–109

Webster J (2005) *Animal Welfare: Limping towards Eden.* Blackwell, Oxford

Wiseman-Orr ML, Nolan AM, Reid J *et al.* (2004) Development of a questionnaire to measure the effects of chronic pain on health-related quality of life in dogs. *American Journal of Veterinary Research* **65**, 1077–1084

Wiseman-Orr ML, Scott EM, Reid J *et al.* (2006) Validation of a structured questionnaire as an instrument to measure chronic pain in dogs on the basis of effects on health-related quality of life. *American Journal of Veterinary Research* **67**, 1826–1836

4

Fear, anxiety and conflict in companion animals

Rachel Casey

Introduction

Until recently, there has been a tendency to consider the behaviour of animals as being separate from, and even immaterial to, their physical health. However, there is now strong evidence that the emotional state of both human and veterinary patients not only influences their behaviour (McGaugh, 2000), but also has a profound influence on the onset of, and recovery from, disease (McEwen, 2000; De Kloet et al., 2005). Understanding how and why behavioural signs are shown, and identifying the types of situations that may cause negative emotional states, is therefore crucial to caring for the veterinary patient in the context of palliation, rehabilitation or supportive care.

Negative emotional states

Emotions can be considered to be either positive or negative and, therefore, events can be associated with a 'good' feeling or a 'bad' feeling. This is adaptive (i.e. biologically useful) in an evolutionary sense, because it enables animals to associate situations or events with different outcomes and to change their behaviour accordingly.

- If an animal associates a particular situation with a *positive* emotional state, it will show behaviours aimed at trying to reach that goal; any behaviours found to be successful will become reinforced (i.e. more likely to be used again).
- Where a particular situation becomes associated with a *negative* emotional state, the animal will show behaviours aimed at trying to avoid that situation and any such behaviour that is successful will become reinforced.
- The other *negative* emotional state to consider is what might be termed 'frustration', which arises when a behaviour that an animal anticipates should be successful at either achieving a positive goal or avoiding an anticipated negative event no longer succeeds.

Fear and anxiety

'Anxiety' is often used non-specifically and inaccurately. The use of the term 'separation anxiety' to describe all dogs that show a behavioural response when left by their owners is an example of this misuse. In fact, different emotional states may underlie similar behavioural signs shown when dogs are left alone. There is also the tendency to use 'anxiety' synonymously with 'fear' when discussing behavioural responses. Looking more closely at how responses are generated in the brain allows a clearer picture of how behaviours associated with negative emotional states develop in dogs and cats, as well as how best to prevent and resolve them.

Essentially, anxiety is best considered as an 'alert state', where an animal is not sure what might happen next or what they might do about it. Dogs and cats prefer their environment to be as predictable as possible so that they know what will happen next. Much of the processing power in the brain is taken up with chaining together events and stimuli that occur closely together in time and space, so that the animal has a 'mental map' of what should occur where and when. For example, a cat that has an established territory in its neighbourhood will develop an expectation of where other local cats' territories are, what time they are likely to be there, and how they are likely to respond in encounters. It will have developed strategies for dealing with the situations that it regularly encounters: it might avoid going to an area at times when another cat is active; or it might divert its path on days when the human in the neighbouring garden, who habitually chases the cat away, is working outside. This means that the cat has some control over its environment: it not only knows what is likely to happen where, but also has an established response to deal with these situations. If an unexpected event happens, such as a completely new cat moving into the neighbourhood, the resident cat is likely to experience anxiety. It does not know how the other cat is likely to respond, where it will go or when it will be around. It is therefore in a state of 'high alert' so that it is ready for whatever might happen. Although anxiety tends to be thought of as a 'bad thing', this type of response is highly adaptive. It makes sense for the brain and body to be alert in unpredictable situations, as this enables the individual to identify all the cues in the environment that might help it identify the best action to take.

In contrast, it is best to think of a *fear* response as an immediate response to a stimulus that is perceived to be aversive by an individual. Unlike the whole-brain activation involved in anxiety, fear responses are thought to be rapid responses that pass through the phylogenetically older parts of the brain. Some events are thought to be innately fear-provoking for a species; i.e. exposure to these stimuli induces a fear response in a significant proportion of the population without any prior learning. Fear responses to these stimuli are, from an evolutionary perspective, adaptive (the common human fears of snakes or heights). The majority of fear responses, however, are learnt through experience. For example, a dog might learn that an owner's angry facial expression and outstretched hand reliably predicts a bad outcome, and show a fear response to this specific collection of cues, such as running off and hiding under the table.

Generally:

- An animal will be anxious if it doesn't recognize a situation or doesn't know how best to respond
- If the animal can work out which cues predict an aversive outcome, and how the situation is likely to turn out, and also learns what behaviour works best to resolve the situation, it shows a fear response.

Hence, when a dog *first* comes into a veterinary practice it is likely to be anxious, because the environment is novel and the animal doesn't know what to expect. This will lead to a high state of arousal and the animal will rapidly pick up any cues that might indicate what will happen and identify the best way to respond. Some dogs may stay in a highly anxious state and are not able to work out any routine or establish how they can regain control of their environment throughout the time they are in the practice. Others may start to learn what is likely to happen in response to different cues, and develop behaviours that enable them to cope. For example, they may learn that people putting a hand into their kennel predicts a painful consequence, which cannot be avoided by withdrawal. With repeated experience, the dog may learn that growling works, at least momentarily, to get the hand to withdraw; this behaviour therefore becomes reinforced. Once the dog learns that this is the most effective strategy for avoiding a perceived threat, it will gradually become more confident in showing the behaviour, hence appearing progressively more aggressive and starting to respond to events that might predict the aversive event, such as people approaching the kennel (Figure 4.1).

Frustration

Frustration is the emotion felt when an expected event does not occur. There are two broad causes of frustration:

- Animals can be in a negative emotional state because they are not able to display species-specific behaviours. These are behaviours that animals are motivated to show because they were adaptive for survival in their evolutionary past. For example, many cats will show signs of frustration if unable to show any predatory (or predatory-type play) behaviour over a prolonged period

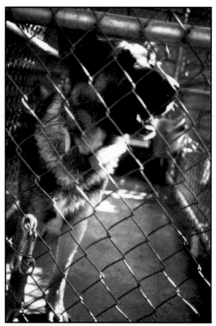

4.1 Dogs will become more confident in showing aggression as a strategy to avoid a perceived aversive consequence. (Courtesy of John Bradshaw)

- Individual animals can become frustrated if they are unable to show behaviours that they have previously learnt are successful at achieving desired goals or avoiding perceived threats. For example, a dog that has learnt that whining is successful at achieving the attention of their owner at home is likely to become frustrated if this behaviour no longer 'works' when in a kennel at the clinic.

Frustration often results in animals trying harder to achieve the desired goal, at least for a short period of time. Individuals vary in how persistent they will be in showing frustration responses. This variation is related both to individual differences in temperament and also to previous learning experiences; for example, a dog who learns that whining for a prolonged period eventually works to achieve owner attention will be more persistent. Hence, some animals may show apparent signs of frustration for prolonged periods when there is no consequence to their behaviour, whereas others 'give up' relatively quickly. Although those that give up quickly are often noticed less, their lack of behavioural signs does not necessarily indicate that they are in a positive emotional state. Many animals will 'give up' trying if behaviours no longer achieve an expected goal – such animals may be in a behaviourally depressed state and should be considered as being as much at risk from the effects of prolonged stress as those showing persistent frustration responses. Animals will usually 'give up' responding in the context in which the behaviour has not been successful, initially, but continue to show the behaviour in other contexts. This is not to be confused with the behaviourally depressed state where animals neither avoid punishment nor seek reward (sometimes called 'learned helplessness').

When considering the influence of frustration on emotional state and behaviour, therefore, it is necessary to ask:

- What are the behavioural needs for this species?
- What are the expectations of this individual animal?

Emotional conflict

Emotional conflict occurs where an animal has two or more conflicting emotional states associated with a particular context or action. This is a very common state in domestic dogs and cats, as owners are often unaware of how they are making the environment inconsistent and confusing for their pets. A common example is where a puppy's behaviour is reinforced with attention for jumping up to greet owners when they return home. The puppy quickly learns to jump up with the expectation of a positive outcome. However, some such dogs are subsequently punished for the same behaviour, particularly if the owners are dressed up to go out, or the dog has muddy paws. This results in an animal that is motivated to show the behaviour but uncertain about the outcome. This can lead to a range of behavioural consequences, such as an over-excited leaping up response, or approaching but then showing aggression, or a displacement activity (completely different behaviour) such as tail chasing.

Awareness of the behavioural signs of emotional conflict is important, because animals may show apparently friendly behaviours, such as tail wagging in dogs or rubbing in cats, but become anxious and possibly aggressive on further contact where they have conflict about close interaction with people.

Behavioural signs

The actual behaviour shown by an animal in response to an aversive stimulus will be one of a range of 'possible strategies' in that species. Animals that are uncertain about their environment (i.e. are anxious) often 'switch' between different behaviours, and also show signs of an activated stress response, such as elevated heart rate, panting or sweating paws. Animals that have previously learnt that a particular behavioural strategy 'works' and gives them control in a particular situation are more likely to show this response straight away. The types of behaviour that may be shown by dogs and cats are shown in Figure 4.2.

When in a state of anxiety, an animal will try a range of different behavioural strategies to attempt to resolve the unexpected situation. A dog that is put into a kennel in the veterinary clinic is likely to be anxious, particularly if it has either not been in the clinic before or associates being there with a painful previous experience. This anxious state will not only enable the dog to identify what might happen next but will also cause it to show behaviours to try to resolve the situation, such as barking or whining, or scratching at the door to try to get out. If one of these behaviours works to resolve the situation (e.g. somebody comes to check the dog), the level of anxiety will decrease rapidly and the animal will be more likely to use that behavioural strategy the next time it is left alone.

The behavioural response that is successful for an animal may vary in different contexts. For example, a dog may associate an outstretched hand with pain when it is in the kennel, but may respond positively to an approaching hand whilst out for exercise.

Dogs	Cats
Responses to uncertainty ('anxiety')	
Trying different avoidance responses (e.g. switching between pulling away, vocalizing and growling) to try to find a successful strategy	Trying different avoidance responses (e.g. switching between moving away, hissing and struggling) to try to find a successful strategy
Freezing	Freezing
Signs of high levels of arousal and vigilance (e.g. alert, tense, noticing changes, not resting)	Signs of high levels of arousal and vigilance (e.g. alert, tense, becoming alert at any noise or movement, not resting or sleeping)
Signs of activated peripheral stress response (e.g. panting, elevated heart rate, dilated pupils)	Signs of activated peripheral stress response (e.g. sweaty paws, dilated pupils, piloerection)
Established responses to perceived threats ('fear responses')	
Withdrawal (moving away from threat, e.g. hiding under furniture or pulling to back of the pen)	Withdrawal (moving away from threat, e.g. hiding on high shelf or squashing into the back of the pen)
Aggression (e.g. barking, growling, snapping, lunging)	Aggression (e.g. hissing, yowling, lashing out)
Soliciting social attention (e.g. howling, whining)	Soliciting social attention (less common than in dogs but may occur in cats that highly value human contact)
Appeasement behaviour (behavioural signs to diffuse social conflict; e.g. ears back, eyes averted, twisted muzzle)	

4.2 Behavioural signs associated with anxiety and fear responses in dogs and cats.

The behavioural response to pain or fear may also vary with context. A dog may learn that, when it is in the kennel and sees the predictive cues, appeasement and avoidance are not successful, but that aggression works well to avoid an anticipated painful event. This response will therefore become reinforced and the dog will become progressively more confident that this is the best response to show in this context. However, if the dog experiences the same cues in the consulting room, it may learn that struggling and wriggling are more successful to avoid pain in this context. Therefore, when investigating the development of a given behaviour, it is important to not only look at a 'presenting sign' but also to evaluate the emotional state that is eliciting that sign. In this example, rather than considering the reason why the dog showed 'aggression to people' in the kennel and 'avoidance of people' in the examination room, investigation should centre on the reason why the dog was fearful of people in both contexts (e.g. due to the anticipation of pain).

The stress response

The term 'stress' is used in everyday language to mean different things. Problems of definition arise because the same term is used to describe: the event that precipitates a response; the emotional response caused; and the peripheral physiological consequences of the event.

- The term 'stress response' will be used here to describe the physiological response that occurs associated with the different emotional and motivational changes described above.
- The term 'stressor' will be used to describe an event or situation that has either an acute or a chronic impact on an individual, and which precipitates a 'stress response'.

Stressors include extremes of environmental conditions, such as heat or cold, as well as the variety of psychological stressors that are of most interest in this chapter. Because the response to most stressors is likely to involve some form of activity, the autonomic and endocrine activity in the stress response are broadly catabolic, in order to mobilize the body's energy reserves.

Although most often discussed with respect to its negative consequences, it is important to understand that the stress response is a normal and highly adaptive mechanism in all animals. It initiates changes that provide the individual with the resources for some form of immediate activity, which may either be skeletal activity or an internal event such as the response of the immune system to an internal challenge. Hence, on exposure to a novel event, an animal is anxious, the brain is trying to identify predictive cues and the peripheral stress response is getting the body ready for action. Once a successful behavioural strategy has been found, both the anxiety and peripheral stress response reduce, returning the animal to a normal or resting state.

Physiology

The peripheral stress response system has different elements, but cumulatively they initiate the changes familiarly associated with the 'fight or flight' response. Sympathetic nervous system activation leads to increased heart rate, increased stroke volume, increased respiratory rate, pupillary dilatation, and vasodilatation of vessels supplying the heart, lungs, skeletal muscles and brain. In addition, sympathetic stimulation of the adrenal medulla results in the production of adrenaline (epinephrine) and noradrenaline (norepinephrine). Adrenaline stimulates glycolysis and both hormones act to increase heart rate and blood pressure, and give rise to other sympathomimetic actions. Noradrenaline is also an important neurotransmitter within the central nervous system: it is the main transmitter within the locus coeruleus and its connections to limbic and cortical regions, and is also released from the hypothalamus and frontal cortex. The locus coeruleus plays a central role in the efferent pathways of the fear response; hence noradrenaline is an important transmitter in the activation of behavioural responses to stressors.

The stress response also includes activation of the hypothalamopituitary–adrenal (HPA) axis, resulting in increased cortisol production from the adrenal cortex (Figure 4.3). The neurons of the paraventricular nucleus in the hypothalamus secrete a peptide, corticotropin-releasing hormone (CRH), which stimulates the anterior pituitary to produce adrenocorticotropic hormone (ACTH). The ACTH is released into the circulation and stimulates cortisol production and release from the adrenal cortex. As this is a negative feedback system, increased levels of cortisol result in a decreased release of CRH and ACTH. CRH is also secreted in other parts of the brain and is important in those systems involved in the formation of emotional

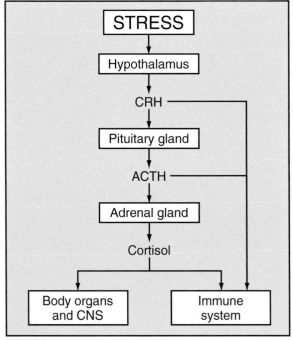

4.3 The hypothalamopituitary–adrenal (HPA) axis. (Reproduced from the *BSAVA Manual of Canine and Feline Behavioural Medicine, 2nd edition*)

responses, such as the locus coeruleus and amygdala. Cortisol has a profound effect on glucose metabolism: blood glucose levels are increased to provide a supply of energy for muscular activity through the breakdown of carbohydrates, proteins and fats. Almost every cell in the body of animals has receptors for cortisol, therefore it has a wide-ranging effect on the metabolic processes of the body.

There are large individual differences in the reactivity of the stress response to external events. These differences are partly genetically determined, but experience also has a powerful effect. Maternal levels of cortisol influence the relative levels of activity of the HPA axis in the developing fetus (Kofman, 2002), but the system also retains some plasticity throughout life (Lynch, 2004), such that the extent to which each animal is exposed to stressors will influence the relative response of the HPA axis.

Chronic stress
Whilst the stress response system is useful to animals, stress responses become problematic when they become chronic or prolonged; for example, where the animal is unable to escape from a perceived threat or achieve a necessary resource, despite showing an appropriate behavioural response. In such cases, the animal will remain anxious, alert and vigilant, because it is adaptive for it to keep trying to work out a way of resolving the situation. The peripheral stress response system will also remain activated, keeping the body in a state of readiness for anticipated activity.

There are different outcomes for animals in this state of prolonged or repeated anxiety (or frustration) and activated stress response. Some individuals may continue trying different behavioural strategies, until eventually identifying a behaviour or combination of behaviours that resolves or improves the situation in some way. This behaviour will be strongly reinforced because it results in the cessation of the negative state, and hence the animal will be likely to show this behaviour more rapidly on subsequent exposures to the same stressor. Either a normal behaviour or an 'abnormal' behaviour (i.e. outside the normal repertoire for the species) can become reinforced in this circumstance. Where an abnormal response successfully results in a reduced level of anxiety and stress, this will become reinforced, with the potential of ultimately developing into what is sometimes described as 'compulsive behaviour'.

For some individuals, no behavioural solution to the situation can be identified. Although these animals may not appear to the observer to be as 'distressed' as those that show extreme or repetitive behaviours, the physiological and welfare implications of having a prolonged 'unresolved' stress response can be profound. Although elevated cortisol for short periods is adaptive in preparing the body for activity, a prolonged catabolic effect can have serious metabolic consequences, such as increased blood pressure, steroid diabetes, infertility, growth inhibition and the inhibition of inflammatory processes. High levels of cortisol can also result in changes to the regulation of the stress response system in the brain, and damage to parts of the brain involved in the storage and retrieval of memories, resulting in decreased attention span and poor ability to remember previously learnt commands.

Emotional state, stress and disease

In human medicine stressful life events have been recognized for some time as influencing or precipitating the occurrence of a range of chronic disease conditions, such as rheumatoid arthritis, irritable bowel syndrome and interstitial cystitis. In addition, stressors can influence rates of postsurgical recovery, and increase susceptibility to infectious agents such as cold and 'flu viruses. Awareness of the importance of stress in the development, prevention and treatment of conditions in veterinary medicine is also increasing. For example, recent research has suggested that exposure to potentially stressful environmental circumstances acts as a flare factor for idiopathic cystitis in cats (Seawright *et al.*, 2008). This may present as pain on urination, straining, haematuria, frequent urination attempts, change in urination locations, distress prior to urination, altered interactions with owners, and grooming of the caudal abdominal region (Figure 4.4).

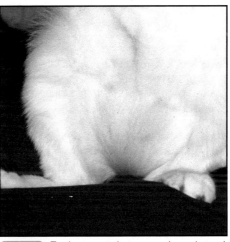

4.4 Environmental stressors have been identified as important flare factors in bouts of idiopathic cystitis in cats. This may present as grooming of the caudal abdominal region.

Clearly, not every animal exposed to a potentially aversive circumstance develops somatic disease and, in those that do, pathology can occur in a number of different functional systems. The relationship between emotional state, stress and occurrence of disease is therefore not a simple one and remains to be fully elucidated (De Kloet and Derijk, 2004).

Adaptation of the stress response system
As discussed earlier, individual differences in temperament influence the type of response that animals show to stressors. This 'predisposition' interacts with the environment that the animal experiences as the stress response system is very 'plastic' (Korte *et al.*, 2005). In general, somatic disease is precipitated where a persistently, or recurrently, adverse environment leads to dysregulation of the stress response

system. For example, a cat in a multi-cat household, where one or more other cats within the household are perceived as a threat but the environment precludes active avoidance strategies, would increase the risk of stress-related somatic disease. Similarly, a dog may be unable to predict the outcome of interactions with a highly inconsistent owner, and be unable to learn which behaviours are successful at achieving social contact. Although these are common examples of situations likely to cause prolonged stress responses in companion animals, the particular circumstances will be unique to each individual animal.

Once an animal has experienced an environment that leads to dysregulation of its normal responses to stressors, other, apparently minor, events can precipitate an excessive physiological and/or behavioural response. Hence, a change in owner routine, or the arrival of visitors, despite not being a chronic, unpredictable or uncontrollable stressor, may well result in physiological changes that seem extreme in relation to the event.

Negative emotional states in dogs in the veterinary practice and in long-term care

Recognizing where animals are in a negative emotional state, and how they respond to this, are important considerations both when animals are admitted to a veterinary hospital or clinic, and where longer-term palliative care is carried out in the clinic or by owners in the home environment. As well as recognizing specific behavioural signs that may indicate negative emotional states, it is useful to consider aspects of the environment that are *likely* to have a negative impact on dogs, so that each animal can be carefully monitored and any adverse consequences picked up rapidly. Species-specific behaviours and needs, and also the previous learning experiences of each individual animal need to be taken into consideration.

The practice environment

Social behaviour
The ancestor of the domestic dog was the grey wolf; like the wolf, the dog is a highly social species. Dogs have a strong motivation to retain contact with familiar individuals, whether these are other dogs or people. It is therefore normal for puppies to show some response to separation when first socially isolated, such as whining or barking to regain vocal contact, or scrabbling and trying to escape to re-establish physical contact. This response can be modified readily in puppies, but in many cases this does not occur adequately and adult dogs remain anxious about social isolation. This is an important consideration when dogs enter the veterinary clinic. They will be separated from familiar family members, which will particularly cause anxiety in individuals that have retained a high level of dependence on their owner's attention or physical presence. In some cases, dogs will never have learnt to be separated from owners overnight, in which case isolation in kennels will cause additional anxiety.

The highly social nature of dogs also makes them very good at reading changes in human facial expression, tone of voice or posture. An important characteristic of social living is the ability to show changing emotional state with facial expression and body posture, such that other members of the social group can 'read' changing states and alter their behaviour accordingly. Where dogs develop with people, they learn to identify even subtle changes in human characteristics, such as pupillary dilatation, where these changes have significance for them. Hence, a dog that has learnt that an angry facial expression predicts a punishment is likely to respond on identifying these characteristics by showing signs of anxiety, or an established avoidance response. Where owners are anxious about their pet, or staff are stressed by a busy day, changes in expression are likely to influence the emotional state of dogs.

The notion that dogs show many behaviours because of a motivation to gain dominance is outdated (Figure 4.5) and based on flawed interpretations of wolf behaviour (Bradshaw *et al.,* 2009). It often leads to the use of punishment- and coercive-based training, which has been associated with the occurrence of undesired behaviours in the dog, such as aggression (Blackwell *et al.,* 2008). Careful assessment of the causes of each unwanted behaviour, including medical causes, avoids the danger of putting every dog in this artificial category of 'dominant' and using inappropriate treatment.

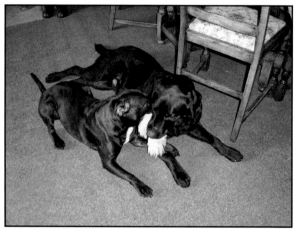

4.5 It is important to have a good understanding of the normal ethology of the dog. For example, relationships between dogs tend to be fluid and not a fixed 'hierarchy' as previously thought. (Courtesy of Sara Jackson)

Physiological effects
Sources of pain influence behaviour: dogs will learn to avoid situations in which a painful event predictably occurs. Pain will also have a less specific effect on behavioural responses, generally reducing the threshold for reacting to new events, and increasing the likelihood of the development of fear responses, including aggression, developing.

Other physiological changes influence the threshold for behavioural changes, making dogs appear to behave uncharacteristically. Pyrexia, for example, may lead to heightened sensitivity or hyperaesthesia, and high levels of oestrogen can result in established behavioural responses occurring at a lower threshold of stimulus.

Changes in routine

It is also important to consider what are the normal routines for each individual dog. Most owners have a reasonably predictable daily routine; dogs expect things to happen at particular times, and they can get anxious or frustrated if things do not happen as usual. A common example of previous learning that might cause anxiety in the kennel situation is that of toilet training. Most dogs have a strong preference for toileting on grass, and many have been punished for toileting on other substrates. Because of this, some will be unwilling to toilet in the kennels or in concrete runs, trying to 'hold on' for considerable periods for a suitable substrate. Normal patterns of eating and activity will also influence hormonal diurnal rhythms in dogs, so it is important to consider how feeding at different times or changed/reduced exercise routines may have direct influences on physiology, as well as potentially causing anxiety.

Experience

Previous experience of kennelling has been found to be an important factor in how dogs respond to entering a kennel environment, with those having had previous experience of being in a kennel adapting faster to the experience (Hiby *et al.*, 2006). However, this is likely to vary with the quality of the previous experience: individuals that have had a particularly aversive experience previously are more likely to be sensitized to entering the practice or being put in a kennel.

Reducing the risk

Preventive measures

In general, making the experience of entering the veterinary clinic as positive as possible for dogs whenever they come in helps to prevent negative associations developing when a dog is in pain or anxious. 'Puppy parties' or socialization classes are a good way of starting this process, as they will ensure that a puppy's first experience of the practice will tend to be a positive one (Figure 4.6).

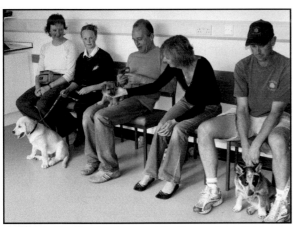

4.6 Running 'puppy socialization parties' gives dogs a positive experience of the practice from an early age. (Courtesy of Emily Blackwell)

Even where dogs first visit a practice as adults, ensuring that their first experience is a positive one, with social attention and rewards, will help prevent subsequent negative associations. Other techniques include:

- Prudent use of perioperative analgesia (especially at routine neutering, which is often the time that dogs who were previously relaxed to enter the clinic become anxious)
- Giving time to anxious animals before examining or performing procedures
- Delaying potential painful procedures, such as microchipping in puppies, until the second vaccination or later.

The practice routine

Once dogs enter the clinic, or are admitted to kennels, it is good practice to ensure that the routine is as predictable as possible for them so that they can learn as quickly as possible what to expect. In practice, this means having the same one or two people looking after a particular animal and keeping the routine of the day as standard as possible. Finding out from the owner what each dog's normal daily routine would be like may help in the anticipation of possible problems or of periods when the dog is particularly likely to become frustrated.

Bearing in mind that many dogs will have learned to be anxious about raised voices and angry or stressed human facial expressions, keeping the kennel area as calm and relaxed as possible is ideal. Where unpredictable noises occur in other areas of the practice, having a radio to mask sounds may help.

Giving dogs short spells of interaction throughout the day, so that they are not left isolated for long periods, is generally preferable to fewer longer periods of interaction. Dogs are more likely to learn that someone coming to the kennel predicts a positive event if they get regular 'fuss' and social contact, rather than only seeing people when a painful dressing change is needed, or a drip needs untangling.

Monitoring

It is important to monitor dogs for behavioural as well as physical signs on a regular basis.

It is helpful to ask owners if there are any specific events to which the dog has an existing fear response. For example, a dog that is fearful of unfamiliar dogs would be better placed in an end kennel, or in one where there is no direct visual contact with other dogs; use of an isolation area may be useful in such a case. Dogs with a fear of noises can be placed in a quieter end of the ward, away from any clanging metal bins.

In addition, monitoring how the dog responds to specific events will help identify contexts in which it is anxious. Identifying that a dog shows appeasement behaviours as its lead is clipped on to take the dog out should be noted as a warning that the dog is worried about this situation. Changing its perception of handling at this point, by associating contact with a positive consequence, is much easier and quicker than when the dog starts to develop defensive aggression in this context.

Where dogs show frustration responses, such as whining in the kennel, or banging at the kennel door, it is important not to reinforce this response with attention. Shouting at a dog that is making a lot of noise may *appear* to reduce the behaviour in the short term, but is counterproductive in the long term. Either the dog will still be motivated to seek attention and try something else, or it may become anxious about the person who shouted, or it may see the shouting as a good consequence and make more noise next time! The dog needs to learn that this behaviour has no consequence, and that other behaviours (such as sitting quietly) *do* work to get positive attention. It is a good idea to speak to dogs, or stop briefly to say 'Hello' when regularly passing through the kennels, as long as they are being quiet, as this will give them some social contact, and reduce the likelihood of attention-seeking behaviours.

Exercise restriction

With the restricted exercise and mental stimulation associated with longer-term care, dogs are more likely to start developing behaviours associated with frustration. In some cases, frustration can be worse where dogs are looked after in their owner's home, as events in this context are often associated with aspects of their normal routine. For example, a dog may have learnt that when the owner gets home from work, they always greet the dog, play with it in the garden, watch a particular programme on TV and then get up to take the dog for a walk as the theme tune finishes. Hence, the occurrence of the owner getting home, and the distinctive TV theme tune that have always before predicted exciting events are likely to cause frustration when the owner has been told to restrict the dog's exercise.

Specific manipulations (see Chapter 9) carried out as part of medical care but which cause anxiety can lead to avoidance responses, including aggression. Where any action that causes anxiety is repeated, dogs will often become progressively more sensitized, and react more over time. It is therefore important to identify the more subtle signs of anxiety and change the dog's perception of that stimulus or activity as soon as possible. Owners may also become angry at the consequences of the specific disease state, e.g. if a dog with diarrhoea fouls the carpet. Ensuring that owners are aware of the consequences of their own responses on the wellbeing of their dog is an important part of explaining the pet's ongoing care needs.

Restrictions during palliative care

It is important to recognize that undesired behaviours such as vocalization or jumping up may occur because of frustration. Being clear and consistent about the new routine, and avoiding particular events that have previously reliably predicted exercise or other exciting events, will help to reduce frustration. Short, regular periods of interaction help to keep the dog interested in its environment. These could include:

- Directing the dog's energy into other activities, the nature of which will depend on the degree of restriction required
- Short regular periods of calm interaction and soothing; these will help with dogs that are very sick or immobile
- For those that have some movement, training exercises that engage the dog's mind without too much movement, e.g. training them to discriminate between particular objects, or teaching a new trick
- Where appetite is normal, stuffing the dog's food ration into a food ball or similar toy will mean that it will take longer to eat the same ration than if just presented with a bowl of food
- Playing hide and seek with food or toys if the dog cannot or should not run for its favourite ball
- If the dog is sociable with people, ensuring it has visitors or is taken to see the people it likes
- Putting the dog in the car and taking it to different places to keep it stimulated, rather than restricting exercise to the same walk around the block.

Negative emotional states in cats in the veterinary practice and in long-term care

Social behaviour

The domestic cat developed from a species (the African wild cat) that evolved as a solitary hunter in a savannah environment. Home ranges tended to only overlap marginally with other adult cats to reduce competition over prey, and olfactory signals were an important method of orientation and communication. Since the domestication of cats occurred a relatively short period of time ago in evolutionary terms, and over that period reproductive activity has been controlled to a much lesser extent than in other domesticated species, modern-day cats retain many of the behavioural characteristics of their ancestors. Of particular importance is the limited ability of the cat to show complex visual signalling. For animals living in a social group, being able to display their emotional state using facial and body posturing is important, as it enables group members to identify how others are likely to react and to change their own behaviour accordingly. Because of their solitary ancestry, such behaviour is limited in cats, making it more difficult for them to live successfully in close proximity with others.

Over the process of domestication, cats have developed some ability to live together in certain circumstances. In the feral or farm situation, social groups are generally made up of related individuals, and the size of groups is limited by the availability of food resource. Because each cat hunts individually, and the number of cats in the group is matched to the amount of food available, there is no need for competition for resources in these groups, nor for cats to wait to access resources, making group living possible. Problems arise, however, for cats in the domestic environment, where cats living together are often unrelated and first introduced as adults, resulting in individuals living in close proximity with others that they do not regard as part of the same social group. This can cause anxiety and, often, the development of one or more avoidance responses. In addition, competition for resources is created in households through the provision of all resources within the same area (such as a line of food bowls in the kitchen; Figure 4.7).

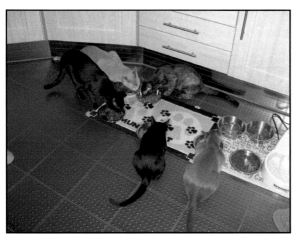

4.7 Cats living in close proximity with others that they do not consider as part of the same social group can become chronically stressed, particularly where individuals cannot easily avoid each other. (Courtesy of Anne Seawright)

Cats may live for many years in the same household as other cats *without* being in the same social group. Each cat learns to avoid the other, for example by one being active when the other is outside, or going to eat when the other is asleep. As a general rule, cats in a household are unlikely to see each other as part of the same social group unless they spend time actively rubbing on or grooming each other, and choose to sleep actually touching each other. Cats living alone in households can also be subject to anxiety about cats from other households in areas of high cat population density. Many cats are worried about going outside or show urine spraying as a consequence of anxiety about the presence of other cats in the area.

The characteristics of cats as a species are likely to make aspects of entering the veterinary clinic a negative experience.

- Close proximity to unfamiliar cats will cause anxiety in most individuals.
- Unfamiliar olfactory cues are also likely to cause anxiety, especially as continuity of scent (which cats prefer) will be difficult where kennels are thoroughly cleaned and disinfected regularly.
- The unfamiliarity and unpredictability of the new environment will cause cats to be anxious. As they start to learn the routine, get to know the staff and know what to expect, levels of anxiety will decline, although this rate of decline varies significantly between individuals (Casey and Bradshaw, 2005).

Cats may also have varying previous experiences of people. Where cats have had limited contact with people during the first weeks of life, they are more likely to show fear behaviour towards people as adults (Casey and Bradshaw, 2008). They may also have had mixed experience of people and show signs of emotional conflict, such as approaching but then becoming tense on closer contact.

The practice environment
Measures can be implemented to reduce the risk of negative emotional states developing in cats entering the veterinary clinic.

- Blocking visual access between cats helps to reduce the perceived threat from other cats, for example by designing pens such that they do not directly face each other, or covering over the front of pens when occupied.
- Although cleaning pens is important for infectious disease control, some continuity of scent can be achieved by using two beds and, if possible, only removing one for cleaning each day, so that the other carries the cat's scent from one day to the next.
- Having separate cat waiting areas reduces the chance of cats being frightened by dogs whilst in a carrying basket, and separate kennelling areas are also helpful in ensuring a quiet area in which cats will start to adapt to the new environment more rapidly.

The other important aspect of reducing anxiety in cats is enabling them to show a normal coping behaviour within the kennel environment. If provided with a simple box cats can hide away, thus effectively reducing levels of measurable stress (Kry and Casey, 2007). Some practices avoid the use of boxes because it is considered difficult to remove cats that are hidden and cats can be difficult to check without disturbing. However, a box placed upside down in the pen can be easily lifted off the cat, and cutting arched holes in the front and side enables rapid inspection (Figure 4.8).

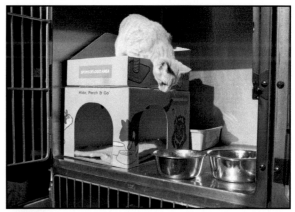

4.8 Environmental enrichment for a shelter cat. This 'Hide, Perch & Go' box (devised by the British Columbia SPCA) serves as a method of stress reduction by offering a hiding place and perch. The box transforms into a carrier when the cat is adopted. (Courtesy of Sheila Segurson. Reproduced from the *BSAVA Manual of Canine and Feline Behavioural Medicine, 2nd edition*)

Synthetic feline facial pheromones may also be useful for reducing anxiety in cats entering the kennels (Griffith *et al.*, 2000). However, they should be regarded as an adjunct to environmental considerations, rather than a panacea for dealing with 'stress' alone. Pheromone therapy is more likely to be effective when used as cats arrive in the new environment – to help reduce their anxiety – rather than once cats have developed a fear response to specific events.

Exercise restriction

Frustration is likely to occur in cats kept restricted for prolonged periods. This will include both frustration of species-specific behaviours (e.g. the motivation to show predatory behaviour) and also the frustration of previously learnt responses. Where outdoor cats are restricted indoors, they can show extreme signs of frustration, such as throwing themselves at the catflap.

Where cats are restricted in an indoor kennel, it is important that other cats in the household are not able to access the area in which they are kept, particularly where feline members of the household do not see each other as part of the same social group. Being 'trapped' in an open cage when threatened by another cat would be an extremely stressful experience for the patient.

Restrictions during palliative care

Cats can be directed into other activities, depending on their degree of movement restriction:

- Short periods of play will help reduce frustration
- Short regular periods of interaction are helpful for cats that like close human attention
- Food enrichment is also effective, to increase the proportion of the time budget engaged in acquiring food (Figure 4.9).

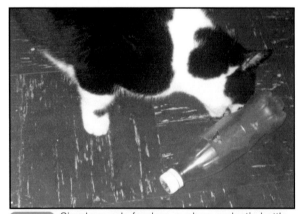

4.9 Simple puzzle feeders, such as a plastic bottle with holes slightly larger than biscuits, keep cats entertained for longer than eating from a bowl. (Courtesy of Anne Seawright)

With the restricted movement of the patient, other cats will have changed their patterns of behaviour and may have occupied the patient's home range area. When the resident becomes active again, encounters between the patient and other cats are more likely. Owners should be warned about the possibility that cats which previously regarded each other as part of the same social group may no longer do so when the patient returns home after hospitalization. This is likely to occur because of the changed olfactory signals from the hospitalized cat; therefore, rubbing the returning cat with a towel from home with the scent of the other resident cat may help the transition period. Where loss of social bonds occurs it may be transient, but can also result in a permanent breakdown of the relationship.

Other tools for reducing negative emotional states in dogs and cats

Reducing the impact of negative emotional states on individual animals requires an individual rather than prescriptive approach. There is no 'magic cure' for stress, nor a single technique that is a panacea for all animals.

The most important aspect of dealing with stress is to identify the specific cause of stress for each individual, and either modify the environment, or change the animal's perception of the stressor. However, in some cases additional therapy may be needed, for example where the threshold of response to specific events is very low, or where it is impossible for the animal to avoid a situation or context which causes high levels of anxiety. The different psychoactive medications that may be considered in such cases are described in the *BSAVA Manual of Canine and Feline Behavioural Medicine*. It is important to consider the contraindications to these agents in sick animals, or possible interactions with other mediations.

Cats may learn avoidance responses associated with handling or the giving of medication where these are considered aversive. It is useful to associate these events with a positive outcome, such as a tasty treat or grooming or stroking, from the start to prevent difficulties later.

Pheromones have been widely suggested to reduce 'stress' in dogs and cats, although robust (i.e. randomized placebo-controlled trials) evidence for efficacy is currently very limited (e.g. Gaultier *et al.*, 2009). As discussed earlier, pheromones are theoretically more likely to influence the perception of animals first entering a new context, rather than altering an existing fear response.

The nutraceutical alpha-casozepine, a tryptic hydrolysate of the milk protein casein, is marketed for use in animals to reduce 'stress' non-specifically. Some evidence for an anxiolytic effect has been demonstrated in one rodent model of anxiety, the defensive burying paradigm (Schroeder *et al.*, 2003), and the postulated action of this compound makes it potentially interesting for further research. However, the strength of evidence supporting use in companion animals is currently very limited (e.g. Beata *et al.*, 2007). Furthermore, although suggested to act at the GABA$_A$ receptor, it is unclear how the effect of this compound is similar to that of benzodiazepines, and with no evidence to date of a retrograde amnesic effect, alpha-casozepine should not be used instead of, or together with, benzodiazepines where a memory blocking function is required.

References and further reading

Beata C, Beaumont-Graff E, Coll V *et al.* (2007) Effect of alpha-casozepine (Zylkene) on anxiety in cats. *Journal of Veterinary Behavior,* **2,** 40–46

Blackwell EJ, Twells C, Seawright A and Casey RA (2008) The relationship between training methods and the occurrence of behavior problems, as reported by owners, in a population of domestic dogs. *Journal of Veterinary Behavior* **3,** 207–217

Bradshaw JWS, Blackwell EJ and Casey RA (2009) Dominance in domestic dogs – useful construct or bad habit? *Journal of Veterinary Behaviour: Clinical Applications and Research* **4,** 109–144

Casey RA and Bradshaw JWS (2005) The assessment of welfare. In: *The Welfare of Cats,* ed. I Rochlitz, pp.23–46. Springer, Dordrecht

Casey RA and Bradshaw JWS (2008) The effects of additional socialisation for kittens in a rescue centre on their behaviour and suitability as a pet. *Applied Animal Behaviour Science* **114,** 196–205

De Kloet ER and Derijk R (2004) Signaling pathways in brain involved in predisposition and pathogenesis of stress-related disease. *Annals of the New York Academy of Sciences* **1032,** 14–34

De Kloet ER, Joëls M and Holsboer F (2005) Stress and the brain: from adaptation to disease. *Nature Reviews Neuroscience* **6,** 463–475

Gaultier E, Bonnafous L, Vienet-Lagué D *et al.* (2009) Efficacy of dog-appeasing pheromone in reducing behaviours associated with fear of unfamiliar people and new surroundings in newly adopted puppies. *Veterinary Record* **164,** 708–714

Griffith CA, Steigerwald ES and Buffington CA (2000) Effects of a synthetic facial pheromone on behavior of cats. *Journal of the American Veterinary Medical Association,* **217,** 1154–1156

Guesdon B, Messaoudi M, Lefranc-Millot C *et al.* (2006) Atryptic hydrolysate from bovine milk Ws1-casein improves sleep in rats subjected to chronic mild stress. *Peptides* **27,** 1476–1482

Hiby EF, Rooney NJ and Bradshaw JWS (2006) Behavioural and physiological responses of dogs entering re-homing kennels. *Physiology and Behavior* **89,** 385–391

Horwitz DF and Mills DS (2009) *BSAVA Manual of Canine and Feline Behavioural Medicine, 2nd edn.* BSAVA Publications, Gloucester

Kofman O (2002) The role of prenatal stress in the etiology of developmental behavioural disorders. *Neuroscience and Biobehavioural Reviews,* **26,** 457–470

Korte SM, Koolhaas JM, Wingfield JC and McEwen BS (2005) The Darwinian concept of stress: benefits of allostasis and costs of allostatic load and the trade-offs in health and disease. *Neuroscience and Biobehavioral Reviews* **29,** 3–38

Kry K and Casey RA (2007) The effect of hiding enrichment on stress levels and behaviour of domestic cats (*Felis sylvestris catus*) in a shelter setting and the implications for adoption potential. *Animal Welfare* **16,** 375–383

Lynch MA (2004) Long-term potentiation and memory. *Physiology Reviews* **84,** 87–136

McEwen BS (2000) The neurobiology of stress: from serendipity to clinical relevance. *Brain Research* **886,** 172–189

McGaugh JL (2000) Memory – a century of consolidation. *Science* **287,** 248–251

Schroeder H, Violle N, Messaoudi M *et al.* (2003) Effects of ING-911, a tryptic hydrolysate from bovine milk alpha-S1 casein on anxiety of Wistar male rats measured in the conditioned defensive burying (CDB) paradigm and the elevated plus maze test. *Behavioral Pharmacology* **14** (S1), 31

Seawright A, Casey RA, Kiddie J *et al.* (2008) A case of recurrent feline idiopathic cystitis: the control of clinical signs with behaviour therapy. *Journal of Veterinary Behavior: Clinical Applications and Research* **3,** 32–38

5

Principles of clinical nutrition

Penny Watson and Daniel L. Chan

Introduction

Clinical nutrition is an often neglected but crucial part of patient management. At a basic level, proper dietary management is aimed at promoting optimal health and maintaining patients in their ideal body condition, preventing either weight loss (which can have adverse metabolic consequences, as outlined below) or weight gain (which can impact negatively on quality of life and predispose animals to other diseases; see Chapter 6). Proper nutrition also has a vital role in preventive medicine, and many commercial diets have been developed to decrease the risk of certain disorders. For example, growth diets designed for large- and giant-breed dogs aim to slow the rate of rapid growth, whilst providing adequate protein and calcium; these factors are believed to decrease the risk of developmental orthopaedic disorders.

Dietary manipulations have the potential to do much more than this, however. Diets could be considered as potential 'drugs', and the same amount of understanding and care should be used in their prescription as would be used in prescribing drug therapies. In some cases, the correct diet can be as effective, or more effective, than drug therapy, whereas the incorrect diet can have severe, sometimes life-threatening, consequences. For example, appropriate use of 'renal diets' can, on average, double the life expectancy of dogs and cats with chronic renal disease, and is the single most effective therapeutic intervention in these cases (Elliott *et al.*, 2000; Jacob *et al.*, 2002; Ross *et al.*, 2006). However, inappropriate use of high-fat diets formulated for dissolution of urinary calculi in a dog prone to pancreatitis could trigger a severe, even fatal, bout of pancreatic inflammation. In other cases dietary manipulations are supportive rather than directly therapeutic: tube feeding a dog that is unable or unwilling to eat its caloric requirements is as important a part of supportive care as is administering fluid therapy to a dog that is dehydrated and/or unwilling to drink.

The relationship between nutritional status and good health is well established:

- Malnutrition has been linked with compromised immune function, increased risk of surgical wound breakdown and increased risk of postsurgical complications
- When adequate energy substrates, protein, essential fatty acids and micronutrients are provided, the body can support wound healing, immune function and tissue repair
- In some illnesses metabolic derangements can lead to catabolism of lean body tissue; these processes may be reversed through provision of nutritional support.

When managing hospitalized patients, clinicians face several challenges to providing optimal nutritional support. These include: inappetence; nausea; gastrointestinal motility disorders (e.g. ileus); and vomiting and diarrhoea. There is a temptation to use appetite stimulants in patients with poor food intake, but appetite stimulants are generally ineffective in optimizing food intake and may increase the risk of certain complications, such as sedation.

The focus of clinical nutrition for the hospitalized patient has shifted to:

- Using the most appropriate diet for the condition at hand
- Implementing more effective means of nutritional support than simply stimulating appetite; this may include the use of feeding tubes or parenteral nutrition.

This chapter will highlight strategies for improving nutritional support and expand on how certain nutritional approaches can aid in the management of several common disorders.

Nutritional requirements in illness and after surgery

Why, when and how much to feed

Provision of adequate nutrition is a vital part of patient care and may have a profound effect on recovery times. Early enteral feeding in appropriately selected populations (i.e. patients that are stable cardiovascularly) has been shown to speed up recovery and reduce septic complications in human patients and in experimental canine models in a wide variety of situations, including acute pancreatitis (Meier and Beglinger, 2006) and after gastrointestinal tract surgery (Sungurtekin *et al.*, 2004). It is very important to keep good records of how much the patient eats and when to ensure that it is receiving optimal nutrition; this can be as important as fluid therapy and treatment records. Laxity in maintaining good nutrition records is likely to be a major contributor to the problem sometimes referred to as 'in-hospital starvation', whereby the nutritional needs of patients are overlooked, leading to malnutrition. Some basic rules for inpatient feeding are summarized in Figure 5.1.

- ANY ANIMAL THAT IS ILL AND NOT EATING SHOULD BE FED AS SOON AS POSSIBLE UNLESS THERE IS A SPECIFIC CONTRAINDICATION. This advice to feed as early as possible includes dogs and cats recovering from gastrointestinal surgery and pancreatitis
- The earlier nutritional support is initiated, the better it is for the animal. Try to anticipate the need for nutritional support rather than wait until the animal is visibly debilitated, by which time many potentially deleterious effects on the immune system, gut wall and barrier function will already be present
- Correct fluid and electrolyte deficits first (acutely), then introduce nutritional support gradually over 2–3 days:
  - o Energy is the next most important factor after fluids/ electrolytes
  - o Then protein
  - o Minerals and vitamins are the last thing to consider. *Vitamin injections or vitamins in the fluids are not a substitute for feeding and it is not practical to supply an animal's daily caloric requirements with dextrose fluids alone.*

5.1 Some basic rules for inpatient feeding.

When to consider nutritional support

Special nutritional support (i.e. a change to a high-calorie/high-protein diet and/or assisted (tube) feeding) should be considered in cases of:

- **Recent weight loss:** Has the dog or cat lost >10% of its bodyweight not due to dehydration or obvious fluid shifts (e.g. diuresis)?
  - o This is relevant even in obese animals – weight loss in an obese, sick animal will predominantly be attributed to loss of lean body mass, and not fat, and this is undesirable. Weight loss and anorexia in an obese cat are particularly worrying because of the risk of hepatic lipidosis
- **Partial or complete anorexia for >3 days:** Has the dog or cat eaten <85% of its calculated resting energy requirement (RER) for the last 3 or more days?
- **Animal already in catabolic state or at risk of overt malnutrition:**
  - o Does the animal have: severe burns; draining sepsis, such as pyothorax or septic peritonitis; malabsorption or protein-losing enteropathy; or nephropathy?
  - o If so, is it receiving enough calories and/or protein?
  - o Is there an obvious loss of weight or lean body mass to suggest it is not?

Monitoring and record keeping

In order to assess whether a hospitalized animal requires extra support, it is important to have a record of how much it is eating every day. This can be achieved by using a simple kennel sheet, recording when food is offered and the proportion actually eaten (Figure 5.2). This becomes even more important if there are frequent changes in nursing

staff, or inadequate intake (refusing all food given) may go unnoticed. The bodyweight and body condition score (BCS) of the animal should also be monitored regularly (preferably daily) during hospitalization, and the energy intake adjusted to maintain stable bodyweight and prevent protein–calorie malnutrition.

Meeting energy requirements

Determining the *exact* energy requirements of individual patients is difficult and, indeed, unfeasible in clinical practice. A more practical and sensible approach for assessing whether an animal's daily food intake is adequate is to calculate its resting energy requirement (RER), which corresponds to the number of calories per day needed to meet the basic needs of the animal, and to compare this with the number of calories consumed. The estimation of energy requirements of hospitalized animals (and people) is an inexact science. Studies using bedside indirect calorimeters have shown that the energy requirements of sick hospitalized human and canine patients vary widely between individuals (as do energy requirements of healthy animals and humans). The studies also show, perhaps surprisingly, that there is not a great increase in energy requirement associated with trauma, sepsis or major surgery in dogs (Walton *et al.*, 1998; O'Toole *et al.*, 2004). **The RER is now used as the 'baseline' energy recommendation for hospitalized dogs and cats, regardless of the disease or surgery.**

There are a number of equations used to estimate RER. The simplest are shown below:

$$RER \text{ (kcal)} = 70 \times \text{bodyweight (kg)}^{0.75}$$

or

$$RER \text{ (kcal)} = 30 \times \text{bodyweight (kg)} + 70$$

To convert kcal (Cal) to kilojoules (kJ) multiply by 4.185

The RER can then be divided by the caloric density of the diet to calculate the amount to be fed. It is worth noting that EU petfood labelling regulations prohibit the inclusion of the caloric density of diets on the tin or bag. However, such information can be obtained from product guides or by contacting the manufacturer.

The RER should be viewed as a starting point and the amount fed may be adjusted upwards (if continued weight loss is apparent) or downwards (if the patient cannot tolerate this amount, e.g. it vomits).

Meeting protein requirements

If using a balanced dog or cat diet, protein requirements are typically met when the calculated calories are fed. However, as a general guideline, estimated protein requirements for hospitalized dogs and cats are:

- Dogs: 5–7.5 g protein per 100 kcal fed
- Cats: 6–9 g protein per 100 kcal fed

DAILY INPATIENT NURSING		Sheet Number	

Patient name:	Owner name:	Reason for admission:
Hosp no:	Breed:	
Clinician:	Age: / Sex:	Day case ☐
Admission weight:	Temperament:	
Today's weight:	Kennel no:	Date:

Diet	Times fed and Quantity eaten (1=little 10=all eaten)				

Fluid therapy

Type		Additives
Rate		VTBI

Time	Temp.	Pulse	Resp.	Per os fluids 1= little 10=all	Urine	Faeces N=norm D=dia	Walk	Other

Procedures for the day	Clinical pathology
	Clipping instructions
Signature	

5.2 Example of a simple kennel sheet that allows daily recording of food consumed. A new sheet is used every day.

Feeding schedule

Note that calculated food intake should not be given immediately on the first day but introduced gradually over 2–3 days to allow the animal's metabolism and gastrointestinal tract the time to adapt. This is particularly important if using feeding tubes. The stomach's capacity may reduce by up to 50% after as little as 48 hours of anorexia. In addition, reduced gastric tone and emptying are features of anorexia, along with changes in gastrointestinal flora and metabolic changes, all of which need time to adapt to the new diet.

Effects of anorexia

Anorexic animals with concurrent injury, infection or neoplasia may be effectively suffering from a complicated, or 'stressed', form of starvation, with many of the physical changes outlined in Figure 5.3. Because of the metabolic changes that occur, fat and protein rapidly become the main energy sources as glycogen stores are depleted. Peripheral insulin resistance may also develop in many disease states, further interfering with the use of carbohydrates as the main energy source. In these circumstances, provision of high-glucose diets (or

Effects of protein–calorie malnutrition
Breakdown of body protein
<ul><li>Catabolism of 'metabolically labile' portion of body protein occurs first (approx. 50% of body protein). This includes plasma proteins, visceral proteins and muscle</li><li>Major loss of protein occurs in the first 2–3 days and primarily involves liver protein. There is a marked reduction in hepatic protein synthesis (all albumin and fibrinogen, and 80% of globulins – but not gamma-globulins as these are not synthesized by the liver)</li><li>Catabolism of structural proteins (bones, ligaments, cartilage) is generally spared until late starvation</li></ul>
Gastrointestinal tract
<ul><li>Great reduction in the mass of villi</li><li>Flattening of villi, with reduced brush border enzyme activity – this affects carbohydrate- and fat-digesting enzymes more than protein-digesting enzymes</li></ul>
Immune system
<ul><li>Reduced ability to synthesize antibodies (especially IgA) and interferon</li><li>Reduced cell-mediated immunity and total lymphocyte counts (due to fewer T cells)</li><li>Reduced barrier function of skin and mucosal surfaces, with possible bacterial translocation from the gastrointestinal tract leading to bacteraemia ± septicaemia</li><li>Reduced inflammatory response</li><li>Reduced levels of most complement proteins except C4</li><li>Reduced leucocyte mobility and bactericidal activity</li></ul>
Renal system
<ul><li>The kidney is less able to control acid/base balance (particularly because this requires glutamine metabolism)</li><li>Kidney also shows obligate high calcium and phosphate excretion</li><li>Little loss of kidney mass</li></ul>
Skeletal muscle
<ul><li>Reduced synthesis and increased degradation of muscle proteins</li><li>Changes in skeletal muscle occur slowly, so there could be quite significant changes in clotting factors, immune system and the gastrointestinal tract before obvious muscle wastage (Dionigi *et al.*, 1977)</li></ul>
Terminal changes
<ul><li>Occur as fat stores are used up and protein becomes the primary energy source once again</li><li>Result in thinning of small intestine wall, and failure of intercostal and diaphragm muscle in severely malnourished people</li><li>Experimental studies in dogs using severe models of starvation have also shown a significant reduction in cardiac function (Abel *et al.*, 1979), although this has not been appreciated clinically</li></ul>
Additional effects of illness or injury
<ul><li>Fibroblasts use glucose, metabolizing it inefficiently and anaerobically to lactic acid, especially early in wound repair</li><li>Because of increased protein and amino acid requirements for wound healing and tissue repair, there is potential for increase in wound dehiscence after surgery, which could be particularly significant if considering gut biopsy in cases of protein-losing enteropathy (PLE), although evidence in small animals is limited</li><li>There is a marked direct protein loss in haemorrhage, PLE, protein-losing nephropathy, persistent vomiting, draining wounds (including pyothorax and chylothorax) or severe burns. The patient's protein intake and blood albumin concentrations should be carefully monitored in these circumstances and the intake of protein increased if necessary</li><li>Fever increases energy requirements by 13% per degree C temperature rise</li><li>Critical illness may, paradoxically, reduce basal energy requirements; coupled with increased energy expenditure due to certain disease processes, this may lead to near normal or resting energy requirements</li><li>Endogenous pyrogens (e.g. interleukin 1) increase proteolysis of muscle protein; cytokines such as tumour necrosis factor (released in both neoplasia and congestive heart failure) are said to contribute to cachexia in these conditions (Freeman *et al.*, 1998)</li><li>Endotoxins from Gram-negative bacteria may have profound effects on carbohydrate metabolism, leading to hypo- or hyperglycaemia and lactic acidosis</li><li>Neoplastic tissue may compete with the host for energy and nitrogen. Tumours often use glucose inefficiently and anaerobically because they have a poor blood supply</li></ul>

5.3 Physiological changes that occur with anorexia in sick, hospitalized patients.

intravenous dextrose solutions) may result in glucos-uria and/or hyperglycaemia.

It is worth noting that, generally speaking, healthy dogs can adapt to a whole range of protein, fat and carbohydrate intake for energy but, during stressed starvation, dogs are less adaptable and need more protein and fat, and less carbohydrate. Studies in normal fasting dogs (i.e. simple or unstressed starvation) demonstrate a significant increase in fat and protein oxidation, with a decrease in carbohydrate oxidation (Himwich and Rose, 1927). Cats are even less able to down-regulate protein catabolism in the face of low protein intake, explaining their higher protein requirements. The metabolic profiles of critically ill cats have been less defined than those of dogs, but studies suggest a shift towards fat oxidation (Chan *et al.*, 2006).

Muscle protein loss occurs more slowly than other changes (Figure 5.3); by the time malnutrition is clinically obvious, other physiological changes are well underway.

Selecting diets for sick animals

> **WARNING**
> Before nutritional interventions are initiated, the patient must be cardiovascularly stable and have fluid, electrolyte and acid–base abnormalities addressed.

The next consideration is energy requirement. This requires provision of protein and fat, as well as carbohydrates, because of changes in substrate metabolism (see above).

Following this provision, a supply of amino acids for other functions apart from energy (e.g. tissue repair, protein synthesis) must be given, particularly in animals whose protein requirements are markedly increased (see Figure 5.3). Specific amino acids may be needed in some conditions. For example, glutamine is now considered a 'conditionally essential' amino acid in human critical illness, particularly when there is associated gastrointestinal inflammation. The small intestine predominantly uses glutamine for its energy requirements and this requirement increases during critical illness. Supplementation of glutamine in certain species and certain conditions has been associated with the growth and repair of the small intestine, maintenance of intestinal immune function, reduced risk of bacterial translocation, and attenuation of villous atrophy (Melis *et al.*, 2004). This is discussed further in Chapter 7.

Feeding a restricted-protein food to sick, hospitalized dogs and cats is inappropriate unless there is a very specific indication (hepatic encephalopathy or severe uraemia). It is usually more appropriate and easier to use a critical care diet specifically formulated for dogs and cats. However, such diets are high in fat, so animals with gastrointestinal disease (particularly acute pancreatitis) would be better maintained on a lower-fat diet, such as one formulated for gastrointestinal disease.

The consistency of the diet is also an important consideration. For naso-oesophageal tube feeding, liquid diets are better, as thicker diets tend to clog the tube. Thicker 'gruel' can be used with oesophagostomy or gastrostomy tubes. The food should be warmed to body temperature before feeding, as cold food can induce either vomiting or rapid gastric emptying (may cause diarrhoea). It is important to remember to introduce new diets gradually.

Methods of feeding hospitalized animals

There are a few important general rules for feeding hospitalized animals.

- IF THE GUT WORKS, USE IT (this applies to the vast majority of patients).
- If only PART of the gut works, use THAT part of the gut.
- When feeding enterally, use the simplest route possible that avoids stress to the animal.

Enteral nutrition

There are a number of advantages of feeding animals enterally, which is why every effort should be made to feed animals in this way. The approach outlined below is designed to ensure that every hospitalized animal is fed enterally unless some contraindication is identified. It is important to emphasize that, regardless of the method involved, feeding should never be stressful to the animal.

Coaxed feeding

This approach is most appropriate for animals that have reduced, but still present, appetite. The palatability of the diet can be improved by warming or wetting it, or by choosing a food with a strong aroma. Some animals will eat only their usual diet and it is best to discuss this with the owner, as it may involve their bringing from home the food to be fed. Hand-feeding can improve intake in some animals. Firm stroking, assuming that the animal enjoys human contact, or providing some area of privacy (e.g. by hanging a towel over the door of the cage) may work for some cats.

Appetite stimulants

To date, there have been no published studies documenting the effectiveness of appetite stimulants in animals as a means of ensuring adequate food intake. Therefore, their role in treating inappetent animals remains unclear, but they are perhaps best used during the recovery phase of disease, ideally once the animal has been discharged. In the authors' experience, appetite stimulation is of very limited benefit in an animal that is totally anorexic as it very rarely, if ever, stimulates a meaningful increase in energy intake in these animals.

Pharmacological stimulation of appetite is not without risks (e.g. sedation, hypotension, behavioural changes) and therefore the use of these agents should not occur without careful consideration. They should *not* be used repeatedly as an alternative to assisted feeding unless they result in the animal eating a significant proportion of its RER, so it is important to monitor food intake carefully when using them.

Appetite stimulants that might be used in cats are listed in Figure 5.4. In general, appetite stimulants are ineffective in dogs. A possible exception is propofol, which has been reported to incite a short-lived appetite stimulation effect on recovery in both dogs (Long and Greco, 2000) and cats. Animals briefly anaesthetized with propofol (e.g. for a bandage change or wound debridement) may therefore display great interest in eating, and food should perhaps be made available soon after recovery.

Note that:

- There is no evidence that anabolic steroids are effective for appetite stimulation
- Vitamin B supplementation has only been shown to stimulate appetite in animals suffering from B vitamin depletion.

Drug	Dose	Comments
Diazepam	0.5 –1.0 mg/kg i.v. once	**No longer recommended in cats** because of reported cases of fatal hepatic necrosis associated with repeated oral use (Center *et al.*, 1996). A single intravenous injection may be safe but the owner should be warned of the potential serious side effects The effect is very rapid and short-lived, so a food bowl should be available immediately when the drug is injected
Midazolam	0.05–0.1 mg/kg i.v.	No reports of hepatotoxicity to date
Cyproheptadine	0.1–0.5 mg/kg orally q8–24h	A serotonin antagonist and antihistamine that can cause sedation and lower the seizure threshold
Mirtazapine	3.75 mg/cat orally every 3 days Can also be used in dogs (dose depends on bodyweight): <10 kg: 3.75 mg/dog orally q24h 10–15 kg: 5–7.5 mg/dog orally q24h 15–20 kg: 7.5 mg/dog orally q24h 21–60 kg: 15 mg/dog orally q24h >60 kg: 30 mg/dog orally q24h. The dose may be increased from these starting points if no response is seen in 24–48 hours; **maximum** 0.6 mg/kg orally q24h	Antidepressant (alpha-2 antagonist) that increases CNS noradrenaline and serotonin; reported to increase appetite in humans as side effect. Anecdotally reported as effective as an appetite stimulant in dogs and cats and rapidly becoming the preferred agent in these species, but only recently used so no extensive pharmacokinetic and safety data available Significant renal and hepatic clearance; avoid in renal/hepatic disease or use with caution and at 30% of usual dose Serotonin syndrome (increased heart rate, shivering, dilated pupils, high blood pressure) potential side effect if CNS serotonin levels get too high, but this should only occur if combined with serotonin-increasing medications such as tramadol, tricyclic antidepressants (e.g. clomipramine) and monoamine oxidase inhibitors (selegiline)

5.4 Potential appetite stimulants for use in cats. Note that these are of limited usefulness (see text) and none is authorized for this use in the UK.

Force-feeding

Much practice time is expended, rather unproductively, attempting to force-feed anorexic dogs and cats by syringe. This method may occasionally be helpful to start a mildly inappetent animal eating, especially with cats, puppies and kittens, but it is usually poorly tolerated and very stressful for the animal. Care must be taken to avoid aspiration, especially in very depressed animals. **Syringe-feeding should *never* be used in comatose or moribund cases; nor in animals with significant neuromuscular, oropharyngeal disease or dyspnoea, as they are much more likely to aspirate the food.** The stress associated with force-feeding, especially in cats, may be a major contributor to food aversion, which then complicates using the newly introduced diet for long-term management. It is important to monitor the amount of food being given when force-feeding; if a significant amount of the daily RER is not delivered, it is best to change to some form of feeding tube instead.

Tube feeding

The options for tube feeding are:

- Naso-oesophageal or nasogastric
- Oesophagostomy
- Gastrostomy (via laparotomy or percutaneous (PEG) or 'blind' gastrostomy)
- Jejunostomy.

Figure 5.5 outlines the advantages and disadvantages of each.

Feeding tube	Duration	Advantages	Disadvantages
Naso-oesophageal	Short term (<5 days)	Inexpensive Easy to place No anaesthesia required	Requires liquid diet Some animals will not eat voluntarily with tube in place
Oesophagostomy	Long term	Inexpensive Easy to place Can use calorically dense diets (caloric density >1.3 kcal/ml) Animals can be sent home with tube in place	Requires anaesthesia Cellulitis is major complication seen
Gastrostomy	Long term	Can use calorically dense diets Animals can be sent home with tube in place Allows gastric decompression, e.g. after gastric surgery Allows use of standard tinned diets liquidized to facilitate feeding	Requires anaesthesia and/or surgery Potential patient interference and dislodgement of tube (uncommon)
Jejunostomy	Long term	Bypasses stomach and duodenum Can be used in patients with pancreatitis, although gastric feeding may also be safe in some	Requires anaesthesia and laparotomy, although nasal placement using fluoroscopy, and placement through a gastrostomy tube, have been described in dogs Requires continuous rate infusion of a liquid diet Not suitable for homecare with tube in place

5.5 Feeding tube selection.

Materials

Most modern feeding tubes are made of polyurethane or silicone. Silicone is softer and more flexible than other tube materials, with a greater tendency to stretch and collapse. However, the flexibility and decreased internal diameter of silicone tubes may lead to clogging or kinking of the tube. Polyurethane is stronger than silicone, allowing for thinner walls and thus a larger internal diameter, in a tube of equivalent size. Neither polyurethane nor silicone will rapidly fragment or disintegrate *in situ* and can therefore remain in place for prolonged periods of time. PVC or red rubber tubes are the least expensive, but PVC tubes may harden within 2 weeks of insertion and cause irritation at the insertion site.

Tube placement

Placement of a naso-oesophageal tube and surgical placement of an oesophagostomy tube are described and illustrated in Figures 5.6 and 5.7. Correct positioning in the distal oesophagus (rather than the stomach) is facilitated by careful measurement before placement, marking the tube with a pen or piece of tape:

- Distal oesophagus: 7th intercostal space, or 75% of distance from nose to last rib if animal is so obese it is not possible to count the ribs accurately
- Nasogastric: 10th intercostal space, or 90% of the distance from the nose to the last rib.

> **WARNING**
> Incorrect tube placement resulting in feeding into the airways could lead to severe pneumonia.

Patient preparation and positioning

- The procedure should be performed with the animal conscious or under light sedation.
- The patient can be positioned standing, or in lateral or sternal recumbency.
- The animal's head should be placed in a 'neutral' position (i.e. not too flexed or extended).

Technique

1. Instil topical anaesthetic drops into one nostril.
2. Measure the distance from the nose to the 7th intercostal space and mark this on the tube with a piece of tape.

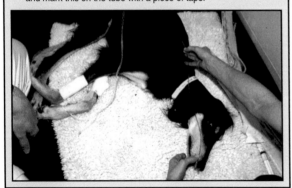

Technique (continued)

3. Lubricate the tube with anaesthetic gel to aid insertion.
4. Aim the tube ventromedially (toward the base of the opposite ear) so that it will pass into the ventral meatus of the nasal cavity. The nasal planum can be pushed dorsally to direct the tube ventrally.

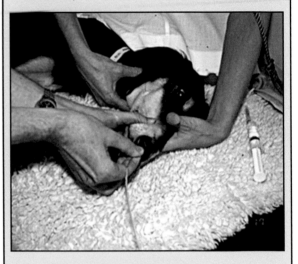

5. Pass the tube until it reaches the predetermined position (nose to 7th intercostal space). It is very important to check its position carefully. If the tube is in the oesophagus, there should be negative pressure when suction is placed on the tube using a 5–10 ml syringe.
6. Confirm correct placement:
   o Radiographic confirmation is best. Modern feeding tubes have a radiodense strip that allows visualization within the oesophagus. With older types of feeding tube, a small amount of *iodine*-containing contrast medium should be instilled first (this would be safe if the tube were inadvertently placed in an airway, whereas barium would not)
   o Attaching the end of the feeding tube to an end-tidal carbon dioxide monitor should elicit a reading of zero

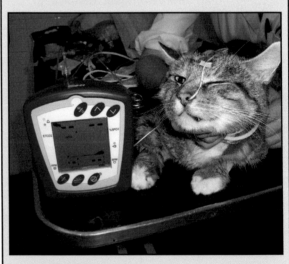

   o Instilling a small amount of fluid and then air into the tube should give a gurgling sound if listening with a stethoscope over the stomach.
7. Make two butterfly tape strips using 25 mm wide adhesive tape and attach these to the tube.
8. Suture or tissue glue these tape strips to the dorsal aspect of the muzzle and the top of the head.
9. Place an Elizabethan collar.

5.6 Naso-oesophageal tube placement. (Adapted from *BSAVA Guide to Procedures in Small Animal Practice*)

Patient preparation and positioning

- General anaesthesia is required.
- The patient is placed in right lateral recumbency.
- Aseptic preparation from the dorsal to the ventral aspects of the neck is required over an area from the angle of the jaw to the shoulder.

Technique

1. Insert curved forceps through the mouth and into the oesophagus, to the mid-cervical region.
2. Turn the tip of the forceps laterally and make a 5–10 mm skin incision over the point of the tips.

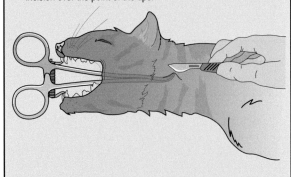

3. Bluntly dissect through the subcutaneous tissues and make an incision into the oesophagus over the tips of the forceps.
4. Push the tips of the forceps outwards through the incision to the external surface.
5. Measure the oesophagostomy tube from this point to the 7th intercostal space (distal oesophagus) and mark the tube with a piece of adhesive tape.
6. Open the tips of the forceps and grasp the distal end of the feeding tube.

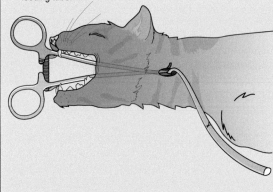

7. Draw the end of the tube through the oesophagostomy incision and rostrally into the pharynx to exit the mouth.

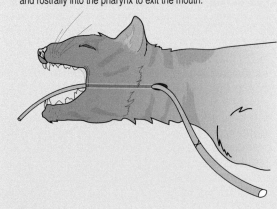

5.7 Oesophagostomy tube placement. (Adapted from *BSAVA Guide to Procedures in Small Animal Practice*) (continues) ▶

Technique (continued)

8. Disengage the tips of the forceps, and curl the tip of the tube back into the mouth and feed it into the oesophagus.
9. Visually inspect the oropharynx to confirm that the tube is no longer present in the oropharynx.
10. The tube should slide easily back and forth a few millimetres, confirming that it has straightened.

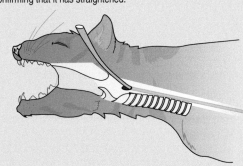

11. Secure the tube by placement of a Chinese finger-trap suture.
12. Take a thoracic radiograph to confirm correct tube placement: the tip of the tube should be in the distal oesophagus, not the stomach.

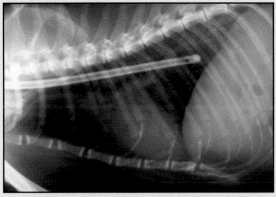

13. Cover the tube site with a sterile dressing and place a soft, padded, loose, neck bandage.

5.7 (continued) Oesophagostomy tube placement. (Adapted from *BSAVA Guide to Procedures in Small Animal Practice*)

Preparing the feed

Before feeding via any tube, it is important to ensure that the diet chosen can be administered easily enough via the tube: thick gruel diets will clog naso-oesophageal and most oesophageal tubes. It is important to make sure that the tube chosen can be used with the diet required.

When diluting diets with water, it is crucial to be able to calculate the new caloric density. If a tin of food contains 450 g of food with a caloric density of 475 kcal per tin, adding 100 ml of water would certainly dilute the calories and reduce the caloric density. To determine the new caloric density, it is necessary to measure the new volume of the gruel (using a measuring jug); this will enable calculation of the new caloric density in kcal/ml. As water does not add to calories but does contribute to the new volume, this simple approach can be used with any diet.

Some diets require addition of a large amount of water (e.g. 200 ml or more) to achieve a consistency that would allow the diet to be used in 5 Fr naso-oesophageal feeding tubes. This may be volume-limiting, especially when feeding small animals like cats, and this should all be considered carefully before choosing the diet and tube. Larger feeding tubes (e.g. 28 Fr PEG tubes) can accommodate thicker, more energy-dense gruels, such as liquidized tinned foods.

Giving the feed
Regardless of the feeding tube chosen, one should start gradually, with the goal of reaching target feedings over 2–3 days.

- Start with a third to half of the calculated required daily amount of food and gradually increase each day.
- As a general guideline, most critically ill patients do not tolerate more than 10–20 ml/kg total volume per feeding. This amount can be gradually increased and some animals (usually healthy ones with structural reasons for not being able to eat voluntarily, e.g. jaw fractures) can tolerate up to 50 ml/kg volume per feeding, but this is unusual.
- Whilst hospitalized, an animal may be fed 4–6 times a day. However, by the time of discharge, most clients will not be able to do more than 3 feedings per day, so it would be wise not to send the patient home until it can tolerate the required volume.

Clients and nursing staff should be trained in exactly how to administer feeds to improve compliance and minimize complications:

- Every feeding should be non-stressful
- The food should be warmed to body temperature
- Each feeding should take 10–15 minutes
- The tube should be flushed with lukewarm water *before and after every feed*.

Gastrostomy tubes should be aspirated before feeding; if there is a residual volume of more than a third of the previous meal, the feed should be delayed until the next scheduled time. Continued problems with stomach emptying should prompt patient reassessment and the potential use of a gastric prokinetic, such as ranitidine, to encourage emptying. If the residual volume is less than a third, it is reasonable to feed at that time, but reduce the amount given accordingly.

Potential complications
Dislodging of the tube can occur with any type of feeding tube; the seriousness of this depends on the location of the tube.

- Premature (<14 days post-placement) dislodgement of PEG and jejunostomy feeding tubes will require surgical exploration because peritonitis is a likely sequel.
- Dislodgement after stoma formation (>14 days) does not require surgical intervention, but does represent a loss of feeding access, although it is possible to replace gastrostomy tubes if this is done rapidly.

- Surgically placed gastrostomy tubes are safer than PEG and jejunostomy tubes, and rarely result in peritonitis after patient interference, even soon after surgery, because the stomach is sutured to the body wall.
- Dislodgement of naso-oesophageal and oesophagostomy tubes does not require surgical intervention, but, again, feeding access is lost.

Clogging of tubes is perhaps the most common problem if the appropriate precautions are not taken:

- The feeding tube should be regularly and carefully flushed
- The tube and diet should be optimized, choosing the right size of feeding tube for the food chosen and enlarging the hole at the tip if necessary
- The gruel must be prepared correctly to ensure that it can pass freely through the tube.

If a tube does get occluded with food, infusing 10–15 ml of carbonated soft drink, letting this sit in the tube for 10 minutes and then forcibly flushing the tube can often dislodge the obstruction.

Cellulitis or infection at the exit incision site of oesophagostomy, gastrostomy or jejunostomy tubes is common and must be addressed appropriately upon detection.

- If a discharge is found, frequent bandage changes and cleaning of the site is necessary.
- With obvious infections the feeding tube may need to be removed.
- Reasons to remove the tube include: purulent discharge with degenerate neutrophils or bacteria; systemic signs, such as pyrexia; and haematological changes compatible with systemic inflammation.

Hyperglycaemia and electrolyte disturbances are potential complications of tube feeding, but usually only occur with enterostomy feeding or in cats with serious metabolic disturbances such as occur in hepatic lipidosis. A more serious metabolic complication related to feeding involves acute and significant drops in serum phosphate and often also potassium. This potentially fatal and rare complication is referred to as 'refeeding syndrome' and is seen when severely debilitated and malnourished animals, particularly cats, are fed too rapidly. Upon refeeding a severely debilitated animal, the surge in blood insulin leads to rapid entry of potassium and phosphate into cells and then consumption of phosphate in the formation of high-energy bonds in ATP, thereby leading to a hypophosphataemic and hypokalaemic crisis. It is therefore important to monitor plasma phosphate and potassium carefully in animals at risk and supplement as necessary.

Diarrhoea may occur, particularly if animals are fed too much, too quickly, or if food is cold as that can lead to rapid stomach emptying. Feeding monomeric enteral diets or other hyperosmolar diets could result in osmotic diarrhoea; diluting such diets with water may be an option, but reduces caloric density.

Withdrawal

Ideally, the animal should be tube-fed until it is voluntarily eating >85% of its calculated RER daily. Most animals are supported via tube feeding for 1–3 weeks.

Tube feeding should be withdrawn gradually, just as it was introduced gradually, to allow the necessary gastrointestinal and metabolic adjustments. Priority should be centred on ensuring adequate nutritional intake, and not 'when to transition' to voluntary feeding. Therefore, simply withholding tube feeding so that the animal 'becomes hungry and eats', may not be appropriate.

Parenteral nutrition

- In situations where there is 'gut failure' or severe gastrointestinal dysfunction, a patient may be supported via parenteral nutrition (PN).
- When PN is administered to supplement some form of enteral nutrition, or only partially meets the patient's nutritional needs, this is referred to as partial parenteral nutrition (PPN; Figure 5.8).
- In severely malnourished patients, PN is aimed at meeting all of the patient's energy and protein requirements and this is referred to as total parenteral nutrition (TPN). Discussion of the formulation and use of TPN is beyond the scope of this Manual.

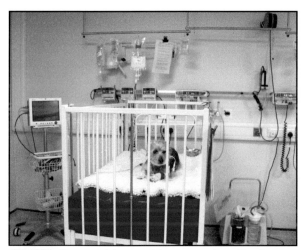

5.8 Dog receiving partial parenteral nutrition in an intensive care setting.

Whilst it is tempting to view PN as a convenient means of providing nutritional support, there are a number of reasons why it must be reserved only for those patients that have an absolute contraindication for enteral feeding:

- PN is associated with a high rate of complications, is rather difficult to formulate and compound, requires special equipment for compounding and administration, and is significantly more expensive than enteral nutrition
- Major concerns with PN include the development of hyperglycaemia, lipaemia, sepsis, and gut atrophy. Enterocytes are almost entirely dependent on intestinal contents for their nutrition (enteral nutrition) and therefore are deprived of nutrition when PN is used. Patients on PN without concurrent enteral nutrition therefore have hypoplastic, hypofunctional enterocytes with altered intestinal myoelectrical activity.

There are few true indications for PN in dogs and cats. PN is *truly* indicated only:

- If there is a severe inability to absorb enteral nutrients
- If the patient cannot tolerate enteral feeding at all (i.e. where there is intractable vomiting or diarrhoea despite adequate drug therapy).

Other examples of cases where PN *might* be indicated include: severe acute (non-surgical) pancreatitis; and extensive small intestinal resection.

The timeframe of when PN becomes necessary is controversial, and some authors state that a patient may need to demonstrate a week of severe gastrointestinal dysfunction before PN should be instituted.

PN solutions

Formulation of a PN solution involves calculating the animal's energy and protein requirements, whilst ensuring that the safe limits of lipids, dextrose and fluid volume are not exceeded. Compounding requires strict aseptic technique and is ideally performed with specialized equipment. Ready-made solutions are commercially available (Figure 5.9) and facilitate PN use in practice in the form of PPN. One of the major differences between PPN and TPN is the lower osmolarity of PPN solutions, which allows them to be administered via peripheral veins. However, they also supply only approximately 50% of the calories needed by the patient. An example protocol for use with one such ready-made solution is given in Figure 5.10.

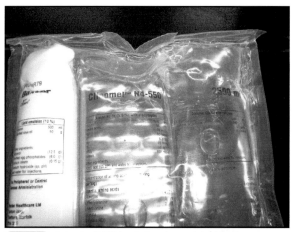

5.9 A typical PPN solution formulated for humans but which can be used in dogs. The white emulsion is lipid; the middle section contains an amino acid solution; and the right hand portion contains dextrose. The fluids have a long shelf life while separated like this. When they are administered, the internal seals between the bags are broken and the solutions mixed.

This parenteral nutrition solution has a relatively low osmolality and thus can be administered via a peripheral catheter. Strict asepsis should be adhered to when delivering the solution. The solution contains **20 mmol/l potassium chloride**, thus adjustments to supplementation rates may be necessary.

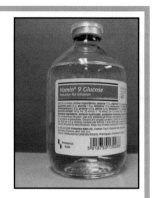

1. Calculate resting energy requirement (RER)

RER = 70 x (current bodyweight in kg)$^{0.75}$
or for animals 2–30 kg, RER = (30 x current bodyweight in kg) + 70

RER = ____ kcal/day

2. Calculate protein requirement

	Dogs (g/100 kcal)	Cats (g/100 kcal)
Standard	4	6
Reduced (hepatic encephalopathy/renal failure)	2–3	3–4
Increased (excessive protein losses)	6	7–8

(RER ÷ 100) x ____ g/100 kcal = ____ g protein required/day
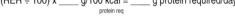

3. Calculate rate of Vamin® 9 Glucose required

Vamin® 9 Glucose is a 5.9% amino acid solution (9% nitrogen) and thus has 0.059 g protein/ml.

PPN rate required = ____ g protein/day ÷ 0.059 g prot/ml ÷ 24 hours = ____ ml/h of PPN

WARNING
Make sure this rate of infusion is clinically appropriate for the patient.

4. Calculate proportion of RER provided at this rate

Vamin® 9 Glucose contains 0.65 kcal/ml of energy.

Energy provided by PPN = 0.65 kcal/ml x ____ ml/h of PPN x 24 hours = ____ kcal/day

Proportion of energy from PPN = ____ PPN energy ÷ ____ RER x 100 = ____ %

5. Calculate rate of glucose infusion at calculated PPN rate:

Vamin® 9 Glucose is a 10% glucose solution, i.e. 100 mg/ml

Glucose infusion rate = ____ ml/h PPN ÷ 60 min x 100 mg/ml ÷ kg bodyweight
= ____ mg/kg/min

WARNING
Glucose infusion rate should not exceed 4 mg/kg/min, as this may cause hyperglycaemia. It may be necessary to decrease the infusion rate and recalculate.

5.10 How to calculate the infusion rate required for PPN using Vamin® 9 Glucose. PPN should ideally provide 40–70% of RER and should not be continued beyond 5 days.

PN administration

- The administration of PN requires a catheter solely used for PN; this catheter must be placed under strict aseptic technique.
- Once PN is delivered via this catheter, it must remain a 'closed system' as much as possible. The line must *not* be unnecessarily disconnected (e.g. when the dog is walked or taken for diagnostic procedures) *nor* used for any other purpose (e.g. blood sampling, intravenous drug administration). Observing such strict protocols is necessary to keep rates of catheter infection very low.
- For TPN the preferred route is via central lines (using either single or multilumen catheters).
- PPN can be administered peripherally (see Figure 5.8) (e.g. cephalic vein in dogs, femoral vein in cats).
- Catheters used for PN must be inspected daily for any sign of infection; if this complication is suspected, the catheter should be removed and submitted for bacteriological culture.

Nutrition in specific diseases

Dietary manipulations are an important part of the treatment in many diseases in dogs and cats, and have the potential to improve both outcome and quality of life. There are many prescription diets available from a variety of manufacturers for a number of diseases in dogs and cats, so it could be tempting just to reach for the tin with the correct name without understanding their ingredients, the rationale for their use, and the indications and contraindications. Some 'clinical diets' are only appropriate in certain circumstances, whilst many diseases can be treated with more than one diet. It is also important to recognize that some diets can be used to manage more than one abnormality, whilst there are some circumstances where no commercial diet is suitable to meet the patient's nutritional needs. Where there are no suitable commercial diets, or the animal or client refuses commercial diets, complete and balanced home-made diets can be formulated, but this usually requires the aid of a veterinary nutritionist.

Regardless of the type of diet chosen, a good understanding of what dietary manipulations are indicated and likely to be most beneficial to the patient is essential to optimal management. An easy way to consider dietary management of a patient is to consider, for each case, the following questions:

- Do I need to alter: protein, fat, carbohydrate, fibre, vitamins or minerals in this case?
- Does this patient need a reduction in calorie intake? (see Chapter 6)
- Are any nutraceuticals indicated in this case? (see Chapter 7)

Nutritional management of renal disease

Correct dietary management in chronic renal failure can be the single most important feature in prolonging life expectancy and quality of life in both dogs and cats. For this reason, dietary manipulation is as important (and exciting!) as drug therapy in this disease. Early recommendations were extrapolated from work on rodents and in people, but recent research in both experimental and naturally occurring renal disease in dogs and cats has further increased understanding of the dietary management of renal disease in these species.

Objectives
- Meet energy and nutrient requirements.
- Alleviate clinical signs of uraemia in order to increase quality of life.
- Minimize electrolyte, vitamin and mineral disturbances.
- Slow the progression of disease and prolong life expectancy if possible.

Nutrient manipulations
The clinically most important manipulations in canine and feline renal diets are phosphate and protein restriction. In one study, dogs fed a 'renal diet' had a median survival time three times longer than those not fed a renal diet. They also showed a 70% reduction in uraemic crises, were free of uraemia 2.5 times longer, and their renal function declined more slowly than dogs not fed the diet (Jacob *et al.*, 2002). In separate studies, cats fed a renal diet survived more than twice as long as cats not fed the diet and showed a reduced risk of uraemic crises and renal-related death (Elliott *et al.*, 2000; Ross *et al.*, 2006). In Elliott's study, cats fed the diet had a median survival time of 633 days, compared with 264 days in those not fed the diet. The challenge is often to get the patients, especially cats, to accept the new diet, but these remarkable increases in survival times mean that it is worth persevering by trying a variety of manufacturers' renal diets, both dried and moist, before giving up. It is unclear which of the manipulations in the renal diets produces this prolongation in life expectancy, but it is suspected to be largely due to the phosphate restriction.

A 'typical' renal diet for dogs and cats would have the following features.

Protein: Protein should be moderately restricted. This has clinical benefits, particularly in more severe disease, because it reduces uraemia and its associated clinical signs (such as vomiting and depression) and therefore improves quality of life. However, there is no convincing evidence that protein restriction actually reduces the progression of disease in dogs and cats, although it does slow progression in rats. There are clear benefits of moderate protein restriction in dogs with renal failure, but a mixture of positive and negative effects with either marked protein restriction or a high-protein diet (Kronfeld, 1993). Paradoxically, in protein-losing nephropathy, moderate protein restriction is recommended on the basis of evidence in humans, and some limited evidence in dogs, that this reduces the magnitude of proteinuria, presumably by reducing glomerular damage by excessive filtering of proteins (Burkholder *et al.*, 2004; Lees *et al.*, 2004).

Phosphorus: Phosphate restriction also imparts clear benefits and is believed to be the most important contributor in slowing disease progression in chronic renal failure (Barber and Elliott, 1998; Barber *et al.*,1999; Elliott *et al.*, 2000). The hyperphosphataemia of chronic renal failure results from reduced renal excretion and leads to reciprocal hypocalcaemia and subsequent hyperparathyroidism. Later in the disease progression, the parathyroids may become relatively autonomous and may continue to secrete parathyroid hormone (PTH) even in the presence of normal or elevated calcium; this is termed renal secondary hyperparathyroidism (Figure 5.11). PTH is an important uraemic toxin, contributing to anaemia, neurotoxicity, and soft tissue and renal calcification. There are high levels of PTH receptors in renal cells; these promote calcium uptake, further worsening kidney damage. Therefore, restricting phosphorus in the diet (with or without additional phosphate binders) reduces PTH levels, leading to clinical benefits.

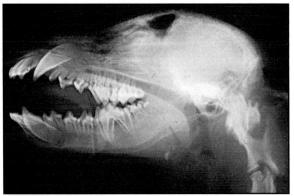

5.11 Lateral skull radiograph of a puppy with juvenile nephropathy and renal secondary hyperparathyroidism. Note the marked reduction in the bone density of the skull in the mandible particularly, which gives the appearance of the teeth 'floating' in very little bone. (Courtesy of the Diagnostic Imaging Department, Queen's Veterinary School Hospital, University of Cambridge)

Calcium and vitamin D: Some authors recommend supplementing vitamin D in renal disease in order to increase calcium and thus reduce the hyperparathyroidism (Nagode *et al.*,1996). However, others contend that this is not necessary (Barber *et al.*,1999) and that it is important to avoid either calcium or vitamin D supplementation, unless the patient is confirmed to be hypocalcaemic and serum phosphate is normal. If the phosphate is elevated, supplementation of calcium and /or vitamin D runs the risk of causing soft tissue calcification, including in the kidneys. Calcium concentrations are therefore kept normal in renal diets.

Fat: Fat is usually increased in renal diets to increase energy density and palatability, on the assumption that most animals with renal failure have some degree of inappetence and therefore require a high-calorie diet. However, care must be taken if the animal is already overweight or is fat-intolerant. Most notably, the use of renal diets can be dangerous in animals prone to bouts of acute pancreatitis. In these cases, the relative risks of triggering a potentially fatal bout of acute pancreatitis must be weighed against the benefits of the renal diet in prolonging life expectancy. Most renal diets also have increased levels of omega-3 fatty acids. These fatty acids are proposed to be beneficial, particularly in glomerular disease (see Chapter 7).

Fibre: Some renal diets incorporate an increased amount of fermentable fibre. There is a logical argument for increasing fermentable fibre in the diet to act as a 'nitrogen trap' in the gut. Colonic bacteria metabolize dietary soluble fibre and, in the process, incorporate nitrogen into their cells. This nitrogen comes from any undigested dietary protein in the gut and (more importantly in renal failure) from free diffusion of urea across the gut wall from the bloodstream. Theoretically, this effect could lead to a reduction of uraemia in renal failure. This has not been demonstrated to date in renal cases, although diets with increased fermentable fibre have been shown to lower postprandial plasma urea in normal Beagles (Diez *et al.*,1997).

Sodium: Sodium has traditionally been restricted in renal diets on the assumption that this will help to reduce the hypertension associated with renal failure. However, there is no experimental evidence on which to base this recommendation, and the fractional excretion (i.e. loss) of sodium via the kidneys is actually increased in renal failure. One recent study showed that sodium restriction in cats acting as experimental models of renal failure lowered glomerular filtration rate and encouraged hypokalaemia (Buranakarl *et al.*, 2004); so the current recommendations are to feed normal levels of sodium in the diet until more work is done.

Potassium: Blood potassium concentrations may be low (particularly in cats with chronic renal failure) or high (particularly in acute and acute-on-chronic renal failure) so the potassium levels in the formulated diets are kept normal, allowing the clinician to supplement as necessary on an individual basis.

B vitamins: B vitamins are supplemented in renal diets to compensate for proposed increased renal losses in polyuric patients.

Nutritional management of gastrointestinal disease and pancreatitis

The gastrointestinal tract (including exocrine pancreas) is central to the digestion and absorption of food. Therefore, not only are dietary manipulations important for treatment of gastrointestinal and pancreatic diseases, but dietary components themselves may be involved in the pathogenesis of disease. Food affects not only faecal consistency, gut wall and pancreatic inflammation, but also motility, particularly rates of gastric emptying and intestinal transit time; all these effects can be useful therapeutically. Crucially, the small and large intestine obtain a large amount of their energy requirements from the products of intraluminal digestion (glutamine metabolism by small intestinal enterocytes and butyrate metabolism by colonocytes). It is therefore increasingly recognized that starvation is inappropriate in many gastrointestinal diseases. Early feeding improves gut wall integrity and speeds recovery in a variety of diseases, including acute pancreatitis.

Objectives
- Address any dietary cause of the gastrointestinal disease.
- Provide adequate, high-quality, digestible nutrition – ideally, if possible, via the enteral route to provide intraluminal nutrition for enterocytes and thus speed recovery and reduce the risk of breakdown of gut wall integrity and translocation of bacteria.
- Help manage clinical signs by beneficially altering gastric motility and intestinal transit times, and reducing undigested nutrients in the gut lumen.

Nutrient manipulations

Consistency and frequency: Feeding a highly digestible diet 'little and often' is often beneficial in gastrointestinal disease. It reduces the demands on the diseased intestinal tract, thereby reducing undigested nutrients remaining in the lumen to cause secondary osmotic diarrhoea. It also reduces gastric stretch, which is beneficial in gastritis where the normal receptive relaxation of the stomach wall during filling is disrupted.

Changing the consistency of the food has a profound effect on gastric emptying times; liquidizing foods speeds gastric emptying, when compared with tinned or dried food of the same nutrient profile, so liquidized food is preferred in gastritis and functional gastric outflow obstructions. Dogs with functional motility disorders causing rapid intestinal transit (e.g. nervous working breeds) may, conversely, benefit from a dried diet.

Protein: Protein is essential for turnover of enterocytes and brush border enzymes, and for immunity. In the small intestine, glutamine is the major nutrient for enterocytes. However, there are also potential negative effects of protein in the gastrointestinal tract: high-protein diets cause increased gastric acid secretion; and intestinal protein is one of the stimuli for cholecystokinin release and thus pancreatic enzyme secretion (although fat is a more potent stimulus for both this and gastric acid secretion; see below). Proteins are also the major cause of gastrointestinal 'allergy' and any dog or cat with inflammatory bowel disease should have food allergy ruled out with a well designed novel or hydrolysed protein diet trial if possible.

Fat: Fat is often 'the enemy' in gastrointestinal disease, with a wide variety of potential deleterious effects, especially in dogs. The effects of dietary fat levels in gastrointestinal disease in cats have not been well investigated and it is often stated that such cats can be fed normal fat concentrations.

Fat is an important source of calories (particularly in large-breed dogs with high calorie requirements), and some dietary fat is necessary to supply essential fatty acids and fat-soluble vitamins. However, high-fat foods delay gastric emptying; therefore, low-fat foods are indicated in gastritis. Fat reduces gastro-oesophageal sphincter tone, so predisposing to reflux. Low-fat foods are therefore indicated in hiatal hernia, gastro-oesophageal reflux and functional delayed gastric emptying (including after surgery for gastric dilatation volvulus), as more rapid gastric emptying and increased gastro-oesophageal sphincter tone is desirable in all of these cases.

Low-fat food is also indicated in many cases of canine small intestinal diarrhoea because fat absorption has been shown to be reduced in small intestinal disease; in instances of small intestinal bacterial overgrowth there is deconjugation of bile acids, which reduces fat digestion. Unabsorbed fat reaching the large intestine is metabolized by bacteria to highly irritant hydroxyl fatty acids, which cause a secondary secretory colitis.

Low-fat foods should logically also be indicated in pancreatic disease, as fat digestion is reduced in these conditions, particularly in exocrine pancreatic insufficiency (EPI) where there is a deficiency of lipase. However, studies in dogs with EPI due to pancreatic acinar atrophy (PAA) have shown no deleterious effects of feeding normal dietary fat levels with enzyme supplementation, and the benefits of supplying sufficient calories to affected large-breed dogs outweigh the risk. High-fat diets should certainly be avoided in EPI. In canine pancreatitis, feeding a low-fat diet reduces postprandial pain and, therefore, low-fat diets *are* indicated in EPI caused by end-stage chronic pancreatitis rather than PAA.

Dietary fat should also be specifically restricted in lymphangiectasia to reduce the flow of lymph. In these cases, extra calories can be supplied by supplementing the diet with medium-chain triglycerides (MCTs) (such as coconut oil) which are not digested by lipase and are absorbed directly into capillaries. However, these triglycerides cannot carry fat-soluble vitamins and do not supply essential long-chain fatty acids, so some dietary fat is still required. MCTs are also poorly tolerated by cats, so are not used in this species. There may be some benefit to feeding extra omega-3 fatty acids in inflammatory intestinal disease (see Chapter 7).

Carbohydrate: There are no specific requirements for carbohydrate in most gastrointestinal diseases. The carbohydrate used should be digestible in order to reduce gut work. Many hypoallergenic diets avoid wheat gluten and use rice or potato instead. However, wheat gluten sensitivity is very unusual in dogs (apart from Irish Setters with gluten enteropathy) and it is also of note that all cereals have some type of gluten – so rice gluten allergy is also possible, and recognized in some dogs.

Fibre: Fermentable and non-fermentable fibre have different activities and benefits, and a mixture of the two is beneficial in colitis. Butyrate, from fermentation of soluble fibre, is a major nutrient for colonocytes. Fermentable fibre encourages beneficial bacterial growth and improves faecal consistency by absorbing water; non-fermentable fibre stretches the colonic muscle, helping to normalize motility. However, it is best to avoid high-fibre foods in gastritis, and in pancreatic and small intestinal disease. Fibre interferes with pancreatic enzyme activity and with nutrient absorption in the diseased small intestine. In the stomach, fermentable fibre delays gastric emptying. Non-fermentable fibre may be helpful in gastritis as it speeds gastric emptying and has a buffering action, but more work is needed to assess its benefits before recommending its use in gastric disease. Generally, therefore, high-fibre diets are avoided in small intestinal and pancreatic diseases. The use of high-fibre diets in cats is controversial.

Vitamins and minerals: Fat maldigestion, when marked, can result in deficiency of fat-soluble vitamins. This is particularly the case in cats and dogs with severe diffuse infiltrative intestinal disease, EPI or lymphangiectasia. Deficiencies of vitamin D (with subsequent reductions in ionized calcium) and vitamin K can be particular problems in these situations and may require supplements. Oral supplementation with more water-soluble analogues may be possible or (in the case of vitamin K), parenteral supplementation may be necessary. Vitamin B12 deficiency is not uncommon in EPI in both dogs and cats (because intrinsic factor, necessary for its absorption, is produced solely by the pancreas in cats and mainly by the pancreas in dogs) and may also be seen in disease of the ileum (because it is absorbed in the ileum). In these cases, supplementation by injection is important because B12 deficiency can contribute to intestinal disease and appears to be a poor prognostic indicator in canine EPI (Batchelor *et al.*, 2007). There are no specific indications for mineral supplementation in gastrointestinal disease but it should be noted that minerals often affect gastrointestinal motility when supplemented in other diseases: for example, zinc supplementation can cause vomiting; iron supplementation often results in constipation.

Nutritional management of liver disease

The liver is central to the metabolism of protein, carbohydrate, lipid, vitamins and minerals, and therefore diet is important in both the cause and treatment of liver disease in dogs and cats. The liver also has an important detoxifying role, including the detoxification of the contents of the portal blood (such as ammonia from glutamine metabolism by enterocytes and from colonic bacterial activity). Cats have very different metabolism and liver diseases from dogs, so their dietary requirements in hepatic diseases are also very different from dogs.

Objectives

- Reduce the detoxification and excretion workload of the liver.
- Provide adequate, high-quality nutrition to prevent deleterious catabolic changes and allow hepatic regeneration.
- Contribute to the management of the clinical signs or complications of the disease, particularly hepatic encephalopathy in congenital and acquired portosystemic shunts, and gastroduodenal ulceration and ascites in animals with cirrhosis and portal hypertension.
- Treat the underlying disease if possible. For example, in copper storage disease in dogs or hepatic lipidosis in cats, dietary management is the primary treatment modality.

Nutrient manipulations

Feed little and often; this is an important manipulation for reasons outlined below.

Protein: Protein restriction has long been advocated in canine liver disease, but is now recognized to be rarely necessary and potentially damaging. The current advice is to feed moderate to normal amounts of high-quality (all essential amino acids), highly digestible protein (so none is left in the colon for bacteria to break down to ammonia). Both excessively high-protein and excessively low-protein

diets are to be avoided. The traditional rationale for restricting dietary protein in animals with hepatic encephalopathy (HE) associated with congenital and acquired portosystemic shunts (PSS) was flawed, since most of the postprandial ammonia in the portal blood in these animals originates from enterocyte metabolism of glutamine as an energy source (which is unavoidable) and not, as previously suggested, from fermentation of dietary protein by bacteria in the colon (Shawcross and Jalan, 2005). The most effective way to reduce this postprandial ammonia burst is therefore to feed little and often.

Dietary protein restriction is very rarely indicated in cats with liver disease, although there is a potential requirement for it in cats with congenital PSS (Figure 5.12). For cats suffering from hepatic lipidosis, protein levels should be high. In cholangitis, a highly digestible novel protein source is often chosen because of the high prevalence of concurrent inflammatory bowel disease.

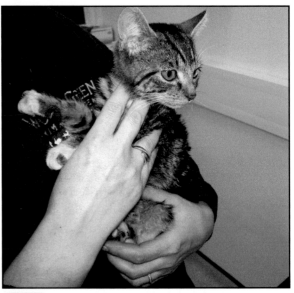

5.12 A kitten with a portosystemic shunt (note the copper-coloured irises which are commonly seen in cats with PSS). This is the only liver disease in cats where dietary protein restriction would be considered.

Fat: In spite of impaired carbohydrate and fat metabolism in liver disease, there is no special advice for dietary fat or carbohydrate levels in hepatic disease, and normal levels are therefore given. Complete biliary tract obstruction would interfere with fat digestion by preventing fat emulsification by bile salts, but very rarely occurs in feline and canine liver disease.

Fibre: A mixture of fermentable and non-fermentable fibre has traditionally been recommended in dogs with liver disease, particularly to reduce HE in animals with congenital or acquired PSS. Fermentable fibre is broken down to short-chain fatty acids in the colon; these are proposed to trap ammonia as ammonium ions and also to increase nitrogen incorporation into bacteria by encouraging their growth. However, doubt has recently been cast on the efficacy of fermentable fibre in reducing HE in humans

(Shawcross and Jalan, 2005) and its true efficacy in dogs is unknown. Non-fermentable fibre prevents constipation, a potential predisposing factor for the development of HE (increases contact time for colonic bacteria to produce ammonia from faeces).

The use of increased dietary fibre in cats is controversial and there is no evidence that it helps with liver disease in this species; therefore a low-residue diet is often used.

Minerals: Restriction of dietary copper and increased dietary zinc in dogs genetically predisposed to copper storage disease will stop development of hepatitis. In animals with established copper storage disease, copper restriction is indicated together with chelation, but zinc supplementation should not be implemented until chelation therapy has stopped (otherwise the chelator will also chelate the zinc). Zinc supplementation is also recommended in any canine chronic hepatitis because it is used in metalloenzymes involved in ammonia metabolism and may also reduce collagen lay-down in the liver, although evidence for its efficacy in dogs is currently very limited.

Copper storage disease is very rare in cats and there is no current advice about minerals in this species.

Vitamins:

- Vitamin E supplementation may be cytoprotective, especially in copper toxicity. Vitamin E neutralizes free radicals and some authors supplement it in any case of chronic hepatitis (dose rate: 400–600 IU q24h in medium-sized dogs).
- Vitamin K supplementation may be necessary if clotting times are prolonged, especially in cats and especially if considering biopsies.
- Vitamins A and D should *not* be supplemented: vitamin A can cause hepatic damage; and vitamin D supplementation can cause calcification in tissues.
- B vitamins should be supplemented because there is an increased loss through polydipsia and polyuria associated with liver disease. It is recommended that dogs and cats with liver disease receive a double dose of B vitamins.
- Vitamin C should *not* be supplemented, as ascorbate can increase the tissue damage associated with copper and iron in liver disease.

Nutritional management of cardiac disease

The role of nutrition in the management of patients with cardiac disease is not without controversy. Certain nutrient deficiencies, such as taurine, are known to lead to cardiomyopathies in both dogs and cats. However, this problem is not common because commercial diets typically have more than adequate quantities of this amino acid. Other components of the diet, such as salt content, are also believed to play a role in the pathogenesis of advanced cardiac disease and have traditionally been a target of nutritional modulation. However, a major challenge in managing animals with advanced cardiac disease is

that they often have a decreased appetite and this makes the introduction of therapeutic diets, which may be reduced in sodium, very difficult. There are also limited data on the long-term effects of dietary manipulations on the course of cardiac disease; most studies relating to diet and progression of heart disease focus on short-term changes, such as left atrial size and hormonal changes. Despite these challenges, there are several nutritional principles that may aid in the management of cardiac disease.

Objectives

- Synergistically work with drug therapy in alleviating clinical signs such as pulmonary congestion and peripheral oedema.
- Reduce blood sodium concentration and minimize water retention.
- Decrease the workload of the heart.
- Maintain lean body mass and restore the animal to normal bodyweight.

Nutrient manipulations

Depending on the type and severity of cardiac dysfunction, diets designed for dogs and cats with heart disease may involve the following alterations.

Increased energy density: Cardiac failure elicits a chronic inflammatory state which increases overall energy demands and promotes various other metabolic changes such as altered substrate metabolism and oxidative stress. At the same time, many animals with cardiac disease will have a reduction in appetite. This leads to lean body wasting, which is sometimes referred to as cardiac cachexia (Figure 5.13). A recent study demonstrated a relationship between maintenance of bodyweight during the course of heart disease and longer survival, highlighting the importance of nutritional status in heart disease (Slupe *et al.,* 2008).

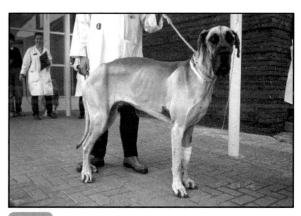

5.13 A Great Dane with cardiac cachexia.

Supplementation with certain fatty acids, such as omega-3 fatty acids, may be beneficial in certain types of cardiomyopathies through modulating the inflammatory response, increasing the caloric density of the diet, and even potentially increasing survival (Freeman *et al.,* 1998; Slupe *et al.,* 2008). Omega-3 fatty acids play an important role in dampening inflammation and may reduce the rates of certain tachyarrhythmias, such as arrhythmogenic right ventricular cardiomyopathy in Boxers (Smith *et al.*, 2007). Some research has also demonstrated that omega-3 fatty acids may enhance appetite in certain canine patient populations (Freeman *et al.*, 1998).

Avoidance of sodium excess: In heart failure, sodium, chloride and water are retained by the body following activation of the aldosterone–angiotensin cascade. This may lead to oedema, ascites, pulmonary congestion and coughing. These deleterious effects are exacerbated by consuming diets with high salt content, which is typical of many maintenance diets. Most treats are also very high in sodium and should be avoided in patients with congestive heart failure. Feeding a diet that is restricted in sodium (less than minimum requirements) is not usually necessary, and in fact may accentuate activation of the aldosterone–angiotensin system. A gradual reduction in sodium levels (or avoidance of sodium excess) in the diet, especially if the animal has formerly been fed a diet high in sodium, is preferred over actual sodium restriction. Furthermore, restricting sodium reduces the palatability of the diet, which is undesirable in this condition. Appreciating the difference between avoidance of sodium excess and sodium restriction is an important point in the dietary management of patients with cardiac disease; clinicians should carefully consider the sodium content of prescription cardiac diets and the needs of their particular patient before prescribing such diets.

Additional B vitamins and magnesium: The use of diuretic agents increases the requirements for water-soluble vitamins and therefore supplementation of these may be necessary, although deficiencies leading to clinical manifestations are uncommon.

Additionally, diuretics increase the requirement for magnesium. If hypomagnesaemia develops, this could lead to an increased risk of cardiac arrhythmias. The risk for the development of cardiac arrhythmias due to hypomagnesaemia may be ameliorated with diets enriched in magnesium.

Optimal potassium intake: Body potassium may also be depleted by the use of diuretics, notably furosemide. For this reason, diets designed for patients with cardiac disease are fortified with potassium to compensate for increased requirements. In animals with a tendency for potassium depletion, the use of potassium-sparing diuretics, such as spironolactone, may be preferable to furosemide. Animals concurrently receiving angiotensin-converting enzyme (ACE) inhibitors usually do not need potassium-supplemented diets.

Nutritional management of lower urinary tract disease

Management of animals with a propensity for forming certain uroliths or cystoliths requires long-term nutritional management. Not all forms of urinary stones respond to dietary manipulation, and identification of the exact type of stone is necessary before attempting nutritional management. It is important to recognize that there may be other risk factors (e.g. urinary tract infection in dogs with struvite urolithiasis) that could present suitable targets for therapy.

Objectives
- Dissolve certain uroliths (e.g. struvite; Figure 5.14).
- Prevent the formation of new uroliths.
- Promote diuresis (encourage increased urination to decrease urine retention and specific gravity of urine).

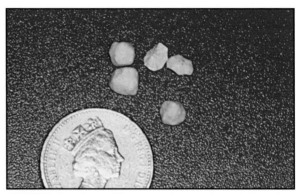

5.14 Struvite uroliths passed spontaneously from the bladder of a female Dachshund. Any struvite uroliths remaining in this dog's bladder could be dissolved and recurrence prevented using a combination of dietary and antibiotic management, provided owner and patient compliance with both were good.

Nutrient manipulations

Calculolytic properties: Dissolution of uroliths through dietary modification may be achieved in some cases (e.g. struvite, urate) but not with all types of urolith. Concurrent antibiotic treatment is also important in dogs with struvite calculi as these are usually caused by bladder infection. Consumption of calculolytic diets may produce alterations in urine pH and urine composition that promote dissolution of calculi. Currently there are no calculolytic diets for calcium oxalate or cysteine stones. In cases where the exact type of calculi is unknown, the use of calculolytic diets is not indicated.

Promote increased water intake: Increasing water intake promotes greater urine output and reduces urine saturation. This is perhaps the most important factor in *preventing* uroliths in both cats and dogs. This may be achieved by using wet diets, adding water to dry diets, or increasing salt intake. It is important to have follow-up in these cases and, ideally, to check the specific gravity of the urine before and after dietary change (particularly in cats) so that clients know whether further changes are required (e.g. adding more water) to achieve a dilute urine. This is particularly important in small-breed dogs and cats that are fed dried diets, as they tend to produce more concentrated urine than when fed tinned food; large-breed dogs fed on dried food tend to drink enough water to produce urine of the same specific gravity as when they are fed moist food (Stevenson *et al.*, 2003).

Promote a specific urinary pH: Urine pH can influence the formation and dissolution of certain uroliths and crystals. For example, struvite uroliths may dissolve in acidic urine. Recommendations for urinary pH for animals with struvite uroliths range from 5.9 to 6.1 (cats) and from 5.8 to 6.2 (dogs) for dissolution, and from 6.2 to 6.4 (dogs and cats) for prevention of recurrence. However, acidic urine may promote formation of calcium oxalate crystals. In animals with calcium oxalate crystals urinary pH targets are approximately 6.8 in cats and 7.1–7.7 for dogs. Dogs with urate stones should also have a urinary pH target above 7.1. Guidance for the expected urinary pH for dogs and cats on a given therapeutic diet can be obtained from product guides or by contacting the manufacturer.

Altered protein content and composition: Certain uroliths composed of urates or cysteine form when there are metabolic abnormalities that lead to excretion of inappropriate calculogenic precursors. For urate stones (most commonly seen in Dalmatians) accumulation of uric acid instead of allantoin in the urine is the major problem. A rare genetic defect in reabsorption of dibasic amino acids in the renal proximal convoluted tubules leads to cysteinuria and calculi formation in some dogs. Significantly lowering the protein and purine content of the diet can therefore lower the risk of both urate and cysteine urolith formation. Some Dalmatians require allopurinol and potassium citrate (urine alkalinizing agent) supplementation in addition to dietary change.

References and further reading

Abel RM, Grimes JB, Alonso D, Alonso M and Gay WA Jr (1979) Adverse hemodynamic and ultrastructural changes in dog hearts subjected to protein-calories malnutrition. *American Heart Journal* **97**, 733–744

Abood SK, McLoughlin MA and Buffington CA (2006) Enteral nutrition. In: *Fluid, Electrolyte, and Acid-Base Disorders in Small Animal Practice, 3rd edn*, ed. SP DiBartola, pp.601–620. Saunders Elsevier, St. Louis

Barber PJ and Elliott J (1998) Feline chronic renal failure: calcium homeostasis in 80 cases diagnosed between 1992 and 1995. *Journal of Small Animal Practice* **39**, 108–116

Barber PJ, Rawlings JM, Markwell PJ and Elliott J (1999) Effect of dietary phosphate restriction on renal secondary hyperparathyroidism in the cat. *Journal of Small Animal Practice* **40**, 62–70

Batchelor DJ, Noble PJ, Taylor RH, Cripps PJ and German AJ (2007) Prognostic factors in canine exocrine pancreatic insufficiency: prolonged survival is likely if clinical remission is achieved. *Journal of Veterinary Internal Medicine* **21**, 54–60

Buranakarl C, Mathur S and Brown SA (2004) Effects of dietary sodium chloride intake on renal function and blood pressure in cats with normal and reduced renal function. *American Journal of Veterinary Research* **65**, 620–627

Burkholder WJ, Lees GE, LeBlanc AK *et al.* (2004) Diet modulates proteinuria in heterozygous female dogs with X-linked hereditary nephropathy. *Journal of Veterinary Internal Medicine* **18**, 165–175

Center SA, Elston TH, Rowland PH *et al.* (1996) Fulminant hepatic failure associated with oral administration of diazepam in 11 cats. *Journal of the American Veterinary Medical Association* **209**, 18–25

Chan DL and Freeman LM (2006) Nutrition in critical illness. *Veterinary Clinics of North America: Small Animal Practice* **36**(6), 1225–1241

Chan DL, Freeman LM, Rozanski EA and Rush JE (2006) Alterations in carbohydrate metabolism in critically ill cats. *Journal of Veterinary Emergency and Critical Care* **16**(S1), S7–S13

Diez M, Hornick JL, Baldwin P and Istasse L (1997) Influence of a blend of fructo-oligosaccharides and sugar beet fiber on nutrient digestibility and plasma metabolite concentrations in healthy beagles. *American Journal of Veterinary Research* **58**(11), 1238–1242

Dionigi R, Ariszonta, Dominioni L, Gnes F and Ballabio A (1977) The effects of total parenteral nutrition on immunodepression due to malnutrition. *Annals of Surgery* **185**, 467–474

Elliott J, Rawlings JM, Markwell PJ and Barber PJ (2000) Survival of cats with naturally occurring chronic renal failure: effect of dietary management. *Journal of Small Animal Practice* **41**, 235–242

Freeman LM and Chan DL (2006) Total parenteral nutrition. In: *Fluid, Electrolyte, and Acid-Base Disorders in Small Animal Practice, 3rd edn*, ed. SP DiBartola, pp.584–600. Saunders Elsevier, St. Louis

Freeman LM, Rush JE, Kehayias JJ *et al.* (1998) Nutritional alterations and the effect of fish oil supplementation in dogs with heart failure. *Journal of Veterinary Internal Medicine* **12**, 440–448

Himwich HE and Rose MI (1927).The respiratory quotient of exercising muscle. *American Journal of Physiology* **81**, 485–486 [abstract]

Jacob, F, Polzin D, Osborne CA *et al.* (2002) Clinical evaluation of dietary modification for treatment of spontaneous chronic renal failure in dogs. *Journal of the American Veterinary Medical Association* **220**, 1163–1170

Kronfeld (1993) Dietary management of chronic renal disease in dogs: a critical appraisal. *Journal of Small Animal Practice* **34**, 211–219

Lees GE, Brown SA, Elliott J, Grauer GF, Vaden SL (2004) Assessment and management of proteinuria in dogs and cats: 2004 ACVIM forum consensus statement (small animal). *Journal of Veterinary Internal Medicine* **19**, 377–385

Long JP and Greco SC (2000) The effect of propofol administered intravenously on appetite stimulation in dogs. *Contemporary Topics in Laboratory Animal Science* **39**, 43–46

Meier RF and Beglinger C (2006) Nutrition in pancreatic diseases. *Best Practice in Research and Clinical Gastroenterology* **20**, 507–529

Melis GC, ter Wengel N, Boelens PG *et al.* (2004) Glutamine: recent developments in research on the clinical significance of glutamine. *Current Opinion in Clinical Nutrition and Metabolic Care* **7**(1), 59–70

Nagode LA, Chew DJ and Podell M (1996) Benefits of calcitriol therapy and serum phosphorus control in dogs and cats with chronic renal failure: both are essential to prevent or suppress toxic hyperparathyroidism. *Veterinary Clinics of North America: Small Animal Practice* **26**(6), 1293–1330

O'Toole E, Miller CW, Wilson BA *et al.* (2004) Comparison of the standard predictive equation for calculation of resting energy expenditure with indirect calorimetry in hospitalized and healthy dogs. *Journal of the American Veterinary Medical Association* **255**, 58–64

Ross SJ, Osborne CA, Kirk CA *et al.* (2006) Clinical evaluation of dietary modification for treatment of spontaneous chronic kidney disease in cats. *Journal of the American Veterinary Medical Association* **229**, 949–957

Shawcross D and Jalan R (2005) Dispelling myths in the treatment of hepatic encephalopathy. *Lancet* **365**, 431–433

Slupe JL, Freeman LM and Rush JE (2008) Association of body weight and body condition with survival in dogs with heart failure. *Journal of Veterinary Internal Medicine* **22**, 561–565

Smith CE, Freeman LM, Rush JE, Cunningham SM and Biourge V (2007) Omega-3 fatty acids in Boxer dogs with arrhythmogenic right ventricular cardiomyopathy. *Journal of Veterinary Internal Medicine* **21**, 265–273

Stevenson AE, Hynds WK and Markwell PJ (2003) Effect of dietary moisture and sodium content on urine composition and calcium oxalate relative supersaturation in healthy miniature schnauzers and labrador retrievers. *Research in Veterinary Science* **74**, 145–151

Sungurtekin H, Sungurtekin U, Balci C, Zencir M and Erdem E (2004) The influence of nutritional status on complications after major intra-abdominal surgery. *Journal of the American College of Nutrition* **23**, 227–232

Walton RS, Wingfield WE and Ogilvie GK (1998) Energy expenditure in 104 postoperative and traumatically injured dogs with indirect calorimetry. *Journal of Veterinary Emergency and Critical Care* **6**, 71–79

6

Obesity and weight management

Alex German

Introduction

Current estimates suggest that approximately 40% of pets in the UK are either overweight or obese (Cope, 2008). Obesity is recognized to be an important medical disease, because it may predispose to a variety of other disorders including osteoarthritis, cardiorespiratory problems, diabetes mellitus, constipation, dermatitis, anaesthetic risk and reduced life expectancy. The condition is now the most common medical disorder of companion animals (Cope, 2008) and a major welfare concern. Not only do veterinary surgeons have an ethical obligation to be proactive in the management and prevention of obesity, but they also now have a legal obligation, as owners have been successfully prosecuted for not adequately addressing obesity in their pets. This chapter will review: how obesity is defined in companion animals; expected disease associations; and methods whereby obesity can be managed and prevented.

Defining obesity

Obesity is defined as a disease where excess body fat has accumulated such that health may be adversely affected.

In humans, epidemiological data demonstrate that both morbidity and mortality risk correlate with increasing body fat mass. Body mass index (BMI = weight (kg) / [height (m)^2]) is most commonly used to quantify human adiposity. Recent epidemiological studies suggest that the optimal BMI for average non-smoking adult Caucasians is 20–25. Additionally, epidemiological data confirm that disease risk and mortality risk progressively increase for people classified as 'overweight' (BMI 25–30), 'obese' (BMI 30–40) and 'morbidly obese' (BMI >40). However, BMI cannot be applied to 'non-average' humans, such as sports players who have greater muscle mass such that a ratio based upon height and weight no longer reflects body fat mass accurately.

BMI cannot be applied to dogs because differences in height and lean:fat ratios between breeds renders it far too variable (see below).Companion animal information is more limited than medical data and, in the most commonly applied definitions:

A dog or cat is considered to be:

- 'overweight' when bodyweight is >10–15% above optimal
- 'obese' when bodyweight is >20% above optimal.

As is the case with human studies, epidemiological data support the use of these definitions in companion animals, and an increased risk of associated diseases is seen with increasing levels of adiposity.

Measuring body composition in companion animals

All objective measures of adiposity involve defining body composition, or the 'relative amounts of the various chemical components of the body'. The main conceptual division is between fat mass (FM; the triglyceride component in adipose tissue representing the energy storage depot) and lean body mass (LBM; the metabolically active part of the body encompassing the tissues most affected by adverse nutrition or disease). Assessment of FM and LBM provides valuable information about the physical and metabolic status of the individual.

Various techniques are available to measure body composition and these differ in applicability to research, referral veterinary practice and first-opinion practice. Dual-energy X-ray absorptiometry (DEXA) has recently been shown to be a precise and reliable method for repeated analysis, and can be used to monitor weight loss in a referral setting. However, for first-opinion practice, there is a need for quick, cheap and non-invasive methods of body composition measurement. The most widely adopted quantitative procedures for clinical measurement of body composition include morphometry (zoometry), bioelectrical impedance measurement and body condition scoring.

Morphometry
By combining a measure of length (e.g. head, thorax and limb), which correlates with LBM, and a measure of girth, which correlates with FM, equations can be generated to predict different body components. The best example of such a measure is the feline body mass index:

$$FBMI = \left[\frac{(Ribcage / 0.7067) - LIM}{0.9156}\right] - LIM$$

- *Ribcage* = thoracic circumference measured at 9th rib
- *LIM* (limb index measurement) = distance between the patella and calcaneus of the left hindlimb
- All measurements are made in centimetres
- Measurements are made with a tape measure
- The cat should be in a standing position, with the legs perpendicular to the ground and the head upright

The main limitation is the accuracy of measurements made by tape measure. Also, correlation with adiposity is usually worse than for body composition scoring (see below).

Although a BMI has been suggested for dogs, it has not proved possible to develop a universal system, given the diversity in size and shape across the multitude of breeds.

Biolectrical impedance

Bioelectrical impedance analysis assesses body composition by measuring the nature of the conductance of an applied electrical current in the patient. Body fluids and electrolytes are responsible for conductance and, since adipose tissue is less hydrated than lean body tissues, a greater proportion of adipose tissue results in lower conducting volume and hence larger impedance to current passage. A new hand-held bioimpedance monitor has recently been validated for dogs. However, although this method correlates with other measures of adiposity such as DEXA, a systematic discrepancy exists whereby this bioimpedance monitor under- and over-estimated higher and lower body fat percentages, respectively (German *et al.*, 2010). Further, the degree of correlation with DEXA is weaker than between DEXA and body condition scoring.

Body condition scoring

Body condition scoring remains the most practical method of assessment of body composition in general practice. A body condition score (BCS) is a subjective semi-quantitative method of evaluating body composition. Various schemes have been devised, with either a 5-point or a 9-point scheme being the most widely accepted. All such systems assess visual and palpable characteristics, which correlate with subcutaneous fat, abdominal fat and superficial musculature (e.g. ribcage, dorsal spinous processes, and waist). When used by trained individuals, scores correlate well with body fat mass determined by DEXA.

A new 7-point algorithm-based approach has recently been developed which was designed to be more objective. Good correlation is seen between this system and body fat measurements made by DEXA and there is excellent agreement between experienced operators.

Some examples of BCS schemes can be found at the end of this chapter.

Pathological consequences of obesity

In humans, the medical importance of obesity lies in its effect on mortality and predisposition to other diseases. Similarly, obesity has detrimental effects on health and longevity of dogs and cats.

Pathogenetic mechanisms

Obesity may predispose to other diseases as a result of either 'mechanical' or 'endocrine' effects of excessive white adipose tissue (WAT) deposition. The 'mechanical' effects of excess deposition include: excessive weightbearing by joints and bones (exacerbating orthopaedic disease); constriction of collapsible structures (exacerbation of upper respiratory tract disorders and urinary incontinence); inability to groom; and reduced heat dissipation, due to the insulating effect of fat (exacerbating heat stroke).

Disturbance of the normal endocrine function of WAT is also recognized as a major pathogenetic mechanism. WAT is now known to secrete a range of chemical factors that can have a regulatory effect on many body systems. In humans, obesity is characterized by a state of chronic mild inflammation. Increases in the production of certain 'inflammatory' adipokines have been causally linked to the development of metabolic syndrome and other disorders linked to the obese state. Inflammatory adipokine gene expression has recently been documented in canine WAT samples (Eisele *et al.*, 2005; Ryan *et al.*, 2008). Furthermore, plasma leptin concentrations have been shown to be independently associated with insulin sensitivity in lean and overweight cats, suggesting that similar pathogenetic mechanisms to those in humans may exist in companion animals.

Effects on longevity

It has long been known that calorie restriction without malnutrition can increase longevity in a wide variety of species, from nematode worms to humans. Although the reason for such an effect has not been clearly established, possible mechanisms include: adaptation of neuroendocrine systems (e.g. the insulin/insulin-like growth factor 1 (IGF-1) signalling pathway); prevention of inflammation; hormetic response (a process whereby a low-intensity stressor increases resistance to a more intense stressor); and protection against damage from oxidative stress.

A colony-based canine research study compared lifelong *ad libitum* feeding with energy restriction (restricted dogs were fed ~75% of the calorie intake of the *ad libitum*-fed dogs for the duration of their lives) (Kealy *et al.*, 2002). *Ad libitum*-fed dogs were overweight (mean BCS 6.8/9) compared with energy-restricted dogs (mean BCS 4.5/9), and lifespan was significantly shorter in the *ad libitum* group compared with the energy-restricted dogs (median lifespan 11.2 years and 13.0 years, respectively). Such findings provide a compelling reason why owners should strive to maintain their pets in an ideal body composition throughout their lives, in addition to reducing any known or proposed obesity-associated diseases.

Diseases associated with obesity

Obesity is reported to be a risk factor for a variety of disorders (Figure 6.1).

Diabetes mellitus and insulin resistance

Cats: An association between obesity and diabetes mellitus has been reported in cats (Lund *et al.*, 2005). Diabetic cats most often suffer from an 'insulin-resistant' form of diabetes mellitus, and there are similarities with 'type II' diabetes in humans. As is also the case for humans, weight loss in cats improves insulin sensitivity, thereby reducing (and occasionally eliminating altogether) the requirement for exogenous insulin therapy.

Dogs: Diabetes is also a common endocrine disorder in dogs but there is limited evidence for a canine equivalent of human type II diabetes. Rather, the disease in dogs is usually characterized by an absolute insulin deficiency associated with progressive loss of pancreatic beta cells (Davison *et al.*, 2005; Fall *et al.*, 2007), such that affected dogs require exogenous insulin therapy and display a tendency to develop ketoacidosis. Although the pathogenesis of beta cell loss is poorly understood, pancreatitis and auto-immune-mediated beta cell destruction are thought to play a role. Nonetheless, a recent epidemiological study has identified an association between obesity and diabetes mellitus in dogs (Lund *et al.*, 2006), and having a lifelong history of being overweight may be particularly important (Cope, 2008). An epidemiological association, however, does not necessarily prove causality, i.e. that obesity directly causes diabetes mellitus. The association may be coincidental, e.g. another factor predisposes to both conditions.

Assuming a genuine causal link did exist, its nature would be likely to be different from that seen in humans and cats because type II diabetes mellitus has not been proven to occur in dogs. Pancreatitis is one possible association, since some studies have revealed obesity to be a risk factor for this condition (Hess *et al.*, 1999; Lund *et al.*, 2006) although others have failed to find a link (Watson *et al.*, 2007). Alternatively, obesity may act as a facilitator, unmasking or aggravating a case caused by something else. If this were so, insulin resistance would be a likely pathogenetic mechanism, and this can be induced experimentally (along with other components of the metabolic syndrome) in dogs through weight gain caused by dietary manipulation (Gayet *et al.*, 2004). Further, insulin sensitivity and glucose tolerance are worse in dogs that are fed *ad libitum* throughout their lives compared with dogs that are energy restricted throughout life (Larson *et al.*, 2003). Moreover, a recent study of naturally occurring obesity in dogs has demonstrated that the percentage of body fat correlates with the degree of insulin resistance, and insulin sensitivity is improved significantly upon successful weight loss (German *et al.*, 2010). Finally, in dogs, there is also a positive correlation between IGF-1 and weight gain; given that IGF-1 inhibits insulin secretion, it may contribute to the insulin-resistant state seen in canine obesity (Gayet *et al.*, 2004). Further work is needed in order to clarify this.

Disease category	Cats	Dogs
Orthopaedic	Increased lameness	Cruciate ligament disease; osteoarthritis; humeral condylar fractures; intervertebral disc disease; hip dysplasia
Endocrine	Diabetes mellitus	Hypothyroidism; hyperadrenocorticism; diabetes mellitus; metabolic syndrome (experimental only)
Lipid disorders	Hepatic lipidosis	Mild hypercholesterolaemia, hypertriglyceridaemia, increased plasma NEFA and triglyceride concentrations (experimental) associated with insulin resistance
Alimentary	Oral cavity disease; increased gastrointestinal disease risk; predisposition to diarrhoea	Oral cavity disease; pancreatitis
Urogenital	Urinary tract disease	Urinary tract disease: urethral sphincter mechanism incompetence; calcium oxalate urolithiasis; transitional cell carcinoma; glomerular disease (experimental) Dystocia
Cardiorespiratory		Tracheal collapse; effect on cardiac function; expiratory airway dysfunction; hypertension (doubtful clinical significance); portal vein thrombosis; myocardial hypoxia
Integumental	Increased risk of dermatoses	
Oncological	Increased neoplasia risk	Variable neoplasia risk (increased in some but not all studies); transitional cell carcinoma
Other		Increased anaesthetic risk Decreased heat tolerance

6.1 Reported disease associations in canine and feline obesity. These associations have been published in peer-reviewed studies but, given the nature of epidemiology, a cause and effect relationship has not been established in all cases. NEFA = non-esterified fatty acids.

Orthopaedic disorders

Dogs: Obesity is a major risk factor for orthopaedic diseases in dogs, with a higher prevalence of both traumatic and degenerative orthopaedic disorders in obese animals, e.g. humeral condylar fractures, cranial cruciate ligament rupture, and intervertebral disc disease (Brown *et al.*, 1996). There are also reported associations with hip dysplasia (Kealy *et al.*, 1992) and osteoarthritis (Kealy *et al.*, 2000), whilst weight reduction can lead to a substantial improvement in degree of lameness in dogs with hip osteoarthritis (Impellizeri *et al.*, 2000). The reason for such an association is not clear: it is not known whether obesity simply causes increased joint loading and, therefore, increased pain in a pre-existing condition, or whether obesity leads to disease progression. An effect upon disease progression might be implied for developmental disorders, such as hip dysplasia, which was found to be more prevalent in the *ad libitum*-fed group in the canine lifelong feeding study described above (Kealy *et al.*, 1992). However, more work is required to elucidate the reasons for these associations.

Cats: Obesity may also be a risk factor for orthopaedic disease in cats, with one study suggesting that obese cats were five times more likely to limp than cats of normal body condition (Scarlett and Donoghue, 1998). However, not all reports have confirmed this association (Lund *et al.*, 2005). Nonetheless, the apparent absence of an association in this latter study might relate to the fact that orthopaedic disease is under-recognized in cats, given that signs are subtle in this species. Indeed, a recent study identified the most prominent signs of osteoarthritis were a reduction in the ability to jump and decreased height of jumping (Clarke and Bennett, 2006), which could easily be overlooked by owners.

Cardiorespiratory disease and hypertension

Obesity in dogs can have effects on respiratory system function, as shown by a recent experimental study (Bach *et al.*, 2007). Although higher body condition score did not influence airway function during normal breathing, airway resistance was markedly greater during hyperpnoea. Further, there was a tendency towards a lower functional residual capacity in markedly obese dogs compared with other dogs. Such effects are similar to those seen in humans and may help to explain the anecdotal links between obesity and certain respiratory diseases in dogs, most notably tracheal collapse, laryngeal paralysis and brachycephalic airway obstruction syndrome.

Although obesity is a risk factor for cardiovascular disease in humans, a link between obesity and cardiac disease has not been established in dogs (Slupe *et al.*, 2008). Similarly, although obesity may predispose to hypertension in dogs, the effect is relatively minor and unlikely to be of clinical significance in most cases (Bodey and Mitchell, 1996).

Neoplasia

Some epidemiological studies in both cats and dogs have reported an increased risk of neoplasia in animals that are obese (Lund *et al.*, 2005, 2006) although, in these studies, different types of neoplasia were not assessed individually. Further, whilst some studies have reported an association between canine mammary carcinoma and obesity (Sonnenschein *et al.*, 1991), others have not (Perez Alenza *et al.*, 2000a,b). Being overweight or obese increases the risk of dogs developing transitional cell carcinoma of the bladder (Glickman *et al.*, 1989).

Urinary system disease

An association between obesity and some cases of canine urethral sphincter mechanism incompetence (USMI) has been reported. Although the risk of developing calcium oxalate urolithiasis is increased in obese dogs, this may be related to dietary factors other than calorie excess (Lekcharoensuk *et al.*, 2000).

Other disorders

Obese cats have been reported to be at increased risk of oral cavity disease, dermatological disorders and diarrhoea (Lund *et al.*, 2005). However, the reasons for such associations are not clear.

Risk factors for obesity

Rare single-gene defects are an occasional cause of obesity in humans, but no such disorders have yet been described in dogs or cats, although breed is a risk factor (see below) and this suggests some genetic element. The main reason for development of obesity is a positive mismatch between energy intake and energy expenditure (Figure 6.2).

Various factors can influence the ease with which adipose tissue is gained or lost:

- Individual factors that have been identified include neutering status, sex, age and breed

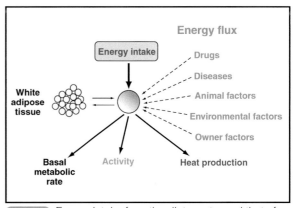

6.2 Energy intake from the diet must equal that of energy expenditure in order for bodyweight to remain stable. Excessive or insufficient energy intake leads, respectively, to expansion or contraction of white adipose tissue. Numerous factors can influence the ease with which energy is stored or mobilized (see text).

- Other studies have implicated owner factors and feeding behaviour as risk factors for overweight and obesity in cats
- Environmental factors predisposing to obesity include type of accommodation and the feeding of certain types of diet
- Additionally, some factors may be the product of both individual and environmental influences, e.g. inactivity.

A number of epidemiological studies have examined risk factors for obesity in dogs and cats, and these are summarized below.

Age
Most studies would suggest that the prevalence of obesity in cats rises sharply after 2 years of age and is most prevalent in middle-aged cats. Similarly, middle-aged dogs are at most risk of developing obesity. It is important for practising veterinary surgeons to be aware of such data, since they suggest that prevention strategies, if instigated early (e.g. around 2 years of age) might have the greatest impact on satisfactory management of the condition (see later).

There is evidence in humans that obesity in youth can significantly increase risks of certain diseases in later life, and there is emerging evidence that the same is true in dogs: obesity in dogs less than a year old has been shown to predispose to developmental bone disease, some types of neoplasia and also to reduce lifespan (see earlier). This provides support for active intervention to prevent and address obesity even in the young animal.

Neutering status and gender
Neutering is an important risk factor for obesity in both cats and dogs, and this is currently thought to be due to effects on behaviours which cause calorie mismatch (e.g. increased food intake in combination with decreased physical activity), particularly in animals fed *ad libitum* (Harper *et al.,* 2001; Hoenig and Ferguson, 2002).

Females are over-represented in some canine studies, whereas a recent feline study suggested that male cats might be over-represented.

Breed
Breed is known to be a major risk factor for development of obesity in dogs; a recent report suggested that Cocker Spaniels, Beagles, Labrador Retrievers, Golden Retrievers, Shetland Sheepdogs, Rottweilers and mixed-breed dogs were most at risk (Lund *et al.,* 2006).

In feline obesity, mixed-breed cats appear to be at greater risk than purebred cats. Anecdotal information has suggested that Siamese cats may be predisposed, but this has not been supported by published reports. Breed relationships are likely to reflect complex genetic interactions with the environment, as described for people, which predispose to calorie mismatch.

Environment and activity
Both indoor dwelling and living in an apartment have been shown to predispose to obesity in some, though not all, feline studies. One study identified cats living either alone or in houses with only one other cat to be more at risk than those living in multi-cat households (Robertson, 1999) but the reasons for this association are not known. Finally, one study demonstrated that the presence of dogs in the household significantly reduced the odds of cats developing obesity (Allan *et al.,* 2000), possibly due to the behavioural traits of the cats, dogs or their owners.

Dietary factors
The type of diet fed (prepared petfood *versus* homemade) does not predispose to obesity, but the cost of food may do. In this respect, obese dogs are more likely to have received inexpensive ('grocery store') diets than more expensive foods (Kienzle *et al.,* 1998), whilst some studies suggest feeding premium petfoods may increase the risk of feline obesity (Lund *et al.,* 2005). The latter is most likely due to the potential for a higher fat (and therefore energy) content in premium foods. However, this finding has been contradicted by other studies where no association was found with a particular type of diet (Robertson, 1999). Although there have been many anecdotal suggestions that feeding a high-carbohydrate diet to cats predisposes to obesity and diabetes mellitus, there is currently no evidence to support this assertion. In fact, a recent study has suggested that increased dietary fat, rather than carbohydrate, predisposes to weight gain in cats (Backus *et al.,* 2007).

One study also found that overweight dogs were more likely to have more than two meals per day (Kienzle *et al.,* 1998), although this was contradicted by another study in which an association with once-daily feeding was noted (Robertson, 2003). In addition, canine obesity has been associated with the animal being present when owners prepared or ate their own meal (Kienzle *et al.,* 1998). Further, some (Russell *et al.,* 2000) but not all (Donohue and Scarlett, 1998) studies have shown that obese cats more commonly have free choice of food intake. Finally, studies in both species have shown that the addition of fresh meat and table scraps to the regular food increases the likelihood of obesity (Robertson, 1999, 2003; Allan *et al.,* 2000; Russell *et al.,* 2000).

Owner factors and behaviour
Owner factors also influence the risk of obesity in their pet. Compared with cats in ideal condition, the owners of obese cats have a closer relationship with their pet, over-'humanize' them and rely more on the cat as a substitute for human companionship (Kienzle and Bergler, 2006). Over-humanization was also associated with overweight in a similar canine study, but a close human–dog relationship was not found to be a factor (Kienzle *et al.,* 1998). Owners of overweight cats also spend less time

playing with their pet and reward with food rather than extra play. Owners of both overweight cats and dogs observe their pets more closely during eating, are less interested in preventive health, and are more likely to be overweight themselves. However, unlike the owners of overweight dogs, who tended to have a lower income, there were no demographic differences amongst owners of overweight and normal-weight cats (Kienzle and Bergler, 2006).

Behavioural factors also play a part in the development of obesity, especially in cats. Factors implicated include: anxiety; failure to establish normal feeding behaviour (see below); and failure to develop control of satiety. The human–animal relationship is also of importance, and appears to be more intense in owners of obese cats (Heath, 2005).

Misinterpretation of feline behaviour on the part of the owner is a critical factor in feline obesity, with owners misreading behaviour signals with regard to eating. In the wild, excluding the Big Cats, most cat species (and most importantly, those from which the domestic cat is thought to be descended) are 'trickle feeders', typically consuming many (10–15) small meals each day. Despite this, many owners choose to feed their cats two or three large meals per day. Further, cats do not have an inherent need for social interaction during feeding times. When the cat initiates contact, owners often assume that it is hungry and asking for food when it is not. Nevertheless, if food is provided at such times, the cat soon learns that initiating contact results in a food reward. Offering either large volumes or high energy-dense foods can then predispose to excessive food intake and obesity. Another misconception is that play is only of interest to juvenile cats when, actually, it is necessary throughout life. Dog owners are usually conditioned to provide regular exercise through both walks and play; in contrast, options for increasing activity for cats are largely limited to stimulating play, but most owners do not engage in play sessions with their pets.

Co-existing health problems

A number of conditions may affect energy balance, either by increasing energy intake (e.g. by increasing appetite) or by reducing energy expenditure (e.g. by decreasing physical activity or slowing the basal metabolic rate), or through a combination of these factors. Diseases that can predispose to obesity in these ways include:

- Endocrinopathies, such as hypothyroidism and hyperadrenocorticism, which have effects on both activity and appetite
- Conditions leading to reduced activity levels, such as orthopaedic and cardiorespiratory diseases
- Conditions requiring a medical or surgical intervention which might predispose to weight gain, such as treatment with drugs that increase appetite (e.g. glucocorticoids or anticonvulsants) and therapeutic neutering (see above).

Therapeutic options for weight management

Surgery

Liposuction is a common cosmetic surgery technique in people and is aimed at reducing adipose tissue mass. However, only subcutaneous fat is removed, which contributes little to metabolic risk in humans. Liposuction also does not modify dietary behaviour. It is therefore not an adequate treatment for obesity. A single canine case study reported the use of liposuction for the treatment of a large subcutaneous lipoma (Bottcher et al., 2007) but it is unlikely that this technique would be an ethically justifiable option in companion animals.

Bariatric surgery describes surgery for the management of obesity through the control of food intake. One of the most successful approaches in people is the Roux-en-Y gastric bypass, which both reduces the stomach volume and allows a rapid delivery of the stomach contents to the small intestine. Compulsory restriction of meal size, decreased digestibility and changes in endocrine signals of the gut contribute to the weight loss. A high rate of complications is encountered; problems include gastric outlet obstruction, vomiting, gastric dumping, gastric leaks and wound infections, and dietary deficiencies from malabsorption. Whilst bariatric surgery is the most successful treatment for obesity in people, it is not a viable therapy for companion animals because of ethical concerns, the complexity of surgical procedures, the expense and the risk of complications.

Pharmaceuticals

Recently, two drugs have been authorized in Europe for management of obesity in dogs, **but they are neither authorized nor safe in cats**. The drugs cause a reduction in caloric intake via two mechanisms:

- **Inhibiting the action of membrane transfer proteins.** MTPs link triglyceride molecules to apolipoprotein B (ApoB) to form lipoproteins, which can then cross cell membranes to be transported in the lymph and blood. Inhibiting MTPs in intestinal epithelial cells blocks the assembly of lipoproteins. The effect is lipid malabsorption when the epithelial cells are shed. It is rare to see signs of lipid malabsorption (e.g. steatorrhoea) in treated animals, most likely because the degree of malabsorption is mild and the lipid remains packaged within enterocytes
- **Release of an unknown satiety signal** from the gastrointestinal tract (possibly peptide YY), which has a central effect (at the 'satiety centre') that reduces appetite and therefore voluntary food intake. This action is useful where negative behaviours associated with dietary restriction (e.g. increased begging and scavenging) lead to poor owner compliance.

Dirlotapide (Slentrol; Pfizer) is authorized for use in dogs in both the European Union and North America, and evidence of efficacy has been provided in peer-reviewed publications (Gossellin *et al.*, 2007). The drug is used as sole therapy (e.g. no initial need to change diet or lifestyle) for a continuous period of up to 12 months. Initially a low dose is administered, doubled after 2 weeks. The dose is further increased if the rate of bodyweight loss slows to <0.75% of starting bodyweight per week between rechecks.

Mitratapide (Yarvitan; Janssen) is authorized for use in dogs in the European Union only, and peer-reviewed publications are lacking. Although similar to dirlotapide, it is used in a different way. Rather than long-term continuous treatment, mitratapide is administered for two 3-week periods, interrupted by a 14-day period off the medication when dietary adjustments are made. The manufacturer's data indicate an expected 5–10% reduction in bodyweight when using the drug. To complete weight loss, a conventional diet-oriented programme is then implemented.

WARNINGS
- Neither drug should be used in: pregnant dogs; dogs under 18 months of age; dogs where there may be concern over liver function; dogs that are obese due to a concomitant systemic disease; diabetic animals; or dogs with hyperadrenocorticism.
- These drugs are not authorized or recommended for use in cats, due to risk of hepatic lipidosis.

Although both drugs are generally well tolerated, gastrointestinal side effects can occur, most typically vomiting but also diarrhoea, in up to 20% of patients. These adverse effects are usually infrequent and occur during the first few weeks of administration. If owners are forewarned about the potential for side effects, then these problems may be better accepted. Reversible decreases in serum albumin, globulin, total protein, calcium and alkaline phosphatase, and increases in alanine aminotransferase, aspartate aminotransferase and potassium may occur. In addition, some owners report reduced appetite as a concern, since it changes the interaction they have with their pet; most notably, their dog may be reported to be less affectionate because of the decrease in interaction with the owner through begging.

Alongside drug therapy, it is essential that a complete nutritionally balanced diet is fed to avoid the development of deficiency states. In addition, because MTP inhibitors are less effective when a low-fat diet (5% fat on a dry matter basis) is fed, it is best not to attempt to use them concurrently with a weight loss diet.

Finally, shortly after the drug is discontinued, appetite will return and, unless other strategies (feeding and behavioural) are implemented, a rapid and predictable rebound in bodyweight will occur. Thus, strategies other than drug therapy are essential to insure long-term success.

Diet

When drugs are not being used, it is recommended that a purpose-formulated diet for use during weight loss be used; these products typically have the following characteristics:

- **Reduced energy density**, usually through a reduction in fat content
- **Increased micronutrient (vitamin and mineral) content** relative to energy content. This ensures that malnutrition does not occur when energy intake is restricted
- **Increased protein content** relative to energy content. As with micronutrients, this ensures that protein malnutrition does not occur when energy intake is restricted, and that lean tissue loss is minimized. Increasing protein content may also promote satiety in dogs
- **Supplemented with L-carnitine**. This is a co-factor of lipid oxidation and assists in the transport of long-chain fatty acids into mitochondria. Thus, it facilitates fatty acid oxidation, maximizing the amount of fat (and thus minimizing amount of lean tissue) lost on a weight management programme
- **Fibre supplementation**. Most weight loss diets have an increased dietary fibre content. Higher dietary fibre content increases the bulk of the diet and improves satiety. In addition it allows the owner to feed more volume without adding calories
- **Altered diet characteristics.** Volume of the diet can also be increased by adding extra 'air' in the extrusion process or water in wet products.

Amount to feed

When calculating energy allocation for weight loss, it is essential to base the calculations on the target bodyweight (see later) and not the current weight. The exact allocation will vary depending upon the characteristics of the dog or cat, the chosen diet and other factors (amount of and ability to exercise, etc.). However, the general principles of initiating a diet-based strategy and calculating initial allocation are detailed in Figure 6.3.

The initial allocation is only a starting point; during the weight loss programme, the level of allocation often requires modification, usually by decreasing the amount given (usually by 5–10% at a time) if the animal is not losing weight. Weighing the daily food ration on electronic scales is strongly recommended, since other methods of determining the amount to feed (e.g. measuring cups) are unreliable.

If possible, no additional food should be given by the owners or scavenged by the dog. Healthy treats may be allowed, provided that they are taken into in the overall allocation and provide <5% of total daily requirements. Liquids (e.g. milk) and food used to facilitate oral administration of medications can also be a source of significant caloric intake and should be avoided.

1. Determine the target weight of the animal (see text).

2. Calculate required energy intake. [a]

DOGS:

Calculate maintenance energy requirement (MER) at target bodyweight (TBW)

$$\text{MER (kcal)} = 132 \times \text{TBW (kg)}^{0.73}$$

Decide upon the degree of caloric restriction for the animal, based upon sex and neuter status

e.g. Entire male: 60% of MER
Entire female: 55% of MER
Neutered male: 55% of MER
Neutered female: 50% of MER

CATS:

Estimated starting energy intake (kcal) for weight loss is usually 35–40 x TBW (kg). [b]
If necessary, adjust the degree of restriction based upon individual circumstances:

Consider additional restriction if:
Reduced activity level (e.g. concurrent orthopaedic disease; owner lifestyle allows limited time for initiating play activity)

Consider a lower degree of restriction if:
Very active dog
Owner desires a more gradual weight loss programme (e.g. to minimize the impact of possible begging activity)

3. Take account of owners' wishes to feed 'treats' [c]

4. Calculate the equivalent amount of food for the desired energy intake (in grams for dried food; in sachets or tins for wet food)

5. Decide upon the feeding strategy:

e.g. Number of meals
Use of a feeding toy
Use of a proportion of the food as treats

6. Switch to the new diet gradually, over a few days if necessary.

6.3 General principles of initiating a diet-based weight loss strategy. [a] This energy equation and degree of restriction is appropriate for weight-loss diets from one manufacturer only (i.e. Royal Canin) and is used for illustrative purposes only. Whilst the principles may be similar, different diets may use different equations and restriction factors. It is the responsibility of the clinician to ensure that they are aware of the equations and restriction factors used for the diet they choose. [b] This equation already takes account of a degree of energy restriction and is equivalent to feeding approximately 60% of maintenance requirements at target weight. [c] Although it is preferable to avoid feeding any treats, some owners are resistant to this. Treats will not unbalance an otherwise balanced weight-loss diet, provided the amount given is <5% of daily energy intake. However, the energy intake from this additional food must be taken into account, i.e. by reducing the amount of diet food fed by an appropriate amount.

Lifestyle alterations

Alterations in lifestyle include changes designed to: increase energy expenditure (e.g. increasing physical activity); improve quality of life (e.g. regular play activity in cats); and control caloric intake (e.g. accurate measuring and recording of daily food intake and avoiding uncontrolled feeding of extras).

Dogs

Increasing physical activity is a useful adjunct to weight reduction and, when used in combination with dietary therapy, it prevents loss of lean body mass. Increasing exercise may also help prevent a rapid regain in weight after successful weight reduction. The exact exercise strategy must be tailored to the individual, taking into account any concurrent medical concerns and existing capabilities (e.g. dependent upon breed and age of the patient), as well as the age, health and lifestyle of the owner.

Recommended physical activity will vary depending upon the individual but might include:

- Controlled exercise, e.g. lead walking
- Non-restricted exercise, e.g. activity off-lead
- Swimming and hydrotherapy (see Chapter 10)
- Treadmill exercise.

Cats

Activity can be increased in cats by play sessions using cat toys (e.g. fishing rod toys and motorized units). Cats can also be encouraged to 'work' for their food by using feeding toys.

The benefits of exercise go beyond the fact that it burns calories. It builds muscle mass and increases resting metabolic rate, improves mobility, is beneficial for the cardiovascular system in general, enhances the pet/owner bond by developing a relationship based on play rather than on food, provides mental stimulation, and generally improves welfare and quality of life. It also enhances compliance and improves outcomes for weight loss programmes.

Identifying an effective strategy

Many veterinary surgeons believe that obesity is simply a disease that is caused by bad behaviour on the part of the owner (e.g. over-feeding), and that weight management must therefore be easy, and all that is required is to inform an owner that they should feed less. However, such an opinion is oversimplistic: weight management can be immensely challenging in cats and dogs.

Obesity is typically multifactorial in origin, and success of weight management in any given case requires an understanding of the specific inciting causes for that animal. In addition, since a complex relationship usually exists between owner and pet, a significant amount of time should be devoted to owner education and counselling. Most importantly, feeding behaviour is often intimately involved in the owner–pet bond (e.g. it is often used as a means of expressing affection by owners), and it can often prove difficult to break the habits that may have contributed to weight gain in the first place. Adopting a sympathetic approach (incorporating patience, support and encouragement) is usually more successful than being judgemental or aggressive, since this is likely to be counterproductive and may mean that the owner refuses to take any action at all.

In the opinion of the author, success correlates directly with input from the veterinary practice; so it is strongly recommended that each veterinary practice has an organized strategy towards weight management, which involves all members of the veterinary team from receptionists through to veterinary surgeons. The most successful practices run busy weight management clinics, often supervised by a veterinary nurse but with active input from veterinary surgeons. A detailed discussion of setting up and running weight management clinics is outside the scope of this chapter, but more details can be found in the *BSAVA Manual of Canine and Feline Advanced Veterinary Nursing, 2nd edition.*

Rather than simply reducing bodyweight, the main aims of weight management are:

- To improve quality of life
- To reduce associated disease risk.

This should be stressed to the owner from the outset. It is vital that a healthier relationship develops between the pet and its owner, or the weight reduction programme will fail in the long term.

The recommended rate of weight loss remains a controversial issue in veterinary medicine: excessively rapid weight loss can have deleterious consequences (e.g. hepatic lipidosis in cats (Biourge *et al.*, 1993), excessive lean tissue loss in both dogs and cats (Butterwick and Hawthorne, 1998)), whilst an overly slow rate of weight loss extends the duration of the programme and increases the risk of failure. Recent work in overweight pet dogs and cats suggests that ~1% bodyweight reduction per week is a realistic goal (German *et al.*, 2007, 2008). Nonetheless, the exact rate should be tailored to the exact needs of each individual case, and slower rates of weight reduction are acceptable if tolerated by client, pet and veterinary surgeon.

The traditional approach to obesity management has been based upon dietary caloric energy restriction, coupled with increasing energy expenditure by increased exercise and play activity (see above). However, the recent licensing of drug therapies for weight loss in obese dogs (see earlier) has increased options for management (Figure 6.4).

The use of drug therapies for weight loss in dogs is a recent development, so specific studies to underline recommendations on when to choose diet therapies and when to use drugs are lacking. No clinical trials yet exist directly comparing the two, although similar success and rates of weight loss are reported with both strategies (German *et al.*, 2007; Gossellin *et al.*, 2007). Moreover, whilst logic might suggest that combining dietary and drug therapy would have an additive effect, concurrent use of a weight loss diet may in fact reduce drug efficacy and is not recommended by the drug manufacturers (see earlier). Thus, unless there is an absolute contraindication for using drug therapy, the clinician and client should agree on using *either* diet *or* drugs from the outset, and consider switching strategies if weight management fails. The advantages and disadvantages of using drug therapies for weight loss are detailed in Figure 6.5.

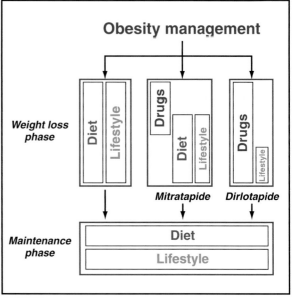

6.4 Broad strategies for weight management in dogs. For the weight loss phase, a conventional approach (left side) involves dietary caloric restriction and changes in lifestyle, including increasing activity via exercise and play sessions. Mitratapide (middle) is designed to 'kick-start' a conventional weight management programme, since it can only be used for the first 8 weeks. In contrast, dirlotapide (right side) can be used continuously for a period of up to 12 months and this may be sufficient for the dog to reach target weight. Only dietary advice and lifestyle changes should be used in the weight maintenance phase.

Advantages of drug therapy
Safe and effective. Side effects are generally mild
No need to change diet or lifestyle at the outset, so may be easier for an owner
Tackles a major reason for failure of conventional weight programmes, namely excessive hunger when caloric restriction is applied
A medical solution for a medical disease
Some clinicians may find therapy easier to implement since no nutritional knowledge is required?
Cost-effective? [a]
Can be used when it is not possible to change the current diet, e.g. diet-responsive skin disease
As an authorized treatment, detailed information exists on safety and efficacy, and many studies have been published in peer-reviewed journals
Weight loss drugs are already licensed for human use and have set a precedent: they typically provide a modest overall benefit to patients (mild weight loss, reduced disease risk)

6.5 Pros and cons of drug therapy for canine weight management. [a] Whether or not the drug is deemed to be cost-effective depends on: price of the drug and weight loss diets set by the practice; size of dog; exact dose requirement; and duration of therapy. In addition, if weight rebound occurs then, by definition, a drug cannot be cost-effective. (continues) ▶

Disadvantages of drug therapy
Side effects are still a concern for some owners
Does not 'cure' the disease: lifestyle changes and dietary management are still required for long-term success
The effect of the drug only lasts whilst drug is given; when the drug is discontinued any effect on satiety is rapidly lost leading to concerns with weight rebound
Some owners, and indeed veterinary surgeons, are uncomfortable with the principle of using a drug for the management of obesity
Knowledge of nutrition is still required for the maintenance phase or rebound will occur
Not cost-effective? a
Diet and lifestyle changes are still required for weight maintenance
Only authorized for use in dogs but NOT cats, and cannot be used where a contraindication exists
Although mechanisms of action differ, and canine drugs are reportedly more effective than human drugs, some owners may be discouraged due to knowledge of concerns with human obesity drugs

6.5 (continued) Pros and cons of drug therapy for canine weight management. a Whether or not the drug is deemed to be cost-effective depends on: price of the drug and weight loss diets set by the practice; size of dog; exact dose requirement; and duration of therapy. In addition, if weight rebound occurs then, by definition, a drug cannot be cost-effective.

Calculating target weight

Calculating target weight is *critical* to success of the weight management programme. The two most appropriate methods are as follows.

- **Using historical patient records**. If the practice policy is to measure and record bodyweight and BCS regularly (e.g. at every visit to the surgery), the animal's own medical records can be used to set target weight. In this instance, the veterinary surgeon should be able to identify a historical bodyweight and BCS from a time when the patient had reached adult bodyweight (e.g. 2 years of age) and was known to be in ideal condition (BCS 5/9). This is the most accurate method for determining optimal weight for that individual.
- **Calculating from current bodyweight and body condition**. In the absence of historical information, an estimate of ideal weight can be made from the current bodyweight and condition, by assuming that each point above ideal BCS on the 9-point BCS scale correlates with ~10% excess bodyweight.

The target weight is only ever a guide, and the final endpoint for weight loss may need to be adjusted depending upon actual response. Further, it may not be appropriate to aim for target weight in some patients, e.g. elderly patients, or patients with an incurable and life-threatening disease such as cancer. In such cases, a modest degree of weight loss may be all that is needed to improve quality of life sufficiently.

The six components of a successful weight management strategy

1. Initial assessment
Upon initial presentation, the patient should be examined thoroughly, with the aim of:

- Quantifying the level of obesity
- Identifying the individual animal's predisposing factors for weight gain (e.g. endocrine disease, drug therapy)
- Determining current health status. *For this the clinician must identify all concurrent diseases, whether they are obesity-associated or unrelated.*

The clinician can thus decide whether or not it is appropriate to instigate a weight management plan. If weight loss is advised, the clinician can also then determine an appropriate target weight and choose the safest and most effective approach for weight loss. Other investigations, such as diagnostic imaging and blood tests, may be indicated on this initial visit: the exact tests performed (if any) will depend upon the individual patient. They are indicated both to identify predisposing factors for obesity (such as endocrine disease) and to identify concurrent diseases that would benefit from weight loss (such as orthopaedic disease).

History
This should include details of environment, lifestyle, and diet and exercise regimes, as well as a complete medical history including previous or current therapy.

Physical – including orthopaedic – examination
Associated diseases causing or contributing to weight gain, or present as incidental findings, can be identified.

Weight measurement and body condition score
A single set of electronic weigh scales should be used at each visit and regularly calibrated for precision and accuracy. For this, an object of known weight should be used, e.g. a bag of dry petfood.

Assessing BCS is the key practice tool for establishing degree of obesity (see above and examples at the end of this chapter).

2. Establishing owner understanding and commitment
Successful treatment of obesity is primarily dependent upon client motivation and compliance with the weight loss programme. In deciding upon how to approach a particular case, the clinician should consider the reason for presentation since the level of client motivation will vary. There are three main scenarios:

- **Presentation for obesity.** Here, client management is likely to be easiest since such owners should already be motivated. However, in practice, this is the least common presentation

- **Presentation for an obesity-associated disease**. The patient presents with a condition potentially related to, or made worse by, obesity, e.g. an orthopaedic disease. This scenario is more common, and it should still be relatively easy to motivate the client, provided the veterinary surgeon can successfully make the link between the medical condition and excess weight
- **Presentation for an unrelated reason**. Obesity is most commonly an incidental observation during a consultation for an unrelated reason, e.g. annual vaccination or routine health check. Initiating discussion in these cases can be problematical because the reaction of the owner is unpredictable. Some may refuse to believe that a problem exists, whilst others may believe that they are being blamed for the problem developing. In addition, some clinicians are reluctant to discuss obesity if the client is also overweight; in these circumstances, it is best to focus on the health of the cat or dog, using sensitive language, and not discuss human obesity directly. If the owner believes that their pet is currently healthy and an obvious co-morbidity does not exist, they may not be convinced by an argument structured around the potential for future health problems. Rather, it may help to focus on the more general detrimental effects of obesity on current quality of life, e.g. fitness, physical activity, grooming. Testimonials from previous clients, highlighting the health benefits of weight loss, may help in convincing these owners.

Some owners may still not be convinced of the need for intervention at the initial consultation, and may require several visits before the argument is accepted. Since owner motivation and compliance are essential prerequisites for successful weight management, there may be little point in embarking upon a weight reduction programme without them.

There is also a real possibility that an owner addressed too 'aggressively' about the problem may fail to return to the practice, preventing further opportunities for persuasion. However, providing information leaflets and then later contacting the owner by phone may help to improve the chances of recruiting them.

3. Setting and managing owner expectations
Once the veterinary surgeon is happy that the owner is fully committed, treatment of obesity can be commenced. There are two phases of the programme:

- **Weight loss** – can take many months
- **Maintenance** – involves lifelong stabilization of bodyweight.

Given that successful weight loss depends on owner commitment, it is vital to ensure that the owner has realistic expectations from the outset. The timescale of treatment, expected rate of weight loss,

estimated cost of therapy, potential side effects, behavioural changes in the pet, time commitment, and any other potential pitfalls should be discussed. The aim should be to ensure that the owner is fully informed and has no unexpected surprises. Problems encountered during weight loss programmes include:

- Difficulty in the pet adapting to the new diet (palatability)
- Difficulty in the pet adapting to a new (reduced) amount of food
- Behavioural problems in the pet related to the first two, with inopportune vocalizing, aggressiveness and/or stealing of food
- Unexpectedly slow rate of weight loss
- Side effects of drug therapy.

4. Intervention
Possible options, described above, include:

- Pharmaceutical intervention (dogs)
- Dietary management (dogs and cats)
- Lifestyle alterations (dogs and cats).

The main aim of all therapies is to reduce adipose tissue mass, either by reducing energy intake or by increasing energy expenditure. Although increasing physical activity provides some benefit, it is rarely successful when used as the sole component of a weight loss programme.

5. Monitoring progress
For any intervention to be successful, close monitoring of bodyweight is vital, particularly during the initial period, since this is when problems are most likely to be encountered. Re-checks at the weight management clinic provide opportunities to verify compliance, deal with any owner concerns (e.g. begging behaviour; Figure 6.6), and provide feedback, encouragement and support to the owner.

- Gradual transition to new weight loss regime (e.g. over 5–7 days)
- Consider using a diet with optimal balance of dietary fibre and protein
- Divide the ration over a number of meals rather than just 1–2 meals per day
- Reserve a portion of the daily diet for use as treats
- Make use of novel feeding strategies that slow intake and stimulate activity, e.g.
  o Puzzle feeders
  o Scatter food or hide food so that the dog or cat must search to find it
  o Use food to stimulate play activity
- Use rewards that are not food-related, e.g. play sessions, walking, grooming, petting

6.6 Some suggestions for tackling increased hunger during weight management.

Initially, rechecks every 2 weeks are recommended, but the interval can be extended if consistent weight loss is achieved. If revisits occur less frequently than every 4 weeks, compliance with the programme might slip. Bodyweight is the principal outcome measure and is used to determine changes to the plan; using the same set of calibrated scales will minimize variability among measurements.

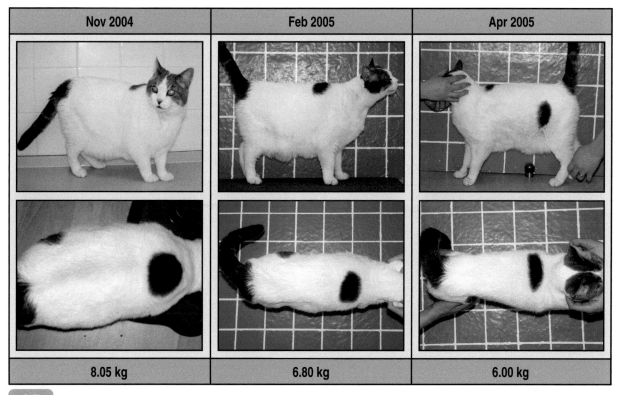

Nov 2004	Feb 2005	Apr 2005
8.05 kg	6.80 kg	6.00 kg

6.7 Periodic photographs can be used to illustrate changes in bodyweight.

BCS can also be monitored, but since more gradual changes are expected it is not essential to record this at every visit. Morphometric measurements (e.g. thoracic and abdominal circumference) can also be used to relay success in terms that the owner will understand. Periodic photographs, preferably taken in a standardized manner, also provide an excellent visual demonstration of success (Figure 6.7).

Between visits, owners should be encouraged to record the pet's food intake in a diary, and this information can also be reviewed. Owner motivation is the key to a successful outcome. Incentives, such as 'slimmer of the month' awards or achievement certificates are motivational tools in human slimming programmes, and are also worth considering for pets. Proactive follow-up with phone calls, for example by a veterinary nurse, is an excellent way of checking on progress, enhancing compliance and addressing any problems as early as possible. The involvement of other members of the veterinary team is a good way to boost success and make owners appreciate the commitment of the whole practice.

6. Maintenance

Although the main medical benefit of weight loss is reduced adiposity, permanently changing to a healthy lifestyle is arguably more beneficial. Thus, success depends on reaching target weight *and* avoiding rebound. Pharmaceuticals can be used for weight reduction in dogs, but not for maintenance, which currently can only be achieved through long-term dietary modification and lifestyle change. A permanent change in the attitude and behaviour of the owner is required to ensure that any weight reduction is maintained in the long term.

Once the target weight is reached, regular rechecks should continue, along with regular support and encouragement. Food intake should be gradually increased to maintenance levels, e.g. by increasing the amount fed by 10% every 2 weeks until weight is stable. Rechecks should continue until the clinician is satisfied that weight is being maintained. Thereafter, the interval between rechecks can gradually be extended but should not be more than 6 months.

For maintenance, any balanced diet can be fed, although low-energy diets (e.g. reduced fat), and those that promote satiety (e.g. high-fibre) may be preferable. Dogs on weight loss drug therapy typically experience a sudden increase in appetite shortly after the medication is stopped, and owners must be forewarned of this. Extensive support should be provided to educate the clients in ways to avoid rebound weight gain. Given that problems associated with excessive appetite (e.g. begging) will not have been evident whilst on the medication, maintenance can be more challenging than if a diet-oriented strategy were used from the outset.

Prevention of obesity

In the author's opinion, the health and welfare of companion animals will be more markedly improved by preventing the development of obesity, rather than by its subsequent treatment. Veterinary surgeons should be proactive in their approach to obesity and should provide adequate client education from the first visit for puppy vaccination throughout life, especially in susceptible breeds. A strategy for obesity prevention is given in Figure 6.8.

The sooner you intervene the better
<ul><li>Prevents a developing problem from becoming serious</li><li>The sooner a cat or dog starts losing weight, the longer it will have to enjoy the benefits</li><li>Minimizes the time spent in the obese state and hence the risk of developing associated diseases</li><li>The problem is less difficult to solve; e.g. intervening at BCS 6/9 and returning to 5/9 is quicker and easier than going from 9/9 to 5/9</li><li>Habits of the obese cat or dog (inactivity, begging behaviour) will be less entrenched</li></ul>
Intervene in early adulthood if possible
<ul><li>Major at-risk populations are 5–10 years of age</li><li>The sooner a cat or dog loses weight, the longer it has to enjoy the benefits</li><li>The animal spends as little time as possible in the obese state</li></ul>
Target neutered animals to prevent weight gain
<ul><li>Monitor proactively with regular weight checks after neutering</li><li>Forewarn owners of risk of weight gain after neutering and the need to reduce caloric intake</li></ul>
Target new pet owners who may not be aware of the concerns over obesity
<ul><li>Such owners will be highly motivated and may be more receptive to advice</li></ul>
Promote awareness of energy balance

6.8 A strategy for obesity prevention.

- **Perform weight and BCS assessments at every visit.** Unwanted increases in bodyweight or BCS can be identified early on and rectified, whilst subtle weight loss (suggestive of occult disease) may also be noted and investigated.
- **Client education.** Advice on healthy eating and physical activity should be included at initial puppy/kitten consultations, and discussion of bodyweight and BCS built in to every subsequent routine check-up.
- **Prevent weight gain after neutering**. Since neutering may predispose to obesity in both dogs and cats, owners must be educated about how to prevent it. It is advisable to schedule two or three weight checks in the first 6–12 months after neutering to identify animals at risk and correct it before it becomes a problem.
- **Prevent weight gain in middle-aged pets.** Cats and dogs aged 5–10 years are most predisposed to obesity and should be closely monitored (e.g. 6-monthly). Proactively targeting young adult cats and dogs ensures that intervention occurs when the benefits to the pet are maximal.
- **Promote a healthy lifestyle for all pets.** This includes awareness of energy balance (Figure 6.9), encompassing accurate recording of food intake, avoiding feeding extra food (treats and table scraps), and promoting regular physical activity through exercise and play sessions. Ideally, all practice staff should be encouraged to promote these concepts, and waiting room literature and other forms of education and support should be available to all owners.

- **Target new pet owners.** People who have only recently acquired their first pet are likely have to limited experience with pet ownership and may also have received bad advice from other sources (e.g. breeders, friends, Internet). Therefore, veterinary practices should ensure that new owners are given the support necessary to prevent obesity developing in their new arrivals. As with other owners, this includes information on responsible pet ownership and the benefits of maintaining a healthy lifestyle.

Regulation of food intake
<ul><li>A feeding guide is only a 'guide': tailor individual intake based upon response (e.g. weight gain or loss)</li><li>Feed a balanced diet appropriate to life stage</li><li>Weigh daily food ration; avoid measuring cups, which can be unreliable</li><li>Minimize feeding of supplemental food (see below)</li><li>Advise caution when switching brands (adapt intake to the diet)</li><li>Maintain a diary of food intake (and activity) in an animal prone to weight gain</li><li>In multi-pet households, feed animals separately or supervise feeding to ensure individual needs are met and excess intake avoided</li></ul>
The need for regular activity
<ul><li>Walks (dogs)</li><li>Play sessions (cats and dogs)</li><li>The use of indoor environmental enrichment (cats)</li><li>Encouraging activity at meal times (cats and dogs): spread kibbles over large area; move food bowl and encourage pet to follow; use a food puzzle; use kibbles to stimulate a play session</li></ul>
Adapt food intake to energy expenditure
<ul><li>Feed more on more active days, e.g. weekend, holidays</li><li>Reduce food intake for inactive periods, e.g. weekdays for working owners, times of bad weather</li><li>Adapt food intake to periods of illness, e.g. lameness may reduce activity</li><li>Reduce food intake when the pet is kennelled</li></ul>
Responsible 'rewarding' of pets
<ul><li>Educate all owners and friends</li><li>Only use healthy (ideally low-fat) treats, e.g. kibble food or dental treats</li><li>If necessary, put aside a portion of the daily ration for treats</li><li>Take account of the treats in daily energy calculation</li><li>Minimize the size of the treat (it is the act of giving which is important, not the amount)</li><li>Consider other methods of reward, e.g. play session, walk, attention</li></ul>
Weigh and condition score the cat or dog regularly to ensure that energy balance is maintained

6.9 Awareness of energy balance.

References and further reading

Allan F, Pfeiffer DU, Jones BR, Esslemont DHB and Wiseman MS (2000) A cross-sectional study of risk factors for obesity in cats in New Zealand. *Preventive Veterinary Medicine* **46**, 183–196

Bach JF, Rozanski EA, Bedenice D *et al.* (2007) Association of expiratory airway dysfunction with marked obesity in healthy adult dogs. *American Journal of Veterinary Research* **68**, 670–675

Backus RC, Cave NJ and Keisler DH (2007) Gonadectomy and high dietary fat but not high dietary carbohydrate induce gains in body weight and fat of domestic cats. *British Journal of Nutrition* **98**, 641–650

Biourge V, Pion P, Lewis J, Morris JG and Rogers QR (1993) Spontaneous occurrence of hepatic lipidosis in a group of laboratory cats. *Journal of Veterinary Internal Medicine* **7**, 194–197

Bodey AR and Mitchell AR (1996) Epidemiological study of blood pressure in domestic dogs. *Journal of Small Animal Practice* **37**, 116–125

Bottcher P, Kluter S, Krastel D and Grevel V (2007) Liposuction – removal of giant lipomas for weight loss in a dog with severe hip osteoarthritis. *Journal of Small Animal Practice* **48**, 46–48

Brown DC, Conzemius MG and Shofer FS (1996) Body weight as a predisposing factor for humeral condylar fractures, cranial cruciate rupture and intervertebral disc disease in Cocker Spaniels. *Veterinary Comparative Orthopedics* **9**, 75–78

Butterwick RF and Hawthorne AJ (1998) Advances in dietary management of obesity in dogs and cats. *Journal of Nutrition* **128**, 2771S–2775S

Clarke SP and Bennett D (2006) Feline osteoarthritis: a prospective study of 28 cases. *Journal of Small Animal Practice* **47**, 439–445

Cope PJ (2008) *Prevalence of Canine Obesity in England and Wales, and its Associations with Diabetes Mellitus and Osteoarthritis.* MPhil thesis, University of Cambridge

Davison LJ, Herrtage ME and Catchpole B (2005) Study of 253 dogs in the United Kingdom with diabetes mellitus. *Veterinary Record* **156**, 467–471

Donoghue S and Scarlett JM (1998) Diet and feline obesity. *Journal of Nutrition* **128**, 2776S–2778S

Eisele I, Wood IS, German AJ et al. (2005) Adipokine gene expression in dog adipose tissues and dog white adipocytes differentiated in primary culture. *Hormone and Metabolic Research* **37**, 1–8

Fall T, Hamlin HH, Hedhammar Å, Kampe O and Egenvall A (2007) Diabetes mellitus in a population of 180,000 insured dogs: incidence, survival, and breed distribution. *Journal of Veterinary Internal Medicine* **21**, 1209–1216

Gayet C, Bailhache E, Dumon H et al. (2004) Insulin resistance and changes in plasma concentration of TNFα, IGF1, and NEFA in dogs during weight gain and obesity. *Journal of Animal Physiology and Animal Nutrition (Berlin)* **88**,157–165

German AJ (2006) The growing problem of obesity in dogs and cats. *Journal of Nutrition* **136**, 1940S–1946S

German AJ, Holden SL, Bissot T et al. (2007) Dietary energy restriction and successful weight loss in obese client-owned dogs. *Journal of Veterinary Internal Medicine* **21**, 1174–1180

German AJ, Holden SL, Bissot T et al. (2008) Changes in body composition during weight loss in obese client-owned cats: loss of lean tissue mass correlates with overall percentage of weight lost. *Journal of Feline Medicine and Surgery* **10**, 452–459

German AJ, Holden SL, Morris PJ et al. (2010) Inaccuracies when using bioimpedance for non-invasive estimation of body fat mass in dogs. *American Journal of Veterinary Research* **71**, 393–398

German AJ, Holden SL, Moxham GL et al. (2006) A simple reliable tool for owners to assess the body condition of their dog or cat. *Journal of Nutrition* **136**, 2031S–2033S

Glickman LT, Schofer FS, McKee LJ, Reif JS and Goldschmidt MH (1989) Epidemiologic study of insecticide exposures, obesity, risk of bladder cancer in household dogs. *Journal of Toxicology and Environmental Health* **28**, 407–414

Gosselin J, McKelvie J, Sherington J et al. (2007) An evaluation of dirlotapide to reduce body weight of client-owned dogs in two placebo-controlled clinical studies in Europe. *Journal of Veterinary Pharmacology and Therapeutics* **30**, 73–80

Harper EJ, Stack DM, Watson TD and Moxham G (2001) Effects of feeding regimens on bodyweight, composition and condition score in cats following ovariohysterectomy. *Journal of Small Animal Practice* **42**, 433–438

Heath S (2005) Behaviour problems and welfare. In: *The Welfare of Cats*, ed. I Rochlitz, pp.91–118. Springer, London

Henegar JR, Bigler SA, Henegar LK, Tyag S and Hall JE (2001) Functional and structural changes in the kidney in the early stages of obesity. *Journal of the American Society of Nephrology* **12**, 1211–1217

Hess RS, Kass PH, Shofer FS, Van Winkle TJ and Washabau RJ (1999) Evaluation of risk factors for fatal acute pancreatitis in dogs. *Journal of the American Veterinary Medical Association* **214**, 46–51

Hoenig M and Ferguson DC (2002) Effects of neutering on hormonal concentrations and energy requirements in male and female cats.

American Journal of Veterinary Research **63**, 634–639

Impellizeri JA, Tetrick MA and Muir P (2000) Effect of weight reduction on clinical signs of lameness in dogs with hip osteoarthritis. *Journal of the American Veterinary Medical Association* **216**, 1089–1091

Kealy RD, Lawler DF, Ballam JM (2000) Evaluation of the effect of limited food consumption on radiographic evidence of osteoarthritis in dogs. *Journal of the American Veterinary Medical Association* **217**, 1678–1680

Kealy RD, Lawler DF, Ballam JM et al. (2002) Effects of diet restriction on life span and age-related changes in dogs. *Journal of the American Veterinary Medical Association* **220**, 1315–1320

Kealy RD, Olsson SE, Monti KL et al. (1992) Effects of limited food consumption on the incidence of hip dysplasia in growing dogs. *Journal of the American Veterinary Medical Association* **201**, 857–863

Kienzle E and Bergler R (2006) Human-animal relationship of owners of normal and overweight cats. *Journal of Nutrition* **136**, 1947S–1950S

Kienzle E, Bergler R and Mandernach A (1998) Comparison of the feeding behaviour of the man-animal relationship in owners of normal and obese dogs. *Journal of Nutrition* **128**, 2779S–2782S

Larson BT, Lawler DF, Spitznagel EL and Kealy RD (2003) Improved glucose tolerance with lifetime restriction favorably affects disease and survival in dogs. *Journal of Nutrition* **133**, 2887–2892

Lekcharoensuk C, Lulich JP, Osborne CA et al. (2000) Patient and environmental factors associated with calcium oxalate urolithiasis in dogs. *Journal of the American Veterinary Medical Association* **217**, 515–519

Lund EM, Armstrong PJ, Kirk CA et al. (2005) Prevalence and risk factors for obesity in adult cats from private US veterinary practices. *International Journal of Applied Research in Veterinary Medicine* **3**, 88–96

Lund EM, Armstrong PJ, Kirk CA et al. (2006) Prevalence and risk factors for obesity in adult dogs from private US veterinary practices. *International Journal of Applied Research in Veterinary Medicine* **4**, 177–186

McLeod HL (2008) Nursing clinics. In: *BSAVA Manual of Canine and Feline Advanced Veterinary Nursing*, ed. A Hotston Moore and S Rudd, pp.302–312. BSAVA Publications, Gloucester

Perez Alenza MD, Pena L, del Castillo N and Nieto AI (2000a) Factors influencing the incidence and prognosis of canine mammary tumours. *Journal of Small Animal Practice* **41**, 287–291

Perez Alenza MD, Rutteman GR, Pena L, Beynen AC and Cuesta P (2000b) Relation between habitual diet and canine mammary tumors in a case-control study. *Journal of Veterinary Internal Medicine* **12**, 132–139

Robertson ID (1999) The influence of diet and other factors on owner-perceived obesity in privately owned cats from metropolitan Perth, Western Australia. *Preventive Veterinary Medicine* **40**, 75–85

Robertson ID (2003) The influence of diet and other factors on owner-perceived obesity in privately owned cats from metropolitan Perth, Western Australia. *Preventive Veterinary Medicine* **40**, 75–85

Russell K, Sabin R, Holt S, Bradley R and Harper EJ (2000) Influence of feeding regimen on body condition in the cat. *Journal of Small Animal Practice* **41**, 12–17

Ryan VH, German AJ, Wood IS et al. (2008) NGF gene expression and secretion by canine adipocytes in primary culture: upregulation by the inflammatory mediators LPS and TNFα. *Hormone and Metabolic Research* **40**, 861–868

Scarlett JM and Donoghue S (1998) Associations between body condition and disease in cats. *Journal of the American Veterinary Medical Association* **212**, 1725–1731

Slupe JL, Freeman LM and Rush JE (2008) Association of body weight and body condition with survival in dogs with heart failure. *Journal of Veterinary Internal Medicine* **22**, 561–565

Sonnenschein EG, Glickman LT, Goldschmidt MH and McKee LJ (1991) Body conformation, diet, and risk of breast cancer in pet dogs: a case-control study. *American Journal of Epidemiology* **133**, 694–703

Watson PJ, Roulois A, Scase T et al. (2007) Prevalence and breed distribution of chronic pancreatitis at post mortem in first opinion dogs. *Journal of Small Animal Practice* **48**, 609–618

▶ Examples of body condition scoring schemes

Nestlé PURINA
BODY CONDITION SYSTEM

TOO THIN

1 Ribs, lumbar vertebrae, pelvic bones and all bony prominences evident from a distance. No discernible body fat. Obvious loss of muscle mass.

2 Ribs, lumbar vertebrae and pelvic bones easily visible. No palpable fat. Some evidence of other bony prominence. Minimal loss of muscle mass.

3 Ribs easily palpated and may be visible with no palpable fat. Tops of lumbar vertebrae visible. Pelvic bones becoming prominent. Obvious waist and abdominal tuck.

IDEAL

4 Ribs easily palpable, with minimal fat covering. Waist easily noted, viewed from above. Abdominal tuck evident.

5 Ribs palpable without excess fat covering. Waist observed behind ribs when viewed from above. Abdomen tucked up when viewed from side.

TOO HEAVY

6 Ribs palpable with slight excess fat covering. Waist is discernible viewed from above but is not prominent. Abdominal tuck apparent.

7 Ribs palpable with difficulty; heavy fat cover. Noticeable fat deposits over lumbar area and base of tail. Waist absent or barely visible. Abdominal tuck may be present.

8 Ribs not palpable under very heavy fat cover, or palpable only with significant pressure. Heavy fat deposits over lumbar area and base of tail. Waist absent. No abdominal tuck. Obvious abdominal distention may be present.

9 Massive fat deposits over thorax, spine and base of tail. Waist and abdominal tuck absent. Fat deposits on neck and limbs. Obvious abdominal distention.

The **BODY CONDITION SYSTEM** was developed at the Nestlé Purina Pet Care Center and has been validated as documented in the following publications:

Mawby D, Bartges JW, Moyers T, et. al. *Comparison of body fat estimates by dual-energy x-ray absorptiometry and deuterium oxide dilution in client owned dogs.* Compendium 2001; 23 (9A): 70

Laflamme DP. *Development and Validation of a Body Condition Score System for Dogs.* Canine Practice July/August 1997; 22:10-15

Kealy, et. al. *Effects of Diet Restriction on Life Span and Age-Related Changes in Dogs.* JAVMA 2002; 220:1315-1320

Nestlé PURINA

9-point body condition scale for dogs. (© Nestlé Purina PetCare and reproduced with their permission)

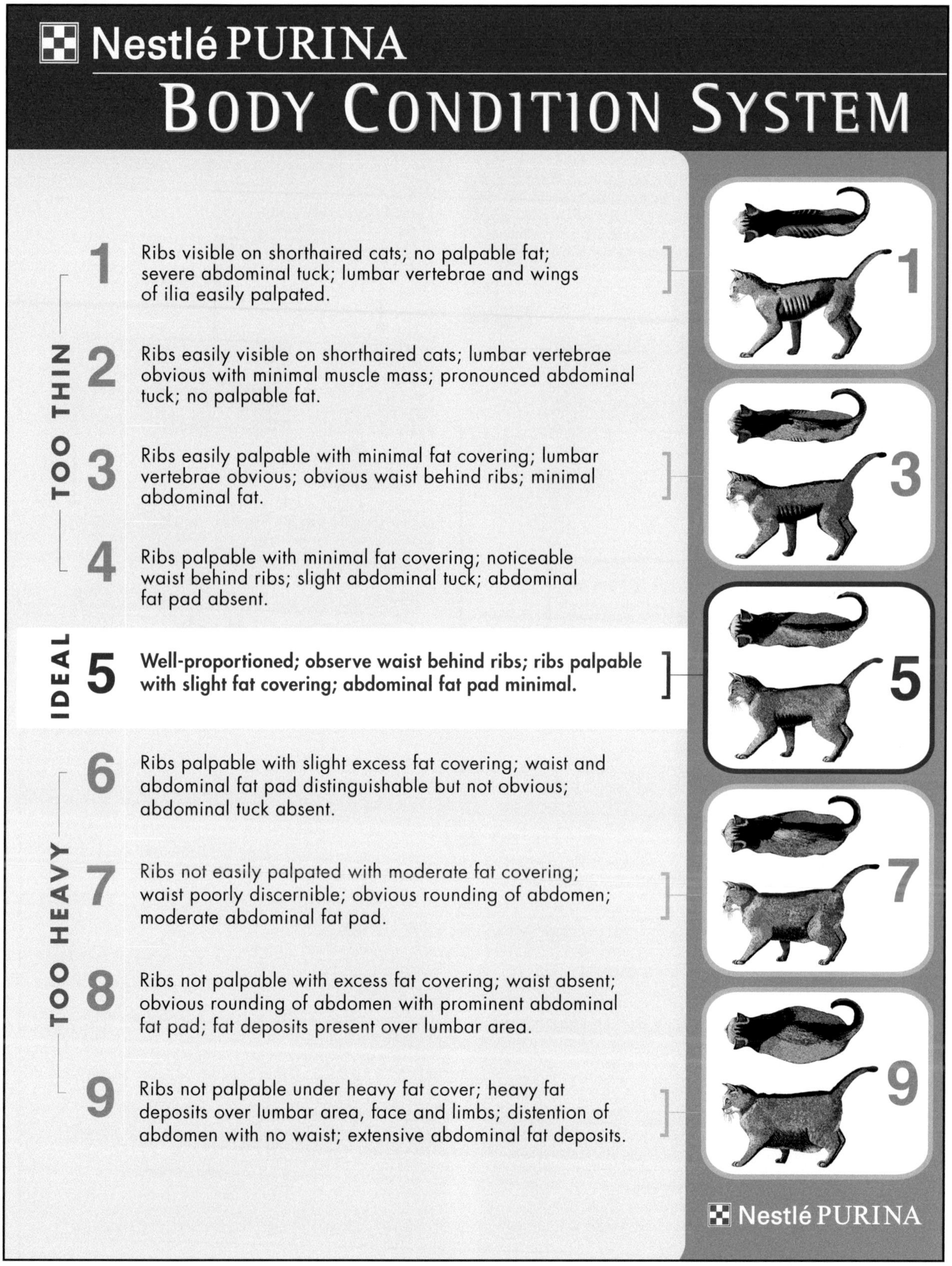

☒ Nestlé PURINA

BODY CONDITION SYSTEM

1 Ribs visible on shorthaired cats; no palpable fat; severe abdominal tuck; lumbar vertebrae and wings of ilia easily palpated.

TOO THIN

2 Ribs easily visible on shorthaired cats; lumbar vertebrae obvious with minimal muscle mass; pronounced abdominal tuck; no palpable fat.

3 Ribs easily palpable with minimal fat covering; lumbar vertebrae obvious; obvious waist behind ribs; minimal abdominal fat.

4 Ribs palpable with minimal fat covering; noticeable waist behind ribs; slight abdominal tuck; abdominal fat pad absent.

IDEAL

5 Well-proportioned; observe waist behind ribs; ribs palpable with slight fat covering; abdominal fat pad minimal.

TOO HEAVY

6 Ribs palpable with slight excess fat covering; waist and abdominal fat pad distinguishable but not obvious; abdominal tuck absent.

7 Ribs not easily palpated with moderate fat covering; waist poorly discernible; obvious rounding of abdomen; moderate abdominal fat pad.

8 Ribs not palpable with excess fat covering; waist absent; obvious rounding of abdomen with prominent abdominal fat pad; fat deposits present over lumbar area.

9 Ribs not palpable under heavy fat cover; heavy fat deposits over lumbar area, face and limbs; distention of abdomen with no waist; extensive abdominal fat deposits.

☒ Nestlé PURINA

9-point body condition scale for cats. (© Nestlé Purina PetCare and reproduced with their permission)

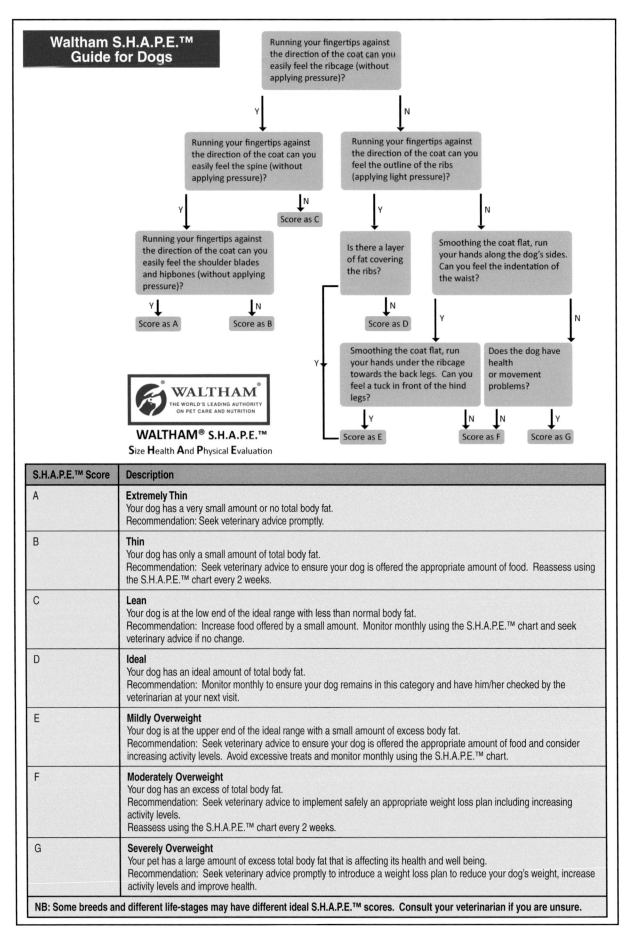

S.H.A.P.E.™ Score	Description
A	**Extremely Thin** Your dog has a very small amount or no total body fat. Recommendation: Seek veterinary advice promptly.
B	**Thin** Your dog has only a small amount of total body fat. Recommendation: Seek veterinary advice to ensure your dog is offered the appropriate amount of food. Reassess using the S.H.A.P.E.™ chart every 2 weeks.
C	**Lean** Your dog is at the low end of the ideal range with less than normal body fat. Recommendation: Increase food offered by a small amount. Monitor monthly using the S.H.A.P.E.™ chart and seek veterinary advice if no change.
D	**Ideal** Your dog has an ideal amount of total body fat. Recommendation: Monitor monthly to ensure your dog remains in this category and have him/her checked by the veterinarian at your next visit.
E	**Mildly Overweight** Your dog is at the upper end of the ideal range with a small amount of excess body fat. Recommendation: Seek veterinary advice to ensure your dog is offered the appropriate amount of food and consider increasing activity levels. Avoid excessive treats and monitor monthly using the S.H.A.P.E.™ chart.
F	**Moderately Overweight** Your dog has an excess of total body fat. Recommendation: Seek veterinary advice to implement safely an appropriate weight loss plan including increasing activity levels. Reassess using the S.H.A.P.E.™ chart every 2 weeks.
G	**Severely Overweight** Your pet has a large amount of excess total body fat that is affecting its health and well being. Recommendation: Seek veterinary advice promptly to introduce a weight loss plan to reduce your dog's weight, increase activity levels and improve health.
NB: Some breeds and different life-stages may have different ideal S.H.A.P.E.™ scores. Consult your veterinarian if you are unsure.	

A recently developed algorithm-based body condition scoring scheme for dogs. (Reproduced by permission of **WALTHAM™** Centre for Pet Nutrition; © 2005 Mars, Inc.)

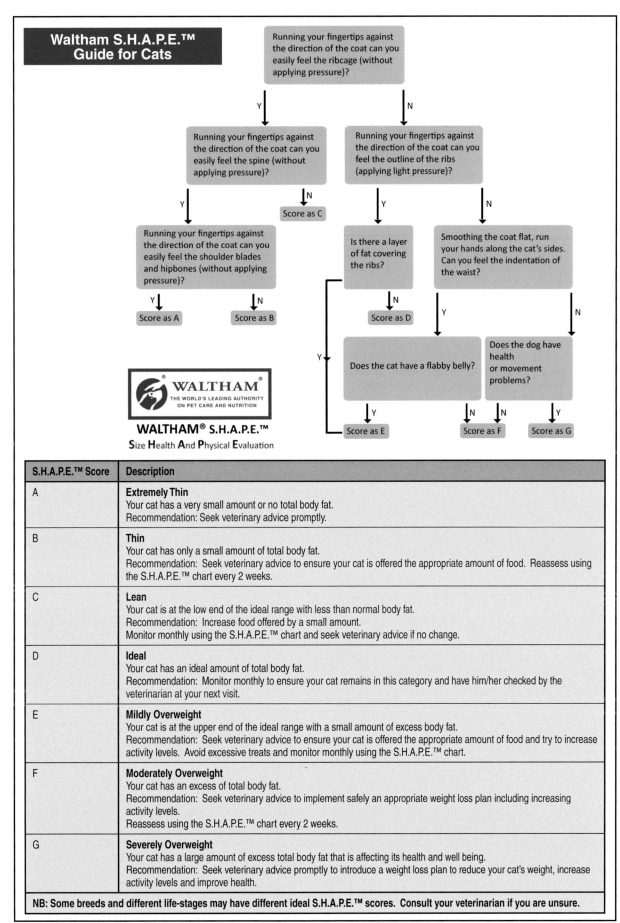

S.H.A.P.E.™ Score	Description
A	**Extremely Thin** Your cat has a very small amount or no total body fat. Recommendation: Seek veterinary advice promptly.
B	**Thin** Your cat has only a small amount of total body fat. Recommendation: Seek veterinary advice to ensure your cat is offered the appropriate amount of food. Reassess using the S.H.A.P.E.™ chart every 2 weeks.
C	**Lean** Your cat is at the low end of the ideal range with less than normal body fat. Recommendation: Increase food offered by a small amount. Monitor monthly using the S.H.A.P.E.™ chart and seek veterinary advice if no change.
D	**Ideal** Your cat has an ideal amount of total body fat. Recommendation: Monitor monthly to ensure your cat remains in this category and have him/her checked by the veterinarian at your next visit.
E	**Mildly Overweight** Your cat is at the upper end of the ideal range with a small amount of excess body fat. Recommendation: Seek veterinary advice to ensure your cat is offered the appropriate amount of food and try to increase activity levels. Avoid excessive treats and monitor monthly using the S.H.A.P.E.™ chart.
F	**Moderately Overweight** Your cat has an excess of total body fat. Recommendation: Seek veterinary advice to implement safely an appropriate weight loss plan including increasing activity levels. Reassess using the S.H.A.P.E.™ chart every 2 weeks.
G	**Severely Overweight** Your cat has a large amount of excess total body fat that is affecting its health and well being. Recommendation: Seek veterinary advice promptly to introduce a weight loss plan to reduce your cat's weight, increase activity levels and improve health.

NB: Some breeds and different life-stages may have different ideal S.H.A.P.E.™ scores. Consult your veterinarian if you are unsure.

A recently developed algorithm-based body condition scoring scheme for cats. (Reproduced by permission of **WALTHAM™** Centre for Pet Nutrition; © 2005 Mars, Inc.)

7

Immune-modulating dietary components and nutraceuticals

Daniel L. Chan

Introduction

Until recently, nutritional strategies have largely focused on altering the composition of foods in order to alleviate stresses on certain organ systems (e.g. protein restriction to reduce the amount of urea that has to be excreted by the kidneys in renal disease; see Chapter 5). However, arguably the most exciting development in clinical nutrition has been the appreciation that certain nutrients have pharmacological effects and can directly modulate pathophysiological processes and thus affect the outcome of some diseases.

In human patients, critical care nutrition is a particular focus of intensive research, because there is mounting evidence that certain nutrients, such as glutamine, omega-3 fatty acids and antioxidants, can have a positive impact on both morbidity and mortality in severely affected populations. A greater understanding of how these nutrients impart such beneficial effects should lead to developments of novel strategies for modulating disease not only in people, but also in small animals.

The term 'nutraceutical' was originally coined to refer to 'any substance that is not a drug and that can be orally administered to promote good health.' Although there is no strict legal definition for 'nutraceuticals', more technical definitions have been devised, such as:

A nutraceutical is a non-drug substance, that is produced in a purified or extracted form and administered orally, to provide agents required for normal body structure and function, with the intent of improving the health and wellbeing of animals.

More recently, certain agents that might be considered as 'nutraceuticals' have also been used more specifically for their modulatory effects on the immune and inflammatory response, and these are referred to as 'immune-enhancing diets'. Interestingly, some of these agents have also been administered parenterally (e.g. glutamine, omega-3 fatty acids, vitamin C) and therefore no longer fulfil the criteria for nutraceuticals. Furthermore, as research continues to uncover the cellular mechanisms by which these agents work, it is becoming increasingly difficult to classify some of these agents as 'non-drug'. Nevertheless, an understanding of how these agents interact with various responses (e.g. inflammatory, immune) can be helpful in deciding whether these agents should be used therapeutically.

Immune-enhancing diets

Formulating diets to modulate the host immune response has led to the concept of 'immune-enhancing diets' (IEDs), and this is a major focus of current nutritional interventions in critically ill human patients. IEDs contain nutrients known to play important roles in ensuring that the host is able to deal with pathophysiological processes such as inflammation and oxidative stress. Such nutrients include glutamine, arginine, omega-3 fatty acids and antioxidants. These supplements are usually supplied as powders that can be easily dissolved in the patient's drink or enteral formula, and are therefore very convenient for clinical practice.

Omega-3 fatty acids

Because inflammation plays a crucial role in many diseases, manipulation of the inflammatory cascade through changing the composition of inflammatory precursors has become an important target of therapy. Omega-3 fatty acids may be supplemented in an attempt to reduce the inflammatory response.

Omega-3 fatty acids are polyunsaturated fatty acids, where the first double bond is on the third carbon from the omega end (carbon with methyl group) of the molecule, whereas omega-6 fatty acids have the first double bond on the sixth carbon from the omega end (Figure 7.1). Both these groups of fatty acids are incorporated into cell membranes.

Omega-6 fatty acids are metabolized to arachidonic acid, which is further metabolized to potent proinflammatory eicosanoids, leucotrienes, and thromboxanes of the 2 and 4 series. Omega-3 fatty acids are metabolized to eicosapentaenoic acid and docosahexaenoic acid, which are then used to produce less inflammatory eicosanoids of the 3 and 5 series (Figure 7.2). Provision of omega-3 fatty acids in the diet, or as supplements, is aimed at displacing and substituting omega-6 fatty acids in membranes, and thereby reducing the potential and magnitude of the inflammatory response.

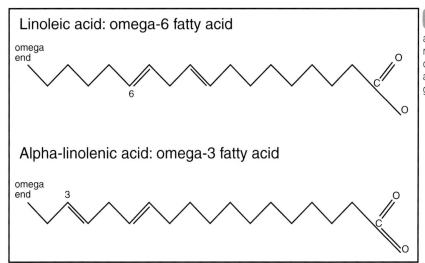

Chemical structures of linoleic and alpha-linolenic acid. The designation omega-6 relates to the presence of the first double bond on the sixth carbon away from the omega end (methyl group) of the molecule.

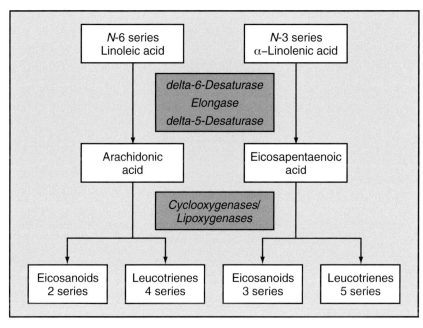

7.2 Metabolic pathways of conversion of polyunsaturated fatty acids (omega-6 and omega-3) into prostaglandins and leucotrienes.

Antioxidants

Oxidative stress is recognized to be a prominent and common feature of many disease processes, including neoplasia, heart disease, trauma, burns, severe pancreatitis, sepsis and critical illness. During various pathophysiological states, particularly those typified by an inflammatory response, cells of the immune system (e.g. neutrophils, macrophages, eosinophils) substantially contribute to the production of reactive oxygen species (ROS). With the depletion of normal antioxidant defences, the host is more vulnerable to free radicals and prone to cellular and subcellular damage (e.g. DNA and mitochondrial damage). Replenishment of antioxidant defences attempts to lessen the intensity of the injury caused by oxygen free radicals.

Antioxidants within the body can be classified into three different systems:

- Antioxidant proteins, such as albumin, haptoglobin and coeruloplasmin
- Enzymatic antioxidants, such as superoxide dismutase, glutathione peroxidase and catalase
- Non-enzymatic or small molecule antioxidants, such as ascorbate (vitamin C), alpha-tocopherol (vitamin E), glutathione, selenium, lycopene and beta-carotene.

N-Acetylcysteine is an effective precursor of glutathione and has been associated with positive results in human patients, including reduced hospitalization time, reduced risk of new organ failure and improved survival in several patient populations. Treatment with N-acetylcysteine not only scavenges ROS but also enables continual production of glutathione and even blocks transcription of inflammatory cytokines. In cats, N-acetylcysteine can be an effective treatment in paracetamol toxicity (Webb *et al.,* 2003; Hill *et al.,* 2005).

Other antioxidants that have been demonstrated to have positive effects on outcome in human patients and in experimental animals include vitamins C and E, lycopene, beta-carotene, allopurinol and S-adenosylmethionine.

There are also instances where antioxidant supplementation appeared to be harmful to people. In a controversial study, long-term high-dosage (>400 IU/day) vitamin E supplementation was linked to possible increases in all-cause mortality (Miller *et al.*, 2005). Confirming previous data, a large study also suggested that long-term supplementation of beta-carotene, retinol, lycopene and luteine may possibly increase risk of lung cancer in smokers (Satia *et al.*, 2009). Even *N*-acetylcysteine has been demonstrated to have deleterious effects in some populations, where it was found that supplementation was associated with increased blood loss and increased blood product utilization during cardiac surgery (Wijeysundera *et al.*, 2009).

Amino acids

Amino acids fulfil a vast array of functions in the body. They primarily serve as building blocks for protein synthesis and participate in chemical reactions. Certain amino acids also serve as an energy source for certain cells, perhaps the most pertinent example being glutamine, which is the preferred fuel source for small intestinal enterocytes and cells of the immune system. During disease states, the body undergoes marked alterations in substrate metabolism that could lead to a deficiency in amino acids. In the response to stress, there may be a dramatic increase in demand by the body for particular amino acids, such as arginine and glutamine. These amino acids are adequately synthesized by the body when it is healthy. However, during periods following severe trauma, infection or inflammation, the demand for these amino acids cannot be met; they become 'conditionally essential' and must be obtained from the diet. In response to acute inflammation, rapidly dividing cells of the gastrointestinal and immune systems consume large amounts of glutamine, whereas activation of nitric oxide synthase leads to depletion of arginine for the synthesis of nitric oxide. Given the importance of these amino acids, the sudden depletion in these important substrates in disease states led to the hypothesis that dietary supplementation of these amino acids during disease would improve clinical outcomes.

An exciting development has been the demonstration that supplementation of amino acids such as glutamine yielded positive results beyond restoration of normal levels. Indeed, it has been recognized that glutamine must possess pharmacological attributes because positive responses have been demonstrated to be dose-dependent and to occur in the absence of deficiency in both humans and experimental animal models. Glutamine supplementation decreased rates of postoperative infection, decreased intensive care unit hospitalization, improved gastrointestinal function and integrity, and even improved survival (O'Dwyer *et al.*, 1989; Gianotti *et al.*, 1995; Wischmeyer *et al.*, 2001). It also appears that these effects are improved when higher dosages are used, and when glutamine is administered parenterally (Bongers *et al.*, 2007; Wischmeyer, 2008).

These findings have generated interest in exploiting the potential for using nutrients to modulate disease. An obvious target for this approach are those serious diseases where nutritional intake is poor and dysregulation of the immune response is present. Enterocytes gain a large amount of their energy requirements from the products of intraluminal digestion rather than from the bloodstream. With decreased enteral nutrition in disease, enterocytes are deprived of the luminal nutrients they require. This leads to gut atrophy and disruption of the gastrointestinal barrier, which in turn leads to the possibility of bacterial translocation or gut-derived sepsis. As the gastrointestinal tract is the largest immune organ in the body, dysregulation of the immune response further compromises the patient and can lead to multiple organ dysfunction. Given the relation between critical illness and gut atrophy, supplementation with the gastrointestinal tract's preferred energy source, glutamine, is an attempt at restoring the integrity and function of this vital organ system.

Despite the important role of glutamine in health and disease, trials evaluating the therapeutic use of glutamine have yielded mixed results in both humans and animals. A possible reason for conflicting results may relate to the form of glutamine used in the various trials. The most consistent positive effects have been associated with glutamine administered parenterally to critically ill surgical patients. Although there are beneficial effects associated with enteral glutamine supplementation, the only cells that appear to benefit from enteral glutamine are surface enterocytes, which have a tremendous capacity to absorb glutamine, but have very short lifespans and are soon sloughed, taking away the absorbed glutamine (Wischmeyer, 2008). When glutamine is administered *parenterally*, usually supplied as a dipeptide, there is greater uptake by the deeper layers of the intestine (i.e. crypts of the villi); as these cells mature and make their way to become surface enterocytes, they are more resistant to stresses such as oxidative stress and can survive longer, thereby preserving gastrointestinal barrier function (Wischmeyer, 2008).

Veterinary data

To date, there is a paucity of information evaluating the role of nutrients used specifically to modulate disease in small animals. Whilst correction of particular deficiencies can have positive effects (e.g. correcting taurine deficiency in cats can prevent and reverse dilated cardiomyopathy), the use of IEDs in animals has not been well documented.

Omega-3 fatty acids

The use of omega-3 fatty acid supplementation has been evaluated in dogs with chronic inflammatory diseases, such as atopy (Bond and Lloyd, 1992; Scarff and Lloyd, 1992), but this approach has not been evaluated in dogs with acute and serious diseases, such as acute kidney failure, acute lung injury and sepsis.

A recent trial did demonstrate a marked improvement of arrhythmias in asymptomatic Boxers with arrhythmogenic right ventricular cardiomyopathy when the dogs were supplemented with omega-3 fatty acids (Smith *et al.*, 2007).

Antioxidants

Despite the clear importance of oxidative stress in various diseases in companion animals, investigations evaluating the effect of antioxidants on disease processes in these species are limited. Positive results have been demonstrated in experimental and natural models of oxidative stress in both cats and dogs, including congestive heart failure (Amado et al., 2005), acute pancreatitis (Marks et al., 1998), gastric dilatation–volvulus (Badylak et al., 1990), renal transplantation (Lee et al., 2006), gentamicin-induced nephrotoxicity (Varzi et al., 2007), and paracetamol toxicity (Webb et al., 2003; Hill et al., 2005). Recent studies evaluating antioxidants in naturally occurring disease, such as chronic valvular disease (Freeman et al., 2006) and renal insufficiency (Plevraki et al., 2006; Yu and Paetau-Robinson, 2006), have also been positive and support the need for further evaluation. In many of these studies, positive effects included improvement in measures of antioxidant capacity, reduction of inflammatory markers, improvement of organ transplant viability and even improvements in survival (Badylak et al., 1990; Marks et al., 1998; Lee et al., 2006; Plevraki et al., 2006).

However, not all studies demonstrate positive results. In a recent study, administration of N-acetyl-cysteine before performing hemilaminectomies in dogs offered no beneficial effects on neurological recovery nor a reduction in markers of oxidative stress (urinary 15-F2t-isoprostane concentrations) (Baltzer et al., 2008). Studies evaluating antioxidant therapy in cats have also yielded mixed results. Supplementation of vitamin E alone did not prevent oxidative injury (development of Heinz body anaemia) in cats fed onion powder or propylene glycol, but the same group of investigators later showed that supplementation of vitamin E with cysteine in cats decreased the production of methaemoglobinaemia following paracetamol challenge (Hill et al., 2005).

Glutamine

Currently, there are only two published trials that have evaluated the use of glutamine in dogs and cats. In a trial of cats treated with methotrexate, enteral glutamine offered no intestinal protection in terms of reducing intestinal permeability (Marks et al., 1999). Another trial evaluating the effects of enteral glutamine on plasma glutamine and prostaglandin E_2 concentrations in radiation-induced mucositis in dogs showed no measurable benefit (Lana et al., 2003). Possible reasons for the apparent failures in both of these trials could be: glutamine does not work; doses used were inadequate; or glutamine perhaps needs to be given parenterally rather than enterally.

Other nutraceuticals and use in veterinary medicine

Various nutraceuticals are commonly used in veterinary medicine for reasons other than immune enhancement. Some of the more pertinent ones will now be discussed.

Osteoarthritis

Dietary supplements that have been critically evaluated for use in the management of osteoarthritis in dogs include green-lipped mussels (*Perna canaliculus*), chondroitin sulphate and P54FP (extract of Indian and Javanese turmeric) (Aragon et al., 2007). Many dietary supplements (e.g. glucosamine, chondroitin sulphate) are believed to be chondromodulating agents, which have a positive effect on cartilage matrix synthesis and on hyaluronan synthesis by synovial membranes, as well as an inhibitory effect on catabolic enzymes in osteoarthritic joints. Glucosamine is a precursor for glycosaminoglycans and it is proposed that its supplementation may help rebuild cartilage. More recently, a combination of chondromodulating agents with omega-3 fatty acids and antioxidants has emerged as a promising approach.

With regard to evidence for the efficacy of such agents, there are conflicting results. Some in vitro work suggests some positive effects for omega-3 fatty acids, whilst clinical trials have sometimes not demonstrated clinical benefit. It is also important to recognize that the various studies performed have varying degrees of quality (some lacked adequate wash-out periods, relied solely on subjective endpoints, lacked appropriate controls) and therefore some caution is warranted in interpreting their results.

- Three prospective placebo-controlled double-blinded clinical trials that included information on dogs treated with green-lipped mussels for treatment of osteoarthritis showed a positive effect (Bierer and Bui, 2002; Bui and Bierer, 2003; Hielm-Bjorkman et al., 2009). There were improvements in pain, swelling and crepitus, and an increase in range of motion compared to controls.
- A study evaluating P54FP showed some improvement on assessment via force plate analysis. However, clients were not able to note a clinical improvement (Innes et al., 2003).
- Studies evaluating chondroitin sulphate have documented a small positive effect (McCarthy et al., 2007).
- A small clinical benefit was attributed to the use of polysulphated glycosaminoglycans (de Haan et al., 1994).
- A negative effect was found associated with hyaluronan use in one study: intra-articular injections of hyaluronan in dogs with experimental osteoarthritis actually reduced proteoglycan synthesis in cartilage, suggesting a possible harmful effect (Smith et al., 1998).

Gastrointestinal disease

Prebiotics

Prebiotics are non-digestible food ingredients that have a beneficial effect through their selective metabolism within the intestinal tract. Prebiotics must fulfil three criteria:

- They must be resistant to gastric acidity and digestive enzymes, and must not be absorbed

from the gastrointestinal tract in their pre-fermented form
- They must be used by intestinal microflora for fermentation
- They must lead to selective stimulation of the growth and/or activity of beneficial intestinal bacteria.

Prebiotics have been incorporated into petfood in order to increase levels of gut bacteria believed to be major contributors to the microbial barrier to infection.

- Prebiotics are purported to reduce small intestinal bacterial overgrowth, improve colonic bacterial profile, decrease faecal putrefactive compounds, and affect faecal characteristics and nutrient digestibility (Gibson *et al.,* 2004).
- The most common of these 'beneficial bacteria' are believed to be lactobacilli and bifidobacteria. Although controversy exists regarding whether lactobacilli and bifidobacteria are in fact truly beneficial in dogs and cats, there have been studies documenting their presence in the gut of healthy dogs and cats (although in much lower numbers than in people) and studies have also demonstrated positive effects associated with prebiotic use (Terada *et al.,* 1992; Sparkes *et al.,* 1998; Swanson *et al.,* 2002; Rastall, 2004).
- For example, the use of oligofructose and mannose oligosaccharides in feeds has been shown to increase faecal bifidobacteria and ileal lactobacilli, with a concomitant decrease in clostridia in dogs (Terada *et al.,* 1992). The same study also demonstrated that prebiotic use was associated with decreased faecal odour and faecal bacterial toxin levels.
- In cats, the use of oligofructose was demonstrated to increase lactobacilli numbers, with decreases in clostridia and *Escherichia coli* (Sparkes *et al.,* 1998).

Probiotics

Probiotics are live microorganisms that, when ingested in sufficient amounts, have a positive effect on the health of the host. They are not, strictly speaking, 'nutraceuticals' but they will be mentioned here for completeness, as they are proposed to have similar benefits to prebiotics. Some of the benefits purportedly conferred by probiotic use include: reduced production of toxic bacterial metabolites; increased production of certain vitamins; enhanced resistance to bacterial colonization; and reinforcing host natural defences. Probiotics are therefore believed to have a role in balancing gut microflora and increasing resistance to pathogenic bacteria.

Microorganisms approved for use in animal feeds within the EU include strains belonging to *Bacillus, Enterococcus* and *Lactobacillus* bacterial groups. Some of the concerns with probiotics are: they may not work; the organisms may themselves lead to sepsis; and there is a risk that certain microorganisms, such as enterococci, may harbour transmissible antibiotic resistance determinants (i.e. plasmids).

- In a study using lactobacilli as a probiotic in dogs, investigators demonstrated good viability of lactobacilli in faeces, decrease in clostridial numbers, increased serum IgG, increased monocyte and neutrophil counts, decreased nitric oxide metabolism, and improvement in red cell osmotic fragility, which were all suggestive of a positive effect on gut microbiology and systemic immune response (Baillon *et al.,* 2004).
- A prospective placebo-controlled probiotic trial using a canine-specific probiotic cocktail containing three different *Lactobacillus* spp. strains, in addition to novel protein diet for the treatment of food-responsive diarrhoea, was able to demonstrate a dramatic improvement in clinical signs after dietary change, but no extra benefit attributed to the addition of the probiotic (Sauter *et al.,* 2006).
- Another study demonstrated that supplementation with *Enterococcus faecium* (SF68) improved faecal IgA concentration and antibody response to canine distemper virus vaccination (Benyacoub *et al.,* 2003).
- A randomized double-blinded placebo-controlled trial of a probiotic cocktail in dogs with acute vomiting and diarrhoea found that the time from initiation of treatment to the last abnormal stool was significantly shorter in the group given probiotics (Herstad *et al.,* 2010).
- Although some studies demonstrate positive effects, there are studies which fail to demonstrate benefits (Veir *et al.,* 2007; Marsella, 2009; Simpson *et al.,* 2009); further studies are warranted.

Interstitial cystitis

The transitional epithelium of the urinary bladder is covered by a glycocalyx composed of hydrated glycoproteins and glycosaminoglycans (GAGs). These GAGs minimize the adherence of microorganisms and crystals to the bladder epithelium and also limit movement of urine proteins and other solutes from the bladder lumen into surrounding tissues. Defects in surface GAGs and subsequent increased epithelial permeability have been hypothesized to be a causative factor in feline idiopathic cystitis. Compared with normal cats, some cats with idiopathic cystitis appear to have decreased bladder mucosal surface GAG expression and decreased urinary GAG excretion. In humans with interstitial cystitis, oral administration of pentosan polysulphate sodium (a semi-synthetic GAG analogue) appears to reduce the severity of symptoms in *some* patients. Although it initially seemed to be that interstitial cystitis in humans and in cats shared a similar pathogenesis, and therefore might respond similarly, results of a randomized placebo-controlled clinical trial of oral glucosamine (a GAG precursor) did not result in any significant difference between the severity of clinical signs in cats treated with glucosamine and those treated with placebo (Gunn-Moore and Shenoy, 2004). Therefore, currently there is no evidence supporting the use of GAG precursors in cats with idiopathic cystitis.

Conclusions

Despite the many pitfalls discussed, nutritional modulation of diseases appears to be a potentially useful strategy for companion animals. However, until trials can elucidate which specific nutrients and what dosages confer beneficial effects to particular patient populations, a certain degree of scepticism is advised. Of particular concern is the distinct possibility that significant species differences may reduce the usefulness of some of these approaches in veterinary patients. Before general recommendations for the use of IED or nutraceuticals in veterinary patients can be made, many questions must be answered.

Central issues of safety, purity and efficacy in regards to nutraceuticals must be addressed. Unfortunately, the fact that nutraceuticals are not subject to the same licensing regulations as pharmaceuticals means that substances of unknown or unproven efficacy can be marketed. In addition, there is no requirement for the manufacturer to prove that their particular formulation is absorbed intact. The user of a nutraceutical preparation should therefore remain critical and obtain as much information about efficacy of that product as they can.

However, as understanding of the interactions between nutrients and disease processes grows, a particular cocktail of nutrients may be identified that could modulate even serious diseases. Based on the progress being made in the area of clinical nutrition, it is quite evident that there should be a greater appreciation for the role nutrients play in ameliorating diseases, and how treatment strategies for certain conditions in companion animals may one day heavily depend on nutritional therapies.

References and further reading

Amado LC, Saliaris AP, Raju SV *et al.* (2005) Xanthine oxidase inhibition ameliorates cardiovascular dysfunction in dogs with pacing induced heart failure. *Journal of Molecular and Cellular Cardiology* **39**, 531–536

Anadon A, Martinez-Larranaga MR and Martinez MA (2006) Probiotics for animal nutrition in the European Union: regulation and safety assessment. *Regulatory Toxicology and Pharmacology* **45**, 91–95

Aragon CL, Hofmeister EH and Budsberg SC (2007) Systematic review of clinical trials of treatments for osteoarthritis in dogs. *Journal of the American Veterinary Medical Association* **230**, 514–521

Badylak SF, Lanz GC and Jeffries M (1990) Prevention of reperfusion injury in surgical induced gastric dilatation volvulus in dogs. *American Journal of Veterinary Research* **51**, 294–299

Baillon MLA, Marshall-Jones ZV and Butterwick RF (2004) Effects of probiotic *Lactobacillus acidophilus* strain DSM13241 in healthy adult dogs. *American Journal of Veterinary Research* **65**, 338–343

Baltzer WI, McMichael MA, Hosgood GL *et al.* (2008) Randomized, blinded, placebo-controlled clinical trial of *n*-acetylcysteine in dogs with spinal cord trauma from intervertebral disc disease. *Spine* **33**, 1397–1402

Bartges JW, Budesberg SC and Pazak HE (2001) Effects of different n6:n3 fatty acid ratio diets on canine stifle osteoarthritis. *Proceedings, Orthopedic Research Society 47th Annual Meeting, San Francisco* p.462 [Abstract]

Bastian L and Weimann A (2002) Immunonutrition in patients after multiple trauma. *British Journal of Nutrition* **87**, S133–S134

Bauer JE (2001) Evaluation of nutraceuticals, dietary supplements, and functional food ingredients for companion animals. *Journal of the American Veterinary Medical Association* **218**, 1755–1760

Bauer JE, Markwell PJ, Rauly JM, Rawlings JM and Senior DE (1999) Effects of dietary fat and polyunsaturated fatty acids in dogs with naturally developing chronic renal failure. *Journal of the American Veterinary Medical Association* **215**, 1588–1591

Benyacoub J, Czarnecki-Maulden GL, Cavadini C *et al.* (2003) Supplementation of food with *Enterococcus faecium* (SF68) stimulates immune function in dogs. *Journal of Nutrition* **133**, 1158–1162

Berger MM (2006) Antioxidant micronutrients in major trauma and burns: evidence and practice. *Nutrition in Clinical Practice* **21**, 438–449

Bierer TL and Bui LM (2002) Improvement of arthritic signs in dogs fed green-lipped mussel (*Perna canaliculus*). *Journal of Nutrition* **132** (Suppl.2), 1634S–1636S

Bond R and Lloyd DH (1992) A double-blind comparison of olive oil and a combination of evening primrose oil and fish oil in the management of canine atopy. *Veterinary Record,* **131**, 558–560

Bongers T, Griffiths RD and McArdle A (2007) Exogenous glutamine: the clinical evidence. *Critical Care Medicine* **35** (9 Suppl), S545–S552

Brown SA, Brown CA, Crowel WA *et al.* (1998) Beneficial effects of chronic administration of dietary omega-3 polyunsaturated fatty acids in dogs with renal insufficiency. *Journal of Laboratory Clinical Medicine* **131**, 447–455

Bui LM and Bierer LM (2003) Influence of green lipped mussels (*Perna canaliculus*) in alleviating signs of arthritis in dogs. *Veterinary Therapeutics* **4**, 397–407

Chan DL, Rozanski EA and Freeman LM (2009) Relationship between plasma amino acids, C-reactive protein, illness severity and outcome in critically ill dogs. *Journal of Veterinary Internal Medicine* **23**, 559–563

Codner EC and Thatcher CD (1990) The role of nutrition in the management of dermatoses. *Seminars in Veterinary Medicine and Surgery* **5**, 167–177

Curtis CL, Harwood JL, Dent CM and Caterson B (2004) Biological basis for the benefit of nutraceutical supplementation in arthritis. *Drug Discovery Today* **9**, 165–172

de Haan JJ, Goring RL and Beale BS (1994) Evaluation of polysulfated glycosaminoglycan for the treatment of hip dysplasia in dogs. *Veterinary Surgery* **23**, 177–181

Elliott DA (2006) Nutritional management of chronic renal disease in dogs and cats. *Veterinary Clinics of North America: Small Animal Practice* **36**, 1377–1384

Freeman LM, Rush JE, Khayias JJ *et al.* (1998) Nutritional alterations and effect of fish oil supplementation in dogs with heart failure. *Journal of Veterinary Internal Medicine* **12**, 440–448

Freeman LM, Rush JE and Markwell PJ (2006) Effects of dietary modification in dogs with early chronic valvular disease. *Journal of Veterinary Internal Medicine* **20**, 116–126

Gianotti L, Alexander JW, Gennari R, Pyles T and Babcock GF (1995) Oral glutamine decreases bacterial translocation and improves survival in experimental gut-origin sepsis. *Journal of Parenteral and Enteral Nutrition* **19**, 69–74

Gibson GR, Probert HM, Loo JV, Rastall RA and Roberfroid MB (2004) Dietary modulation of the human colonic microbiota: updating the concept of prebiotics. *Nutrition Research Reviews* **17**, 259–275

Gunn-Moore DA and Shenoy CM (2004) Oral glucosamine and the management of feline idiopathic cystitis. *Journal of Feline Medicine and Surgery* **6**, 219–225

Henderson A and Hayes P (1994) Acetylcysteine as a cytoprotective antioxidant in patients with severe sepsis: potential use for an old drug. *Annals of Pharmacotherapy* **28**, 1086–1088

Herstad HK, Nesheim BB, L'Abée-Lund T, Larsen S and Skancke E (2010) Effects of a probiotic intervention in acute canine gastroenteritis – a controlled clinical trial. *Journal of Small Animal Practice* **51**, 34–48

Heyland DK and Dhaliwal R (2005) Immunonutrition in the critically ill: from old approaches to new paradigms. *Intensive Care Medicine* **31**, 501–503

Hielm-Bjorkman A, Tulamo RM, Salonen H and Raekallio M (2009) Evaluating complementary therapies for canine osteoarthritis. Part 1: Green-lipped mussel (*Perna canaliculus*). *Evidence-based Complementary and Alternative Medicine* **6**, 365–373

Hill AS, Rogers QR, O'Neill SL and Christopher MM (2005) Effects of dietary antioxidant supplementation before and after oral acetaminophen challenge in cats. *American Journal of Veterinary Research* **66**, 196–204

Innes JF, Fuller CJ, Grover ER, Kelly AL and Burn JF (2003) Randomised, double-blind, placebo-controlled parallel group study of P54FP for the treatment of dogs with osteoarthritis. *Veterinary Record* **152**, 457–460

Kruger JM, Osborne CA and Lulich JP (2008) Changing paradigms of feline idiopathic cystitis. *Veterinary Clinics of North America: Small Animal Practice* **39**, 15–40

Lana SE, Hansen RA, Kloer L *et al.* (2003) The effects of oral glutamine supplementation on plasma glutamine concentrations and PGE2 concentrations in dogs experiencing radiation-induced mucositis. *Journal of Applied Research Veterinary Medicine* **1**, 259–265

Lantz GC, Badylak SF, Hiles MC *et al.* (1992) Treatment of reperfusion injury in dogs with experimentally induced gastric dilatation–volvulus. *American Journal of Veterinary Research* **53**, 1594–1598

Lee JI, Son HY and Kim MC (2006) Attenuation of ischemia-reperfusion injury by ascorbic acid in the canine renal transplantation. *Journal of Veterinary Science* **7**, 375–379

Marks JM, Dunkin BJ, Shillingstad BL *et al.* (1998) Pretreatment with allopurinol diminishes pancreatography-induced pancreatitis in a canine model. *Gastrointestinal Endoscopy* **48**, 180–183

Marks SL, Cook AK, Reader R *et al.* (1999) Effects of glutamine supplementation of an amino acid-based purified diet on intestinal mucosal integrity in cats with methotrexate-induced enteritis. *American Journal of Veterinary Research* **60**, 755–763

Marsella R (2009) Evaluation of *Lactobacillus rhamnosus* strain GG for the prevention of atopic dermatis in dogs. *American Journal of Veterinary Research* **70**, 735–740

McCarthy G, O'Donovan J, Jones B *et al.* (2007) Randomized double blind, positive controlled trial to assess the efficacy of glucosamine/chondroitin sulfate for the treatment of dogs with osteoarthritis. *Veterinary Journal* **174**, 54–61

Miller ER, Paston-Barruso R, Dalal D *et al.* (2005) Meta-analysis: high-dosage of vitamin E supplementation may increase all-cause mortality. *Annals of Internal Medicine* **142**, 37–46

O'Dwyer ST, Smith RJ, Hwang TL and Wilmore DW (1989) Maintenance of small bowel mucosa with glutamine-enriched parenteral nutrition. *Journal of Parenteral and Enteral Nutrition* **13**, 579–585

Plevraki K, Koutinas AF, Kaldrymidou H *et al.* (2006) Effects of allopurinol treatment on the progression of chronic nephritis in canine leishmaniosis (*Leishmania infantum*). *Journal of Veterinary Internal Medicine* **20**, 228–233

Rastall RA (2004) Bacteria in the gut: friends and foes and how to alter the balance. *Journal of Nutrition* **134**, 2022S–2026S

Ristow M, Zarse K, Oberbach A *et al.* (2009) Antioxidants prevent health-promoting effects of physical exercise in humans. *Proceedings of the National Academy of Science* **106**, 8665–8670

Roush JK, Cross AR, Renberg WC *et al.* (2005) Effects of feeding a high omega-3 fatty acid diet on serum fatty acid profiles and force plate analysis in dogs with osteoarthritis. *Veterinary Surgery* **34**, E21 [Abstract]

Satia JA, Littman A, Slatore CG, Galnko JA and White E (2009) Long-term use of beta-carotene, retinol, lycopene, and lutein supplementation and lung cancer risk: results from the VITamins And Lifestyle (VITAL) study. *American Journal of Epidemiology* **169**, 815–818

Sauter SN, Benyacoub J, Allenspach K *et al.* (2006) Effects of probiotic bacteria in dogs with food responsive diarrhoea treated with an elimination diet. *Journal of Animal Physiology and Animal Nutrition* **90**, 269–277

Scarff DH and Lloyd DH (1992) Double blind, placebo-controlled, crossover study of evening primrose oil in the treatment of canine atopy. *Veterinary Record* **131**, 97–99

Simpson KW, Rishniw M, Bellosa M *et al.* (2009) Influence of *Enterococcus faecium* SF68 probiotic on giardiasis in dogs. *Journal of Veterinary Internal Medicine* **23**, 476–481

Smith CE, Freeman LM, Rush JE, Cunningham SM and Biourge V (2007) Omega-3 fatty acids in Boxer dogs with arrhythmogenic right ventricular cardiomyopathy. *Journal of Veterinary Internal Medicine* **21**, 265–273

Smith GN, Myers SL, Brandt KD and Mickler EA (1998) Effect of intraarticular hyaluronan injection in experimental canine osteoarthritis. *Arthritis and Rheumatism* **41**, 976–985

Sparkes AH, Papasouliotis K, Sunvold G *et al.* (1998) Effect of supplementation with fructo-oligosaccharides on fecal flora of healthy cats. *American Journal of Veterinary Research* **59**, 436–440

Swanson KS, Grieshop CM, Flickinger EA *et al.* (2002) Supplemental fructo-oligosaccharides and mannanoligosaccharides influence immune function, ileal and total tract nutrient digestibilities, microbial populations, and concentrations of protein catabolites in the large bowel of dogs. *Journal of Nutrition* **132**, 980–989

Terada A, Hara H, Oishi T *et al.* (1992) Effect of dietary lactosucrose on fecal flora and fecal metabolites of dogs. *Microbiology and Ecology in Health and Disease* **5**, 87–92

Varzi HN, Esmailzadeh S, Morovvati H *et al.* (2007) Effect of silymarin and vitamin E on gentamycin-induced nephrotoxicity in dogs. *Journal of Veterinary Pharmacology and Therapeutics* **30**, 477–481

Veir JK, Knorr R, Cavadini C *et al.* (2007) Effect of supplementation with *Enterococcus faecium* (SF68) on immune functions in cats. *Veterinary Therapeutics* **8**, 229–238

Webb CB, Twedt DC, Fettman MJ and Mason G (2003) S-Adenosylmethionine (SAMe) in a feline acetaminophen model of oxidative injury. *Journal of Feline Medicine and Surgery* **5**, 69–75

Wijeysundera DN, Karkouti K, Rao V *et al.* (2009) N-Acetylcysteine is associated with increased blood loss and blood product utilization during cardiac surgery. *Critical Care Medicine* **37**, 1929–1934

Wischmeyer PE (2008) Glutamine: role in critical illness and ongoing clinical trials. *Current Opinion in Gastroenterology* **24**, 190–197

Wischmeyer PE, Kahana M, Wolfson R *et al.* (2001) Glutamine induces heat shock protein and protects against endotoxin shock in the rat. *Journal of Applied Physiology* **90**, 2403–2410

Yu S and Paetau-Robinson I (2006) Dietary supplements of vitamin E, and C and beta-carotene reduce oxidative stress in cats with renal insufficiency. *Veterinary Research Communications* **30**, 403–413

8

An introduction to physical therapies

Samantha Lindley

Introduction

The chapters on Physiotherapy (9), Hydrotherapy (10) and Acupuncture (11) which follow deal with interventions that involve a physical interaction with the patient as an integral part of the therapy. These therapies have been selected for inclusion in this Manual because there is some evidence for the claims made about their effectiveness. The critical reader may conclude that the evidence presented is less than robust in some cases. It is important to remember, however, that these are emerging fields in veterinary medicine; until there is a reasonable body of experience with these therapies in a practical setting, it can be difficult to formulate the kinds of research questions that can give useful results. There are also specific difficulties in designing research studies to evaluate therapies that include a physical component, and these challenges are discussed below.

The purpose of this short chapter is to introduce some ideas and concepts that may help the veterinary practice to evaluate realistically the possible effects *and* effectiveness of such therapies.

Evidence-based medicine

The evidence hierarchy is outlined in Figure 8.1.

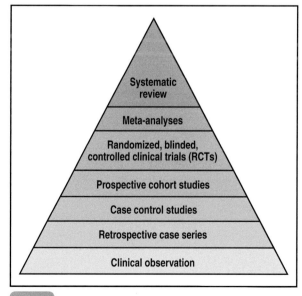

8.1 The evidence base hierarchy.

Clinical observation is what excites clinicians (and convinces owners – 'it works because it worked for my dog!'), but there are many factors that may have made it appear that an intervention applied to a given condition resulted in a successful outcome. These non-specific effects include:

- Natural history of the disease
- Coincidence/chance
- Non-specific effects of the treatment.

Non-specific effects of a treatment include, but are not limited to, the placebo effect, and are discussed in detail below.

Controlled trials allow for non-specific effects of a therapy (because these will apply to both treated and untreated groups), but bias can mean that it is possible, even unconsciously, to select the patients that are most likely to respond to the intervention under question and put them in the active group, whilst the rest go into the 'control' group. Randomizing the selection of patients removes this particular bias. In a 'blind' study, neither the patients (important for human trials) nor the clinician (or assessor) knows which group each patient belongs to, which should mean that there will be the same level of expectation of effect in both groups. Thus, *randomized controlled trials* (RCTs) are generally considered to be the first level of 'best testing' for a given therapy.

Meta-analysis takes a number of RCTs and analyses the results in a way that gives more confidence in the outcome.

Systematic reviews are considered to offer the highest level of evidence, because they look at all studies within their scope, quantify the value of each study (i.e. they do not all get equal weighting) and analyse the overall outcome.

Efficacy *versus* effectiveness

For the purposes of this discussion:

- **Efficacy** is the effect of a treatment compared with 'placebo'
- **Effectiveness** is the effect of a treatment compared to either an active or an inactive comparator.

Efficacy studies attempt to demonstrate the specific effects of a treatment, e.g. whether it is the needle penetrating the skin in an acupuncture treatment that results in analgesia, rather than the non-specific effects of needling (see below). This is important when an intervention carries some risk or significant financial cost. The question may then be: 'Is there a specific effect of inserting a needle through the skin?' If so, the treatment should be compared with an inactive intervention that looks and feels the same as the 'real' therapy. There are various ways of doing this with acupuncture, depending on the site of needling (see Chapter 11), but for hydrotherapy and physiotherapy it is difficult to apply an *inactive* hydrotherapy or physiotherapy treatment that looks and feels like the real thing.

Effectiveness studies are a pragmatic device to help indicate whether one treatment is better than, or at least as good as, another; or whether the combination of two treatments is better than one alone. Such studies do not make allowance for non-specific effects. This is less important in most veterinary trials, e.g. of non-steroidal anti-inflammatory drugs, where a new drug is often tested against one whose efficacy is established. If all the other aspects of differences between the two medications are controlled for (i.e. the 'blinding' of the study is adequate), then if both medications produce equally good effects one may be reasonably sure that drug A is as useful as drug B in controlling the pain and/or inflammation under test.

For physical therapies, the approach is usually to compare one intervention (e.g. hydrotherapy) against another (e.g. the normal graduated exercise plan for post-orthopaedic surgery patients). If the outcome is improved in the hydrotherapy group compared with the exercise group, this is a useful pragmatic result. However, it does not mean that hydrotherapy 'works' as a specific intervention, because there are lots of aspects to hydrotherapy (e.g. physical contact, attention, enjoyment) that are not *specific* to a hydrotherapy session but that may have influenced the outcome. Does this matter? Sometimes it does not, but if the client has to take a day off work and drive 50 miles to the nearest pool, it would be useful to know that there are specific benefits of the treatment.

Non-specific effects

Non-specific effects of therapies are all those effects that occur over and above the specific effect of a given treatment.

Natural history of the disease

Diseases tend to wax and wane in their severity but help is often sought when the disease reaches a peak of severity. It may be expected, for many diseases, that clinical signs will reach a peak and there will then be a natural improvement, though the condition may worsen again later. Any intervention given at the time of improvement will be naturally judged to be successful, usually by the owner and often by the practitioner.

Chance

It is always possible that an intervention was given just at the time when the condition was going to resolve anyway.

The therapeutic relationship

The so-called 'working alliance' between human patients and their therapists is important for the outcome of treatment (Fuertes *et al.*, 2007). The owner of a pet is also likely to have a more positive attitude to their pet's problem and the likely outcome if they have confidence in the veterinary team and the therapy employed (this is sometimes referred to as the 'owner placebo effect'). Is it also possible that veterinary patients themselves can be convinced to 'feel better' (and actually become better in demonstrable ways) by a positive therapeutic relationship with the veterinary surgeon or nurse; if so, is this not 'just' placebo?

The placebo effect

The placebo effect represents actual, potent neurophysiological changes. It is real and not imagined. The body has a remarkable ability to provide pain relief and healing; the placebo effect exploits this. Yet it is often dismissed as 'only' placebo.

Placebo technically means 'pleasing the patient', and veterinary surgeons may argue that many of their patients would feel more pleased if they never had to see the inside of a veterinary clinic again. However, as well as referring to the expectation of a patient to be healed, which may be stretching the actual cognitive abilities of veterinary patients, placebo can also be used to refer to some of the non-specific effects of interacting positively with the animal.

It has been postulated that one reason why placebo is perceived as such a pejorative term is that it was originally a mistranslation of a phrase used to refer to vespers sung for the dead in the fourteenth century. Since the practice of paying large sums for these vespers to be sung was not quite in the spirit of usual religious observance, the term started off with a negative connotation (Spiro, 1986). This may have been maintained by Cartesian ideas of body and mind being seen as separate entities and not able to influence each other. Placebo *is* 'all in the mind', but since the brain has potent effects on the body (and *vice versa*), that is a perfectly reasonable place for it to be in order to have the effects that are now recognized. Pain, after all, according to the International Association for the Study of Pain (IASP), is a psychological state (Merskey and Bogduk, 1994).

The evidence for placebo

From studies by Benedetti *et al.* (2005) it is known that:

- Placebo is a real neurophysiological effect, which can be targeted to a specific area of the body
- Placebo can be blocked by opiate antagonists that can block the targeted effect
- A placebo needle (i.e. not penetrating but looks as though it penetrates) is a more potent stimulator of a placebo effect than is a placebo pill

- Placebo effect can be augmented by an antagonist (proglumide) of the body's natural opiate inhibitor cholecystokinin (CCK).

Nocebo effects also exist, i.e. where an inactive substance or intervention can cause a worsening of symptoms; these are also subject to the kinds of manipulations described above (Benedetti *et al.,* 2005).

Placebo effects are recognized in animals, and so animal studies to determine the efficacy of an intervention must allow for them in the study design.

Physical interactions with animals

There are other effects of positive physical interactions with animal patients; whether these are strictly part of the placebo effect or not, they are physiological and demonstrable. In the words of the late Johannes Odendaal (2002) they are a way to 'open up the drugstore between our [and our patients'] ears'. Some of these effects are described in more detail below.

From the studies of Odendaal and others it can be seen that stroking a dog results in a decrease in blood pressure in both the person and the dog. When the blood pressure has reached a trough in an individual, there is a demonstrable rise in both subjects in the mood-enhancing neurotransmitters endorphins, prolactin, oxytocin, noradrenaline and dopamine (probably also serotonin, but this required urinalysis to determine and was not performed in the Odendaal study). When the dog being stroked belongs to the person doing the stroking, there is a significantly higher rise in prolactin and oxytocin in both subjects than when the dog is unfamiliar to the person. This should not be surprising, since prolactin and oxytocin are hormones associated with, amongst other things, bonding; but it is a gratifying outcome nonetheless to have a quantitative explanation of a common observation – i.e. that both dogs and people get pleasure from the stroking interaction.

Whilst general stroking releases oxytocin, it has been shown that lightly stroking the ventral surface (i.e. the abdomen and chest, probably along the mammary line) of animals (human and otherwise) is an efficient way of releasing this hormone in both males and females. As well as its association with bonding and milk let-down, this versatile hormone also has some sedative, anxiolytic and analgesic properties.

When owners are taught and encouraged to touch and massage their pets these physiological effects are exploited by helping the owners to help their pets feel better. Additionally, such interactions can help give the owner a sense of control over their pet's pain and anxiety.

In the current discussion, this knowledge highlights how complicated matters become when one starts to interact physically with the patient, as the whole veterinary team does on a daily basis. How much of the effect of treatment becomes specific and reliable, and how much is based on physical interaction with the patients once touch is involved?

Conclusions and practical considerations

- Targeting the placebo effect can be a potent method of stimulating the body's own healing and pain-relieving mechanisms (e.g. the periaqueductal grey (PAG) in the brain releases β-endorphin, which is many times more potent than morphine).
- Targeting the placebo effect, however it is done, should be a *safe* method of stimulating such mechanisms. If an intervention is used which cannot be shown to be superior to, or different from, placebo then it should at least be safe. However, if an intervention is not completely safe, efficacy studies should be performed: hence the need for efficacy studies in some of the disciplines discussed here, like acupuncture, for example, which is safe, but not *completely* safe.
- Any intervention that involves pointing at (or pointing *something* at) the area under treatment is likely to have an effect, regardless of any specific efficacy of the pointing device (laser, ultrasound, acupuncture, even non-touch therapies such as Reiki). This was demonstrated in a study showing that a sham needle was more effective than a sham tablet (Kaptchuk *et al.,* 2006).
- All the physical therapies will employ, to a greater or lesser extent, the power of placebo. This is true of any therapy/intervention, but for physical therapies the specific effects are difficult to demonstrate because any convincing placebo in an efficacy study should persuade the patient (and owner) that they have received the real treatment when they have not. This is easy with a pill, but harder with acupuncture, physiotherapy and hydrotherapy, for example, since all involve interactions with the patient. Since the placebo must also involve interactions to convince patient and owner that they have received a real treatment, the effects of these must be accounted for. If it turns out that the interaction with the patient is a significant part of the overall effects of treatment, then it will need a large number of subjects to show a difference between, for example, gently stroking the affected limb (placebo group) and taking it regularly through a passive range of motion (active intervention), always assuming that the owner can be convinced that the former is going to be as effective as the latter.
- Touch in any form that is pleasant to the patient can have a positive and real neurophysiological effect on that patient. However, what is 'pleasant to the patient' will be an individual preference, based not only on the individual and its previous experiences but also on the current state of its nervous system, e.g. a patient with allodynia will not enjoy being stroked over the sensitive area. Touch includes light stroking, massage and grooming. It is likely to be important to adapt the method of touch to suit the individual. Whatever is done should be clearly enjoyed, rather than endured, by the patient, for it to have to optimum effects. Touch should be in non-threatening

places for that individual (Figure 8.2). Massage using the fingertips or kneading actions is best avoided by owners, since a compliant patient will not move away or object to uncomfortable stimuli. The use of flat hand techniques is preferable, where the palm of the hand is held against the skin and the hand and skin moved together over the underlying muscles (Figure 8.3); this technique should be demonstrated to the owner. Grooming should be carried out with a groomer that does not dig into painful areas, but which mimics a massaging action (Figure 8.4).

- Giving the patient attention to which it will react positively is likely to have an overall beneficial effect.

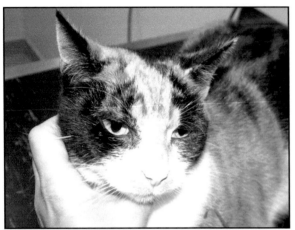

8.2   Stroking animals makes both the animal and the person doing the stroking feel good, but it confuses the assessment of the specific effects of therapies.

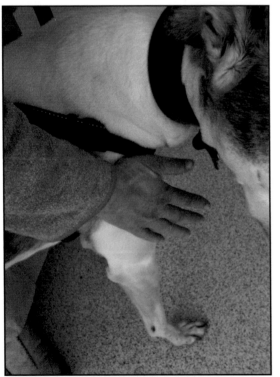

8.3   Flat hand massage should be employed, to avoid exacerbating pain by digging the fingers into underlying tissue.

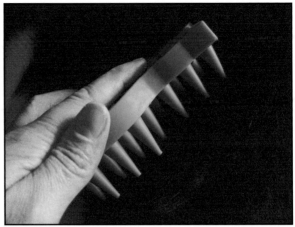

8.4   Grooming is one method of delivering touch and massage to an animal. The groomer used should not dig into painful areas.

Exercise

Exercise (Figure 8.5) has positive effects on wellbeing, mood, musculoskeletal strength and muscle tone, immunomodulation and sleep regulation. At least some of these effects are mediated by endorphins and any physical therapy that mimics exercise will almost certainly produce some of its effects by this mechanism.

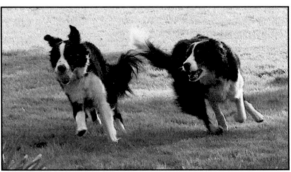

8.5   Exercise has numerous positive effects and is fun.

Hydrotherapy (see Chapter 10) allows the patient to exercise: by fairly vigorous exertion, in the case of swimming; or by moving the limbs through a normal range of motion for ambulation on an underwater treadmill. As well as the usual recognized benefits on muscle tone and bulk, avoidance of concussion on the joints, normal movement of the joints and the consumption of calories, the simple benefits of exercising *per se* are likely to have positive effects over and above anything that is specifically achieved by the therapy.

Assessing the effects of physical therapies

In order to demonstrate that a physical therapy 'works' for a given condition, it should be demonstrated that it has a specific effect, over and above all of the relevant non-specific effects mentioned above.

The problem with looking for *specific efficacy* is that the therapy should be compared to a true placebo effect. Effectiveness studies that have an inactive arm and are therefore leaving a group of patients untreated are subject to Home Office regulations as animal experimentation. Clinical studies must show an 'intention to treat' all subjects and this means, in practical terms, that clinical studies are *effectiveness* studies, i.e. comparing an intervention with the standard treatment. This is a pragmatic approach and useful; after all, in practice, the veterinary surgeon wants to know: 'Is this technique better than the one I am currently using?' or 'If I add this to my current protocol, will I get better results?'.

Specific effects become important when the intervention carries some risk. Acupuncture practitioners often say that it does not really matter whether the effect is placebo or not as long it works for the patient. However, acupuncture stops being *totally* safe when the needle penetrates the skin. If it were possible to achieve the same effects by merely pointing at the affected area or tapping it with something that feels a little sharp on the skin, then there would be no justification for introducing a needle into the body.

Specific effects also become important when someone has to make a decision to pay for the treatment. In human medicine this decision is often guided (but not ultimately made) by the National Institute for Health and Clinical Excellence (NIHCE) who demand not only a high level of evidence that a given therapy works above placebo, but also that the therapy is cost-effective. In veterinary medicine these decisions are made by practices and insurance companies, and ultimately by the owner who must decide, guided by the practice, whether a given treatment is worth not only their financial input, but also the time involved and any potential additional stress to their pet.

The veterinary team is obliged to be aware of the limits to current knowledge of the effects of many therapies and to advise clients accordingly, but 'the baby should not be thrown out with the bath water'. The pessimist may dismiss *all* physical therapies (including the many not included in this Manual) as no more than 'placebo', but the optimist will embrace the value of placebo and realize that many therapies, however implausible some of their mechanisms may sound, can have some merit and real effects. Gradually, the science is emerging that will demonstrate effectiveness (and in some cases specific efficacy) and help to direct these treatments more effectively and to design consistently useful protocols. Until then, existing evidence, common sense and clinical experience will dictate which of the physical therapies have a place in practice. The following chapters discuss the use of and evidence for physiotherapy, hydrotherapy and acupuncture, all of which have some veterinary, experimental and comparative clinical evidence for their use. More evidence is needed, but it should be appreciated that there are unique difficulties in obtaining meaningful results when physical interaction exists as part of the therapy. It should also be remembered that **lack of evidence of effect is not evidence of lack of effect.**

References and further reading

Benedetti F, Mayberg HS, Wager TD *et al.* (2005) Neurobiological effects of the Placebo Effect. *Journal of Neuroscience* **25**, 10390–10402

Fuertes JN, Mislowack A, Bennet J *et al.* (2007) The physician–patient working alliance. *Patient Education and Counselling* **66**, 29–36

Kaptchuk TJ, Stason WB, Davis RB *et al.* (2006) Sham device v inert pill: randomised controlled trial of two placebo treatments. *British Medical Journal* **332**, 391–397

Merskey H and Bogduk N (1994) *Classification of Chronic Pain, 2nd edn.* IASP Press, Seattle

Odendaal J (2002) *Pets and our Mental Health: The Why, the What, and the How.* Vantage Press, New York

Spiro HM (1986) *Doctors, Patients and Placebos.* Yale University Press, Newhaven, CT

Uvnas-Moberg K, Bruzelius G, Alster P *et al.* (1993) The antinociceptive effect of non-noxious sensory stimulation is mediated partly through oxytocinergic mechanisms. *Acta Physiologica Scandinavica* **149**, 199–204

9

Physiotherapy and physical rehabilitation

Brian Sharp

Introduction

Physiotherapy (or physical therapy) is concerned with physical function, and regards movement and optimal function as central to the health and well-being of individuals. A practical healthcare profession, physiotherapy involves the assessment, diagnosis and treatment of disease and disability through physical means. Based upon the principles of medical science, it is regarded as within the sphere of conventional (rather than alternative) medicine. Human physiotherapy is an internationally recognized discipline and the positive benefits of physiotherapeutic intervention in human patients have been well documented (e.g. Ostelo *et al.,* 2002; Moffet *et al.,* 2004).

A range of physical modalities is used to treat and prevent injuries, to restore movement and function, and to maximize physical potential by:

- Reducing pain
- Promoting the healing process
- Increasing and maintaining muscle strength and joint flexibility
- Promoting and restoring normal movement patterns
- Increasing cardiovascular fitness.

Rehabilitation is an integral component of physiotherapy and is the process of helping an individual achieve the highest possible level of function, independence and quality of life following illness or injury.

Physiotherapy in small animal practice

The benefits of physiotherapy are now acknowledged within veterinary medicine (e.g. Millis *et al.,* 1997; Marsolais *et al.,* 2002; Monk *et al.,* 2006). Physiotherapy is complementary to conventional veterinary treatment and is usually more effective when used in collaboration with it. Techniques and protocols that have been developed and successfully used in human healthcare are now being adapted for animal use, creating exciting opportunities for animal care.

Within veterinary care, there are now recognized qualifications relating to the practice of physiotherapy on animals (see Figure 9.2) but these are not specifically identified by law, so the responsibility for approving individuals to carry out physiotherapy rests with the attending veterinary surgeon. Within animal care, physiotherapy has developed in an *ad hoc* way, with many people practising as physiotherapists without any formal physiotherapy qualifications or registration. At present, there is no protection of title for 'animal' or 'veterinary physiotherapists' and this allows anyone to practise under these names. This situation contrasts markedly to human healthcare.

The team approach

In the UK the Veterinary Surgeons Act 1966 provides that (with certain specific exceptions) only veterinary surgeons may carry out acts of veterinary surgery upon animals. 'Veterinary surgery' is defined by the Act as to include the making of a diagnosis, the carrying out of tests for diagnostic purposes, and both medical and surgical treatment. Of the exceptions created by the Veterinary Surgery (Exemptions) Order 1962, one permits the treatment of an animal by physiotherapy: 'provided such treatment is given by a person acting under the direction of a veterinary surgeon who has examined the animal and has prescribed the treatment of the animal by physiotherapy'. In this context, physiotherapy is interpreted as including all kinds of manipulative therapy, including osteopathy and chiropractic, but does not include alternative therapies such as acupuncture and aromatherapy. Although it is the veterinary surgeon's legal responsibility to decide on appropriate physiotherapy intervention, in most cases these decisions are best made through a team approach involving the veterinary surgeon, physiotherapist, nurse and owner.

Veterinary expertise can discover the source and pathology of many conditions, and determine appropriate medical or surgical interventions; *physiotherapy* expertise can identify associated mechanical dysfunctions and develop appropriate treatment plans for restoring mechanical function. Such collaboration between the professions ensures compliance with existing legislation as well as improving treatment and outcomes for patients in their care.

Whilst actual divisions between the roles of the various team members are not precisely defined, all members of the team can participate at different levels, within the limits of their professional training, experience and the legal framework of veterinary medicine (Figure 9.1). There is now a growing

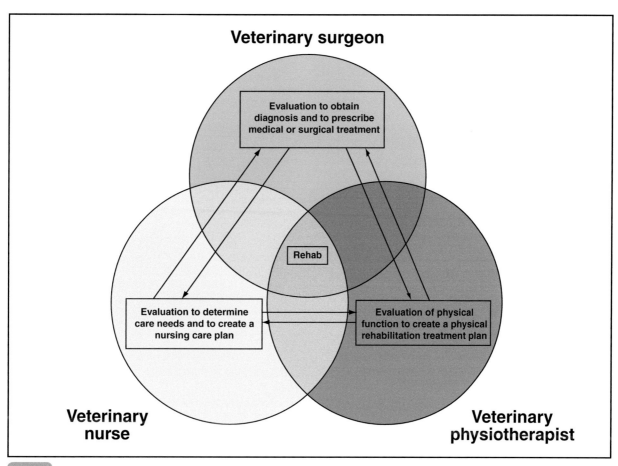

9.1 The overlapping roles of the veterinary team involved in physiotherapy and rehabilitation.

awareness of, and demand for, these services from the general public and from much of the veterinary profession. The non-specialist veterinary surgeon and veterinary nurse can provide simple physiotherapy techniques in-house; having qualified veterinary physiotherapists on site, or available via referral, provides an additional valuable resource to the veterinary team.

The role of the veterinary surgeon

As physiotherapy is not currently included in the training of veterinary surgeons (nor of veterinary nurses) in the UK, it may only be the basic modalities (massage, passive movements and hydrotherapy) that are familiar. If patients do not 'fit' into the category of animals likely to benefit from these approaches, patients that might benefit from physiotherapy could miss out. Because the veterinary surgeon is the primary person responsible for decisions regarding appropriate physiotherapy and rehabilitative care, it is incumbent upon him or her to be aware of the developing role of physiotherapy and of the physiotherapist within small animal practice. In recent years, short-course CPD training in physiotherapy has become available to increase the knowledge and skill base of veterinary surgeons and a growing number of general practices are collaborating with local veterinary physiotherapists to improve outcomes for the animals in their care.

The role of the veterinary physiotherapist

Physiotherapy and rehabilitation within a small animal practice will always benefit from the involvement of a qualified veterinary physiotherapist, as these professionals are appropriately trained, registered and regulated in respect of their animal work. The current lack of legal protection of the title 'veterinary physiotherapist', which allows people to practise physiotherapy on animals without any formal qualification, has wide-ranging implications for the referring veterinary surgeon, who needs to be sure that patients are being treated by properly qualified professionals (Figure 9.2), and also for the owner, who rightly demands the same level of expertise for their pet as they would receive as a human patient. Early assessment by a qualified physiotherapist will ensure that appropriate and effective physiotherapy and rehabilitation plans are devised for each animal.

The role of the veterinary nurse

Notwithstanding the comments above, there is much that can be carried out in-house, particularly by the trained veterinary nurse. Nursing care plans covering the immediate postoperative period should routinely incorporate the basic physiotherapy techniques of massage, passive movements, cold therapy, simple therapeutic exercises and chest care, as appropriate (see case studies chapters). These basic postoperative physiotherapy techniques can easily be carried

Physiotherapist titles
• MCSP (Member of the Chartered Society of Physiotherapy) • HPC Reg (Registration with the Health Professions Council) All physiotherapists with these qualifications have completed a 3-year degree training in physiotherapy, and are legally entitled to practise physiotherapy on humans. Also known as 'chartered physiotherapists', they no longer have to use the term 'chartered' because 'physiotherapist' and 'physical therapist' are now legally protected titles.
Animal Physiotherapist titles
• ACPAT – Category A (Member of the Association of Chartered Physiotherapists in Animal Therapy) ACPAT is a clinical interest group of the Chartered Society of Physiotherapy, and represents the only professionally recognized physiotherapy organization in the UK whose members treat animals through the practice of physiotherapy. This organization was established in 1985 and its members have the widest and most appropriate range of qualifications, skills and knowledge on the subject of animal physiotherapy, are professionally accountable, maintain standards through regular CPD, and have appropriate professional and liability insurance.
Veterinary Physiotherapist titles
• MSc (or PGDip) in Veterinary Physiotherapy All veterinary physiotherapists with these qualifications are qualified human physiotherapists, with a minimum of 2 years' experience with humans, and have also completed a further 2-year higher degree training in veterinary physiotherapy. Most UK practitioners are MSc graduates from the Royal Veterinary College, although there are now equivalent MSc courses in other countries.

9.2 Veterinary physiotherapist qualifications. A physiotherapist with these qualifications is a professional who: has appropriate qualifications, experience and insurance cover; has undergone the best training available; has the widest and most appropriate range of skills/knowledge on the subject of animal physiotherapy; updates their skills regularly; and is professionally accountable.

out by veterinary nurses or nursing assistants who are confident and competent in their use and application. This competence can be achieved by attending appropriate courses to learn and practise the techniques and to develop appropriate decision-making skills around their use. Short courses in basic physiotherapy techniques, as well as in specific modalities such as massage, hydrotherapy and canine rehabilitation, are available. Postoperative physiotherapy and rehabilitation for patients is essential in many cases to achieve a satisfactory outcome and can be a particularly satisfying aspect of the work of the veterinary nurse.

In respect of the veterinary nurse's role in physiotherapy, it remains the responsibility of the veterinary surgeon to be sure that the nurse is capable of carrying out appropriate physiotherapy procedures, but the nurse must also be sure of working within their own sphere of competence. If in doubt, cases should be referred to a qualified veterinary physiotherapist (see later) to ensure the patient is receiving the best possible care.

The role of the owner

In many cases, owners whose pets are having physiotherapy or undergoing a rehabilitation programme are keen to be involved in the process. If the therapist believes that the owner is competent to carry out suitable techniques/exercises, this can be an excellent way of ensuring that the patient receives regular therapy. If owners are taught practical techniques, they must not only be physically able to perform them to a good standard, but also have sufficient time and commitment to be able to carry them out as regularly as required. If this is not feasible then the therapist should arrange to perform the treatments

themselves. Involving owners in the planning of the rehabilitation programme and establishing goals for the treatment helps to improve compliance.

To help further ensure compliance from owners, the therapist should first demonstrate the technique (or exercise) fully to the owner, with a suitable explanation as to the reasons *why* the technique is important. Having an adequate understanding of the reasons for the different components of a rehabilitation programme is a most effective way to achieve compliance. The owner should then practise the technique (exercise) until the therapist is convinced the owner can perform it well. A summary of the techniques (exercises) should be provided to the owner in written form, with accompanying illustrations if possible.

Owner involvement can be highly beneficial to the eventual outcome of the programme, but any therapist teaching techniques to owners has a responsibility to ensure that involvement is suitable, effective and not harmful to the patient.

Providing a physiotherapy service

The provision of a physiotherapy or rehabilitation service within a small animal practice demonstrates a positive, caring image to clients, as well as improving outcomes for animals following injury or surgery (Marsolais *et al.*, 2002; Monk *et al.*, 2006). Integrating physiotherapy into practice can be achieved in several ways.

Referral

Referral to a veterinary physiotherapist can be made at various stages of the treatment/rehabilitative process (Figure 9.3). Earlier referral is likely to be more effective and achieve better outcomes in

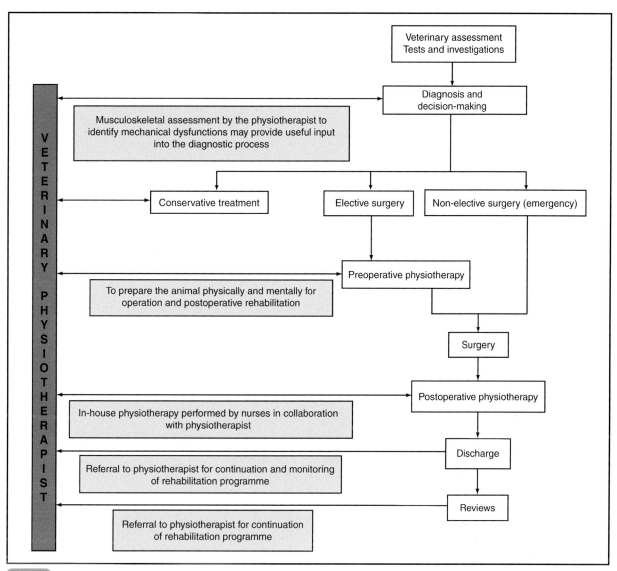

9.3 Stages for possible referral to the veterinary physiotherapist.

most cases. Some physiotherapists are based in hydrotherapy or rehabilitation centres to which the owner has to bring their pet, but most will assess and treat animals in the client's home. The physiotherapist will provide reports and contact the referring veterinary surgeon as required. The referral option requires little expenditure by the practice, and no allocation of space for physiotherapy purposes, yet still provides clients with an adequate service. However, when the physiotherapist is working in isolation from the rest of the veterinary team, there is little opportunity for interdisciplinary discussion, learning or exchange of views.

In-practice clinic
Referrals of appropriate cases can be made directly into the clinic, which can be staffed either by a qualified physiotherapist who is working as an independent practitioner or by one who is a full- or part-time member of the veterinary team. For a group practice, a single physiotherapy clinic may be sufficient for several practices within the group. The practice provides the administration for the clinic and

the physiotherapist is available for new assessments and ongoing treatments. This option encourages much more effective team working, case discussion and interdisciplinary cooperation. It also promotes a positive image of a caring practice to clients.

An *independent* physiotherapist provides the practice with expertise to assess, advise and assist with inpatients and outpatients. Apart from the costs of room provision and administration, there is little monetary outlay required.

A physiotherapist working as a full-time or part-time *member of staff* provides all of the above benefits and has the advantage that physiotherapy expertise is available more frequently. The physiotherapist could then take an active role in the postoperative care of all appropriate in- and outpatients. This scenario would inevitably require more outlay on the part of the practice because of salary costs, but such a service would run well in conjunction with other rehabilitation facilities that may already be available within the practice (such as hydrotherapy), providing a comprehensive physiotherapy and rehabilitation service for clients.

Indications for physiotherapy

In small animal practice, physiotherapy may help with a wide range of orthopaedic, neurological and other conditions (Figure 9.4; see also case studies). Many inpatients requiring physiotherapy will have had orthopaedic or neurological surgery, but in these cases a satisfactory technical outcome of surgery does not always equate to a good functional recovery or adequate return of neuromusculoskeletal control of the limb; therefore appropriate rehabilitation should be considered essential. Inadequate treatment, especially during the early stages of recovery, can lead to excessive discomfort for the animal and delay early use of the limb. This may result in a slow or incomplete return to function, associated muscle atrophy, joint stiffness, cartilage degeneration and joint dysfunction.

Orthopaedic conditions (see Chapter 14)

- Postoperative rehabilitation, e.g. stifle or hip surgery, arthrodesis, amputation, ligament/tendon repair
- Acute and chronic soft tissue injuries, involving muscle, tendon, joint capsule or ligament
- Arthritis – long-term management
- Hip dysplasia and elbow dysplasia – conservative care
- Trauma and wound care
- Sports/working injuries
- Back/neck pain

Neurological conditions (see Chapter 13)

- Postoperative rehabilitation, e.g. decompression surgery
- Disc prolapses – conservative care
- Central or peripheral nerve injuries
- Fibrocartilaginous embolism
- Degenerative myelopathy – management
- Balance/vestibular problems

Other

- Pain management
- Athletic/working dogs – performance problems, improving strength and endurance
- Obesity
- Depression
- Elderly patients

9.4 Conditions that may benefit from physiotherapy.

Typical problems that arise in the postoperative patient and that may benefit from appropriate physiotherapeutic interventions are:

- Pain
- Inflammation
- Swelling/oedema
- Reduced range of motion (ROM)
- Reduced muscle strength
- Reduced balance/proprioception
- Reduced function
- Poor gait
- Hypertonicity/hypotonicity
- Paralysis/paresis
- Muscle spasm/contracture
- Retained chest secretions/inability to cough.

Many different physiotherapy modalities exist that will address these problems; these must be selected appropriately, based on the requirements of the individual animal. Specific protocols are described for many of the major types of surgery (Bockstahler *et al.*, 2004), but each animal's response to, and recovery from, injury and surgery is different, and problem-solving and decision-making must form an integral part of the treatment planning process for each patient. Whilst it may be appropriate for the veterinary surgeon or nurse to provide some of the physiotherapy care, much of it requires specialized intervention from a qualified veterinary physiotherapist.

The physiotherapy process

This includes the following:

1. Assessment
2. Problem identification
3. Treatment goals: short-term; long-term
4. Treatment plans
5. Outcome measures.

Assessment and problem identification

A physiotherapy assessment is a thorough exploration of the musculoskeletal problems of the individual in order to determine appropriate intervention. Effective assessment helps to identify the structures that are causing the problem, whether treatment is appropriate and, if so, what treatment should be given.

Subjective assessment

This involves:

- Signalment (species, breed, age, gender)
- Information about the problems (primary and secondary) from referring veterinary surgeon, nurse, owner, investigations/tests, diagnosis
- Signs (aggravating and easing factors, daily pattern)
- History of present condition (onset, duration, progression, treatments)
- Medication (current and previous)
- Previous medical history (illnesses, surgery)
- Exercise levels (current/previous) and occupation (sporting/working)
- Home environment (other dogs, children, garden, flooring, stairs, food).

SIN

Information gained from the subjective assessment helps to determine the **S**everity, **I**rritability and **N**ature of the animal's signs, to identify structures that require objective testing (joints, muscles, ligaments, tendons, nerves), and to guide the physiotherapist to the most appropriate objective assessment.

- **Severity** is determined by how much the problem is affecting the individual's normal lifestyle, and varies from 'minimal' (little effect on day-to-day activity) to 'maximal' (large impact on daily activity).

- **Irritability** is probably the most important and is determined by how quickly the clinical signs can be brought on, and how they long they take to go:
  - o High irritability: clinical sign can be aggravated very easily and will take a long time to ease
  - o Low irritability: clinical sign requires a lot to aggravate it, and it eases very quickly.
- **Nature** relates to the suspected causative factor, e.g. neuropathic, arthritic, inflammatory.

Objective assessment
This includes:

- Posture/gait (conformation, symmetry, deviations)
- Functional movements (standing, walking, trotting, sit-to-stand, lie-to-sit, circles, steps)
- Analysis of provoking activities
- Active and passive movements (quality and quantity)
- Accessory movements (see later) of all joints being tested (quality and quantity of movement, pain response)
- Muscle activity, primarily via functional movement tests
- Ligament stress tests
- Neural provocation tests: involves positioning of the body and limb segments to create tension on specific peripheral nerves in order to assess the nerve's response
- Palpation of limbs and vertebral column (temperature, swelling, reaction to pressure, muscle bulk and tone)
- Specific tests (e.g. neurological, orthopaedic, cardiovascular, respiratory).

Information gained from the objective assessment helps to determine specific problem areas that need addressing, and to guide the physiotherapist toward the most appropriate treatment options.

Goals and outcomes
Realistic goals should be devised in conjunction with the owner, and progress should be monitored regularly to ensure satisfactory outcomes are achieved.

Outcome measures are essential tools for determining how an animal is progressing, and the effectiveness of the treatment protocol.

Subjective measures
These include:

- **Owner feedback.** This can be an effective and valuable way of determining outcome. Owners can often be very perceptive in gauging their pet's condition and progress
- **Lameness scoring.** Lameness evaluation is normally carried out with the animal walking and trotting. Subsequent comparative scores can determine the level of progress
- **Pain assessment.** The presence of pain can prevent satisfactory progress from being made and its impact on the animal's physical function can be a useful measure to assess progress. However, pain in animals is difficult to assess objectively. Although behaviour changes (including willingness to move or be handled) can often be helpful in determining an animal's level of pain, the tolerance of pain can be very variable between different animals. The use of pain assessment scoring or visual analogue scales can be used to compare pain levels at different stages of treatment to assess the effectiveness of the treatment protocol (see Chapters 2 and 3).

Objective measures
These include:

- Gait analysis:
  - o Force plates (Figure 9.5) measure ground reaction forces acting on the limb during the stance phase of gait (kinetic studies)
  - o Kinematic studies (Figure 9.6) provide information about limb and joint movement and aid the diagnosis of lameness
  - o Pressure mat systems (Figure 9.7) assess foot biomechanics by measuring pressure and force distribution during gait

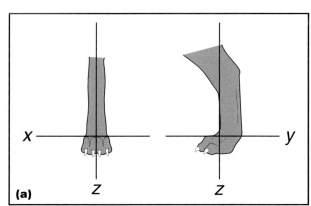
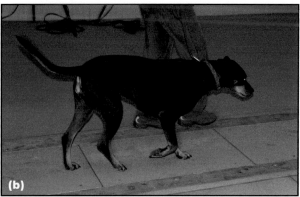

9.5 Kinetic analysis. Force plates measure ground reaction forces acting on the limb during the stance phase of gait. **(a)** The forces are measured in three orthogonal planes: medial–lateral (x), craniocaudal (y) and vertical (z). Measurements obtained include peak forces and impulses, and analysis allows comparisons to be made at different times (same limb), or at the same time (different limbs). **(b)** The dog is led across the force plate by a handler, in a consistent manner and with no interference from the handler. Three satisfactory foot strikes are required to provide adequate data for analysis. (b, courtesy of the Royal Veterinary College)

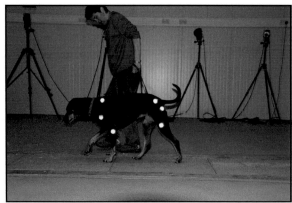

9.6 Kinematic analysis. Reflective markers are applied to specific anatomical landmarks on the animal. The subject is then moved down a runway and the movement filmed by a series of video cameras. The motion of the markers is converted into digital images, allowing analysis of limb and joint movements. Comparisons can be made at different times (same joint) or by comparing equivalent joints on each side. (Courtesy of the Royal Veterinary College)

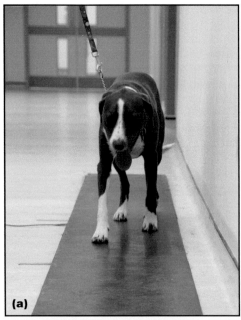

(a)

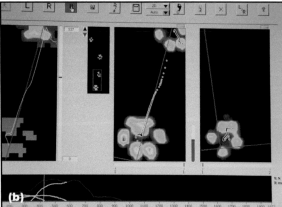

(b)

9.7 Pressure mat scanning systems allow clinicians to collect information about foot biomechanics, gait and balance. The use of pressure plates is a useful way of examining weightbearing through the limb and helps identify specific high/low pressure areas. (Courtesy of the Royal Veterinary College)

o Gait analysis using these techniques can be a useful tool for clinicians and researchers, but they are rarely available in general practice due to the complexities and time constraints of data collection and analysis
o At a more simplistic level, simple video analysis can provide useful information to determine functional joint movement, ease of weightbearing through individual limbs and identification of problem areas.
- Electromyographic analysis:
  o Electromyography (EMG) is used to measure muscle activation; both surface and intramuscular sensors can be used
  o EMG can help to explain the motor performance underlying the kinetic and kinematic findings, but, as with those techniques, it is specialized and rarely found in general practice
- Range-of-motion (ROM) measurements using goniometry (Figures 9.8 and 9.9)
- Circumferential limb measurements (improvements in muscle bulk, oedema, effusion)
- Neurological tests (improvements in reflexes, knuckling, foot placement)
- Accessory movements (improvements in quality, quantity and pain response)

Joint	Joint motions	Normal canine ROM (degrees)
Shoulder	Flexion Extension Abduction Adduction Medial rotation Lateral rotation	30–60 160–170 40–50 40–50 40–50 40–50
Elbow	Flexion Extension	20–40 160–170
Radioulnar	Pronation Supination	40–50 80–90
Carpus	Flexion Hyperextension Radial deviation Ulnar deviation	20–35 190–200 5–15 10–20
Hip	Flexion Extension Abduction (with flexed hip) Abduction (with extended hip) Adduction (with flexed hip) Adduction (with extended hip) Medial rotation Lateral rotation	55 160–165 120 (stifle at 90) 85 65 (stifle at 90) 63 55 50
Stifle	Flexion Extension	45 160–170
Talocrural, tarsocrural	Flexion Extension	40 170

9.8 Canine joint motions and ranges. The straight joint position is regarded as 180 degrees rather than zero. (Data from Millis *et al.*, 2004a)

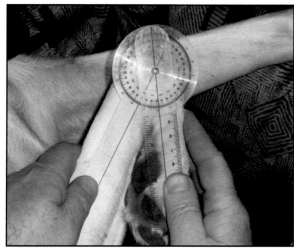

9.9 Measuring carpal joint flexion using a goniometer.

- Palpation of limbs and vertebral column (improvements in temperature, swelling, reaction to pressure, muscle bulk and tone)
- Functional activities (improvements in ability)
- Balance tests (improvements in speed and effectiveness of reaction)
- Stamina tests (exercise and pulse testing).

Physiotherapy treatments

Physiotherapy encompasses a wide variety of techniques and modalities. Some of the simpler techniques can easily be carried out in-house by the non-specialist veterinary surgeon and nurse, but there are many additional specialist modalities that the qualified physiotherapist can provide (Figure 9.10). The selection of appropriate treatments should be based on the assessment findings, diagnosis and prognosis. Often a combination of techniques will be used to maximize outcome and return the patient more quickly to maximum function.

Massage

The practice of physiotherapy has its origins in massage. This comprises a wide variety of different techniques, which also form the basis for additional therapies in human patients (e.g. Rolfing, Alexander, bodywork, reflexology, acupressure). Although there is a paucity of scientific evidence for the benefits of massage, it has been used for centuries to apparent good effect by a wide variety of medical practitioners and is now gradually gaining acceptance within veterinary care (Sutton, 2004). Qualified veterinary physiotherapists are fully trained in the basic massage skills and many have done further training in other soft tissue techniques. Simple massage techniques can be easily learnt by the practising veterinary surgeon or veterinary nurse, and massage can also be performed by owners following appropriate tuition. The techniques selected should be based upon the individual requirements of each patient, i.e. effect required, size of animal, size of area requiring treatment, any pertinent contraindications.

Non-specialist (veterinary surgeons, nurses, and owners after suitable training)
Manual therapies: • Massage • Passive movements • Stretches Thermotherapies: • Heat • Cold Exercise therapy: • Basic exercises for the postoperative orthopaedic and neurological patient • Hydrotherapy (see Chapter 10)
Specialist (qualified physiotherapists)
All of the above, plus Manual therapies: • Joint mobilizations: Maitland mobilizations; natural apophyseal glides (NAGS); sustained natural apophyseal glides (SNAGS); mobilizations with movement (MWMs); traction • Joint manipulations • Soft tissue techniques: soft tissue release; myofascial release; trigger pointing; acupressure; proprioceptive neuromuscular facilitation (PNF); neural mobilizations Electrotherapies: • Ultrasound • Laser • Neuromuscular electrical stimulation (NMES) • Transcutaneous electrical nerve stimulation (TENS) • Pulsed shortwave diathermy (PSWD) Exercise therapy: • Advanced rehabilitation protocols following surgery or injury: strengthening exercises; flexibility exercises; endurance exercises; balance and proprioception exercises • Rehabilitation regimes for sporting and working dogs for return to full function • Gait re-education Other: • Postural management for neurological patients • Positioning and chest care for ICU patients • Maintenance exercises for recumbent patients

9.10 Modalities used in physiotherapy.

Effects of massage

The major effects of massage are:

- Pain relief via:
  - o The 'pain gate'
  - o Removal of noxious chemicals
  - o Release of endogenous endorphins
- Increase in circulation:
  - o Aids healing by improving oxygen supply to tissues and removing metabolic waste products
  - o Increase in venous and lymphatic return
- Mobilization of adhesions, breakdown of scar tissue and restoration of mobility to tissues
- Manual stimulation of the body, improving proprioceptive awareness
- Preparation of muscle for exercise; reduction of muscle fatigue and delayed-onset muscle soreness (DOMS) following exercise
- Reduction of tension and anxiety; aid to relaxation

- Loosening of chest secretions to aid their removal
- Improved bonding between the animal and the professional (or owner) (see Chapter 8).

A summary of the major massage techniques and their specific benefits is given in Figure 9.11.

Massage technique	Major benefits	Other benefits
Stroking (see Figure 9.12)	Accustoms animal to touch; reduces tension and anxiety; lowers muscle tone	Useful to start and finish massage session and as a link between different techniques
Effleurage (see Figure 9.13)	Reduces swelling and oedema	Removes chemical byproducts of inflammation; maintains mobility of soft tissues; stretches muscle
Kneading, picking-up, wringing (see Figures 9.14–9.16)	Increase circulation and lymphatic flow; mobilize soft tissues	Remove chemical byproducts of inflammation; sensory stimulation and invigorating (fast technique); relaxing and lowering of muscle tension (slow technique)
Skin rolling (see Figure 9.17)	Mobilizes skin and scar tissue	
Frictions (see Figure 9.18)	Break down adhesions	Local hyperaemia
Hacking, clapping, beating, pounding (see Figure 9.19)	Increase circulation; loosen chest secretions and stimulate coughing; sensory stimulation	
Shaking, vibration (see Figure 9.20)	Increase circulation; mobilize soft tissues; loosen chest secretions and stimulate coughing	Sensory stimulation; reduce adhesions

9.11 Benefits of massage techniques.

Massage techniques

The following represent the major massage techniques used in small animal treatment.

Stroking techniques: Stroking (Figure 9.12) is primarily used for its calming and soothing effects. This technique is particularly useful with animals that are particularly anxious or stressed due to pain and unfamiliar surroundings (see Chapter 8) and that enjoy human contact. It is best used at the beginning of a treatment session and is an easy technique to teach owners.

Effleurage is a stroking movement generally used to reduce swelling (Figure 9.13). The stroking should be done with even pressure, and each stroke carried to the nearest group of superficial lymphatic nodes, in the axilla (forelimb) or groin and caudal stifle (hindlimb).

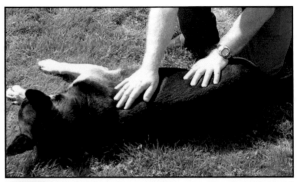

9.12 Stroking involves a gliding movement performed in any direction on the surface of the body, although it usually starts proximally and ends distally.

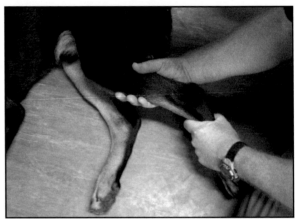

9.13 Effleurage is a stroking movement starting distally and moving proximally in the direction of the flow of the veins and lymphatics. In the limbs the movement starts at the paw. The hand(s) must be relaxed and moulded accurately to the shape of the limb or part being treated.

Pressure techniques (petrissage): These techniques compress and release the muscles and subcutaneous tissues in a rhythmic manner to improve circulation and lymph flow, as well as mobilizing the soft tissues (Figures 9.14 to 9.17).

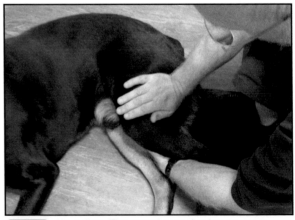

9.14 Kneading. The muscles and subcutaneous tissues are pressed alternately inward and upward by one or both hands. The skin is moved on the underlying tissue, and the hands (or fingers) moved in a circular motion. The hand(s) glides very gently over the area under treatment during the relaxation phase, with small areas being treated with the tips of the fingers or thumb.

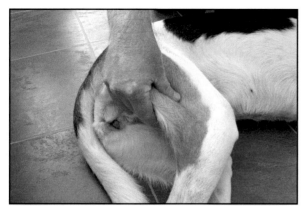

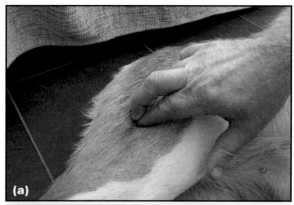

9.15 Picking-up. The muscles are grasped, lifted, squeezed and released. During the lift, the fingers and thumb(s) should be controlled by the intrinsic muscles and the palm(s) must not lose contact with the skin. A good technique for the larger muscles of the fore and hindlimb.

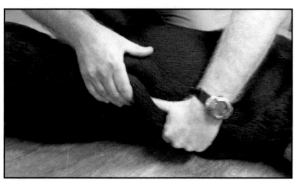

9.16 Wringing. The tissues are grasped with both hands, lifted, and then the hands moved in opposite directions, backwards and forwards across the long axis of the muscles, stretching the tissues. This is a good technique to use on the animal's back and hindquarters.

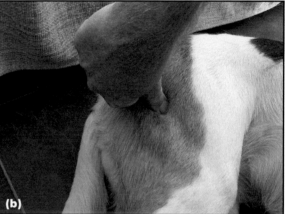

9.18 Frictions are performed by the thumb or fingertips, with the superficial tissues moved on the deeper ones, the depth varying with the structure to be treated. There should be no movement of the finger or thumb on the skin. **(a)** Transverse frictions move across the muscle fibres and maintain even pressure throughout. **(b)** Circular frictions work on one area and progressively increase in depth.

Percussion techniques (tapotement): This is a series of techniques in which the hands strike the body (Figure 9.19). The hands usually work alternately and the wrists are kept flexible so that the movements are springy and invigorating. These techniques are mainly used for musculoskeletal

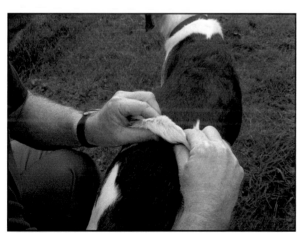

9.17 Skin rolling. The skin and subcutaneous tissues are grasped between the fingers and thumbs of both hands. The tissues are then rolled forwards or backwards against the fingers or thumbs. This is a useful technique for finding adhesions between the skin and deeper structures, and then for treating those adhesions.

Frictions: These are small, accurately localized, penetrating movements performed in a circular or transverse direction, primarily to break down adhesions (Figure 9.18).

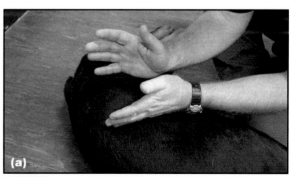

9.19 Percussion. **(a)** Hacking is performed with the ulnar border of the little finger, either alone or supplemented by other fingers. The operator's elbows are flexed to about 90 degrees, the wrists are held in extension, and the fingers are relaxed. The striking movement is one of alternate pronation and supination of the hands/forearms. Hacking is a good technique for the back muscles, and the thicker muscles of the hindquarters. (continues) ▶

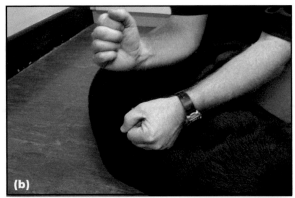

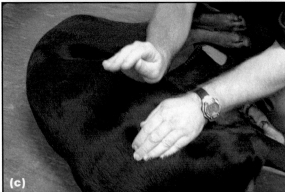

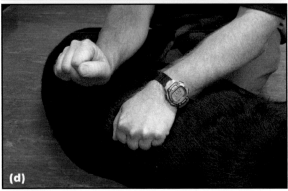

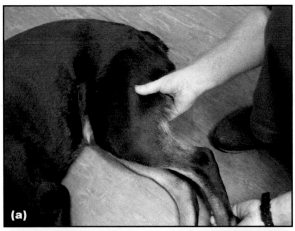

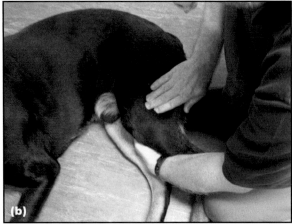

9.20   **(a)** A rhythmic shaking – performed by holding the body part with one or both hands, moving it from side to side, up and down, or in and out to stimulate circulation. **(b)** Vibrations are a finer form of shaking, conveyed through the hands or fingertips for just a few seconds. This technique relaxes the nervous system, is useful over joints and around bony prominences, and near well-healed scar tissue to reduce adhesions. It is generally thought to be more effective in loosening chest secretions than the more vigorous form of shaking.

9.19   (continued) Percussion. **(b)** Pounding uses a similar movement to hacking, with a loosely clenched fist striking the part with the ulnar border of the hand. **(c)** During clapping (coupage) the operator's hands are cupped and the forearms pronated. The elbows are bent, and alternate flexion and extension of the wrists brings the hands sharply into contact with the patient's body, resulting in a deep toned clapping sound. This can be used over most muscular areas, and it is often used over the ribs to loosen secretions. **(d)** Beating is similar to clapping but is performed with a loosely clenched hand so that the dorsal aspect of the fingers and the base of the hand come into contact with the part being treated. Beating should be used only over large muscle groups.

treatment and, because of their stimulatory effects, they are particularly useful for the patient with hypotonicity (flaccidity). Coupage (Figure 9.19c) is also commonly used in chest care of the postoperative or recumbent patient.

Shaking and vibration: These techniques are commonly used in chest care of the postoperative or recumbent patient for loosening secretions, in addition to their role in musculoskeletal treatment (Figure 9.20).

Contraindications and cautions
Massage should **not** be performed on an animal if any of the following apply:

- Acute inflammation
- Infectious diseases
- Pyrexia
- Shock.

Massage should be *avoided* in the area of:

- Infectious skin problems (e.g. ringworm)
- Open wounds
- Unstable fractures
- Acute haematoma
- Neoplasia.

Massage should be undertaken *with care* in the following situations:

- Acute neural conditions such as disc disease, where stimulation may be uncomfortable
- Arthritis, where pressure may be uncomfortable.

Passive movements and stretches

Range of motion (ROM) refers to the full range through which a joint (or muscle) may be moved. Tissues limiting ROM may be normal or pathological and may occur as a common consequence of injury or surgery: joints may develop arthritic changes; wounds and surgical procedures may result in adhesions and fibrosis between tissues; and muscles may shorten because of spasm, contracture or hypertonicity. This loss may be temporary but can become permanent if full ROM is not achieved within 2 weeks (Millis *et al.,* 1997). Loss of range will inevitably limit an animal's functional abilities and create a background for subsequent muscle and joint problems in other body areas due to compensatory postures and gaits. To diminish the effects of disuse and immobilization, joints and muscles must be moved through their available range on a regular basis. This can be carried out by passive or active means.

Passive movements

A passive movement is the movement of a joint by external forces and is generally used when a patient is incapable of moving the joint on its own or when active motion may be injurious to the patient (such as would happen by contracting a muscle soon after surgical repair of that muscle). Passive movements (Figure 9.21) are used to maintain normal range. The most common indications for passive movements in small animal practice are: immediately after surgery; in recumbent animals and those with chronic degenerative conditions; and during recovery from neurological conditions. It is generally appropriate to initiate passive movements as soon after injury as possible, provided there are no contraindications, but movements must be comfortable to the patient and tissues must not be further injured by exceeding the limits of the damaged or repairing tissues. Passive movements *will not* prevent muscle atrophy or increase (maintain) strength.

Stretches

Stretches (Figure 9.22) place more stress on tissues than passive movements, so they are used to improve or regain range of movement that has been lost. They are often carried out in conjunction with passive movements to improve flexibility. Stretches can be more effective following the application of massage or hot packs, and after exercise.

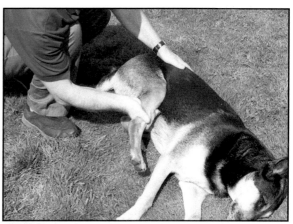

9.22 Stretch applied to hamstrings with hip in flexion and stifle in extension. The muscles are stretched to the point of resistance and held for 30 seconds (range can be increased if resistance eases during this time). The stretch is repeated 2–3 times, and this regime should be performed several times daily.

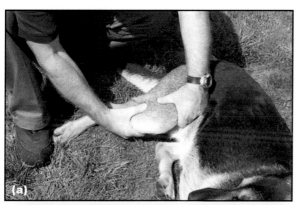
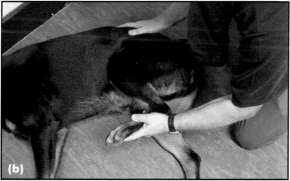

9.21 Passive movements. **(a)** Flexion and extension passive movements performed on the stifle. The joint is moved into flexion to the first point of resistance (or animal reaction), and then similarly into extension. This is repeated in a rhythmic manner 15–20 times, and should be performed several times daily. **(b)** Hindlimb moved in a bicycling motion to simulate normal gait patterning; a useful technique for patients with neurological disease that are unable to walk.

Tightness is a mild shortening of a muscle and has no specific pathology. It is commonly found in muscles that cross two joints (such as biceps brachii and rectus femoris muscles). Stretching exercises can usually restore length to tight muscles.

Contracture is the significant shortening of the muscles and/or other soft tissues around a joint, causing a limit to the joint's range of motion. Contracture is often due to scar tissue, adhesions between different tissues and muscle hypertonicity from upper motor neuron lesions. Contracture is unlikely to be improved through stretching and generally requires surgical intervention to restore range.

There are several different types of stretching, but the following are the most useful within small animal practice:

- *Static stretching* utilizes a low-intensity stretch, which is generally comfortable for the patient, less likely to induce tension in the muscles (through stimulation of muscle spindles and Golgi tendon organs), and less likely to cause damage to the tissues. Low forces applied over a period of time allow collagen fibres to realign (Starring *et al.,* 1988)

- *Prolonged mechanical stretching* is similar, in that a low intensity stretch is applied, but it is held much longer, for a minimum of 20 minutes up to several hours daily. It requires the use of splints (static or dynamic), which can also be used in a serial manner.

Effects of passive movements and stretches

According to Millis *et al.* (2004b), passive movements and stretches:

- Prevent loss of ROM caused by shortening and contracture of soft tissues such as ligaments, tendons and muscles
- Maintain or increase muscle length and flexibility (sarcomere numbers increase with slow, low-load passive stretches)
- Prevent adhesions in articular capsules and joints and therefore maintain joint range
- Improve articular nutrition by increasing synovial fluid production and diffusion
- Maintain mobility between different tissues
- Produce or maintain normal patterns of movement
- Stimulate mechanoreceptors in joints, muscles, skin and other soft tissues and therefore improve proprioceptive awareness
- Reduce the pain caused through tissue shortening
- Increase circulatory and lymphatic return (passive movements).

Contraindications and cautions

Passive movements or stretches should **not** be performed on an animal if any of the following apply:

- Acute injury to a ligament, muscle or tendon, where the repair tissue is not yet strong enough to withstand some stress
- Motion may result in further injury or instability
- Unstable fractures are present.

Passive movements and stretches should be used *with caution*:
- In areas close to any recent fractures
- If there is haemarthrosis
- If there is joint infection
- If there are intravenous catheters in the area being treated
- If the limb has been immobilized for a length of time.

> **WARNING**
> Joints should not be stretched when they are cold.

Joint mobilizations and manipulations

Mobilizations

Mobilizations are passive movements made to joints, used to reduce pain and improve range of motion (ROM) (Figure 9.23). They are performed mainly as

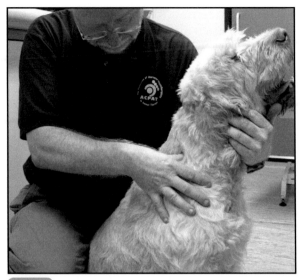

9.23 Mobilizations performed on the cervical spine.

oscillatory movements in either the physiological (able to be performed voluntarily by the individual, e.g. elbow flexion) or accessory (unable to be performed voluntarily, e.g. medial or lateral glide of the patella) range of a joint. Various accessory movements (spins, slides and rolls) occur in joints as a result of the joint anatomy and surrounding musculature (Figure 9.24), but these can sometimes become restricted through injury or disease, thereby limiting the overall range of the joint. Mobilizations help to restore these natural movements and can be performed as low- or high-amplitude movements, in the direction of the joint line, or to achieve compression or distraction of the joint surfaces. Individual joints may be mobilized, or a group of joints can be mobilized synchronously, as with many traction techniques. Some techniques allow mobilizations to be performed alongside active movements of the joint (mobilizations with movement).

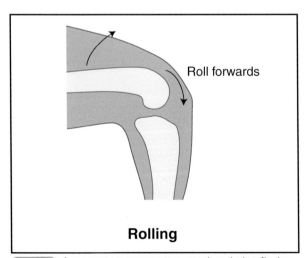

9.24 Accessory movements occurring during flexion to extension movement at the stifle joint. Through the combined movements of rolling, sliding and rotation, the stifle is able to move from flexion to full extension. These movements are reversed when the stifle returns to flexion. Any interference with these accessory movements can result in pain and reduction in range. (continues) ▶

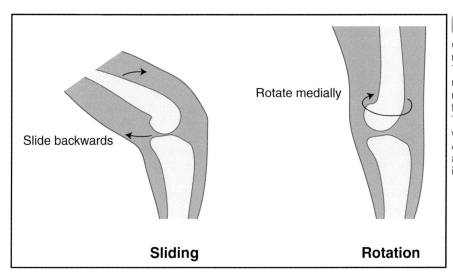

(continued) Accessory movements occurring during flexion to extension movement at the stifle joint. Through the combined movements of rolling, sliding and rotation, the stifle is able to move from flexion to full extension. These movements are reversed when the stifle returns to flexion. Any interference with these accessory movements can result in pain and reduction in range.

Manipulations

Manipulations are low-amplitude, high-velocity thrusts performed at the end of the joint range (Figure 9.25). They can provide pain relief and restoration of joint range, as well as correction of postural asymmetries.

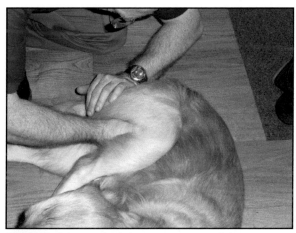

9.25 Joint manipulation to correct a pelvic dysfunction.

Soft tissue techniques

There are a wide range of these used to mobilize and restore extensibility to tissues, improve circulation, and reduce pain. They include: many types of massage; soft tissue release; acupressure; myofascial release and trigger pointing (i.e. treatment of myofascial trigger points, see Chapters 3 and 11); stretching; and proprioceptive neuromuscular facilitation (PNF) (i.e techniques to promote functional movement through facilitation, inhibition, strengthening and relaxation of muscle groups).

Neural mobility (i.e. the ability of nerves to move in relation to their interfaces) can be compromised through injury, surgery and muscle spasm, and can result in pain (localized or referred), paraesthesia and a variety of other sensory aberrations. The status of a nerve's mobility and its neurodynamics in respect of interfaces with surrounding structures such as muscles and bones can be tested by neural provocation tests. The restoration of adequate neural mobility can be achieved through a combination of joint mobilizations, soft tissue release and neural mobilization techniques. Neural mobilizations require detailed knowledge of the course of nerves, and gentle and precise handling of the limbs to effect suitable mobilization of the required nerve (Butler, 1991).

Heat and cold therapies

Heat and cold are simple and effective modalities used in the treatment and rehabilitation of animals. However, their successful use requires a proper assessment of the problems encountered and the effects required (appropriate to the stage of the inflammatory process reached; Heinrichs, 2004).

- Cold should be used in the acute stages of inflammation (during the first 2–3 days).
- Heat is used subsequent to this (days 4–5 onwards), once the acute phase is over.

Heat (thermotherapy)

Heat has been used for centuries as a means of managing acute and chronic conditions.

- *Superficial heating* penetrates to a depth of approximately 1–2 cm.
- *Deep heating* penetrates more deeply (average half value depth – the point in a tissue at which the intensity of heat is half that at the surface – approximately 4 cm).

Superficial forms of heating include hot packs or wraps, hotwater bottles, baths/spas, hosing, heat pads and warm-air driers; the water-based forms (e.g. hotwater bottles or hot packs) allow more effective penetration through the tissues. These are particularly useful in subacute and chronic conditions to relieve pain and as a prequel to passive movements, stretches or exercise. Deep heating can be achieved by the use of electrotherapy modalities such as therapeutic ultrasound, which must only be carried out by operators trained and competent in its use, because of the potential inherent dangers, including tissue burns, tissue destruction, blood cell stasis and endothelial damage.

Hot packs should be applied to the area being treated for 15–30 minutes. They should be wrapped in a towel prior to application, but the number of layers will depend on the temperature of the pack. The therapist should always check the temperature on themselves before applying a hot pack, especially following microwaving. The temperature of the pack should not exceed 75°C. Some commercial hot packs contain a gel, which may be toxic, so patients must be observed to ensure they do not bite the pack. Owners can be taught how to use hot packs at home but must be made aware of the possible dangers: they must understand the importance of ensuring the pack is just comfortably warm, that they should try it on themselves first, and that they should monitor their pet at all times when in use.

Effects of heat: According to Kitchen (2008), heat:

- Reduces pain. Various mechanisms have been suggested for this effect, including: the reduction of secondary muscle spasm; increasing circulation to ischaemic muscle; as a counterirritant; the removal of pain-inducing metabolites or inflammatory byproducts; stimulation of cutaneous thermoreceptors; and the inhibition of pain transmission via the 'pain gate' and, possibly, due to changes in nerve conduction velocity
- Reduces blood pressure
- Reduces muscle spasm and aids muscle relaxation
- Increases local circulation (vasodilatation) and metabolism
- Increases capillary pressure and blood vessel permeability (which can have the negative effect of promoting oedema)
- Increases leucocyte migration into the heated area and accelerates tissue healing
- Improves tissue elasticity
- Increases nerve conduction velocity.

Contraindications and cautions: Heat therapy should **not** be applied in areas affected by the following:

- Acute inflammation
- Active or recent bleeding or haemorrhage
- Open wounds
- Cardiac insufficiency
- Impaired circulation in the area to be treated
- Pyrexia
- Malignancy
- Poor body heat regulation
- Devitalized tissue, e.g. after radiotherapy.

> **WARNING**
> Caution should be exercised in patients that are sedated or have decreased sensation as they are unable to react to burning.

Cold (cryotherapy)

Cold penetrates deeper and lasts longer than heat. It is most effective when used immediately after trauma (accidental or surgical) during the acute phase of inflammation. It will provide analgesia, reduce inflammation, control bleeding, and reduce muscle spasm (Olsen and Stravino, 1972; McMaster, 1977; Chartered Society of Physiotherapy, 2002).

The simplest method of cold application is to wrap a freezer bag containing crushed ice in a thin damp cloth and apply to the area being treated for 10–15 minutes. This can be repeated every 2 hours if necessary (for severe injuries) but for most postoperative indications application should be made every 3–4 hours (i.e. three or four times during the day). Superficial tissues show the most rapid cooling and rewarming effects. Deeper muscle layers respond more slowly and may take as long as 60 minutes to return to baseline temperature after a 10-minute ice application (90 minutes after a 15-minute application). Commercial cold packs may contain a toxic gel, so patients should always be monitored when using these packs to ensure they do not bite them. Packs at temperatures lower than –20°C should not be used. Cold compression units are very effective as they combine cold with compression (Figure 9.26), and most research indicates greater effectiveness of this method over cold packs (Merrick *et al.*, 1993; Glenn *et al.*, 2004).

Ice can also be used to provide sensory input for patients with neurological problems. Ice massage (Figure 9.27) stimulates the local mechanoreceptors and so is useful for stimulating flaccid muscles.

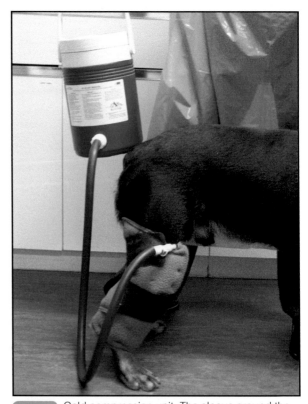

9.26 Cold compression unit. The sleeve around the animal's limb is connected by a hose to a container filled with iced water. Water enters the sleeve by gravitational effect when the container is held above it. The hose can then be disconnected to allow the animal to move around or exercise. At the conclusion of treatment, the hose is reconnected and the container lowered to empty the sleeve.

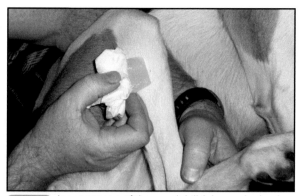

9.27 Ice massage of the cranial tibial muscle. Ice is rubbed over the area using short strokes for 5–10 minutes, parallel to the muscle fibres.

Effects of cryotherapy: According to Heinrichs (2004) and Kitchen (2008), cryotherapy:

- Reduces pain
- Reduces blood flow (vasoconstriction) and haemorrhage
- Reduces inflammation and oedema formation
- Reduces muscle tone (spasticity)
- Reduces metabolism and histamine release
- Reduces nerve conduction velocity
- Increases connective tissue stiffness
- Increases muscle viscosity temporarily (reduced ability to perform rapid movements).

Contraindications and cautions: Cold therapy should **not** be applied:

- In advanced cardiovascular disease
- In acute febrile illness
- To individuals who are cold-sensitive
- In some acute skin conditions, e.g. eczema, dermatitis.

Cold therapy should **not** be applied in areas affected by the following:

- Local areas of impaired peripheral circulation
- Areas of ischaemia; generalized or localized vascular compromise
- History of frostbite or impaired thermoregulation
- Radiotherapy or other ionizing radiations used in the last 6 months
- Open or infected wounds (without appropriate precautions)
- Malignant tissue
- Extensive scar tissue – poor blood supply may lead to cell damage through excessive chilling.

WARNING
- Never apply ice directly to skin (ice massage is an exception).
- Always cover ice packs with a damp towel.
- Take care when applying cold packs directly over superficial metal plates. (The high conductivity of metal allows the effect of the cold to be prolonged, even when the cold pack is removed, thereby potentially preventing healing). Cold compression units are preferable.

Electrotherapy

All electrotherapy modalities should only be performed by operators who have received specialist training and gained a thorough understanding of the indications, contraindications, physiological effects and practical use of each. It is, however, valuable for the veterinary surgeon in general practice to have some knowledge of the types that are commonly used within a physiotherapy treatment programme and the effects they can have, so that referral can be made to trained operators, or training undertaken.

Laser therapy

A laser can be considered a form of light amplifier, providing enhancement of particular properties of light energy. Many different types are available, but for therapeutic purposes Class 3A or 3B lasers are used. Most lasers generate light in the visible red and infrared bands, with typical wavelengths of 600–1000 nm. The treatment device may be a single emitter (or probe) or a group of several emitters (cluster probe) containing a combination of lasers and light-emitting diodes (LEDs). Although much of the applied laser light is absorbed by the superficial tissues, deeper effects can be achieved. Lasers are generally considered to be a non-thermal energy application, but it should be appreciated that delivery and absorption of any energy to the body will result in the development of heat to some extent. The cell membrane appears to be the primary absorber of the energy, which then generates intracellular effects. Laser light irradiation of the tissues therefore acts as a trigger for the alteration of cellular metabolic processes. Research into the clinical effects of laser therapy has concentrated on a few key areas. Most dominant amongst these are the effects on wound healing, inflammatory arthropathies, soft tissue injury and the relief of pain. There is some supportive evidence for the clinical use of lasers in humans (Mester *et al.*, 1985; Anders *et al.*, 2004; Ferreira *et al.*, 2005) but, as with many treatment modalities, evidence of their value in animal care is currently limited.

Ultrasound

Ultrasound therapy, which requires the use of a coupling agent between the transducer and the animal's skin, can be used to produce thermal as well as non-thermal effects. Because of the high protein content of hair, much of the energy transmitted is absorbed by the animal's hair coat; even a thick layer of gel does not improve the situation, so clipping is always recommended. The best absorbing tissues in terms of clinical practice are those with a high collagen content (i.e. ligament, tendon, fascia, joint capsule, scar tissue; ter Haar (1999), Watson (2000)). As it is difficult to know the thickness of tissues in each patient, average half value depths (the point in a tissue at which the intensity of ultrasound is half that at the surface) of 2.0 cm (for 3 MHz) and 4.0 cm (for 1 MHz) are generally employed.

The application of ultrasound during the inflammatory, proliferative and repair phases of tissue healing is of value because it stimulates or enhances the normal sequence of events, and thus increases the efficiency of the repair process. It can also influence the remodelling of scar tissue by enhancing the appropriate orientation of the newly formed collagen fibres and influencing the collagen profile, thus increasing tensile strength and enhancing scar mobility (Nussbaum, 1998). Recent papers have also identified the benefits of using low-intensity pulsed ultrasound for normally healing (fresh) fractures and delayed or non-unions, as well as stress fractures; several of these have included studies on animals (Warden *et al.*, 1999; Tis *et al.*, 2002; Sakurakichi *et al.*, 2004).

Electrical nerve stimulation

Electrical nerve stimulation is widely used in veterinary physiotherapy for muscle stimulation, using NMES (neuromuscular electrical stimulation), and for pain relief, using TENS (transcutaneous electrical nerve stimulation) (see Chapter 3). Models of stimulator that incorporate both functions are available, but in the UK separate machines are generally used. The stimulators utilize a small control unit connected via leads to electrodes that are applied to the patient's skin. With animals, the use of a conductivity gel is recommended to achieve optimum electrode contact. Clipping the hair over the area to be treated will further improve contact.

Neuromuscular electrical stimulation: Stimulation of the motor nerves can be achieved with a wide range of frequencies. Stimulation at low frequencies (e.g. 1 Hz) results in a series of twitches, whilst stimulation at 50 Hz results in a tetanic contraction. Evidence exists for the 'strengthening' effect of NMES, which is particularly useful for animals who cannot generate useful voluntary contraction on demand and for those who find active exercise difficult, such as patients with neurological disease (Selkowitz, 1989; Lake, 1992). There is no evidence that NMES has any significant benefit over active exercise, and the use of such treatment is generally stopped once the animal is able to exercise its muscles actively.

Caution should be exercised when using NMES: it is possible to stimulate the muscle beyond its point of fatigue because the contractions are forced via the motor nerve. Short stimulation periods with adequate rest are required.

Effects of NMES (in animals that cannot exercise actively) are:

- Muscle strengthening and prevention of disuse muscle atrophy
- Muscle re-education and facilitation of muscle control
- Improved sensory awareness
- Decreased spasticity and muscle spasm
- Blood flow changes
- Reduction of oedema.

Transcutaneous electrical nerve stimulation: TENS primarily aims to provide symptomatic pain relief by specifically exciting sensory nerves and thereby stimulating either the 'pain gate' mechanism and/or the endogenous opioid system. Pain relief by means of the pain gate mechanism (Traditional TENS, Hi TENS or Normal TENS) involves activation (excitation) of the Aβ sensory fibres, reducing transmission of noxious stimuli from the C pain fibres, via GABA and presynaptic inhibition in the dorsal horn of the spinal cord. The Aβ fibres respond most effectively at a relatively high rate (90–130 Hz). There does not seem to be a single frequency that works best for every patient, but this range appears to cover the majority of individuals. This method of action is rapid in onset and offset, having a limited carry-over effect once the machine is stopped. An alternative approach (Acupuncture TENS, Lo TENS or AL-TENS) is to stimulate the Aδ fibres which respond preferentially to a much lower rate of stimulation (2–5 Hz). This activates the opioid mechanisms and provides pain relief through the release of endogenous opiates (encephalins) in the spinal cord which, in turn, reduces the activation of the noxious sensory pathways. This has a slower onset and offset, but may have a carry over that lasts several hours.

Positioning of the electrodes is not an exact science and there are many alternatives that have been researched and found to be effective in human patients:

- Either side of the lesion or painful area
- At the appropriate nerve root(s) level
- Along the peripheral nerve
- Over the motor point
- Over trigger point(s) or acupuncture point(s) (see Chapters 3 and 11)
- Over the appropriate dermatome, myotome or sclerotome.

Contraindications to electrical nerve stimulation:

- Patients with implanted pacemakers.
- Patients who have an allergic response to the electrode, tape or gel.
- Patients with skin conditions (e.g. eczema, dermatitis).
- Patients with current or recent bleeding/ haemorrhage.
- Stimulation over infected areas or neoplasms.
- Patients with open wounds, i.e. not near the open wounds, but elsewhere is safe.
- Patients with compromised circulation, e.g. ischaemic tissue, thrombosis and associated conditions.
- Application over:
  o The ventral aspect of the neck or carotid sinus (stimulation of the carotid sinus may lead to an acute hypotensive response via a vasovagal reflex. It may also stimulate laryngeal nerves leading to laryngeal spasm)
  o The heart
  o Lower trunk, abdomen or pelvis during pregnancy
  o The eyes
  o Areas lacking sensation
  o Active epiphyseal regions in growing animals.

> **WARNING**
>
> The use of any electrotherapy modality should only be undertaken by a professional properly trained in its use, to ensure that it is used safely, appropriately and most effectively.

Therapeutic exercise

Therapeutic exercise is the systematic performance or execution of planned physical movements, postures, or activities intended to:

- Prevent long-term physical impairment
- Enhance function
- Reduce risk of injury
- Optimize overall health
- Enhance fitness and wellbeing.

Exercise represents the final element in the process of helping an animal achieve optimum function following injury, surgery or disease and so forms an integral component of any rehabilitation programme. All animals should be given the opportunity to achieve maximum function and, if necessary, referral should be made to a veterinary physiotherapist at discharge for further rehabilitation advice. Effective rehabilitation may make the difference between an animal simply coping with its disabilities or functioning normally.

Therapeutic exercise may be used to improve:

- Aerobic capacity and endurance
- Agility, coordination and balance – static and dynamic
- Gait and locomotion
- Neuromuscular capability and movement patterning
- Postural stabilization
- Joint ROM
- Strength and power.

Types of exercise

There are four main types of therapeutic exercise.

Strengthening (power): Strength is the ability of a muscle or muscle group to produce tension and a resulting force. Exercises to improve strength create an increase in the myofibril content of the muscle and, as a result, increase its cross-sectional area. Strengthening exercises include such activities as running, hill work (uphill and downhill), pulling weights, dancing (Figure 9.28), wheelbarrowing and swimming. Animals with marked weakness may require assistance to stand and walk using 'physio' rolls and harnesses (see Chapter 14).

Endurance (stamina): Endurance is important to those dogs that have to perform prolonged activities, such as long-distance running (e.g. sled dogs, trailhounds), herding and swimming (rescue). Exercises to improve aerobic endurance usually target muscle groups for periods longer than 15 minutes, and are repeated several times each week. Long-term changes occur in muscle, including increased vascularization (which increases the amount of oxygen

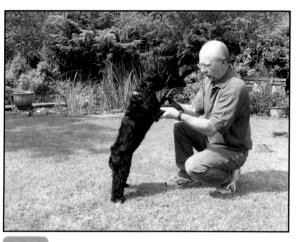

9.28 'Dancing' is a muscle-strengthening exercise.

taken to the muscle), together with decreased resting heart rate and increased stroke volume (which allow greater time for ventricular filling), decreased resting blood pressure, and increased respiratory enzymes (for generating energy quicker). Endurance exercises would include trotting, swimming (Figure 9.29), treadmill activity and sled pulling.

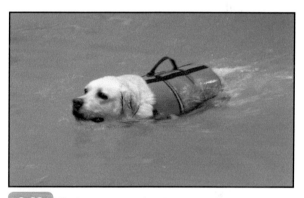

9.29 Endurance exercises include swimming.

Flexibility (suppleness): Flexibility is the ability of the muscles, tendons and ligaments to stretch, allowing the joints to have a larger ROM, and the animal to be able to manoeuvre through awkward spaces. Flexibility helps to protect against injury, and is particularly important in cats and sporting and working dogs, although all animals require good flexibility. Flexibility exercises include any activities that make the animal reach or stretch for something, or flex the vertebral column in different directions. These include crawling under or stepping over obstacles, stair climbing, baiting and weaving (Figure 9.30).

Balance and proprioception: Balance is the ability to adjust equilibrium at a stance (static balance) or during locomotion (dynamic balance), and to take account of changes in direction or ground surfaces. Proprioception is the unconscious perception of movement and spatial orientation originating from the body position. Proprioception decreases with age, and can also be affected by injury or surgery. It is especially affected by neurological pathology. All

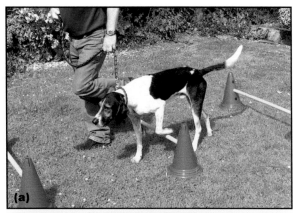

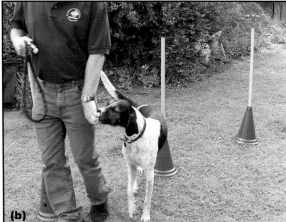

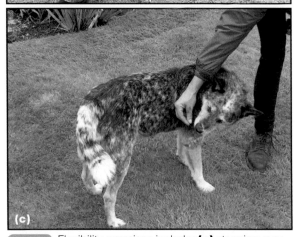

9.30 Flexibility exercises include: **(a)** stepping over obstacles; **(b)** weaving; and **(c)** baiting (here, a treat is used to encourage the animal to move in a certain way, thereby mobilizing its spine and adjusting its balance and weightbearing).

animals need satisfactory balance and proprioception to function normally, but many sporting and working dogs need heightened levels if they are to cope with the demands of their work. Balance exercises include activities requiring rapid responses to changes of the supporting surface, e.g. wobble boards, balance pads (Figure 9.31), trampolines, changes of direction when running, ball-playing, dancing and standing on the gym ball (small dogs and cats). Proprioception exercises include walking in circles or weaving (see Figure 9.30b), walking over obstacles or on different types of surface, and weight shifting.

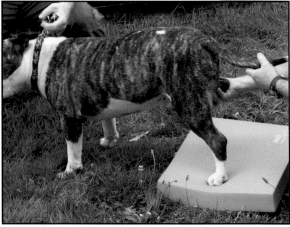

9.31 Balance exercises include activities requiring rapid responses to changes of the supporting surface. Balance pads can be used to achieve these.

Exercise progression

Therapeutic exercise can take several forms:

- **Assisted exercise.** When muscle strength or coordination is inadequate to perform any movement at all, an external force is required to compensate for the deficiency. Passively moving an animal's limb through a normal walking pattern is an example of this.
- **Active-assisted exercise.** When muscle strength or coordination is inadequate to perform a full movement, an external force is required to compensate for the deficiency. As the animal recovers, limb use returns to some extent but may still require some assistance from a therapist.
- **Free active exercise.** Muscle strength and coordination is adequate to perform a movement, but only against the forces of gravity and bodyweight, e.g. sitting to standing.
- **Resisted exercise.** Muscle strength and coordination is adequate to perform a movement against gravity, bodyweight and additional resistance, e.g. using weights.

Animals commencing a rehabilitation programme will be at different points on the exercise scale, depending on their current ability, but will then progress through the other stages as strength and coordination improves:

Assisted → Active-assisted → Free active → Resisted

Basic to any exercise programme are the concepts of overload and specificity.

- *Overload* is the principle of applying increased difficulty to an exercise, so the body gradually adapts to cope with the extra demands placed on it. In the case of strengthening exercises, the resistance applied is gradually increased (by increasing the load, number of repetitions or speed of the activity); in the case of proprioceptive exercises, the stability of the supporting surface is gradually reduced.

• *Specificity* relates to the content of the programme, ensuring that it provides exercises appropriate to the ultimate needs of each individual. For example, a sled dog requires high levels of strength and stamina, whereas an agility dog requires greater flexibility and proprioception.

Rehabilitation

Rehabilitation is an integral component of physiotherapy and is the process of helping an individual who has had an illness or injury to achieve the highest level of function, independence and quality of life possible. The success of many surgeries owes as much to the rehabilitation carried out as to the surgical technique performed (Johnson and Johnson, 1993; Marsolais *et al.*, 2002) and it has been predominantly because of advances in rehabilitation that many human postoperative outcomes have improved so markedly over the last 10 years (Shelbourne and Gray, 1997).

The goal of any rehabilitation programme is to regain symptom-free movement and function. Such an approach generally takes the form of a dynamic programme of prescribed exercise and other techniques for preventing, limiting or reversing the deleterious effects of inactivity, injury or disease processes, while returning the individual to a level of activity as close as possible to their former pre-injury level. Rehabilitation can be effective for patients with neurological dysfunction and respiratory dysfunction, as well as neuromuscular and musculoskeletal disorders. Designing an effective rehabilitation programme requires the ability to assess which components of a movement are not working adequately, whether normal actions can be achieved and how best to achieve them (Figure 9.32).

---

1. Assessment of the animal and identification of its problems:
   • Affected structures and functional limitations
   • Stage of recovery
   • Desired outcome for the owners.
2. Development of a treatment plan, with realistic outcome goals.
3. Design of an exercise programme that will achieve those goals.
4. Continued evaluation of progress:
   • Adjustment of goals.
   • Progression/alteration of exercises.

9.32 Stages in the design of an effective rehabilitation programme.

One of the major aims of a rehabilitation programme is to counteract the effects of immobilization and disuse. Immobilization may be indicated as part of the treatment of many musculoskeletal injuries in order to allow an adequate healing time and environment. However, immobilization has severe detrimental effects on body structures (see below); to counteract these effects, a comprehensive rehabilitation programme should include various types of therapeutic exercise. These include exercises for strength (and power), flexibility, endurance (muscle and cardiovascular), proprioception and skill. However, the process of remobilizing tissues after injury

and immobilization requires a delicate balance between providing sufficient exercise to challenge repaired tissues without overworking them and causing further damage. Effective rehabilitation demands a thoughtful and knowledgeable approach in order to create the best environment for healing and recovery.

Immobilization, disuse and remobilization

Immobilization occurs when a limb is maintained in a fixed position by splints, casts or external fixators. Disuse occurs when a part of the body is not used because of injury, surgery or restriction of mobility (cage rest) and can affect muscle, bone, ligament, tendon and articular cartilage. The importance of exercise and movement in any rehabilitation programme is clear when the effects of immobilization and disuse on body tissues are examined (Figure 9.33).

Muscle

• Decrease in muscle fibre size and number (increase in ratio of connective tissue to muscle fibre); decrease in number of sarcomeres
• Decrease in size and number of mitochondria
• Decrease in total muscle weight (atrophy)
• Increase in muscle contraction time
• Decrease in muscle tension produced
• Decrease in levels of glycogen and ATP
• More rapid decrease in level of ATP during exercise
• Greater increase in lactate concentration during exercise
• Decrease in protein synthesis

Articular cartilage

• Decrease in proteoglycan synthesis and increase in proteoglycan proteolysis
• Softening of articular cartilage (leading to mineralization and thickening of subchondral bone)
• Decrease in articular cartilage thickness (30–50% loss)
• Reduced nutrition of cartilage (due to reduced synovial fluid production and reduced synovial pumping and nutrient diffusion)
• Adherence of fibrofatty connective tissue to cartilage surfaces
• Pressure necrosis at points of cartilage–cartilage contact
• Chondrocyte death

Ligaments and tendons

• Significant decrease in linear stress, maximum stress and stiffness
• Decrease in fibril cross-sectional area, resulting in a decrease in fibril size and density
• Decrease in synthesis and degradation of collagen
• Disorganization of parallel fibre arrangement and haphazard arrangement of new collagen fibres
• Reduction in load- and energy-absorbing capabilities of the bone–ligament/bone–tendon complex
• Decrease in glycosaminoglycan level reducing water content and extensibility
• Increase in osteoclastic activity at the bone–ligament/bone–tendon junction, causing an increase in bone resorption and destruction of ligament/tendon fibres in that area

Bone

• Increase in bone resorption and decrease in bone deposition
• Reduction in cortical and cancellous bone mass
• Reduction in cortical bone density and stiffness
• Bone loss, particularly in the more distal weightbearing bones
• Osteoporosis and osteopenia

9.33 The effects of immobilization on various body tissues.

Articular cartilage

The changes that occur to articular cartilage are due to a combination of decreased joint motion and reduced loading. Although both are important to maintain cartilage integrity, normal loading is particularly important because it also activates those muscles that span the joint and stabilize the limb during weightbearing.

If high levels of stress and repeated loading are applied immediately following a period of immobilization, further damage may be caused to the softened cartilage. Gentle prolonged remobilization has been shown to be more beneficial in restoring normal properties of cartilage in dogs (Palmoski *et al.*, 1979).The effects of immobilization for periods of 6 weeks or less are generally reversible after several weeks of mild remobilization. Longer immobilization periods (11 weeks or more) require much greater periods of remobilization to reverse the deleterious effects, but even 50 weeks of rehabilitation is unlikely to reverse the effects completely. In particular, immobilization of the joints of young dogs may cause permanent changes to articular cartilage, such that joints may be predisposed to degenerative changes as the dog ages (Millis, 2004).

Muscle

Muscles that are most prone to disuse atrophy are the postural muscles that contain a large proportion of type I (slow twitch) fibres and generally only cross one joint (such as vastus medialis and vastus intermedius). The next most vulnerable group are the antigravity muscles that cross multiple joints but are also composed mainly of type I fibres (such as gastrocnemius and rectus femoris). Those that are least susceptible to atrophy are those that are intermittently activated, contain mainly type II (fast twitch) fibres, and cross multiple joints (such as biceps femoris and cranial tibial muscles) (Lieber *et al.*, 1988).

Immobilization results in a decreased cross-sectional diameter of the muscle and a rapid decrease in strength, especially during the first week of immobilization, with up to 50% of the peak force being lost in humans (Musacchia *et al.*, 1988; Appell, 1990). Muscles that are immobilized in a lengthened position generally show less atrophy. Fortunately, most of the changes that occur during immobilization are reversible and it is generally expected that a remobilization period of twice the immobilization period will return limb circumference to normal values (Shires *et al.*, 1982 (dogs); Heerkens *et al.*, 1987 (humans)).

Ligaments and tendons

Injuries to ligaments and tendons often require a period of immobilization to aid the healing process, but this is quite likely to result in an adverse decline in structural and material properties, with the bone–tendon/bone–ligament complex particularly affected. Cage confinement will have less effect than immobilization in a cast. Remobilization returns the mechanical properties to nearly normal over time, but recovery of the bony insertion sites is prolonged compared to the ligament/tendon mid-substance. A remobilization period of three times the immobilization period restores many of the structural properties, but as much as 12 months may be required for complete recovery. In humans, the maintenance of joint ROM and reducing the period of immobilization helps preserve ligament properties, reducing the required period of remobilization (Keira *et al.*, 1996).

Bone

The recovery of mechanical and morphological properties of bone following a period of immobilization depends on:

* The length and type of immobilization
* The type and intensity of remobilization
* The age of the animal.

Recovery is greater in younger dogs, and older dogs have more residual deficits (Jaworski and Uhthoff, 1986). Short periods of immobilization (e.g. 6 weeks) can often achieve good recovery with 2–3 months of remobilization; longer periods of immobilization (e.g. 32 weeks) are likely to result in bone loss of 30–50% despite long periods of remobilization. This limited recovery is probably due to changes that occur in trabecular bone architecture: increases in trabecular bone width are evident but there is no recovery of those trabeculae lost during immobilization. Hence, remobilization adds bone on to existing surfaces, but is unable to restore lost trabeculae.

Preoperative physiotherapy

Preoperative physiotherapy is an often neglected area that can be a major benefit to the eventual outcome of the surgery performed, as described in human studies (Shelbourne and Gray, 1997; De Carlo *et al.*, 1999). While it is not always possible, especially when emergency surgery is required, elective surgeries may benefit from a period of preoperative physiotherapy and rehabilitation.

Preoperative physiotherapy:

* Prepares the animal physically for the forthcoming surgery, by improving muscle strength and joint stability, ROM, balance and proprioception
* Familiarizes the animal with the type of exercises required following surgery. For example, animals familiar with the hydrotherapy pool and surroundings, procedures and staff, are less likely to react negatively when reintroduced to the pool following surgery. This is less likely to result in damage to the surgical site than if the animal is unfamiliar with the surroundings
* Provides owners with a sense of involvement
* In some cases, the animal may improve to such a degree that surgery is no longer required.

Postoperative rehabilitation

Postoperative patients probably represent the major recipients of physiotherapeutic care in veterinary practice and it is likely that most of these will have had orthopaedic or neurological surgery (see Chapters 13 and 14). The value of basic physiotherapy carried out during the first few postoperative days should not be underestimated, and it can have a major impact on the eventual outcome of the surgery (Taylor and Adamson, 2002). Physiotherapy would include treatments such as: effleurage and cold therapy, to control the inflammatory process; passive movements and gentle mobilization, to restore strength and ROM; and simple balance exercises to improve balance, weightbearing and proprioception. Rehabilitation should then be progressed at a speed appropriate to the animal's condition.

Physiotherapy protocols are available in a number of texts (Bockstahler *et al.*, 2004; Millis *et al.*, 2004a; Sharp, 2008a), which provide useful guidance on the appropriate physiotherapy for most orthopaedic and neurological surgeries. In practice, however, all patients are different and will arrive in the clinic with various pre-existing conditions, various levels of fitness and different postoperative recoveries. It is incumbent on the veterinary surgeon (in consultation with the veterinary physiotherapist) to assess the patient's needs fully and select the most appropriate therapeutic modalities for each individual patient at each stage of recovery.

Special considerations

Physiotherapy for cats
In general terms, cats are more protective of their injuries than dogs and, because of their lighter bulk they exert fewer weightbearing stresses on their injured limbs. Although the principles and techniques of physiotherapy described in this chapter are applicable to all species, the feline patient is generally less tolerant of the regular handling involved in physiotherapeutic care than are most canine patients and is less accepting of new activities; therefore, modification of techniques and their application may be required. In cats, the tolerance, and therefore benefits, of leash walking and hydrotherapy are restricted to just a few individuals. To achieve satisfactory results, treatment sessions with cats should be kept short, exercises introduced more gradually, and items familiar to the cat, such as toys, used more frequently.

Manual therapies (Figure 9.34a), electrotherapies and rehabilitative therapies can all be used successfully in cats. Many exercises described above (e.g. dancing (Figure 9.34b), wheelbarrowing, baiting) can be readily adapted. In addition, cats will follow, chase and 'pat' objects such as toys dragged along the floor or waved in the air and these activities will help improve strength, ROM and balance. Beams of light from torches can be guided along the floor and across walls to gain the cat's interest and encourage movement.

Elderly patients
Advances in medical and surgical treatment have increased the lifespan of many dogs and cats. The effects of aging and the presence of multiple comorbidities can often challenge the veterinary surgeon in respect of diagnosis, treatment and management. Muscles tend to atrophy with age, bones lose density

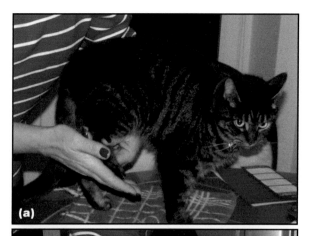

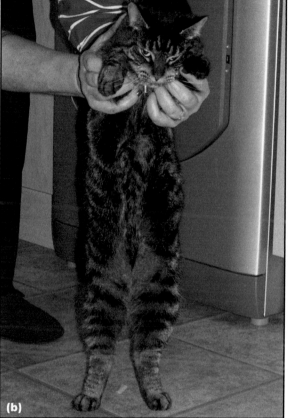

9.34 Manual treatments such as **(a)** massage and passive movements, as well as **(b)** exercises to improve strength and mobility can be used in cats.

and cartilage degenerates. Fractures and soft tissue injuries require longer healing times, and many elderly dogs develop degenerative conditions such as arthritis. Disc disease and conditions such as degenerative myelopathy and neoplasia are more common in older dogs. Respiratory conditions may develop as lungs lose elasticity, fibrosis develops, cough reflex decreases and pulmonary secretions become more viscous. Cognitive dysfunctions may develop and affect the patient's ability to participate in treatment and rehabilitation programmes. The veterinary team has a vitally important role in maintaining the quality of life in elderly patients and, in particular, the physiotherapist can provide valuable input into the management process for this group of patients through the maintenance of mobility and function.

Approach	Benefits achieved	How achieved
Positioning	Improved respiratory function (ventilation/perfusion relationship); prevention of pressure sores; reduced dependent limb oedema; prevention of spastic patterns developing (hypertonic animals)	Regular repositioning (alternation between right, left and sternal recumbency every 2–4 hours) Elevation of limb above heart level Neutral positioning of limbs Calm, gentle handling
Chest care	Maintenance of bronchial hygiene; loosening and elimination of secretions from airways; re-expansion of atelectatic lung segments; improved oxygenation; reduced incidence of pneumonia	Gentle exercise Positioning Postural drainage (10–20 minutes) in conjunction with: massage – coupage (1–2 minutes), vibrations (4–6 breathing cycles, treat on expiration only)
ROM maintenance	Maintenance of joint and muscle range; prevention of contractures	Passive movements Stretches Active exercise
Control of swelling	Quicker recovery time; no loss of range; reduced scar formation	Cryotherapy Effleurage Elevation of limb above heart level
Pain relief	Greater comfort; quicker recovery time; earlier mobilization	Neutral positioning and regular repositioning Passive movements Gentle massage TENS
Progressive exercise	Reduced loss of strength; reduced loss of ROM; reduced loss of balance and proprioception; loosening and elimination of secretions from airways; re-expansion of atelectatic lung segments	Assisted, active-assisted or active standing and walking

9.35 Major physiotherapeutic approaches in critical care patients.

Intensive care patients

Physiotherapy for patients admitted to the ICU is primarily required to offset the effects of immobility, in addition to dealing with the primary reason for the admittance. The enforced reduction in physical activity results in significant changes to the musculoskeletal and cardiovascular systems; in human patients, bed rest for even a week can lead to marked muscle atrophy, loss of ROM, exercise intolerance, increased risk of pressure sores, pulmonary complications and deep vein thrombosis and it has been hypothesized that similar changes occur in animal patients (Dunning *et al.*, 2005). As soon as the animal is stable, rehabilitative procedures should be started to prevent the secondary onset of these changes. A proactive approach to rehabilitation is preferable to a reactive approach to a worsening situation, and even simple physiotherapy techniques (such as positioning, massage, passive movements and stretching) can make a huge improvement to the eventual functional outcome of the patient (Manning, 2004; Sharp, 2008a). The main physiotherapeutic approaches to patients in ICU are given in Figure 9.35. More details are given in some of the case examples later in this Manual.

References and further reading

Anders JJ, Geuna S and Rochkind S (2004) Phototherapy promotes regeneration and functional recovery of injured peripheral nerve. *Neurological Research* **26**, 233–239

Appell HJ (1990) Muscular atrophy following immobilisation: a review. *Sports Medicine* **10**, 42–58

Bockstahler B, Levine D and Millis D (2004) *Essential Facts of Physiotherapy in Dogs and Cats*. BE VetVerlag, Babenhausen, Germany

Butler DS (1991) *Mobilisation of the Nervous System*. Churchill Livingstone, Melbourne, Australia

Chartered Society of Physiotherapy (2002) *Guidelines for the Management of Soft Tissue Injury with PRICE*. Available from: http://www.csp.org.uk/effective practice/clinical guidelines/physiotherapyguidelines.cfm

De Carlo M, Shelbourne KD and Oneacre K (1999) Rehabilitation program for both knees when the contralateral autogenous patellar tendon graft is used for primary anterior cruciate ligament reconstruction: a case study. *Journal of Orthopaedic and Sports Physical Therapy* **29**, 144–159

Dunning D, Haling KB and Ehrhart N (2005) Rehabilitation of medical and acute care patients. *Veterinary Clinics of North America: Small Animal Practice* **35**, 1411–1426

Ferreira DM, Zangaro RA, Villaverde AB *et al.* (2005) Analgesic effect of He-Ne (632.8 nm) low-level therapy on acute inflammatory pain. *Photomedicine and Laser Surgery* **23**, 177–181

Glenn R, Spindler K, Warren T *et al.* (2004) Cryotherapy decreases intraarticular temperature after ACL reconstruction. *Clinical Orthopaedics and Related Research* **421**, 268–272

Heerkens YF *et al.* (1987) Passive resistance of the human knee: the effect of remobilisation. *Journal of Biomedical Engineering* **9**, 69–76

Heinrichs K (2004) Superficial thermal modalities. In: *Canine Rehabilitation and Physical Therapy*, ed. DL Millis *et al.*, pp. 277–288. Saunders, St. Louis

Jaworski ZF and Uhthoff HK (1986) Reversibility of nontraumatic disuse osteoporosis during its active phase. *Bone* **21**, 431–439

Johnson JM and Johnson AL (1993) Cranial cruciate ligament rupture: pathogenesis, diagnosis and postoperative rehabilitation. *Veterinary Clinics of North America: Small Animal Practice* **23**, 717–733

Keira M, Yasuda K, Kanuda K *et al.* (1996) Mechanical properties of the anterior cruciate ligament chronically relaxed by elevation of the tibial insertion. *Journal of Orthopaedic Research* **14**, 157–166

Kitchen S (2008) Thermal effects. In: *Electrotherapy: Evidence-based Practice, 12th edn*, ed. T Watson, pp. 99–114. Churchill Livingstone, Edinburgh

Lake DA (1992) Neuromuscular electrical stimulation: an overview of its application in the treatment of sports injuries. *Sports Medicine* **15**, 320–336

Lieber RL, Fridean JO, Hargens AR *et al.* (1988) Differential response of the dog quadriceps muscle to external skeletal fixation of the knee. *Muscle and Nerve* **11**, 193–201

Levine D, Millis DL, Marcellin-Little DJ and Taylor RA (2005) Rehabilitation and physical therapy. *Veterinary Clinics of North America: Small Animal Practice* **35**, 1247–1517

Manning AM (2004) Physical rehabilitation for the critically injured veterinary patient. In: *Canine Rehabilitation and Physical Therapy*, ed. DL Millis *et al.*, pp. 115–119. Saunders, St. Louis

Marsolais GS, Dvorak G and Conzemius MG (2002) Effects of postoperative rehabilitation on limb function after cranial cruciate ligament repair in dogs. *Journal of the American Veterinary Medical Association* **220**, 1325–1330

McMaster W (1977) A literary review on ice therapy in injuries. *American Journal of Sports Medicine* **5**, 124–126

Merrick MA, Knight KL, Ingersoll CD and Potteiger JA (1993) The effects of ice and compression wraps on intramuscular temperature at various depths. *Journal of Athletic Training* **28**, 236–245

Mester E, Mester AF and Mester A (1985) The biomedical effects of laser application. *Lasers in Surgery and Medicine* **5**, 31–39

Millis DL (2004) Responses of musculoskeletal tissues to disuse and remobilization. In: *Canine Rehabilitation and Physical Therapy*, ed. DL Millis *et al.*, pp. 115–119. Saunders, St. Louis

Millis DL (2006) Postoperative management and rehabilitation. In: *BSAVA Manual of Canine and Feline Musculoskeletal Disorders*, ed. JEF Houlton *et al.*, pp. 193–211. BSAVA Publications, Gloucester

Millis DL, Levine D and Brumlow M (1997) A preliminary study of early physical therapy following surgery for cranial cruciate ligament rupture in dogs. *Veterinary Surgery* **26**, 434

Millis DL, Levine D and Taylor RA (2004a) *Canine Rehabilitation and Physical Therapy.* Saunders, St. Louis

Millis DL, Lewelling A and Hamilton S (2004b) Range-of-motion and stretching exercises. In: *Canine Rehabilitation and Physical Therapy*, ed. DL Millis *et al.*, pp. 228–243. Saunders, St. Louis

Moffet H, Collet JP, Shapiro SH *et al.* (2004) Effectiveness of intensive rehabilitation on functional ability and quality of life after first total knee arthroplasty: a single blind randomised controlled study. *Archives of Physical Medicine and Rehabilitation* **85**, 546–556

Monk ML, Preston CA and McGowan CM (2006) Effects of early intensive postoperative physiotherapy on limb function after tibial plateau levelling osteotomy in dogs with deficiency of the cranial cruciate ligament. *American Journal of Veterinary Research* **67**, 529–536

Musacchia XJ, Steffen JM and Fell RD (1988) Disuse atrophy of skeletal muscle: animal models. *Exercise and Sport Sciences Reviews* **16**, 61–87

Nussbaum E (1998) The influence of ultrasound on healing tissues. *Journal of Hand Therapy* **11**, 140–147

Olsen J and Stravino V (1972) A review of cryotherapy. *Physical Therapy* **62**, 840–853

Ostelo RWJG, de Vet HCW, Waddell G *et al.* (2002) Rehabilitation after lumbar disc surgery. *Cochrane Database Systematic Reviews* **2**, CD003007

Palmoski M, Perricone E and Brandt KD (1979) Development and reversal of a proteoglycan aggregation defect in normal canine knee cartilage after immobilisation. *Arthritis and Rheumatism* **22**, 508–517

Sakurakichi KH, Tsuchiya H, Uehara T *et al.* (2004) Effects of timing of low-intensity pulsed ultrasound on distraction osteogenesis. *Journal of Orthopaedic Research* **22**, 395–403

Selkowitz DM (1989) High frequency electrical stimulation in muscle strengthening: a review and discussion. *American Journal of Sports Medicine* **17**, 103–111

Sharp B (2008a) Physiotherapy and rehabilitation. In: *BSAVA Manual of Canine and Feline Advanced Veterinary Nursing, 2nd edn*, ed. A Hotston Moore and S Rudd, pp. 87–90. BSAVA Publications, Gloucester

Sharp B (2008b) Physiotherapy in small animal practice. *In Practice* **30**, 190–199

Shelbourne KD and Gray T (1997) Anterior cruciate ligament reconstruction with autologous patellar tendon graft followed by accelerated rehabilitation. *American Journal of Sports Medicine* **25**, 786–795

Shires PK, Braund KG, Milton JL *et al.* (1982) Effect of localized trauma and temporary splinting on immature skeletal muscle and mobility of the femorotibial joint in the dog. *American Journal of Veterinary Research* **43**, 454–460

Starring D, Grossman MR, Nicholson GG Jr *et al.* (1988) Comparison of cyclic and sustained passive stretching using a mechanical device to increase resting length of hamstring muscles. *Physical Therapy* **68**, 314–320

Sutton A (2004) Massage. In: *Canine Rehabilitation and Physical Therapy*, ed. DL Millis *et al.*, pp. 303–323. Saunders, St. Louis

Taylor, RA and Adamson CP (2002) Stifle surgery and rehabilitation. In: *Proceedings, 2nd International Symposium on Rehabilitation and Physical Therapy in Veterinary Medicine, Knoxville, Tennessee* pp. 143–146

ter Haar G (1999) Therapeutic ultrasound. *European Journal of Ultrasound* **9**, 3–9

Tis JE, Meffert RH, Inoue N *et al.* (2002) The effect of low intensity pulsed ultrasound applied to rabbit tibiae during the consolidation phase of distraction osteogenesis. *Journal of Orthopaedic Research* **20**, 793–800

Warden SJ, Bennell K, McMeeken JM *et al.* (1999) Can conventional therapeutic ultrasound units be used to accelerate fracture repair? *Physical Therapy Review* **4**, 117–126

Watson T (2000) Masterclass: the role of electrotherapy in contemporary physiotherapy practice. *Manual Therapy* **5**, 132–141

10

Hydrotherapy

Samantha Lindley and Holly Smith

Introduction

Hydrotherapy employs certain properties of water to enable and facilitate the rehabilitation (and sometimes training) of patients who find land-based exercise too difficult or painful.

It has been used for many years for the treatment, rehabilitation, analgesia and general wellbeing of human patients. From human studies, hydrotherapy appears to have potential for helping in the rehabilitation and palliation of orthopaedic and neurological patients in particular. In recent years it has begun to be used in the veterinary profession: first for horses and then for small animals, especially dogs. Dogs are given hydrotherapy more commonly than cats, but some cats will tolerate swimming.

The use of hydrotherapy is largely based on evidence from human studies, but studies on dogs are gradually emerging. The reasons for difficulty in obtaining data on *efficacy* (compared with placebo) are outlined in Chapter 8. *Effectiveness* studies are less problematic; for example, in dogs that have undergone fracture repair surgery, it is possible to compare one group that had simple lead-walking rehabilitation with another group that received hydrotherapy, to try to judge whether one was more effective than the other. These are pragmatic studies and should provide the information that most clinicians actually need, i.e. is it worth adding this treatment in to the rehabilitation programme, and is it worth encouraging an owner to spend the time and money needed to give their pet a course of hydrotherapy?

In common with animal physiotherapy and animal acupuncture, more evidence is required to guide the clinician and owner towards making sensible choices to optimize the patient's welfare.

Principles of hydrotherapy

The principles of hydrotherapy are determined by the basic principles that apply to objects interacting with water and by the inherent properties of water.

Specific gravity

Specific gravity (SG) is the relative density of an object compared to water, i.e. the ratio of the weight of the object to the weight of an equal volume of water. This depends on the object's composition (Figure 10.1).

Constituent/tissue	Specific gravity
Water	1.0
Fat	0.8
Muscle	1.0
Bone	1.5–2.0

10.1 Specific gravity (relative density) of body constituents.

This relative density determines how well an object – or patient – will float on water: when SG>1, the object will tend to sink; when SG<1, it will tend to float. In practice, this means that a lean animal that is not moving in the water will have more of a tendency to sink than an obese animal and may need more support until it learns to move effectively.

Buoyancy and gravity

Buoyancy is the upward thrust of water acting on a body, which creates an apparent decrease in the weight of the body whilst it is immersed. Gravity is also acting on the same body (Figure 10.2). If the centre of gravity and the centre of buoyancy are not in the same vertical plane, the body (or patient) will have a tendency to tilt and tip in order to correct the imbalance (Figure 10.2bc). In practice, this means that incorrectly placed flotation aids can disrupt the patient's balance in the water and decrease the effectiveness of the therapy.

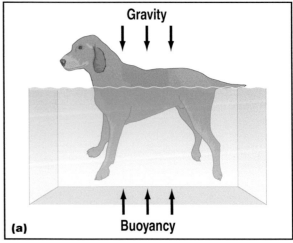

10.2 Buoyancy is the upward thrust of water acting on a body; gravity (downward thrust) is also acting on the same body. (continues) ▶

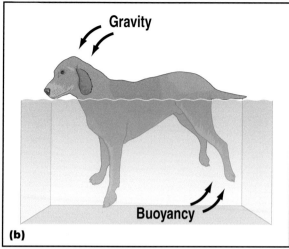

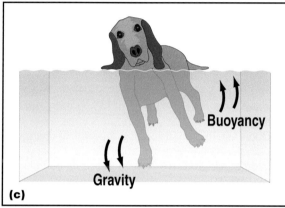

10.2 (continued) Buoyancy is the upward thrust of water acting on a body; gravity (downward thrust) is also acting on the same body. If the centre of gravity and the centre of buoyancy are not in the same vertical plane, the body (or patient) will have a tendency to tip **(b)** or tilt **(c)**. This has implications for the placement of flotation devices.

If the opposing forces of buoyancy and gravity are taken into account, the patient can exercise in an upright position and the weightbearing on joints will be reduced, potentially reducing pain during exercise in the water. In practice, this means that during water treadmill exercising, the affected joint or joints can be 'unloaded' by raising the water level to above these joints (Figure 10.3).

Hydrostatic pressure

Fluid will exert pressure on to an object that is submerged into it and this pressure is directly proportional to the depth and density of the water. Although animals are not completely submerged when they swim or walk on a treadmill, the limbs, or parts of the limbs, will be subject to this pressure, which is exerted over the surface area.

It is hypothesized that this pressure *per se* may help to reduce oedema and local swelling in the limbs and joints, although the actual exertion of walking or swimming may also improve general circulation. If the animal is not fit enough to swim or walk, standing it in an underwater treadmill, filled to the axilla/shoulder level, or on the ramp of a hydrotherapy pool may still help to reduce oedema (Levine *et al.*, 2004).

The hydrostatic pressure of the water applied up to shoulder height has the effect of increasing venous return by:

- Compression of capillary beds in tissue – leading to a decreased filtration of plasma from the arterioles into the extracellular fluid and also an increase in the absorption of extracellular fluid into the lymphatics and venules
- Compression of the venules, veins and lymphatics – causing an increased return of fluid to the circulating volume.

This increased venous return causes atrial stretch and release of atrial natriuretic peptide, which leads to increased blood flow to the glomerulus, increased glomerular filtration rate, and increased loss of sodium and water through the kidneys. The application of 'surgical' or elastic stockings to a human limb would have a similar effect.

Water viscosity, drag and turbulence

Water provides more resistance than air as an object is dragged or moved through it, due to the viscosity of the water. Such resistance has the potential to improve muscle strength and cardiovascular fitness. In addition, viscosity may enable unstable animals to stand for longer periods; as falling will take longer, they will have more time in which to move their limbs to rebalance themselves. Water viscosity is also hypothesized to improve sensory awareness.

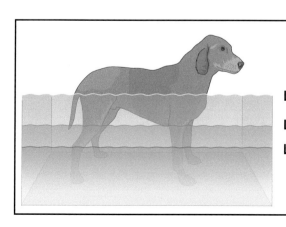

Level of greater trochanter

Level of lateral epicondyle

Level of lateral malleolus of tibia

10.3 Increasing proportions of bodyweight are supported with increasing depth of water.

Increasing turbulence in the hydrotherapy pool will increase the amount of drag and, consequently, the amount of work that has to be done by the patient, without having to increase the length of a session. Underwater jets can also be used to stimulate a patient to move its limbs.

Surface tension

The surface tension of water means that the resistance to working at the surface of the water is greater. In practice, this means that exercises at the surface of the water are more difficult. When working with an animal in an underwater treadmill this can be taken into account and the water level altered, if necessary, for animals that are weaker; greater caution is required when working with weaker animals in swimming pools.

Water temperature

When warmth is applied to muscle tissue it causes: an increase in elasticity of the muscle tissue; increased cell metabolism; increased blood flow; relaxation; and pain relief (Levine *et al.*, 2004). In practice, this contributes to an overall increase in function or performance when in the pool, so more effective and comfortable exercise is possible. Caution should be taken when swimming an animal that is stressed or working hard because hyperthermia can be a risk in these circumstances. A concurrent inflammatory process/condition may be exacerbated by heat, e.g. there could be a flare-up of arthritis, so the animal should be carefully monitored.

Potential benefits of hydrotherapy

A number of potential benefits of hydrotherapy have been postulated. These are extrapolated from human studies, unless stated otherwise:

- Increase in joint flexion and extension. Kinetic studies of canine joints have shown that swimming generally gives better joint flexion (Figure 10.4) than land-based exercise, but that water treadmill walking (Figure 10.5) improves both flexion and extension (Millis and Levine,

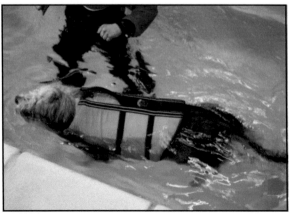

10.4 Swimming aids joint flexion, here of the left hindleg.

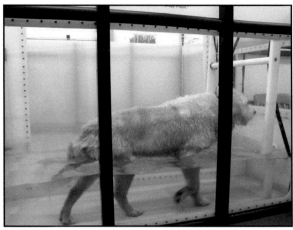

10.5 Underwater treadmill exercise. Note the flexion of the carpus and elbow joints, which is typically greater than when walking over ground. The top of the water level is typically near the elbow. (Courtesy of Darryl L. Millis; reproduced from the *BSAVA Manual of Canine and Feline Musculoskeletal Disorders*)

1997; Marsolais *et al.*, 2003). To achieve this the water level needs to be at, or higher than, the target joint
- Decrease in pain, through a theoretical change in pain perception brought about by the effect of hydrostatic pressure on skin afferents (Geigle *et al.*, 1997)
- Increase in blood circulation
- Increase in sodium excretion by the kidneys and, thus, potential mobilization of oedema (see above)
- Increase in heart rate and oxygen uptake
- Increase in metabolic requirements. Hydrotherapy is often cited as being useful for weight loss, but while this is theoretically true it is not inevitable and often not even likely with some patients swimming or walking for a only few minutes once a week
- Muscle strengthening
- Improvement in proprioception, for patients having underwater treadmill therapy
- A useful transition towards land-based exercise.

Indications for hydrotherapy

In addition to the neurological and orthopaedic problems outlined below, hydrotherapy may be indicated for patients who are generally weak, are reluctant to use a limb or limbs properly, whose proprioception is poor and/or whose joint range of movement is restricted. Hydrotherapy may also be utilized in training of animal athletes but this is outwith the remit of this Manual.

Neurological problems

> **WARNING**
> It is important FIRST to seek the advice of a veterinary neurologist about the safety of hydrotherapy in spinal disease or after spinal surgery.

Paresis

Patients that are paretic are often able to move when supported in the water. With a hydrotherapist or trained staff member in the water (essential for these patients' safety) range of motion (ROM) exercises and stimulation to the limbs can be carried out to aid the correct movement or to encourage preferential use of different limbs/parts of limbs.

Paraparesis

A paraparetic patient can swim normally with the forelimbs but will need help with, and stimulation of, the hindlimbs. This stimulation can be achieved by pushing against the patient's feet, playing with their toes and putting the limbs through a normal ROM, whilst in the pool.

Tetraparesis

Tetraparetic patients will need help with all limbs. They may also need a float under the chin, especially if they have had cervical spinal surgery. They may have a low head carriage, with an associated risk of water aspiration. Also, if the patient has to struggle to hold the head up, this may cause neck pain and deterioration in their condition. Larger patients may need more than one person in the water with them at first, in order to be able to carry out ROM exercises effectively and give them the necessary support.

Orthopaedic problems

Following joint surgery (e.g. cruciate ligament repair, patella luxation correction) or for palliative pain relief (e.g. in osteoarthritis), the buoyancy of water will temporarily relieve the pressure on the joints and will allow greater joint flexion (swimming) and greater flexion and extension (treadmill) than land-based exercise. The increased joint movement may reduce stiffness (so allowing even greater movement), improve muscle strength and bulk, and reduce swelling.

Joint kinetic studies on normal dogs ($n = 13$) and dogs that had undergone surgical cranial cruciate ligament (CCL) repair ($n = 7$) showed that dogs that were swum demonstrated greater joint flexion and range of motion (ROM) in the stifle and tarsal joints, than those that were walked on land (Marsolais *et al.*, 2003), although the normal dogs showed an overall greater ROM in the stifle than those with CCL rupture, regardless of whether they were walked or swum. The authors concluded, with caution, that, *if* increased ROM is a factor in the rehabilitation and recovery of post-CCL rupture surgical patients, then swimming should improve the outcome over walking alone.

From further joint kinetic studies demonstrating greater joint extension in dogs walking on an underwater treadmill than when swimming, it may be suggested, with equal caution, that treadmill rehabilitation *may* be superior to swimming for these patients. However, it should be noted that this study was carried out on normal dogs and not on CCL patients (Jackson *et al.*, 2002).

Anecdotal evidence from clients about their pets' comfort and quality of life suggests that hydrotherapy can reduce the pain of chronic conditions so that doses of some medications, such as non-steroidal anti-inflammatory agents, can be decreased. This is not true for every chronic pain case and it must be emphasized that it is not the primary aim of the treatment. Discussions with both the client and the veterinary surgeon are vital before medication doses are changed, and any change should be done gradually.

The earlier that hydrotherapy can be started, the more effective it may be for chronic problems such as arthritis, although there are no definitive studies showing this. Sessions may start twice weekly, reducing to weekly, then fortnightly, to help the patient become comfortable and mobile. Sessions will need to be continued regularly in the long term for them to be beneficial.

Long-term recumbency

For animals that have undergone long-term treatment in a critical care unit and have been recumbent for a number of days, hydrotherapy may be a useful way to build muscle mass and strength, whilst giving support.

Contraindications and cautions

Fear of water

Dogs that are frightened of water may struggle, panic or become aggressive when first introduced to a treadmill or pool, and may injure themselves or a member of staff. Dogs with a clear history of fear of water (provided by the owner) should not be considered for hydrotherapy, or only under exceptional circumstances.

Prevention of an aversive reaction to the pool setting itself may be helped by introducing a patient to the pool area, staff and water, with some gentle exercises. If this is done prior to planned elective surgery it would have the added benefit of improving muscle strength and fitness prior to surgery, if carried out often enough.

Some dogs who will swim voluntarily in ponds, rivers and lakes may struggle against the controls and limitations imposed upon them in a formal hydrotherapy setting. This reluctance may be overcome by using play and encouragement by the owners, such as getting the owners in the pool with the dog and throwing balls.

Severe pain

If a patient has any signs of central sensitization, i.e. allodynia or hyperalgesia (see Chapter 3), effective analgesia should be administered prior to lifting/ hoisting/holding and subjecting the patient to forced exercise. Whilst pain perception and joint pain may be reduced by the warmth of the water and movement in the water, this will not be sufficient to provide analgesia for a patient in severe pain.

Surgical or open wounds

Ideally, hydrotherapy should not start until wounds are healed and there is no discharge, infection, flap or gaping area. If treatment is started before healing, any wounds must be sealed with a waterproof dressing before the patient can enter the pool. Until there is firm evidence that starting hydrotherapy as soon after surgery as possible gives significantly better results than waiting 10 days or so, until the surgical wound has healed, erring on the side of caution is the most sensible approach.

Cardiovascular problems

Hydrotherapy significantly increases cardiovascular work when compared with land-based exercise, so the fitness of a patient must be evaluated prior to starting aquatic therapy. Hydrotherapy should be avoided in animals with significant cardiovascular compromise. Underwater treadmill therapy is generally less strenuous than swimming and would be safer for unfit and weak patients, who may progress, as their fitness improves, to swimming.

Atopy and dietary sensitivity

Whilst there is no evidence to suggest that atopic animals should not receive hydrotherapy, skin irritation is possible (even in patients with no concurrent dermatological problems). In addition, water is often swallowed, especially in early sessions; animals who have demonstrated intolerance to a wide range of ingested substances may be vulnerable to gastrointestinal disturbances.

Equipment

Hydrotherapy can be carried out using equipment designed specifically for that purpose, such as a pool, an underwater treadmill or a whirlpool; less formally, it can make use of rivers, the sea or even a bathtub or plastic paddling pool.

Hydrotherapy pools and treadmills

The area should be clean, uncluttered and have a non-slip floor. It should also be warm and not smell strongly of chlorine.

There should be easy pool access for ambulatory patients via a ramp (Figure 10.6). An electric hoist (Figure 10.7), with a range of harnesses in a variety of sizes, can be used for larger animals that are unable to walk into the pool or cannot be lifted into the treadmill.

Water temperature

- The hydrotherapy pool or treadmill water should be heated to a temperature of 28–30°C, so that muscles will be kept warm during exercise.
- Higher temperatures are not desirable; even though warmer water may feel 'nice' to the human operator, exercising in water above body temperature can significantly increase cardiovascular demands.
- At lower temperatures (26–28°C) blood pressure and heart rate are reduced. This may be the optimal temperature for training, rather than for rehabilitation (Choukroun and Varene, 1990).

Water treatment

Chlorine/bromine compounds: The water in hydrotherapy pools and underwater treadmills is generally treated with a chlorine- or bromine-based

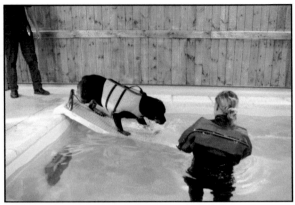

10.6 A ramp with a textured non-slip grip surface allows animals to walk into the pool.

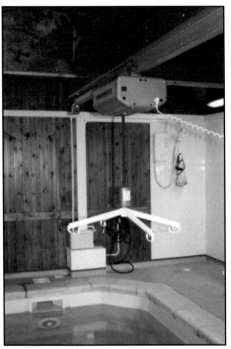

10.7 Electric hoist that goes out over the centre of the pool with a slow and quiet mechanism and has an emergency lowering action, for use if electricity fails.

disinfectant which is safe for human and animal bathers (at correct levels) and effective against bacteria. A hydrotherapy pool or tank is a perfect environment for bacterial growth due to the warm water, moist atmosphere and contaminants from the swimmers, so the water should be treated regularly, as required. This can be done using an autodosing unit, a corrosion feeder, or by hand. The choice of method will depend on cost, space for a plant room and staff training.

Chlorine has been in use as a swimming pool disinfectant since around 1900 and therefore there has been more research into, and experience of, its use than of alternatives. Effective chlorine delivery systems and testing kits are well established. However, the byproducts of chlorine (chloramines) can be both corrosive to equipment and harmful to the skin and eyes. Alternatives to chemical disinfection are ultraviolet light and ozone.

Ultraviolet light: UV radiation kills potential pathogens as the water passes over the light. UV lights are often put into the plant room as an addition to treating the water with chlorine or bromine, to ensure high water quality.

Ozone: Ozone has a short shelf life (20 minutes) and therefore has to be manufactured on site and added to the pool water. It is much more expensive to install an ozone system than to use chlorine or bromine disinfectants, but it is arguably less expensive in maintenance costs as there are no corrosive byproducts. However, filter systems still need to be regularly cleaned and maintained.

Ozone works by reacting with pool water contaminants. If used in combination with chlorine or bromine, it will reduce the amount of chemicals needed to keep the water clean. It can also destroy some of the chloramines produced by chlorine, reducing the potentially harmful byproducts. Ozone also acts as a flocculent on solid particles and therefore increases the pool's efficiency at filtering these out.

Water testing

In-house tests: The pool should be tested a minimum of three times during the day, but, ideally, every 2 hours, especially on days when there is a heavy swim load. The water should be tested for:

- Free chlorine (FC) (active) or bromine
- Total chlorine (TC) (active and used) or bromine
- Combined chlorine (CC comb) (used chloramines calculated as TC minus FC) or bromine
- pH.

A photometer (Figure 10.8a) or comparator should be used to obtain accurate readings of chlorine or bromine levels and pH levels. Every test should be documented and any action taken included on a test sheet (Figure 10.8b).

Free chlorine or bromine should be kept as low as possible but still give effective microbiological quality. In pools with a UV light and ozone in the plant room as part of the water treatment, FC can be as low as 0.5 mg/l (usually 1.5–2.0 mg/l in pools used for human patients). Animal pools benefit from slightly higher levels, such as 2.0–2.5 mg/l, because of the greater amount of hair and dirt in the water. Free bromine levels should be 4–6 mg/l.

The pH level in the pool should be 7.2–7.4. Free chlorine is more efficient at a lower pH and will become less effective as the pH rises. Adding chlorine causes the pH to rise, so an acidic compound such as sodium bisulphate also has to be added to lower it again.

External tests: An independent pool company can be employed to test for 'total dissolved solids with balanced water' and also to service equipment, ensuring that the pool runs correctly and safely. A monthly water sample (from periods of normal use) should be sent for microbiological testing or colony count. This ensures that the disinfection system used is efficient and that there is no serious risk to either patients or personnel from *Escherichia coli, Pseudomonas, Staphylococcus, Cryptosporidium, Giardia* or *Campylobacter*, which are the organisms commonly found associated with such systems.

'DIY' hydrotherapy

Hydrotherapy can be carried out by allowing dogs to swim in naturally occurring water or in plastic paddling pools, or even bathtubs.

Advantages:

- Inexpensive
- Less time-consuming (for the owner, since it usually occurs during normal exercise periods)
- May be better accepted by some dogs.

Disadvantages:

- Strong river currents may be potentially lethal, or may cause injury
- Support and interventions that can be carried out by a therapist in the pool or by using flotation devices in the treadmill (to target different limbs and joints) are absent; thus the dog may not use the limb any better whilst swimming than walking
- It is hard to deliver a consistent or gradually progressive programme.

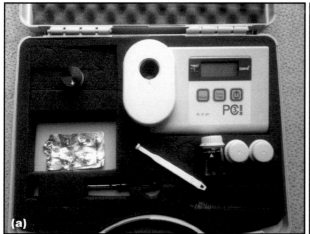
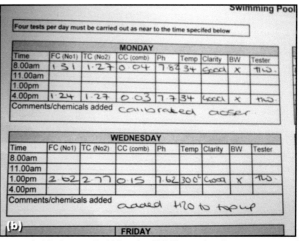

10.8 Water testing. **(a)** Photometer for testing free chlorine, total chlorine and pH levels. **(b)** Example of water test records.

However, if local pools or treadmills are not available, or simply out of the question financially, then a gentle programme could be devised using the principles outlined above. For example, a bathtub may suffice for a small dog if a non-slip surface is laid down, the temperature can be measured and controlled, and the water level can be adjusted according to the targeted joints.

If naturally occurring water is used, the main risks are when the dog enters and leaves the lake or river. Dogs should not be allowed to dive in or scramble out; they should be guided on a lead to a shallow entrance point and encouraged to exit the same way, either by using a long leash or rope to guide them or by commands. The rope, lead or commands should also be used to limit the time they are in the lake or river.

Safe practice

There is currently no legislation or governing body regulating hydrotherapy practice. There are no qualifications required to run a pool or treadmill, therefore anyone can set up a pool offering treatment. However, the Canine Hydrotherapy Association (www.canine-hydrotherapy.org), a self-regulating organization, has endeavoured to set out guidelines for pools and for staff training.

Health and safety considerations

- The animal should be fitted with a buoyancy aid of suitable size (Figure 10.9). This will keep the patient at the surface of the water should there be an emergency, such as the patient becoming exhausted or experiencing respiratory distress or collapse. It also provides the handler with a means of staying in contact with the animal during the session and gives support for weaker patients, keeping the hindquarters higher in the water and the back straighter.
- It is essential that a drysuit or wetsuit is worn by the therapist, both for safety (to protect against scratches) and for hygiene (because animals may contaminate the water).
- When the patient is in a treadmill there should be one member of staff – or the owner – standing in front of the patient to encourage it to move

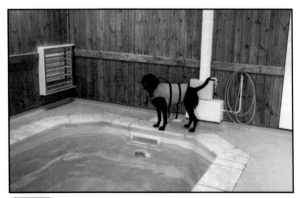

10.9 Patients should be fitted with a buoyancy aid.

forward. For this reason, the front of the tank should not face a blank wall.
- Showers should be available and should be used after the session, particularly if the patient has a concurrent skin problem. Showering the patient off before they go in the pool or treadmill is also beneficial, as it will reduce contaminants in the tank or pool and help to maintain the effectiveness of the disinfectant.
- Drying facilities should be available, such as a blower to direct warm air on to the coat, forcing the water off. Towelling (often time-consuming), static dryers or heated drying kennels are also options. Animals left in drying kennels should be monitored for signs of heat distress.
- A trained medical first aider with access to a first aid kit and an eye wash station (Figure 10.10) should also be available throughout the session.

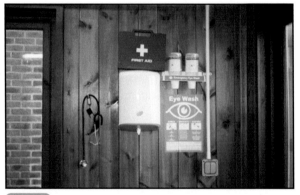

10.10 First aid box and eye wash for staff and clients.

Staff training
Staff should have:

- Good understanding of pool water treatment (a certified course is available)
- Knowledge of, or qualification in, first aid for animals
- Knowledge of how to swim dogs and handle them confidently
- Outline knowledge of common orthopaedic and neurological conditions
- Awareness of when not to swim patients.

Staff should be prepared and trained to work in a pool with the patient, especially in rehabilitation cases such as paraparetic spinal patients. This enables more exercises to be carried out and means that any subtle movements can be felt and the limbs stimulated.

Comprehensive training courses are available in the human sector and these are also appropriate for animal hydrotherapy.

Protocols

These should be devised for the individual patient based on: the principles outlined above; the veterinary surgeon's advice; the therapist's experience; and, most importantly, the patient's response to each session.

- Hydrotherapy should start gently, with very short periods (minutes) of swimming (without jets) or walking.
- The patient should be then assessed for fatigue, but also stiffness or increased pain after subsequent rest, and the therapy time adjusted accordingly.
- Weak or unfit animals appear to benefit from initial underwater treadmill therapy rather than work in a hydrotherapy pool.

Wooster was a 13-year-old Bearded Collie who had undergone previous surgery for a ruptured cruciate ligament, and had since developed osteoarthritis in this joint and a dysplastic hip joint. Wooster was exercise-intolerant, and became stiff and sore after land-based exercise. He abducted his left hindleg when he walked.

Wooster's owner was keen to try supportive physiotherapy treatments before going ahead with proposed surgery (femoral head and neck excision). Hydrotherapy was proposed and had the potential to help Wooster in the following ways:

- He would be able to exercise much more comfortably in the water because he would be supported and the concussive stress on his joints would be relieved
- The resistance of the water might help to strengthen his muscles
- The warmth of the water might reduce pain and allow more efficient exercise
- Swimming might increase range of movement of his joints, through increased flexion
- Swimming might improve cardiovascular fitness.

Assessment and planning

- Animals with osteoarthritis/degenerative joint disease are likely to experience stiffness and pain after swimming sessions if the sessions are too long; this is often much more noticeable after periods of rest, e.g. overnight.
- Tiredness and decreased exercise tolerance may occur due to fatigue after swimming; Wooster was not fit enough to swim for long.
- Owner feedback is always important. Swimming sessions should not be lengthened if they report that their pet is overly tired or has become lame, stiff or sore.

Hydrotherapy sessions

Hydrotherapy sessions took place weekly and swimming was started off very slowly. No underwater resistance jets were used. Wooster was swum in laps around the pool. A veterinary nurse was in the pool to help support and guide him and also to observe the way in which he moved his limbs.

Session 1
1. Started in the pool, swimming for 30 seconds.
2. Rested on the steps; pulse monitored.
3. Waited until pulse had slowed and the patient wasn't panting.
4. Swum for another 30 seconds; then rested again as before.
5. Swum for 30 seconds
6. Ended session.

Observations:
- Nervous initially, but relaxed once in the water.
- Hindlegs moving but left hind abducting rather than going through normal ROM in pool.
- Collapsed on hind legs when got out.

Session 2
Timing as Session 1.

Observations:
- More relaxed this time.
- Increased extension of left hindlimb.
- Crepitus noticed in stifles and hips.
- No collapse after the session this time.

Notes:
- Wooster's pulse rate before the session started was 80 bpm. After the session it was 120 bpm. Monitor pulse rate closely next time.

Session 3
1. Started in the pool, swimming for 1 minute.
2. Rested on the steps; pulse monitored.
3. Waited until pulse had slowed and the patient wasn't panting.
4. Swum for another 30 seconds; then rested again as before.
5. Swum for 30 seconds
6. Ended session.

Observations:
- Coped well with the increased time, relaxed in the water and extending hindlegs well.
- Observed using leg better on exit of the pool, lameness reduced on the left hindlimb and Wooster was less 'wobbly'.

Notes:
- Walks better on grass; owner taking to heath every day now.

Session 4
Timing as Session 3.

Observations:
- Coped well, relaxed in water and extending hindlegs well.
- Using leg better when walking on land.

Session 5
1. Started in the pool, swimming for 1 minute.
2. Rested on the steps; pulse monitored.
3. Waited until pulse had slowed and the patient wasn't panting.
4. Swum for another 1 minute; then rested again as before.

5. Swum for 30 seconds
6. Ended session.

Observations:
• Very relaxed, good ROM with both hindlegs now.
• Owner reports he is weightbearing on the left hind well and seems stronger.

Notes: Wooster's pulse rate before the session started was 80 bpm. After the session it was 100 bpm.

Session 6
Timing as Session 5.

Observations:
• Kicks harder/better on hindlegs.
• Good extension left hind

Notes:
• Wooster's pulse rate before the session started was 96 bpm. After the session it was 120 bpm. Increase times to swim 1 minute, rest 1 minute, swim 1 minute next session.

Results
• By recording Wooster's pulse before and after each session, an increase in fitness can be noted and monitored, although in this case the trend is not definite.
• From the notes made at each swimming session, observations from the owner at home, and from the nurse watching him walk before each session, it was noticeable that Wooster was already weight bearing and using his left hindleg better. He was also not noticeably abducting this leg.
• An improved ROM and extension was evident when Wooster was swimming (Figure 10.11).
• It would be anticipated that continued hydrotherapy would improve Wooster's fitness, exercise tolerance, muscle strength and weight bearing still further.

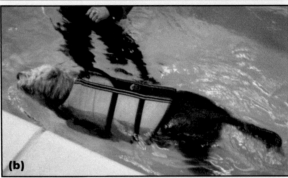

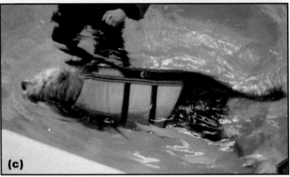

10.11 **(a)** Left hindleg moving cranially in a more normal ROM. **(b)** Left hindleg moving down and caudally. **(c)** Left hindleg in extension.

Outcome assessment

• Outcome measures include both owner assessment and clinician assessment of pain and gait. More sophisticated gait analysis and force plate assessments can also be used if the equipment is available.
• Range of movement (ROM) measurements can be taken accurately with a goniometer.
• More simply, measurement of muscle circumference at predetermined sites is often carried out to assess and demonstrate improvement in muscle mass.

References and further reading

Bockstahler B, Levine D and Millis D (2004) *Essential Facts of Physiotherapy in Dogs and Cats*. BE VetVerlag, Babenhausen, Germany

Choukroun ML and Varene P (1990) Adjustments in oxygen transport during head out immersion in water at different temperatures. *Journal of Applied Physiology* **68**,1475–1480

Geigle PR, Cheek WL, Gould ML *et al.* (1997) Aquatic physical therapy for balance: the interaction of somatosensory and hydrodynamic principles. *Journal of Aquatic Physical Therapy* **5**, 4–10

Jackson AM, Millis DL, Stevens M *et al.* (2002) Joint kinematics during underwater treadmill activity. *Proceedings, 2nd International Symposium on Rehabilitation and Physical Therapy in Veterinary Medicine, Knoxville, Tennessee*, p.191

Levine D, Rittenberry L and Millis D (2004) Aquatic therapy. In: *Canine Rehabilitation and Physical Therapy*, ed. D Millis *et al.*, pp.264–276. Saunders, Missouri

Levine D, Tragauer V and Millis DL (2002) Percentage of normal weight bearing during partial immersion at various depths in dogs. *Proceedings, Second International Symposium on Rehabilitation and Physical Therapy in Veterinary Medicine, Knoxville, Tennessee*

Marsolais GS, McLean SMS, Derrick T *et al.* (2003) Kinematic analysis of the hind limb during swimming and walking in healthy dogs and dogs with surgically corrected cranial cruciate ligament rupture. *Journal of the American Veterinary Medical Association* **222**, 739–743

Millis DL (2006) Postoperative management and rehabilitation. In: *BSAVA Manual of Canine and Feline Musculoskeletal Disorders*, ed. JEF Houlton *et al.*, pp.193–211. BSAVA Publications, Gloucester

Millis DL and Levine D (1997) The role of exercise and physical modalities in the treatment of osteoarthritis. *Veterinary Clinics of North America: Small Animal Practice* **27**, 913–930

11

Acupuncture in palliative and rehabilitative medicine

Samantha Lindley

Introduction

Acupuncture is defined here as:

'the insertion of a solid needle into the body with the purpose of therapy, disease prevention or maintenance of health'
(Acupuncture Regulatory Working Group, 2003)

However, 'the maintenance of health' is often not included in most so-called 'western' approaches to acupuncture (Lindley and Cummings, 2006).

It is worth defining acupuncture at the start of any discussion of its uses, since the term means different things to different people. Whilst a given drug will have the same formula and same accepted dose rate the world over, acupuncture looks – and feels – very different depending upon the training, approach and, sometimes, philosophy of whoever is delivering the treatment. In some cases the skin is not even penetrated by a needle but is stimulated by a small electrical charge. Strictly speaking, this is not 'true' acupuncture, since the word comes from the Latin *acus* (needle) and *punctura* (puncture) or possibly *pungere* (to prick).

Some practitioners use fine needles placed subcutaneously for all insertions. At the other end of the spectrum, needles are repeatedly used to stimulate areas within muscle with a robust 'lift and thrust' technique, or with the aid of an electrical impulse stimulator (electroacupuncture).

The following review of the mechanisms of acupuncture, together with some evidence for its effectiveness/efficacy, and the broad categories of conditions treated, aims to put this intervention into perspective before roles can be defined for acupuncture in palliative and rehabilitative care.

A neurophysiological approach

For the purposes of this Manual, the use of acupuncture is suggested where:

- The evidence supports its use for the given, or a related, condition
- The neurophysiological effects of acupuncture, as they are understood, support its use in a given condition.

Where anecdotal reports have been received of success, and there is a plausible mechanism for its action in that condition, these will be mentioned.

A word on traditional acupuncture

Traditional Chinese Medicine (TCM) is a complex system of diagnosis and treatment based on a number of principles formulated before therapists had any detailed knowledge of neurophysiology, or indeed, physiology. TCM uses many techniques, including herbs and acupuncture, but is not a synonym for acupuncture. It is valid in its own context but becomes problematical when applied directly to a western scientific approach. The names of the acupuncture points and their approximate anatomical positions are maintained for ease of communication between practitioners, and there is a remarkable degree of overlap between practitioners, whether classically or 'western' trained, in the points used to treat similar conditions. Worrying about which approach is 'better' is therefore unnecessary. Acupuncture stimulates the body's own remarkable pain-relieving and healing mechanisms and it can do this whichever approach is adopted.

How acupuncture works

Mechanisms of acupuncture can be classified in different ways, but two of the main categories are: analgesic; and non-analgesic. Acupuncture is often associated in the public mind with three broad uses:

- So-called 'acupuncture anaesthesia' (see Analgesia)
- Pain relief
- 'Cure' of addictions – (see Non-analgesic effects).

Analgesia
'Acupuncture anaesthesia'

'Acupuncture anaesthesia' is not actually anaesthesia but is more correctly termed 'acupuncture analgesia' (AA). AA usually refers to surgical analgesia when described this way. The patient remains conscious and continues to have sensation but with reduced nociception – *if they are sensitive enough to the acupuncture stimulus and can cope with the sensations that they experience*.

Whilst there are some positive studies on AA (e.g. human patients will use less self-administered opiate postoperatively when AA is used than when it is not) and whilst there are obvious potential advantages over conventional anaesthesia for cardiovascular stability (less respiratory depression, less anaesthetic overall) (White, 1998) there are some significant problems which have dampened the initial enthusiasm for AA. For example, it takes around 25 minutes to achieve surgical analgesia with acupuncture *but* the effect depends upon the sensitivity of the patient to acupuncture; an individual may not be sensitive enough for surgery to be performed under acupuncture alone. AA is also time-consuming and potentially takes up space with additional wires and equipment. Additionally, and importantly, after 45 minutes of electroacupuncture, the brain starts to release cholecystokinin (CCK), an opiate antagonist, which then counteracts the endorphin-mediated mechanism of the action of acupuncture. So, whilst AA as surgical analgesia may have a small place as an adjunct to anaesthesia in sensitive and willing human patients, modern anaesthetic drugs and western expectations make it unlikely that surgery performed under acupuncture alone will be anything other than a constant source of amazement to onlookers.

For animal patients, the fact that they would retain sensation and variable nociception makes AA impractical, and probably unethical, except under very special circumstances and with additional pharmacological assistance.

Pain relief

Pomeranz's famous 'sixteen lines of evidence' for acupuncture were based on experimental evidence from laboratory animals, including tail flick latency in rats (Cheng and Pomeranz, 1980). This acute, or physiological, pain is a different picture from the chronic pain that affects most veterinary patients (see Chapters 2 and 3). However, it is likely that most, if not all, of the mechanisms cited below for

acute pain are also involved when acupuncture is used successfully to treat chronic pain conditions.

From Pomeranz's studies we know that:

- Acupuncture requires an intact nervous system (sectioning of nerves and local anaesthetic block the action)
- Acupuncture has humoral and CSF effects (from cross-circulation studies)
- Acupuncture is partly mediated by endorphins and other opiates (opiate antagonists block the effects of acupuncture)
- Acupuncture upregulates messenger RNA for pre-encephalin. Thus, with subsequent treatments acupuncture triggers the body to make more of its own opiates, thus winding down pain. This is believed to be one of the mechanisms for the observed prolonged effects of acupuncture.

Segmental effects: Acupuncture needles are fine, minimally traumatic needles. This means that insertion mainly stimulates fast myelinated fibres (Aδ in skin; type II and III in muscle). These fibres signal actual or potential tissue damage, and cause the body or area damaged to withdraw from the threatening/damaging stimulus. Because potential new damage to the body takes priority over chronic pain in terms of signalling to the brain, the fast pain fibre input takes priority over the slow fibre input in the dorsal horn of the spinal cord where pain is modulated. Fast pain fibres stimulate encephalinergic interneurons, which, in turn, inhibit onward transmission of C fibre (slow pain) signals (Figure 11.1). This is a postsynaptic effect and is distinct from the

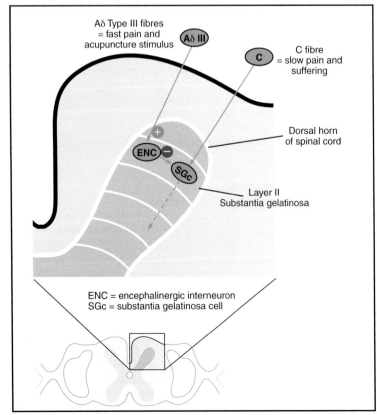

11.1

Segmental acupuncture. Stimulation of Aδ fibres by acupuncture needles stimulates encephalinergic interneurons (ENC) in layer II (substantia gelatinosa) of the dorsal horn of the spinal cord. These interneurons inhibit substantia gelatinosa cells (SGc) from onward transmission of C-fibre pain. Thus, acupuncture 'competes' with C-fibre pain at the dorsal horn.

'pain gate' mechanism (Melzack and Wall, 1965) which is presynaptic.

The presynaptic effect is most potent at the segment stimulated, i.e. when the needle is close to the relevant dorsal horn. Hence, the neurophysiological approach to acupuncture places needles as close as possible to the source of pain (or dysfunction). For a musculoskeletal problem this means putting the needle directly in the area of pain, where it is safe to do so, e.g. avoiding joint spaces but needling around the joint margin, or in local muscles for arthritis. For a visceral condition this would mean needling an area that is innervated by the same spinal nerve as the disordered organ(s) in question.

This is termed *segmental* acupuncture.

Heterosegmental effects: After 'competing' at the dorsal horn, the acupuncture stimulus continues via crossed spinothalamic tracts to the brain and affects areas that include the limbic system, periaqueductal grey (PAG) and nucleus raphe magnus. This stimulus triggers release of beta-endorphins (from the PAG), serotonin and noradrenaline, amongst other neurotransmitters (Figure 11.2), and these have effects both humorally and via the descending inhibitory pain pathways. These pain-relieving effects occur throughout the body but are most potent at the segment stimulated. In some individuals, who are generally referred to as 'sensitive' to the treatment, this heterosegmental effect is very potent.

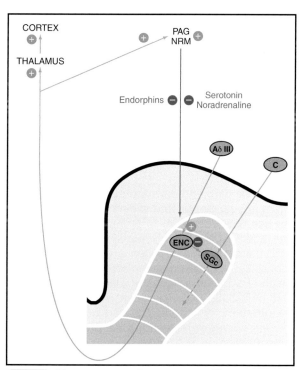

11.2 Heterosegmental acupuncture. The acupuncture stimulus (of Aδ fibres) continues via crossed spinothalamic tracts to the brain. Consequent release of endorphins (from the periaqueductal grey, PAG), serotonin and noradrenaline (from centres including the nucleus raphe magnus, NRM) work (via the descending inhibitory pain pathways and humorally) to inhibit pain at every spinal segment. The effect is most potent at the segment stimulated.

In essence, through both *segmental* and *heterosegmental* effects, the acupuncture stimulus 'fools' the body and brain into reacting as though there had been tissue damage, thus triggering potent pain-relieving and protective mechanisms, whilst causing only microtrauma with the needle insertion (Bowsher, 1998).

From this perspective, insistence on absolute anatomical accuracy of points is not logical: the needle insertion should be as close as possible to the source of pain or at least in the same spinal segment. This chapter does not deal with acupuncture points or meridians because the terms would be meaningless to those who do not practise acupuncture and superfluous to those who do. Point selection (from a 'western' perspective) is based on neurophysiological principles and examination of the patient rather than on standard formulae. Points *are* mentioned as examples in the case studies later in this Manual.

Trigger points: Myofascial trigger points (MTrPs or TrPs) (see also Chapter 3) are dysfunctional areas within muscle that give rise to pain and, sometimes, autonomic dysfunction. These are the 'knots' in muscles that most people experience at some time after muscle strain or in periods of tension. They commonly occur in the neck and upper trapezius muscles; people rub or press them when they are painful and they would be targeted by masseurs during a 'deep massage'. Myofascial trigger points are *not* synonymous with muscle spasms, although muscle spasm may be present in adjacent muscles (Travell, 1976).

Muscle pain is not well recognized in veterinary medicine and often not in human medicine. The phrase 'it's only muscular' sums up the attitude to muscular pain quite well. However, studies show that pain from muscle problems will be referred extensively and that the longer the duration of the pain and the more intense the pain, the more widespread will be the referral (Kellgren, 1938). This means that, in practice, a small area of muscle damage can have marked repercussions for the patient's wellbeing (see Chapter 3).

Trigger points in the body wall have been reported to cause visceral effects such as colic, diarrhoea, vomiting and other functional disturbances (Simons *et al.*, 1999). These are reported in humans, but it would be difficult to prove a relationship between trigger points in the soma of animals and their functional effects.

Conversely, a painful visceral condition, such as pancreatitis or kidney stones, can set up trigger points in the body wall. Even when the visceral condition is resolved, the patient can still feel the pain, which is now coming from the body wall rather than the viscera. Because human patients make the association with the pain and the condition that previously caused it, this association will cause worry and focus on the possibility that the condition has recurred. Such conditions are often the focus of continued medical and even surgical investigations. Since animal patients do not present themselves because they are concerned that they have the same pain that they experienced during the last bout of pancreatitis for example, veterinary surgeons must depend on owner observation of similar behavioural signs, such as excessive stretching or 'praying', and it would be the owner's association and concern that would bring them to the veterinary clinic. There is no physiological reason why such viscerosomatic effects should *not* occur in non-human animals, but it is likely that they will be presented less frequently.

Trigger points are characterized in humans by:

- Taut bands in skeletal muscle (the band is palpable when the muscle is on a slight stretch; in a relaxed muscle these do feel more like knots)
- Pain on compression and more painful than the rest of the muscle ('hyper-irritable')
- Characteristic referral patterns when needled or digitally compressed
- Exhibiting a 'jump sign' (a voluntary movement away from the pain) and a local twitch response (a twitch in the muscle involved).

In human patients the most reliable feature is patient recognition (Gerwin *et al.*, 1997), a term that is often used synonymously with the 'jump sign', but is a little more than this. The human patient recognizes that the pain elicited is 'their' pain, i.e. the one that is bothering them. Although a jump sign is recognizable in animal patients, the veterinary surgeon cannot be sure that the trigger point identified is the one that is bothering the animal, or indeed that it is bothering them at all, unless in some few fortunate cases compression of the trigger point exactly recreates the problem complained about by the owner, e.g. frantic licking of the leg.

Trigger points tend to occur in motor endplate zones. Motor endplates normally release acetylcholine sufficient to cause muscle contraction. If these endplates are damaged (by strain, trauma or age degeneration) then they become 'leaky'. They release just enough acetylcholine to cause the sarcomeres in that endplate zone to bunch up (creating the 'knot' or band within the muscle). This constriction of sarcomeres compromises local blood vessels such that they no longer remove the toxic waste products of muscle metabolism so efficiently. These toxins build up in the endplate zone of the muscle and hypersensitize the local sensory nerves, causing hyperirritability of the trigger point (Hong and Simons, 1998).

Acupuncture is arguably the most efficient way of treating trigger points (Cummings and White, 2001), although non-invasive modalities such as stretch and pressure (massage, acupressure) can also be useful. Currently, the mechanism of action for the relief of trigger points by acupuncture is not agreed; if it were, there would be more confidence about the best approach to treat them. Some therapists advocate subcutaneous needles over, but not in, the trigger point (Baldry, 2001); others state that vigorous needling into the trigger point should continue until the local twitches are abolished (the theory being that

each motor endplate is 'cleaved off' with each twitch) (Gunn, 1998). As always, the middle ground suggests the middle way: moderate needling getting as close to the trigger point as the patient will allow. The kind of vigorous needling described above would only be tolerated by a very few animal patients.

Relief from the pain of trigger points may be mediated by the same mechanism as described above for segmental acupuncture. It may be a mechanical effect – stimulating the motor endplate to release sufficient acetylcholine to cause muscle contraction (the twitch) and thereby 'reset' itself; or the explanation may be more complex.

Non-analgesic effects

Anxiolysis

Acupuncture often has a transient anxiolytic effect on many human and animal patients: they become sedated and relaxed, sometimes for a day or two after treatment. Whether this effect is enough to produce any meaningful change in these patients' attitudes to life and its stressors is questionable, and the evidence for true antidepressant anxiolytic effects of acupuncture in humans is still sketchy (Luo *et al.*, 1985). Although the neurotransmitters released are the same ones associated with mood and that are manipulated with antidepressant medications, a genuine antidepressant effect, as needed by a small proportion of the human (and arguably cat and dog) population at the severe end of the spectrum, takes several weeks of increased levels of serotonin/ noradrenaline and other neurotransmitters to produce the secondary messenger effect that results in 'feeling better' (Scott and Mayhew, 2001). Once-weekly treatment of anxious animals with acupuncture is therefore unlikely to result in such therapeutic changes, but it is possible that there may be other non-specific effects of treatment (see Chapter 8) that will make both owner and animal feel less anxious. It should also be remembered that most animals are *not* in need of potent antidepressant medication.

Wound healing and dermatological conditions

There is both clinical and experimental evidence for the use of acupuncture to promote wound healing. The effect is mediated primarily by the release of local neurotransmitters when a needle is inserted, especially calcitonin gene-related peptide (CGRP) which is a potent vasodilator (Jansen *et al.*, 1989). This so-called antidromic release of neurotransmitter (85–95% of the neurotransmitter released by afferent nerves is released at the periphery) stimulates healing in the same way an injury would. Again, the needle insertion is 'fooling' the body into triggering its healing mechanisms, without causing the damage that would usually have to occur in order to stimulate their action (Lundeberg *et al.*, 1988; Jansen *et al.*, 1989).

Acupuncture has a number of other potential effects in dermatological conditions, although the experimental evidence for these having an effect in clinical conditions is less convincing:

- Pruritus: theoretically, one would expect that itch, transmitted by C fibres, may be modulated in the same way that C-fibre pain is modulated in the dorsal horn. In practice, the effect does not appear to be as convincing as the analgesic effects of acupuncture. This may be because the C fibres that transmit itch are postulated to be different from the C fibres that transmit pain. Recent studies have suggested that itch may be more akin to neuropathic pain, which would explain why it is challenging to treat itch by any modality. Acupuncture does not compete well with pain arising directly from nerve damage or irritation. Having said that, there is a small amount of data (Belgrade *et al.*, 1984) to suggest that acupuncture can have an effect on itch caused by histamine, so one would hope that histamine-mediated pruritus would be moderated by acupuncture.
- Immunomodulation: there is a lot of experimental scientific evidence supporting the effects of acupuncture on the immune system (Zhao and Liu, 1989; Lundeberg *et al.*, 1991; Kashara *et al.*, 1992; Karst *et al.*, 2003). In practice, the results do not appear to reflect the basic science, but there does appear to be a small effect on immune function, possibly similar to the effects produced by optimum levels of exercise and therefore mediated by endorphins. In certain very sensitive individuals, this effect may be enough to 'normalize' immune function in conditions such as atopy (or asthma). There is anecdotal evidence only for immunomodulation in the veterinary species, in which an apparently small subpopulation of atopic animals will respond dramatically well to acupuncture, whilst the remainder do not respond at all.

Anti-emesis/anti-nausea

In human studies there is often no distinction made between anti-emesis and the treatment of nausea, presumably since the feeling of nausea is usually associated with the experience of vomiting. Therefore, it is assumed that if the patient stops vomiting they will no longer be nauseous or, if they are nauseous, they can verbally report this phenomenon. In canine and feline patients, it is more difficult to be confident about nausea and its intensity, since there is no verbal communication about the sensation of nausea. The signs can be subtle and easily overlooked: excessive salivation is the easiest to recognize, although this can also occur with anxiety (and anxiety can be associated with feelings of nausea in humans). Frequent yawning, lip licking, excessive eating of grass and plants, and general dullness may be identified by the more observant owner.

There is good evidence that acupuncture works for post-chemotherapeutic and postoperative nausea in humans (Dundee *et al.*, 1989; Ho *et al.*, 1990). One reason why the evidence is convincing for these conditions, but less so for the morning sickness of pregnancy and travel sickness, is

probably that the treatment needs to be given at the time of the emetic stimulus. This is relatively easy to predict with anaesthesia or chemotherapy and the patients are often on hand to be treated, whereas there are limited numbers of travellers wealthy or foresighted enough to travel with their own personal acupuncturist, and a vomiting mother-to-be is unlikely to want to move far from home whilst experiencing symptoms.

The acupuncture point tested most frequently is the 'famous' PC6 point (where PC refers to the meridian or line called the Pericardium and the 6 is the sixth point described along that line). This point lies on the forearm of humans, between the tendons of flexor carpi radialis and palmaris longus, directly above the median nerve. Traditional Chinese medicine ascribes anti-nauseous properties to this point, hence its use in many studies, and so it is known that PC6 does work for nausea in humans. However, it seems unlikely that humans would have developed one specific tiny area on the body that would have such exclusive properties or that such a point would be anatomically transposable to non-human animals. In practice, it is probably more relevant to use points that can be stimulated strongly, but without aversive pain (Lindley and Cummings, 2006).

Functional disturbances of the viscera

There are a few clinical and experimental findings that support the use of acupuncture to 'normalize' dysfunction in viscera (Sato *et al.*, 1993; Kelleher *et al.*, 1994). Since viscera cannot be needled directly, a structure (usually muscle) innervated by the same spinal nerve as the viscera is selected for stimulation (see Segmental effects, above). In veterinary practice, the most accessible and reliable way of stimulating a spinal segment is by needling the multifidus muscles (Lindley and Cummings, 2006). These muscles lie next to the spinous processes (see Figure 11.4) and are innervated from the spinous process with which they are associated; therefore, needling multifidus at L4 will stimulate the L4 segment of the spinal cord. It is likely that stimulation of ventral segments (from which the viscera arise embryologically) may be marginally more effective for visceral conditions than stimulating dorsal segments, so adding in some ventral points (in rectus abdominus or linea alba) may be helpful, if practical and acceptable to the patient. The acupuncture stimulus still 'competes' at the dorsal horn with the afferent nerves from the viscera, but the 'noise' it creates here is thought to reset the function via an indirect effect on the visceral efferent nerves.

In practice, this means that it should be possible to normalize gut function in some cats with megacolon (presumably only in those animals where some function remains) and also to relieve urethral spasm during urinary tract blockage for example, as well as relieving the pain of cystitis; and there are numerous anecdotal reports to say that this is the case. The problem with treating visceral conditions with acupuncture is that one is not always confident about the cause of the problem, so it is not possible to predict the effects. For example, acupuncture has previously been anecdotally reported to be useful for the treatment of incontinence in bitches, although there is no reason why acupuncture should have an impact on a sphincter mechanism incompetence that responds to oestrogen nor on the physical pressures on an intrapelvic bladder. However, some dogs *and* bitches with mild incontinence have pain on palpation of their lumbar spine and this author has observed an improvement in, or complete cessation of, incontinence when that lumbar pain is treated, whether with acupuncture or conventional medication.

The role of acupuncture in veterinary palliative care and rehabilitative medicine

Pain relief
The primary role of acupuncture will almost always be seen as the provision of analgesia (Figure 11.3). Usually this will be as an adjunct to more conventional analgesic medication (see Chapters 2 and 3), but occasionally as an alternative to NSAIDs where these are contraindicated because of the animal's condition (e.g. inflammatory bowel disease) or because of concurrent medication (e.g. glucocorticoids). However, it should be remembered that, as far as is understood, acupuncture does not have a direct anti-inflammatory effect, so will *not* replace anti-inflammatories where a specific anti-inflammatory action is indicated. It has been postulated that relief of pain (a stressor) may well modify disease, but more evidence is necessary before such a hypothesis could form the basis of treatment.

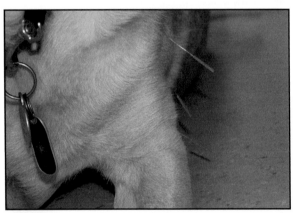

11.3 Pain relief is currently the most common use of acupuncture in veterinary practice. This Labrador has elbow arthritis and has responded well to acupuncture treatment.

Targets
Acupuncture competes with nociception, which is modified at the dorsal horn. Acupuncture does not compete well with neuropathic pain where that pain arises directly from nerve damage or irritation/pressure, although it is not often that such cases are 'purely' neuropathic; there may well be some secondary soft tissue pain that would benefit from being targeted.

Response
Acupuncture does not have the same effect on each individual. Acupuncture is an unusual stimulus, but every individual responds to incoming stimuli in a different way and this is determined by their individual sensitivities and the state of their nervous system at the time. Evidence suggests that differences in populations of opiate receptors between individuals may play a part in this variation in response (Campbell, 1998). There are a few (possibly 10%) individuals who are extremely sensitive to acupuncture: the so-called 'good responders'. In these cases acupuncture may appear to have a more potent effect on pain than do the most potent analgesic drugs.

It is important to remember that, just because pain is relieved with acupuncture, it does not follow that the source of the pain is not serious or life-threatening. Even in good responders, acupuncture should not be able to compete with the pain of, for example, tumour or ischaemia for long, and the signs of pain and dysfunction will return, alerting the clinician to further investigations and treatment.

Anti-emesis/anti-nausea
The role of acupuncture in anti-emesis in palliative care for humans is reasonably well established, supported by clinical and experimental evidence (see above). It is far from being accepted as a part of the treatment for side effects of chemotherapeutic regimes in veterinary practice, but nausea and vomiting not only affect the wellbeing of veterinary chemotherapy patients, but also the attitude of the owner to continuing the treatment. The emphasis, when offering acupuncture as a possible aid to managing such side effects, should be on using knowledge of the individual's previous response to chemotherapy. Using this information, acupuncture treatment should be given at the time the animal would be *expected to start feeling unwell* after the administration of the chemotherapy, which is of course not necessarily the same time as when the chemotherapy is given. Strong but acceptable stimulus in easily accessible points is recommended. *Safety aspects should be considered* (see below).

Wound healing and dermatological conditions
In 'good responders', acupuncture is worth trying in order to relieve the itch and pain of dermatological conditions. Acral lick dermatitis appears to be especially susceptible to needling. Wound healing should be approached by needling as close as possible to the wound edge and/or skin flap base, in healthy tissue, to the depth required (i.e. if the wound includes muscle then the needle should be inserted into muscle), at about 2.5 cm spacing, and repeated every few days or at weekly intervals (Jansen *et al.*, 1989).

Painful and functional problems of the viscera
Acupuncture may be indicated here as an adjunct to standard treatment. Needling may be especially useful if high doses of opiates are confusing the

signs of recovery, i.e. causing dysphoria, sedation or dullness. A segmental approach is recommended, needling at 45 degrees into multifidus muscle next to the spinous process (Figure 11.4), with some ventral points where possible.

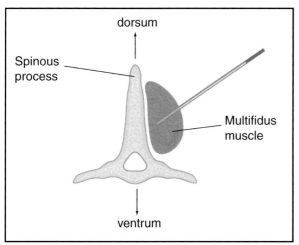

11.4 Segmental acupuncture for visceral conditions is most conveniently achieved in the veterinary species by paraspinal needling. The needle is inserted at an angle of 45 degrees through the epaxial muscles and into the multifidus muscle next to the spinous process.

Clinical considerations

- Initial treatment is usually carried out once a week, although twice-weekly or every 3 days in a hospitalized animal is often preferable if the condition is severe. An increase in frequency of the treatment does not improve the overall outcome, but it is likely to give faster improvement by a rapid 'ramping up' of endorphin release.
- The patient is usually fully conscious, but it may occasionally be necessary to use sedation. Some animals are profoundly sedated by the treatment itself (Figure 11.5).
- Patients are often (though not always) sleepy *after* treatment, sometimes profoundly so, and this usually indicates that they will respond well, assuming acupuncture is appropriate for the condition being treated. However, an absence of sedation does *not* mean that the treatment will be ineffective.
- Cats usually tolerate and respond well to acupuncture (Figure 11.6).
- Four treatments are usually enough to judge whether or not the therapy is working, although one cannot say that acupuncture is not working until electroacupuncture has been tried.
- Electroacupuncture involves using an electrical impulse stimulator to stimulate the needles (Figure 11.7) at alternating frequencies of 2 Hz and 80–100 Hz (usually). Stimulation at 2 Hz is associated with the release of beta-endorphins (Thomas and Lundeberg, 1994) and a longer lasting relief of pain. The higher frequencies release serotonin, metencephalins and dynorphins (White, 1998).

- The choice between manual needling and electroacupuncture is based upon the severity of the clinical signs and the response to needling generally.

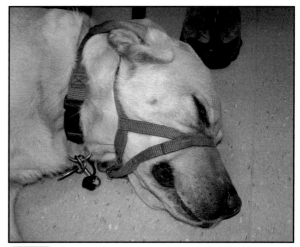

11.5 Some patients are profoundly sedated by acupuncture. This Labrador predictably and consistently lies down and closes his eyes within seconds of needle insertion.

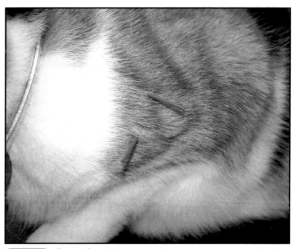

11.6 Cats often tolerate and appear to respond well to acupuncture.

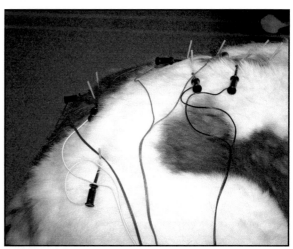

11.7 Electroacupuncture involves stimulating pairs of needles with an electrical impulse stimulator.

Clinical responses

These include:

- **No change.** This may be due to a real lack of response or due to inadequate stimulation, inadequate numbers of treatments, too long a gap between treatments, or the owner/clinician looking for the wrong outcome measures, e.g. a resolution of lameness instead of an improvement in demeanour.
- **A worsening of signs.** This almost always results ultimately in an improvement, before the next treatment, but this subsequent treatment should be modified (fewer needles, finer needles and/or less stimulation of needles) so as not to cause worsening after each session.
- **An improvement.** The first improvement is usually seen in the patient's demeanour, i.e. they appear to be happier and suffering less. This improvement may be short lived and can occur up to 3 days after the treatment. The patient's signs will usually recur but after each treatment the improvement will be greater and longer lasting, until it reaches a plateau. At that point a frequency of treatment can be settled on to keep the signs at bay, e.g. monthly or 6-weekly.

Safety considerations

The introduction of infection is not likely when needling healthy animals, but needling should be avoided into infected skin, tumours, oedema (especially lymphoedema), open wounds and joint spaces. Needle penetration in a severely immunocompromised patient increases the risk of introducing infection (Rampes and Peuker, 1999). This should be discussed with owners of dogs receiving chemotherapy, and the treatment based on review of haematological findings, the need for the treatment and the timing of chemotherapy in relation to the acupuncture.

Aggressive needling in closed fascial spaces (such as the lower limb) should be avoided, especially in animals with bleeding disorders (risk of compartment syndrome). Ventral needling over the abdomen carries a risk of penetrating the peritoneal cavity and it is recommended that needles are angled and not left in place.

The most common serious adverse effect of acupuncture in humans is pneumothorax; because of the shape of the human ribcage it is harder to angle the acupuncture needle to avoid the rib spaces when trying to reach deep muscle layers. There are no recorded cases of pneumothorax following acupuncture in animals, but it is easy to avoid needling between the ribs in cats and dogs, therefore tangential needling, superficial needling or needling close to the spinous processes should be practised, especially when the animal has a chronic respiratory problem.

References and further reading

Acupuncture Regulatory Working Group (2003) *The Statutory Regulation of the Acupuncture Profession – The Report of the Acupuncture Regulatory Working Group.* The Prince of Wales Foundation, London

Baldry PE (2001) *Myofascial Pain and Fibromyalgia Syndromes: A Clinical Guide to Diagnosis and Management.* Churchill Livingstone, London

Belgrade MJ, Solomon LM and Lichter EA (1084) Effect of acupuncture on experimentally induced itch. *Acta Dermato-venereologica* **64**, 129–133

Bowsher D (1998) Mechanisms of acupuncture. In: *Medical Acupuncture: A Western Scientific Approach,* ed. J Filshie and A White, pp. 69–82. Churchill Livingstone, Edinburgh

Campbell A (1998) Methods of acupuncture. In: *Medical Acupuncture: A Western Scientific Approach,* ed. J Filshie and A White, pp. 19–32. Churchill Livingstone, Edinburgh

Cheng RSS and Pomeranz BH (1980) Electroacupuncture analgesia is mediated by stereospecific opiate receptors and is reversed by antagonists of Type I receptors. *Life Sciences* **26**, 631–638

Cummings TM and White AR (2001) Needling therapies in the management of myofascial trigger point pain: a systematic review. *Archive of Physical Medicine and Rehabilitation* **82**, 986–992

Dundee JW, Ghaly RG, Bill KM *et al.* (1989) Effect of stimulation of the P6 antiemetic point on postoperative nausea and vomiting. *British Journal of Anaesthesia* **63**, 612–618

Gerwin RD, Shannon S, Hong CZ *et al.* (1997) Inter-rater reliability in myofascial trigger point examination. *Pain* **69**, 65–73

Gunn CC (1998) Acupuncture and the peripheral nervous system. In: *Medical Acupuncture: A Western Scientific Approach,* ed. J Filshie and A White, pp. 137–150. Churchill Livingstone, Edinburgh

Ho RT, Jawan B, Fung ST *et al.* (1990) Electroacupuncture and postoperative antiemesis. *Anaesthesia* **45**, 327–329

Hong CZ and Simons DG (1998) Pathophysiologic and electrophysiologic mechanisms of myofascial trigger points. *Archives of Physical Medicine and Rehabilitation* **79**, 863–872

Jansen G, Lundeberg T, Kjartsson J *et al.* (1989) Acupuncture and sensory neuropeptides increase cutaneous blood flow in rats. *Neuroscience Letters* **97**, 305–309

Karst M, Scheinichen D, Rueckert T *et al.* (2003) Effect of acupuncture on the neutrophil respiratory burst: a placebo controlled single blinded study. *Complementary Therapy Medicine* **11**, 4–10

Kashara T, Wu Y, Sakurai Y *et al.* (1992) Suppressive effect of acupuncture on delayed type hypersensitivity to trinitrotrochlorobenzene and involvement of opiate receptors. *International Journal of Immunopharmacology* **14**, 661–665

Kelleher CJ, Filshie J, Burton G *et al.* (1994) Acupuncture and the treatment of irritative bladder symptoms. *Acupuncture in Medicine* **12**, 9–12

Kellgren JH (1938) Observations on referred pain arising from muscle. *Clinical Science* **3**, 175–190

Lindley S and Cummings TM (2006) *The Essentials of Western Veterinary Acupuncture.* Blackwell Publishing, Oxford

Lundeberg T, Eriksson SV and Theodorsson E (1991) Neuroimmunomodulatory effects of acupuncture in mice. *Neuroscience Letters* **128**, 161–164

Lundeberg T, Kjartansson J and Samuelson U (1988) Effect of electrical nerve stimulation on healing of ischaemic skin flaps. *Lancet* **1988 (ii)**, 712–714

Luo HC, Jia YK and Li Z (1985) Electroacupuncture vs amitriptyline in the treatment of depressive states. *Journal of Traditional Chinese Medicine* **5**, 3–8

Melzack R and Wall PD (1965) Pain mechanisms: a new theory. *Science* **150**, 971–979

Rampes H and Peuker E (1999) Adverse effects of acupuncture. In: *Acupuncture: A Scientific Appraisal,* ed. E Ernst and A White, pp. 128–152. Butterworth Heinemann, Oxford

Sato A, Sato Y, Suzuki A and Uchida S (1993) Neural mechanisms of the reflex inhibition and excitation of gastric motility elicited by acupuncture-like stimulation in anesthetized rats. *Neuroscience Research* **18**, 53–62

Scott S and Mayhew IG (2001) Guest editorial: Pharmacological treatment in behavioural medicine. *Veterinary Journal* **162**, 5–6

Simons DG, Travell JG and Simons PT (1999) *Travell and Simons' Myofascial Pain and Dysfunction: The Trigger Point Manual. Volume 1, Upper Half of the Body.* Williams and Wilkins, Baltimore

Thomas M and Lundeberg T (1994) Importance of modes of acupuncture in the treatment of chronic, nociceptive low back pain. *Acta Anaesthesiology Scandinavia* **38**, 63–69

Travell J (1976) Myofascial trigger points: clinical view. *Advances in Pain Research and Therapy* **1**, 919–926

Wen HL and Cheung SYC (1973) Treatment of drug addiction by acupuncture and electrical stimulation. *Asian Journal of Medicine* **9**, 138–141

White A (1998) Electroacupuncture and acupuncture analgesia. In: *Medical Acupuncture: A Western Scientific Approach,* ed. J Filshie and A White, pp. 153–176. Churchill Livingstone, Edinburgh

White AR, Rampes H and Ernst E (2000) Acupuncture for smoking cessation. *Cochrane Database Systematic Reviews* **2**: CD000009

Zhao J and Liu W (1989) Relationship between acupuncture induced immunity and the regulation of central neurotransmitter system in rabbits. II. Effect of the endogenous opioid peptides on the regulation of acupuncture–induced immune reaction. *Acupuncture Electrotherapy Research* **14**, 1–7

12

Patients undergoing soft tissue surgery

Edited by Karla Lee

Introduction

The goals of soft tissue surgery in small animals must ultimately be to improve quality of life or to prolong life. However, surgery itself represents a traumatic insult to the patient and, along with anaesthesia, results in disturbances to normal physiology. Therefore preoperative assessment of risk of surgical morbidity and mortality is imperative to determine the best approach to an individual case (Hardie *et al.*, 1995).

For each surgical procedure and surgical disease there will be a set of recognized potential complications. Knowledge of these complications is imperative for appropriate postoperative management and planning. Surgery-specific complications are discussed within individual case studies, but more general considerations will be outlined here.

The postoperative plan

Following the decision to carry out surgery, a plan must be in place to provide appropriate postoperative care. This is important because reported rates of postoperative complications in healthy dogs and cats undergoing elective procedures are substantial, ranging from 14 to 20% (Pollari *et al.*, 1996; Burrow *et al.* 2005). Early detection of complications is important to facilitate treatment and to minimize postoperative morbidity and mortality (Grocott, 2009).

The aims of postoperative care are:

- To minimize the postoperative physiological effects of anaesthesia and surgery
- To speed postoperative recovery
- To detect postoperative complications as early as possible
- To minimize postoperative morbidity and mortality.

To achieve these aims, the postoperative plan should include:

- Management of surgery-induced pain until resolution
- Monitoring and support of the major body systems (including cardiovascular, respiratory, gastrointestinal, neurological and urinary) until normal homeostasis is achieved
- Nutritional support and maintenance of adequate fluid intake, as required
- Management of surgical wounds until healing
- Management of surgical inflammation until resolution
- Continued management of devices placed at the time of surgery to assist with postoperative recovery, e.g. skin staples, surgical drains, cystostomy tubes
- Continued management of the primary problem for which the surgical procedure was performed, and of concurrent medical diseases
- Early detection and management of postoperative complications related to: the surgical procedure; anaesthesia; primary disease for which surgery was performed; or concurrent disease unrelated to the surgical procedure.

Management of surgery-induced pain

Pain management is very important. It is discussed in Chapters 2 and 3, and specific considerations for postoperative patients are considered in the case studies that follow this introduction.

Recovery from anaesthesia

A comprehensive review of the recovery from anaesthesia and, in particular, the impact of perianaesthetic drugs on recovery, is beyond the scope of this chapter but can be found in the *BSAVA Manual of Canine and Feline Anaesthesia and Analgesia*.

The aim should be a rapid but smooth recovery. Excessive excitement characterized by varying degrees of vocalization, aggression, trembling, paddling, vomiting, violent movements and convulsions can adversely affect patient physiology, in particular via stimulation of the sympathetic nervous system (Jimenez Lozano *et al.*, 2009). Abnormalities in thermoregulation, cardiovascular instability and respiratory depression are commonly seen early in the postoperative period and need to be managed appropriately.

Postoperative monitoring

Hypothermia

Hypothermia has been associated with prolonged recovery from anaesthesia in healthy dogs undergoing elective surgeries, may result in bradycardia and cardiac arrhythmias, and may predispose to postoperative complications (Pottie *et al.*, 2007). Active attempts to warm the patient (e.g. with blankets, hot air blankets, warm intravenous fluids, heated accommodation) will therefore speed recovery and may decrease the risk of postoperative complications. However, care must be taken not to overheat the patient. Body temperature should be recorded at least every 30 minutes and active heating techniques switched off once the patient's temperature reaches 37°C.

Hyperthermia

Post-anaesthetic hyperthermia has been reported in cats and has been associated with the use of pure opiates (Niedfeldt and Robertson, 2006). Hyperthermia results in increased metabolic activity and can lead to tissue necrosis in extreme situations. Reduction in body temperature can be promoted by using acepromazine (vasodilation), fans, application of cold blankets and liquids to the body, and application of alcohol to the footpads. Naloxone was also found to be effective in reducing anaesthetic-related hyperthermia in cats with temperatures above 41.6°C.

Postoperative hyperthermia can also be seen in large dogs in which low-flow anaesthesia has been performed, and in rare cases of malignant hyperthermia. For malignant hyperthermia, immediate treatment with dantrolene (2–5 mg/kg i.v. to effect) is required (Holden, 2007).

Cardiovascular system

Heart rate, pulse rate and quality, capillary refill time and, if possible, blood pressure should be monitored until they normalize. Hypotension is commonly seen as a result of perianaesthetic drugs and fluid losses during surgery. Cardiac arrhythmias are also not uncommon, though often do not require specific treatment if normal blood pressures are maintained. Intravenous fluid therapy should be continued into the postoperative period to maintain blood pressures and normovolaemia. The use of specific inotropes and vasopressors to maintain blood pressures is not usually required in healthy animals, but they may be used in animals with pre-existing cardiovascular disease, in animals with systemic disease, or in animals experiencing severe blood loss (Holden, 2007).

Respiration

Respiratory rate and nature and oxygen saturation should be monitored until they normalize. Transient, uncomplicated hypoventilation and hypoxaemia can be seen in postoperative animals as a result of recumbency-induced atelectasis and drug-induced perfusion–ventilation mismatching (Campbell, 2003). Rapid recovery, oxygen therapy, sternal recumbency and encouragement to walk are therefore important. Suspicion of major pulmonary complications should prompt immediate respiratory assessment (see *BSAVA Manual of Canine and Feline Cardiorespiratory Medicine*). Prompt initiation of oxygen therapy and other appropriate treatments, including broad-spectrum antibiosis and respiratory physiotherapy for pneumonia, will reduce overall morbidity and mortality (see Chapter 17).

Urine output

Urine output can be an indicator of cardiovascular stability postoperatively. In cases in which hypotension is a concern and direct blood pressure monitoring is not possible, placement of a urinary catheter and attachment to a closed collection system is useful. In these cases a urine output of 0.5–2.0 ml/kg/h is the aim, and intravenous fluid therapy should be adjusted accordingly.

Postoperative urinary retention has been reported in small animals, primarily associated with epidural analgesia, especially in patients with spinal disorders (Sharp and Wheeler, 2005). Other possible causes of retention include: large perioperative volumes of intravenous fluids, which may result in stretching of the bladder wall and decreased detrusor muscle function; pain, especially in the perineal and pelvic region, resulting in sympathetic stimulation and increased urethral resistance; and anal stimulation, activating the vesicoanal reflex. In addition, voluntary urinary retention may be seen in animals reluctant to urinate in their own kennel/cage or on unfamiliar litter.

Signs of urinary retention include involuntary dribbling of urine in the absence of normal urination and a large distended bladder associated with abdominal discomfort. Monitoring voluntary urination and bladder size, and giving dogs the opportunity to urinate away from their kennels, are recommended. For animals receiving epidural analgesia, the bladder should be emptied (e.g. by manual expression) just prior to recovery from anaesthesia, and bladder size and urination monitored for 24 hours postoperatively. Emptying the bladder by urethral catheterization is usually sufficient to promote return of normal urination in the absence of neurological or urinary disease.

Gastro-oesophageal reflux

Gastro-oesophageal reflux has been reported to occur in up to 60% of dogs undergoing anaesthesia. Associated risk factors include abdominal surgery, a prolonged pre-anaesthetic fast, and choice of drugs for premedication and anaesthesia; it is also recognized after prolonged spinal or orthopaedic procedures. Reflux may predispose to oesophagitis, oesophageal stricture formation, regurgitation and aspiration pneumonia (Wilson and Walshaw, 2004); the incidence of oesophagitis is unknown, but post-anaesthetic oesophageal stricture appears to be rare.

The incidence of regurgitation (the passage of gastric contents through the mouth or nose) during anaesthesia varies in different reports. It is currently difficult to predict which animals will actually experience gastro-oesophageal reflux, so appropriate recognition and treatment may be more important in clinical practice.

Drugs that may decrease the incidence and consequences of gastro-oesophageal reflux are still being investigated in veterinary medicine, but include metoclopramide and omeprazole (Panti *et al.*, 2009). Recommended treatment includes lavage of the oesophagus with water *during anaesthesia* (the cuff of the endotracheal tube must be inflated to protect against aspiration during this procedure) plus a post-anaesthetic course of ranitidine or omeprazole (Panti *et al.*, 2009). Oral sucralfate paste is also recommended after recovery.

Nutritional and fluid support

Nutritional and fluid support are very important. General considerations for nutritional support of postoperative patients are discussed in Chapter 5. It is important in soft tissue surgery patients to try to predict the need for postoperative assisted nutrition where possible. This will avoid repeat sedation or anaesthesia for placement of a feeding tube and avoid delays in providing adequate nutrition.

Continuation of intravenous fluid therapy until voluntary fluid intake is advisable in all cases.

Wound management

The aims of postoperative surgical wound management are uninterrupted wound healing and prevention of postoperative bacterial invasion. Knowledge and recognition of the stages of wound healing are required for appropriate management (see *BSAVA Manual of Canine and Feline Wound Management and Reconstruction*).

Dressings

All open wounds should be covered to decrease the risk of bacterial contamination and to promote healing. For closed surgical wounds, there are no certain guidelines for the need for a postoperative dressing. Covering a wound in the immediate postoperative period may decrease bacterial invasion and will absorb any wound discharge. However, a dressing that becomes wet or soiled with urine or faeces can predispose to bacterial contamination and infection, and a covered wound may hide the presence of complications. For most closed surgical wounds a mildly absorbent dressing is generally appropriate, though adhesive dressings can be irritating to the patient and result in self-damage to the wound in sensitive areas such as the ventral neck of a cat or pinna of a dog.

Prevention of patient-induced complications

Wound healing can be compromised by interference or excessive movement by the patient. Elizabethan collars should be placed on those patients that lick or chew at their wounds, or that show a tendency to rub head wounds. Wound dressings or bandages may also be used as a deterrent to interference.

In addition, rest (with supervised lead exercise only) should be encouraged – at least until after removal of skin sutures or staples. This is especially important where wounds are in areas of high movement, but also prevents inadvertent trauma to other wounds. Longer periods of rest may be advisable for surgical wounds involving tissues with longer healing times than skin. For example, 6 weeks' rest would be recommended for healing of coeliotomy wounds, repairs of hernias or body wall ruptures, or a median sternotomy stabilized with orthopaedic wire.

Seroma and haematoma

Seroma and haematoma formation are associated with extensive soft tissue dissections and/or the presence of dead space. They may occur due to poor operative technique or may be an unavoidable consequence of particular surgeries, such as large oncological resections and limb amputations. In addition, excessive postoperative movement and premature removal of surgical drains may promote or exacerbate seroma and haematoma formation in already susceptible patients. Seroma can lead to delayed wound healing, prolonged discomfort, wound dehiscence and infection; careful monitoring is therefore required. Uncomplicated seroma or haematoma will be resorbed by the surrounding tissues and resolve without specific treatment, usually over 1–2 weeks. The evidence that seroma aspiration speeds seroma resolution is limited; therefore, seroma aspiration in small animals is primarily recommended for diagnostic purposes and must be performed using strict aseptic technique. If seroma is associated with significant morbidity, placement of surgical drains may be required.

Drains

Types, indications for, and placement of wound drains are discussed in the *BSAVA Manual of Canine and Feline Wound Management and Reconstruction*. Key points of drain care are noted below.

- Passive Penrose drains should be covered with an appropriate sterile absorbent dressing, where possible, to allow estimation of fluid volume and to prevent environmental contamination.
- The exit point of active suction drains should be covered.
- Active suction drains may be activated 6 hours after completion of surgery, to allow the cutaneous wound to seal and avoid active suction of environmental air into the wound.
- All wound drains should be assessed regularly (every 4 hours for highly productive wounds; twice daily for less productive wounds) for volume of fluid discharge, the need for replacement of associated dressings/bandages and to ensure that they are still secured in position and functioning.
- Persistent high-volume discharge should prompt investigations to rule out infection.
- Recommendations for timing of drain removal vary. In general, drain removal is indicated: when fluid production has reached a constant low level or is <2–4 ml/kg/24h; or when cytological analysis of drain fluid reveals resolution of previous septic neutrophilic inflammation.

Infection control

Postoperative wound infections occur in every surgical facility. It is therefore important to have an appropriate infection control policy to limit postoperative introduction of bacteria and to permit early detection, diagnosis and treatment of postoperative infections. A model for an infection control plan for veterinary practices was published by the National Association of State Public Health Veterinarians in 2008 and includes attention to hand washing before and after each patient encounter and maintenance of good standards of environmental and personnel hygiene.

Figure 12.1 shows criteria for defining postoperative surgical site infections (SSIs). It is important to recognize subtle signs of infection (e.g. persistent or progressive erythema, swelling, heat), as well as the more overt signs of infection (e.g. purulent discharge, abscess, pyrexia). Where possible, diagnosis of an SSI should be confirmed by cytology and/or culture of wound aspirates.

Treatment includes, as appropriate, removal of inciting or perpetuating factors (including suture material), lavage, debridement, and antibiosis based on the results of culture and sensitivity testing.

Dehiscence

Surgical wound dehiscence may result from: inappropriate or poor operative technique; patient factors, such as concurrent endocrinopathy; wound seroma, haematoma or infection; other wound factors, such as the presence of neoplasia or foreign material; drug therapy; or radiation therapy. In addition, inappropriate exercise and self-trauma to the wound in the postoperative period may promote or exacerbate wound dehiscence. Appropriate exercise restriction and the use of an Elizabethan collar for the first 10–14 days of wound healing are therefore appropriate (see above). It is important to note, however, that self-trauma may reflect a postoperative problem that is causing excessive wound irritation or pain. In treating surgical wound dehiscence, the cause for dehiscence should be identified to prevent recurrence. Healing by second intention, or delayed primary closure, may be preferable to repeating primary closure.

References and further reading

Alwood AJ, Brainard BM, LaFond E, Drobatz KJ and King LJ (2006) Postoperative pulmonary complications in dogs undergoing laparotomy: frequency, characterization and disease-related risk factors. *Journal of Veterinary Emergency and Critical Care* **16**, 176–183

Baxter H (2003) Management of surgical wounds. *Nursing Times* **99**, 66

Brainard BM, Alwood AJ, Kushner LI, Drobatz KJ and King LJ (2006) Postoperative pulmonary complications in dogs undergoing laparotomy: anesthetic and perioperative factors. *Journal of Veterinary Emergency and Critical Care* **16**, 184–191

Brown DC, Conzemius MG, Shofer F and Swann H (1997) Epidemiologic evaluation of postoperative wound infections in dogs and cats. *Journal of the American Veterinary Medical Association* **210**, 1302–1306

Burrow R, Batchelor P and Cripps P (2005) Complications observed during and after ovariohysterectomy of 142 bitches at a veterinary teaching hospital. *Veterinary Record* **157**, 829–833

Campbell VL, Drobatz KJ and Perkowski SZ (2003) Postoperative hypoxemia and hypercarbia in healthy dogs undergoing routine ovariohysterectomy or castration and receiving butorphanol or hydromorphone for analgesia. *Journal of the American Veterinary Medical Association* **222**, 330–336

Eugster S, Schawalder P, Gaschen F and Boerlin P (2004) A prospective study of postoperative surgical site infections in dogs and cats. *Veterinary Surgery* **33**, 542–550

Grocott MPW (2009) Improving outcomes after surgery. *British Medical Journal* **339**, b5173

Hardie EM, Jayawickrama J, Duff LC and Becker KM (1995) Prognostic indicators of survival in high-risk canine surgery patients. *Journal of Veterinary Emergency and Critical Care* **5**, 42–49

Holden D (2007) Postoperative care: general principles. In: *BSAVA Manual of Canine and Feline Anaesthesia and Analgesia, 2nd edn*, ed. C Seymour and T Duke-Novakovski, pp.12–17. BSAVA Publications, Gloucester

Horan TC, Gaynes RP, Martone WJ, Jarvis WR and Emori TG (1992) CDC definitions of nosocomial surgical site infections, 1992: a modification of CDC definitions of surgical wound infections. *American Journal of Infection Control* **20**, 271–274

Jimenez Lozano A, Brodbelt DC, Borer KE *et al.* (2009) A comparison of the duration and quality of recovery from isoflurane, sevoflurane, or desflurane anaesthesia in dogs undergoing magnetic resonance imaging. *Veterinary Anaesthesia and Analgesia* **36**, 220–229

Niedfeldt RL and Robertson SA (2006) Postanesthetic hyperthermia in cats: a retrospective comparison between hydromorphone and buprenorphine. *Veterinary Anaesthesia and Analgesia* **33**, 381–389

Panti A, Bennett RC, Corletto F *et al.* (2009) The effect of omeprazole on oesophageal pH in dogs during anaesthesia. *Journal of Small Animal Practice* **50**, 540–544

Pollari FL, Bonnett BN, Bamsey SC, Meek AH and Allen DG (1996) Postoperative complications of elective surgeries in dogs and cats determined by examining electronic and paper medical records. *Journal of the American Veterinary Medical Association* **208**, 1882–1886

Pottie RG, Dart CM, Perkins NR and Hodgson DR (2007) Effect of hypothermia on recovery from general anaesthesia in the dog. *Australian Veterinary Journal* **85**, 158–162.

Sharp NJH and Wheeler SJ (2005) Postoperative care. In: *Small Animal Spinal Disorders Diagnosis and Surgery, 2nd edn*, pp.339–362. Elsevier, Philadelphia

Weese JS (2008) A review of post-operative infections in veterinary orthopaedic surgery. *Veterinary and Comparative Orthopaedics*

Criterion	Superficial incisional SSI	Deep incisional SSI	Organ/space SSI
Timing	Within 30 days of surgery	Within 30 days of surgery or 1 year if implant in place	Within 30 days of surgery or 1 year if implant in place
Location	Only skin or subcutaneous tissues of the incision	Deep soft tissues (i.e. fascial and muscle layers) of the incision	Any area other than the incision that was opened or manipulated during surgery
Clinical aspects (one or more must be present)	• Purulent discharge • Organisms isolated from an aseptically collected sample of fluid or tissue • One or more of pain or tenderness, localized swelling, redness, heat *and* incision is deliberately opened by surgeon *unless* culture is negative	• Purulent drainage from the deep incision but not organ/space • Deep incision spontaneously dehisces or is deliberately opened when patient has one or more of fever, localized pain or tenderness *unless* culture is negative • Abscess or other evidence of infection on direct examination, during re-operation or by histopathology or radiology	• Purulent drainage from drain that is placed into the organ/space • Organisms isolated from aseptically collected sample from organ/space • Abscess or other evidence of infection on direct examination, during re-operation or by histopathology or radiology • Diagnosis of organ/space SSI by attending clinician

12.1 Criteria for defining a surgical site infection. (Data from Horan *et al.*, 1992)

and Traumatology **21**, 99–105

Wilson DV and Walshaw R (2004) Postanesthetic esophageal dysfunction in 13 dogs. *Journal of the American Animal Hospital Association* **40**, 455–460

Williams JM and Moores A (2009) *BSAVA Manual of Canine and Feline Wound Management and Reconstruction, 2nd edn.* BSAVA Publications, Gloucester

Clinical case studies

A variety of case scenarios in dogs and cats will now be presented to illustrate the considerations to be made and the options available within a specific clinical setting. Information relating to the rehabilitation and palliation of each condition has been contributed to each case by the authors in the first part of this Manual, plus notes on nursing and homecare from Rachel Lumbis RVN. The reader should refer back to the appropriate chapters for further details. Photographs used to illustrate the principles and techniques within the cases do not necessarily feature the original patient.

Case 12.1
Bladder rupture repair in a dog

A timid 8-year-old male neutered crossbreed dog was presented with a 1-week history of pollakiuria, haematuria and apparent stranguria, followed by the acute onset of abdominal pain, depression and reluctance to walk.

Clinical examination revealed tachycardia (140 bpm), a prolonged capillary refill time (CRT), weak peripheral pulses, dehydration and marked abdominal pain. An emergency blood profile demonstrated elevations in packed cell volume, total protein, urea (11.4 mmol/l; reference range 2.5–8.9 mmol/l) and creatinine (323 μmol/l; reference range 70–170 μmol/l). Abdominal radiography revealed free peritoneal fluid. Abdominocentesis yielded a sanguineous yellow fluid, containing 1656 μmol/l creatinine, >8.5 mmol/l potassium and 28.4 mmol/l urea, leading to a diagnosis of uroperitoneum.

Agreed medical/surgical management

Lactated Ringer's solution and pethidine were given after initial clinical examination. Fluid therapy was continued with 0.9% lactated Ringer's. Heart rate decreased to 120 bpm and CRT and pulse quality improved.

Anaesthesia was induced and prophylactic perioperative intravenous cefuroxime administered. A retrograde urethrocystogram was performed, followed by an emergency exploratory laparotomy. A ruptured bladder secondary to a bleeding solitary bladder mass was found. The mass was resected with 1 cm margins, the bladder repaired and the peritoneal cavity lavaged with copious sterile 0.9% saline. Histopathology of the mass gave a diagnosis of bladder leiomyoma with clean surgical margins.

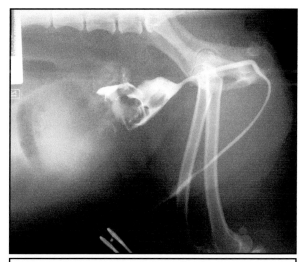

Positive contrast retrograde urethrocystogram demonstrating escape of contrast material into the peritoneal space, an irregular bladder outline, and the possibility of an irregular filling defect within the cranial pole of the bladder.

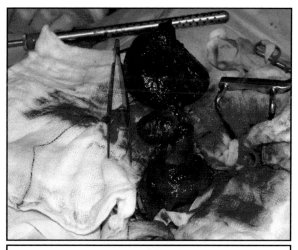

Intraoperative photograph of the bladder (bottom of the photo), demonstrating a tear in the ventral bladder wall, through which a pedunculated bladder mass (middle of the photo) had passed. The smooth deep red mass attached to the bladder mass is an organized haematoma.

A urinary catheter was placed and attached to a closed collection system to monitor urinary output and to prevent bladder distension for 72 hours after surgery. Despite the potential for ascending urinary tract infection, prophylactic antibiotics are not indicated as they may increase the risk of infection with a multi-antibiotic resistant bacterium.

Postoperatively the dog developed peripheral oedema of the distal limbs and muzzle, as well as haematuria and clinical signs of cystitis. Haematuria should self-resolve over a few days in the absence of infection; any signs of urinary tract infection should prompt urine culture and appropriate antibiotic therapy.

As the dog was hypovolaemic, hypoalbuminaemic and anorexic, it was likely that he had a reduced voluntary fluid intake. Preoperatively, azotaemia had resulted from uroperitoneum but a component of pre-renal azotaemia due to hypovolaemia cannot be excluded. Therefore, careful attention to ongoing intravenous fluid therapy is critical in this patient to maintain normovolaemia, renal perfusion and intravascular colloid osmotic pressures, and to correct dehydration. Placement of a jugular catheter with two or three ports would be useful to ensure good intravenous access. Regular monitoring of electrolytes, acid–base status, lactate, haematocrit, total protein, urea, creatinine and glucose should be performed at least every 6 hours for the first 24 hours. With adequate fluid therapy and the absence of pre-existing renal failure or surgical complications, abnormalities in these parameters should resolve. Failure to resolve, particularly in combination with low urine output and/or inappropriate isosthenuria, should prompt consideration of pre-existing renal disease or ongoing uroperitoneum due to leakage from the surgical wounds in the bladder.

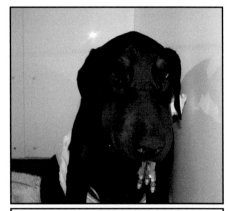

This Dobermann developed postoperative facial oedema secondary to severe hypoalbuminaemia.

Acute/chronic pain management

Perioperative
Perioperative use of non-steroidal anti-inflammatory drugs is contraindicated in hypovolaemia, with any renal pathology, or if uraemia has resulted in gastrointestinal signs; so NSAIDs should not be used in this case. Instead, a full mu agonist, such as morphine, methadone or pethidine (meperidine), should be used for premedication.

Partial agonists such as buprenorphine should be avoided because they may interfere with the action of a full agonist if one is required later in the procedure (e.g. when using fentanyl). It is important to avoid using partial agonists in any preoperative sedation protocol for diagnostic imaging, as this will interfere with the use of full agonists during surgery.

Epidural morphine can be used to provide long-lasting (up to 24 hours) analgesia postoperatively. The use of local anaesthetic in the skin and connective tissue of the midline before incision should be considered. Intraoperative opioids (e.g. fentanyl) may be needed if the epidural is unsuccessful. Lidocaine by CRI, which may be continued postoperatively, could also be considered. A fentanyl patch may be useful for postoperative analgesia, but ideally this would be placed 24 hours before surgery. Otherwise, full mu agonist opioids can be given intravenously or intramuscularly, based on pain assessment.

Chronic pain
If the pain of cystitis continues, NSAIDs may be used, *provided the dog's renal function has recovered postoperatively*. Alternatively, tramadol may be useful for more long-term use. Amitriptyline may be helpful in cystitis, but clearance requires competent hepatic and renal function. Gabapentin is partially metabolized by the liver in the dog and eliminated by the kidneys, so if renal function is impaired, doses should be lowered (5 mg/kg q12h or less).

Fear, stress, conflict concerns

This dog is timid: this may be a specific anxiety about people, or more generalized anxiety about exposure to an unfamiliar and unpredictable environment, or both. With anxiety about handling, the clinic staff should be careful in their approach – talking gently, and getting down to the level of the dog. Reaching over him may increase anxiety. Many dogs are worried about being handled around the collar, so staff should look for signs of appeasement in this context (see Chapter 4).

Making the environment as quiet and predictable as possible is important for a dog that is worried about an unfamiliar environment. Having as few individual carers as possible would be preferable, and giving the dog warning when something is going to happen, such as talking on approach, may help. Consider where he is positioned within the hospital (i.e. away from noisy dogs or procedures). The use of pheromone diffusers or sprays and/or alpha-casozepine may be helpful, although overall efficacy is unclear in these situations (see Chapter 4).

Touch and massage should not be underestimated as a method of relaxing animals. However, even stroking may increase anxiety in a dog that is worried about people, so these techniques should only be used if he does not respond to touch with tension or appeasement behaviours. At home, the owners should develop a bright jolly attitude and not reinforce any anxiety behaviours.

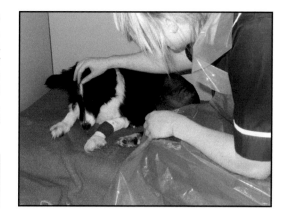

Getting down to the level of the dog may reassure him if he is anxious. (Courtesy of Rachel Lumbis)

Nutritional requirements

Nutritional support and preoperative considerations

Nutritional support may be an important aspect of the treatment strategy. However, before nutritional support can begin, the dog must be stable cardiovascularly and have any major metabolic abnormalities addressed. Therefore, for the first 24 hours and preoperatively, fluid and electrolyte therapy is more important than nutritional support. Thereafter, feeding should be instituted.

In many critically ill dogs recovering from major surgery, the placement of oesophagostomy or gastrostomy feeding tubes greatly facilitates nutritional support (see Chapter 5). As a result of the assessment of the severity and extent of injuries, it may be prudent to place a feeding tube pre-emptively during the original surgery. This would give control of the food intake in the dog and considerably help management of the anorexia.

Postoperative feeding requirements

It is very important to keep adequate records of the dog's daily energy intake, whether he is eating voluntarily or being tube-fed, to ensure that energy requirements are met. It is recommended that feeding is started at 50% of the dog's resting energy requirement (RER; see Chapter 5) on the first day. Suitable diets include gruel-type diets that are high in calories and protein, and easily digestible. Nutritional support may be adjusted to provide more calories, based on the patient's response and tolerance to enteral feeding.

If a feeding tube is NOT paced pre-emptively, postoperative anorexia will need addressing urgently. A naso-oesophageal or oesophagostomy feeding tube might be most appropriate.

Postoperative diets

Nutritional requirements of critically ill dogs have not been clearly defined but may include increased protein requirements. Given this dog's hypoalbuminaemia, provision of higher levels of protein in the diet is recommended. This can be achieved practically by administering a diet formulated for critical care or hospitalized dogs. However, this has to be balanced against considerations of any permanent renal damage sustained as a result of the post-renal failure induced by bladder rupture. If the dog has developed permanent chronic renal failure, a phosphate-restricted diet should be fed long term. Ideally, a diet formulated for renal failure but with only moderate and not marked protein restriction should be chosen.

Nutritional supplements

There has been growing interest in the use of immune-enhancing nutrients, such as glutamine, in critically ill patients. Glutamine may reduce infectious complications by boosting the immunocompetence of the patient and supporting enterocytes. However, although there have been successes with this strategy in other species, there are no positive results from studies evaluating the use of glutamine in dogs (see Chapter 7).

Antioxidants have also been recommended in the treatment of critically ill human patients, but there is limited evidence supporting their use in veterinary critical care. The use of increased omega-3 fatty acids has been recommended in neoplasia in dogs, although evidence for their efficacy is lacking.

This dog has signs of persistent cystitis, so addition of cranberry juice capsules might be beneficial in helping to control this. There is some evidence that cranberry juice protects against infectious cystitis in people (Jepson and Craig, 2008), although evidence of effectiveness in dogs is currently only anecdotal.

Physiotherapy

In this case, peripheral oedema is best managed by a combination of effleurage massage (see Chapter 9) and exercise. Anxiety may be reduced through the inclusion of gentle stroking massage alongside the effleurage. Cold compression can be helpful in many cases when the oedema is caused through injury or surgery to a specific body area that can then be treated to limit the oedema, but is generally less effective when the oedema is more widespread due to hypoproteinaemia, as it seems to be in this case. Encouragement to exercise is a useful way of reducing oedema, and simple walking is adequate. Oedema in the muzzle should be treated by gentle kneading and caudally directed effleurage, although the timidity of the dog may be a difficulty here.

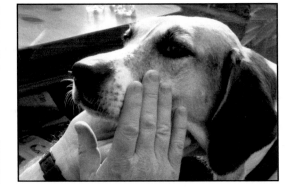

Effleurage of the muzzle to reduce oedema. (Courtesy of Brian Sharp)

Hydrotherapy

This can only be started once the urinary catheter has been removed. Hydrotherapy may help with the distal limb oedema due to the hydrostatic pressure applied to the limbs and the movement in the water (so called 'muscle pump' activity, see Chapter 10). As the dog is nervous, someone will need to be in the pool with him and the owners should be present at the session. Standing the dog in water up to his shoulders, or walking him on an underwater treadmill, may be less stressful in patients that are anxious.

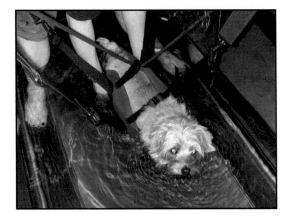

An underwater treadmill, with plenty of support, may be more suitable for a nervous patient. (© Linhay Veterinary Rehabilitation Centre)

Acupuncture

Segmental acupuncture (see Chapter 11) may be helpful in alleviating the pain of cystitis and may also have some mild anxiolytic effects. For this patient, one would select paraspinal points in multifidus muscles from L1 to L4 and S1 to S3. Electroacupuncture may be helpful.

Other nursing and supportive care

Patient comfort
The patient must be kept warm and comfortable and preferably accommodated in a quiet ward. A walk-in kennel may be preferable (see below).

Monitoring
The dog should be monitored closely for worsening abdominal pain, progressive and severe dehydration, hypovolaemia despite intravenous fluid therapy, abdominal distension, discharge from the surgical wound, depression and vomiting.

Blood pressure measurement would be best achieved via an arterial catheter; indirect measurements are less accurate and these inaccuracies will be exacerbated by the peripheral oedema evident in this patient. Mean arterial pressures >80 mmHg are the goal. If direct arterial blood pressures cannot be monitored, a urine output of 0.5–2.0 ml/kg/h, with evidence of renal concentrating function, are suggestive of adequate renal perfusion.

Urination and care of urinary catheter
Postoperatively, the dog must be fitted with an Elizabethan collar to prevent premature removal of the indwelling urinary catheter and to prevent self-mutilation. The indwelling urinary catheter will enable more comfortable urination, which is easier to monitor.

The urine collection bag should be managed to minimize contamination and risk of ascending urinary tract infection:

- The urine bag should be enclosed within a clean transparent bag
- The urine bag is best positioned lower than the dog, to allow urine flow from the bladder by gravity. This means

that the bag is often placed at floor level; it should be on a clean surface, such as an incontinence sheet

- The urine bag and catheter should be handled as far as is possible using aseptic technique: sterile gloves should be worn and the port to empty the urine bag should be cleaned with alcohol before and after use

- The urinary catheter should not be disconnected from the urine collection system unless it is absolutely necessary.

The urine bag should be emptied every 4 hours and urine volume and specific gravity noted to ensure adequate kidney function and normovolaemia. If urine output falls below 1 ml/kg/h, the urinary catheter should be checked to see that it is properly positioned and patent. This will require disconnection of the urinary catheter from the urine collection system. If this is required, sterile gloves should be worn and direct contact with the connection points of the urinary catheter and urine collection system avoided. A catheter tip syringe is attached directly to the urinary catheter and aspirated gently; if negative pressure is present, suggestive of a blockage, the urinary catheter is flushed with saline and reaspirated to ensure patency. If necessary, a new urine collection system should be used. Spraying the connection points with alcohol and air drying prior to reconnection is advisable.

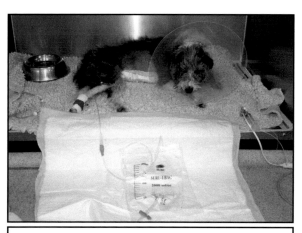

A bitch following urinary tract surgery. An indwelling catheter is attached to a closed urine collection bag. The urine collection bag is contained within a transparent bag and placed on a clean incontinence sheet to decrease contamination. An Elizabethan collar has been fitted to prevent interference with the catheter. The surgical wound is covered with a light dressing. Intravenous fluid therapy is being given via a jugular catheter and direct arterial blood pressures are being monitored via a metatarsal artery catheter. The dog is on comfortable fleecy bedding (a large covering blanket for warmth was removed while the photograph was taken).

Once the indwelling urinary catheter has been removed, it is important to verify the dog's ability to urinate adequately. He should be allowed frequent opportunities for urination, by taking him for walks every 2–4 hours. Note: reduction in bladder size may lead to a need for more frequent urination in the short term. The kennel should be arranged so that the dog can get out of his bed and urinate if he needs to. A walk-in kennel might be more appropriate to allow this and may also be better for a dog that is timid and who may be reluctant to urinate when in close proximity to a stranger.

Care of the surgical wound
The surgical wound should be monitored for: exudates; erythema; haematoma; pain; odour; swelling; and wound breakdown.

Fluid therapy
Hydration status should be checked frequently, by monitoring and recording fluid intake and assessing metabolic state and serum potassium concentrations.

Feeding and tube care
If a feeding tube has been placed, this should be monitored carefully as the majority of complications involve tube occlusion. See Chapter 5 for details of feeding and tube care.

Bodyweight should be monitored daily for patients receiving enteral nutritional support. Food and water should continue to be offered *per os* even if a feeding tube is *in situ,* and the dog should be encouraged to eat voluntarily.

Owner advice and homecare recommendations

Once the dog is at home, he should be strictly rested, with short lead walks for toileting purposes only, for 6 weeks following surgery, as required for healing of the abdominal wall and skin. The owners should maintain a positive attitude toward the dog, so as not to reinforce anxiety behaviours.

Urination
The dog is likely to have increased frequency or urgency to urinate after this type of surgery, so will need frequent access outdoors. Increased frequency of urination associated with reduced bladder size needs to be distinguished from signs of a bacterial cystitis, e.g. depression, non-productive straining, dysuria and haematuria, which should be referred back to the veterinary surgeon.

Follow-up

Owners should be aware of when they need to return for follow-up visits:

- Skin suture or skin staple removal would be advised 10–14 days after surgery
- If a bacterial urinary tract infection has been diagnosed, a 3-week course of an antibiotic will be prescribed; this should be followed by repeat urine culture one week after the end of the course of antibiotics
- Monthly to 3-monthly scans of the bladder would be appropriate to monitor for recurrence of the mass. Bladder leiomyoma is a benign tumour with a good prognosis following complete surgical resection, but it can be difficult to distinguish from leiomyosarcoma, which may have a greater potential to recur locally and metastasize.

References

Jepson RG and Craig JC (2008) Cranberries for preventing urinary tract infections. *Cochrane Database Systematic Reviews* CD001321

Case 12.2
Gastric dilatation–volvulus in a dog

A 4-year-old male neutered Weimaraner was presented with a 4-day history of vomiting a clear frothy liquid, non-productive retching, inappetence and lethargy. Prior to this he had been kennelled for 2 weeks, during which time he was reported to be anxious and continually pacing around his kennel.

Clinical examination revealed depression, weakness, tachycardia (150 bpm), weak peripheral pulses, pale mucous membranes, panting, increased lung sounds bilaterally, pyrexia (39.9°C) and an uncomfortable distended cranial abdomen. Blood biochemistry revealed azotaemia, elevated total protein (90 g/l), hypokalaemia, and mild to moderate elevations in liver enzymes. Haematology revealed a neutrophilia with a left shift and an elevated RBC (9.0 x 10^{12}/l). Thoracic and abdominal radiography demonstrated an alveolar pattern in the ventral lung fields consistent with aspiration pneumonia and gastric dilatation–volvulus (GDV).

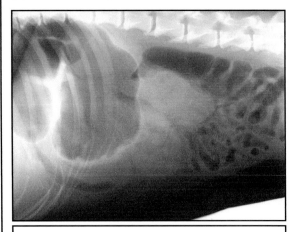

Right lateral abdominal radiograph demonstrating GDV.

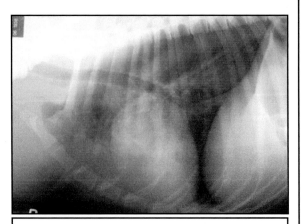

Right lateral thoracic radiograph demonstrating an alveolar pattern in the ventral lung fields, typical of aspiration pneumonia.

Agreed medical/surgical management

Decompensating hypovolaemic shock was initially treated with fluid resuscitation, with 90 ml/kg of lactated Ringer's solution given as quickly as possible after the initial clinical examination. The stomach was partially decompressed by passage of an orogastric tube.

Following successful cardiovascular stabilization, the dog was anaesthetized for an exploratory laparotomy. Prophylactic perioperative antibiotics (intravenous amoxicillin/clavulanate) were administered. The stomach was de-rotated. Organ ischaemic necrosis was not present. An incisional gastropexy was performed to prevent future gastric rotation (though it does not prevent dilatation).

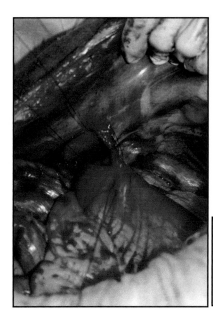

Incisional gastropexy to secure the pyloric antrum of the stomach to the right abdominal wall.

Postoperative medications included antibiosis (amoxicillin/clavulanate and metronidazole) for treatment of aspiration pneumonia.

Ventricular arrhythmias are commonly seen in the postoperative period though they do not usually require treatment. Indications for treatment are: pulse deficits leading to a significant decrease in pulse rate; hypotension due to arrhythmia; or the 'R-on-T' phenomenon. An intravenous lidocaine bolus to restore sinus rhythm should be followed by a CRI.

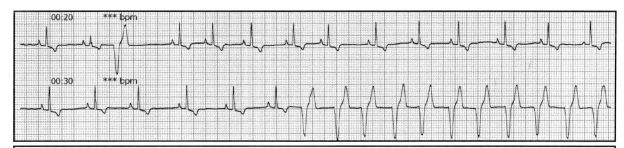

Ventricular premature complexes interspersed with normal PQRS complexes in a dog with GDV. These were seen in the presence of a good pulse quality and normal blood pressures, negating the need for specific therapy. (Courtesy of Simon Dennis)

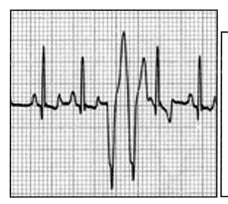

This ECG shows a ventricular couplet (two consecutive ventricular premature complexes, VPCs), with the second VPC occurring on the T-wave of the first VPC. This is referred to as the 'R-on-T' phenomenon. Such patients can be more likely to develop more severe ventricular arrhythmias (ventricular tachycardia, ventricular fibrillation), so there may be a need for anti-arrhythmic therapy. Lead II; paper speed 25 mm/s; gain 1 cm/mV. (Courtesy of Simon Dennis)

Acute/chronic pain management

WARNING
- NSAIDs are contraindicated in the presence of gastric pathology.
- The considerable shock present in GDV with concomitant renal compromise also makes NSAIDs dangerous in this dog.

Perioperative

A full mu agonist, such as morphine, methadone or pethidine, should be used in premedication. Partial agonists such as buprenorphine should be avoided both in premedication and for any sedation for imaging prior to surgery because they may interfere with the action of a full agonist if one is required later in the procedure (e.g. when using fentanyl).

Epidural morphine may provide up to 24 hours' analgesia perioperatively. Local anaesthetic should be placed in the skin and connective tissue of the midline before the incision. Fentanyl by CRI can be used during surgery and can be continued postoperatively. If postoperative fentanyl is not an option, other full mu agonists could be used. Alternatives would include **either** intermittent administration of methadone or morphine, **or** a CRI of morphine.

Lidocaine by CRI can also be used intra- and postoperatively as an adjunct to opioid analgesia. (Lidocaine may also be useful to reduce volatile agent requirement, to minimize reperfusion injury to the stomach, as a prokinetic and as an anti-arrhythmic.)

Chronic pain

Chronic pain should not be an issue in this patient, but should always be borne in mind during subsequent examinations.

Fear, stress, conflict concerns

Since both exposure to stressful events and/or the possession of a generally anxious demeanour have been identified as risk factors for GDV, it is important to investigate carefully any events that cause anxiety in this dog and avoid them in future if possible, or take steps to minimize the stress. In addition to the event that precipitated the current GDV, other stressors should be investigated to reduce the chance of recurrence. Dogs may become anxious in kennels for a number of reasons, so the motivation for the dog's response to kennelling should be investigated by asking about behaviour in other contexts. For example, the dog may generally be anxious about: separation from his owners; social isolation from other dogs; close contact with unfamiliar dogs; or specific noises that occur in the vicinity of the kennels. Once the reason for the anxiety is established, a specific programme of behaviour therapy can be implemented to change the dog's perception of this context. The use of behaviour-modifying medication may be valuable as an adjunct to behaviour therapy in this case to speed up resolution, due to the potentially serious consequences of exposure to stress. However, this will depend also on identifying the specific stressors and the ability of owners to avoid these in the short term (see the *BSAVA Manual of Canine and Feline Behavioural Medicine*).

Nutritional requirements

Food and GDV

There is considerable controversy regarding the potential effect of diet in the pathogenesis of GDV. Studies have identified several risk factors for the occurrence of this disease. The most important of these are genetic and not diet-related, but eating a large meal at one sitting, eating high-fat food and eating from a height have all been implicated as risk factors. One study also identified large food particle sizes as a potential risk factor. Some breeders still persist in feeding susceptible dogs from a height, in the mistaken belief that this reduces the risk of GDV. However, it is important to try to persuade them not to do this, as it actually seems to *increase* the risk, probably because it allows the dog to eat more rapidly. The confusion may possibly have arisen because of concurrent megaoesophagus in some Great Danes, in which feeding from a height *would* be indicated. Some authors have suggested dried food as a risk factor, but studies fail to support this and show no differences in risk with dried, moist or homemade food, or with different proportions of energy supplied as carbohydrate or protein, or with different amounts of soy or cereal in the diet (Glickman *et al.*, 1997; Raghavan *et al.*, 2004, 2006).

Nutritional support

The use of a tube gastropexy (as opposed to the incisional gastropexy performed) would facilitate tube feeding if the dog were unwilling to eat after surgery. Additional benefits of a tube gastropexy in GDV include the ability to decompress the stomach postoperatively, which may be an important consideration especially in dogs that have had repeated episodes of gastric dilatation prior to GDV. Delayed gastric emptying may be present in this patient. Therefore, it is particularly important to check for residual food in his stomach prior to the feeding, by gently aspirating the tube. If a significant amount of the previous feed is still present in the stomach, the feed should be delayed and a prokinetic considered (see Chapter 5). Energy requirements are not very different from those of normal dogs and can be calculated using the resting energy requirement (RER) equations given in Chapter 5.

In GDV cases, rather than bolus feeding (which can result in regurgitation or vomiting) it is often worth trickle-feeding the patient:

- An amount of liquid feed suitable for 12–24 hours is placed into an intravenous fluids bag and giving set, attached to a feeding tube and placed in a pump infusion unit to enable accurate monitoring
- A fresh bag and new solution should be provided every 12–24 hours to prevent bacterial or yeast growth.

Alternatively, the patient can be bolus-fed but the feeds split up into multiple small feeds instead of several bigger ones.

Postoperative diet

It is unclear whether a change in diet affects the risk for future episodes of gastric dilatation. However, it is known that dietary fat and consistency (dried, moist or gruel) have the biggest effects on gastric emptying time (see Chapter 5). Gastric emptying time is increased for days to weeks after GDV surgery, with disruption of the activity of the normal gastric 'pacemaker' in the greater curvature of the stomach. Therefore, a low-fat moist diet would be ideal postoperatively to encourage gastric emptying.

There is a recognized association between GDV and concurrent inflammatory bowel disease (Braun *et al.*, 1996) which could be related to associated delayed gastric emptying. Dietary management postoperatively might include consideration of a novel protein source diet (see Case 22.2). Therefore, the ideal postoperative diet might be one designed for gastrointestinal disease in dogs, i.e. either simple low-fat or low-fat/novel protein.

Feeding should be instituted as soon as possible after surgery. It is no longer believed that a delay in feeding quickens recovery from gastrointestinal surgery. Rather, it appears to be the opposite: a lack of intraluminal food would be expected to delay gut wall healing; and the giant migrating motility complexes of the gut associated with fasting are more likely to disrupt sutures than are the small postprandial peristaltic waves. Therefore, dogs that have gastric resection as part of their surgical treatment for GDV do not require bowel rest and should be encouraged to be fed enterally, as this will promote tissue perfusion and aid in healing.

Gastric wall protection and prokinetics

Although full-thickness gastric wall necrosis was not present, pressure injury to the gastric mucosa is likely. Treatment with sucralfate and agents to increase gastric pH (e.g. H2 receptor anatagonists or proton pump inhibitors) should be considered. Gastric promotility agents (e.g. metoclopramide, ranitidine) are often useful to stimulate return of normal gastric motility and are particularly indicated in dogs that vomit postoperatively. Continuous intravenous infusions of metoclopramide may be more effective than bolus injections in the early postoperative period. Return of appetite and passage of faeces are signs of a return to normal gastrointestinal motility.

Physiotherapy

Physiotherapy is indicated for the aspiration pneumonia (see Case 12.3).

Hydrotherapy

Hydrotherapy is not indicated for this patient.

Acupuncture

There is good experimental (rats) and some clinical (humans) evidence for the use of acupuncture in various visceral functional disorders. Segmental acupuncture (see Chapter 11) may help to restore normal stomach function postoperatively. In this case, paraspinal needling into multifidus muscles in the lower thoracic segments would be appropriate. Ventral needling in the upper rectus abdominus muscles, depending on the wound, may also be helpful in this regard.

Other nursing and supportive care

The patient should be kept warm and comfortable. Patients that are in pain will not appear to be recovering well or may be reluctant to eat. Some may be tachycardic/tachypnoeic.

Postoperative fluid therapy

Fluid therapy must continue in order to maintain intravascular blood volume and blood pressure. A combination of colloids and crystalloids may be required, especially if hypoproteinaemia is present. Electrolyte balance should also be maintained; serum electrolyte concentrations should be checked at least every 12 hours until stable. Hypokalaemia is a common problem, requiring intravenous supplementation (see Chapter 19).

Frequent blood pressure monitoring is also required: at least every 2 hours until it is stable. Placement of an arterial catheter for continuous arterial blood pressure recording is ideal. Alternatively, maintenance of adequate renal perfusion, and thus blood pressure, can be assessed by measuring urine output; this requires an indwelling urinary catheter attached to a closed collection system (see Case 12.1). Urine output should be 1–2 ml/kg/h.

Haemorrhage

Significant blood loss can occur following vessel avulsion, and persistent haemorrhage can be seen due to platelet and clotting factor depletion. Blood loss should be assessed at surgery and postoperatively. A blood transfusion may be required if PCV falls below 15%. A fresh whole blood transfusion will also be a useful source of platelets and clotting factors.

Postoperative monitoring

Monitoring of respiration and oxygenation status by pulse oximetry or arterial blood gas analysis is required due to decreased tissue oxygenation resulting from GDV. In addition this patient has aspiration pneumonia. Oxygen supplementation via nasal prongs or in an oxygen cage may be required (see Chapter 17).

Body temperature should be assessed at least four times a day initially, due to pyrexia at presentation and the aspiration pneumonia. Ongoing pyrexia may suggest that treatment of aspiration pneumonia is not effective or that sepsis has developed.

Monitoring for possible development of septic peritonitis secondary to gastric wall ischaemic necrosis is required during the first 5 days after surgery. Signs of septic peritonitis would include ongoing inappetence, vomiting, abdominal pain, abdominal effusion, hypovolaemic shock and pyrexia. However, thorough assessment of the stomach at initial surgery with partial gastrectomy of ischaemic areas should avoid this late complication.

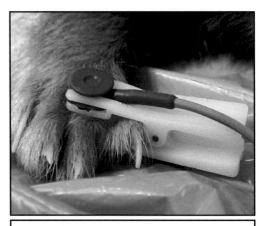

Sensor of a pulse oximeter placed on a non-pigmented toe. (Reproduced from the *BSAVA Manual of Canine and Feline Advanced Veterinary Nursing*)

Care of the surgical wound

The surgical wound should be monitored for: exudates; erythema; haematoma; pain; odour or swelling.

Feeding and tube care

If a feeding tube has been placed, this should be monitored carefully as the majority of complications involve tube occlusion. See Chapter 5 for details of feeding and tube care. An Elizabethan collar to prevent premature removal is less vital with a surgically placed tube and pexied stomach than with a PEG tube, and a collar may not be necessary if the dog is showing no interest in the tube. In this case, a light body bandage may be all that is necessary.

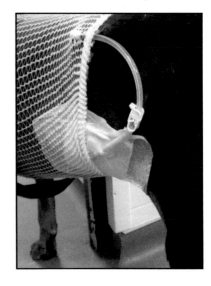

Gastrostomy tube held in place by a light body bandage.(Courtesy of Hilary Orpet)

Addressing anxiety

The GDV patient will have vets and nurses monitoring him closely, thus disturbing him frequently. Additional attention aimed at decreasing anxiety may therefore have the opposite effect. He should be allowed to sleep and recover whenever possible, preferably with the lights turned down and in a quiet area.

Owner advice and homecare recommendations

The client should be advised to rest the dog for 6 weeks following surgery, as required for healing of the abdominal wall and skin. The wound should be monitored carefully and the surgery informed if the wound develops any exudates, swelling, heat or erythema.

Feeding

The owner should be advised about feeding of this dog and also of any other dogs in the household at risk of GDV:

- The dog must not be fed for *at least one hour before or after* exercise
- He should always be fed several small feeds a day rather than one big feed
- Food should either be moist (tinned) or soaked kibbles, not dried.

If the dog is sent home with a feeding tube *in situ*, the client must be fully competent in the provision of tube feeds and caring for the feeding tube.

Follow-up and prognosis

The owners need to be aware of when they need to return for follow-up visits for skin suture/staple removal.

Many dogs with GDV are believed to have an underlying gastric motility disorder and are often prone to recurrent episodes of gastric dilatation. The owner must be warned that these may occur and that the surgery has done nothing to prevent *dilatation*, only to protect against life-threatening *volvulus* by attaching the stomach to the body wall. If the dog has frequent episodes of dilatation, the owner should contact the surgery to discuss further investigation and/or treatment for a medical cause for gastric dilatation/delayed gastric emptying, such as inflammatory bowel disease.

References

Braun L, Lester S, Kuzma AB and Hosie SC (1996) Gastric dilatation-volvulus in the dog with histological evidence of pre-existing inflammatory bowel disease: a retrospective study of 23 cases. *Journal of the American Animal Hospital Association* **32**, 287–290

Glickman LT, Glickman NW, Schellenberg DB, Simpson K and Lantz GC (1997) Multiple risk factors for the gastric dilatation-volvulus syndrome in dogs: a practitioner/owner case-control study. *Journal of the American Animal Hospital Association* **33**, 197–204

Raghavan M, Glickman NW and Glickman LT (2006) The effect of ingredients in dry dog foods on the risk of gastric dilatation-volvulus in dogs. *Journal of the American Animal Hospital Association* **42**, 28–36

Raghavan M, Glickman N, McCabe G, Lantz G and Glickman LT (2004) Diet-related risk factors for gastric dilatation-volvulus in dogs of high risk breeds. *Journal of the American Animal Hospital Association* **40**, 192–203

Case 12.3
Aspergillosis and laryngeal paralysis in a dog

A 10-year-old entire male Golden Retriever of calm temperament was presented for investigation of a 3-month history of progressively worsening, constant, unilateral right-sided, green mucoid nasal discharge associated with sneezing. He had also lost his bark and had short periods of respiratory distress characterized by a marked increase in inspiratory effort. Respiratory distress was noted during mild exertion. The dog had limited his exercise to slow walks with no running.

No active abduction of the arytenoids was seen on examination of the larynx under a light plane of anaesthesia. Thoracic and cervical CT were unremarkable. A clinical diagnosis of laryngeal paralysis was made.

CT of the head demonstrated extensive loss of the nasal turbinates in the right nasal cavity, with fluid accumulation that extended into the right frontal sinus. A bony reaction in the surrounding right maxilla, right frontal bone and right calvarium was evident. Destruction of the nasal turbinates was confirmed by rhinoscopy; it was not associated with a mass lesion. Rhinoscopic biopsy of the right nasal cavity revealed neutrophilic inflammation. Exploration of the right frontal sinus revealed a white fungal plaque consistent with aspergillosis. Culture of this plaque confirmed infection with **Aspergillus fumigatus**.

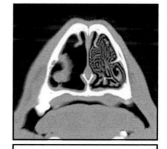

CT scan from a dog with aspergillosis, showing loss of the nasal turbinates in one nasal cavity. (Courtesy of CR Lamb. Reproduced from *BSAVA Manual of Canine and Feline Musculoskeletal Imaging*)

Surgery

Left arytenoid lateralization was performed for treatment of laryngeal paralysis. Prophylactic perioperative antibiosis (intravenous amoxicillin) was administered.

Enilconazole treatments

Topical administration of enilconazole bilaterally into the frontal sinuses and nasal chambers was chosen, due to extensive frontal sinus involvement and the reported success of this treatment (Sharp *et al.*, 1993). Tubes for topical administration of the enilconazole were placed surgically during the surgical anaesthesia. The tubes (sections of wide-bore intravenous extension tubing) were placed via right and left frontal sinusotomies: two tubes were placed in each sinus, one to instil medication into the sinus and one into the nasal chamber. The tubes were secured with Chinese finger-trap sutures and left open to the air to prevent excess build-up of pressures in the sinuses and nasal cavities. An Elizabethan collar is used to prevent the dog removing the treatment tubes. This collar must be kept clean and dry; in particular, any enilconazole that drips on to this collar must be removed. Care must be taken to ensure that the collar does not interfere with the surgical wound from the arytenoid lateralization.

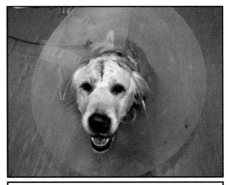

Golden Retriever with apergillosis undergoing daily local enilconazole treatment. Bilateral nasal discharge, worse on the left, is evident. The Elizabethan collar is cleaned regularly, but a small amount of discharge is still present.

Enilconazole treatment was due to start the day after tube placement but was delayed due to the development of aspiration pneumonia. Treatment with intravenous ampicillin and enrofloxacin, and oxygen therapy via nasal prongs was initiated. Clinical improvement and improved oxygenation permitted initiation of enilconazole treatment 5 days later. Antibiotics for aspiration pneumonia should be continued for at least 1 week beyond the resolution of visible radiographic changes.

Care is required during enilconazole treatment to avoid aspiration and to encourage the flow of enilconazole along the nasal chambers and out through the nostrils. Treatment is ideally performed outside and the dog should be made to feel relaxed. The Elizabethan collar should be removed while the drug is administered, and it is best if the dog is sitting upright or standing. The dog's nose should be pointed downwards during treatment and for approximately 10 minutes afterward. The tubes are flushed with 10 ml of air before and after treatments to avoid blockage.

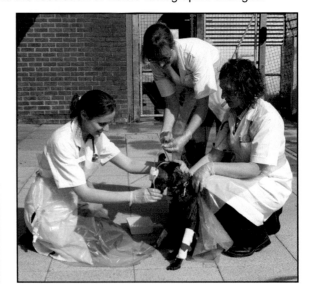

Enilconazole treatment being performed outside. This dog's Elizabethan collar has been removed for treatment and he has been made to feel relaxed. Enilconazole is being administered via four tubes placed via bilateral frontal sinusotomy into the frontal sinuses and nasal chambers. The dog is sitting with his nose pointing downwards to allow the enilconazole to drain through the nostrils.

Perioperative

Analgesics to be incorporated into premedication include: full mu agonist opioid (e.g. methadone, morphine, pethidine); medetomidine (NB medetomidine should not be used if there is any underlying cardiovascular disease); and NSAIDs, provided the dog's renal function is good. Local anaesthetic should be placed in the skin and subcutaneous tissue down to the periosteum before the incision is made. Fentanyl can be used intraoperatively as required as an intermittent bolus or CRI. Opioids should be continued postoperatively for 1–2 days as necessary, based on frequent pain assessment.

Tube flushes

The dog may become distressed with tubes in his nose. The use of local anaesthetic at the time of surgery may be helpful; and EMLA cream applied before each tube flush may help later if this distress continues. NSAIDs should be continued postoperatively for as long as the tubes need to be flushed, and as necessary based on further pain assessments.

Chronic pain

If assessments indicate that the dog is still experiencing discomfort, tramadol may be helpful in addition to NSAIDs. Tramadol can cause dysphoria and dullness, which may be mistaken for depression due to the pain and disease; also, vomiting occasionally occurs with tramadol. If other analgesics are not tolerated, acupuncture may have a role in relaxing the patient and providing some general analgesia (see below).

Fear, stress, conflict concerns

The patient may become anxious with increasing difficulty in breathing. There is good evidence in dogs (and in rats and humans) that gentle stroking of the chest and abdomen releases oxytocin, along with other neurotransmitters, and that this has mild anxiolytic, analgesic and sedative effects (see Chapter 8). These may help prevent the positive feedback cycle of dyspnoea and anxiety.

It is of note that this dog has a calm temperament. It would be difficult to administer the enilconazole treatment described to an aggressive dog or one that resents handling. It is important to provide this dog with a reassuring and stress-free environment to maintain his amenable nature throughout treatment.

Nutritional requirements

Challenges

Inappetence is a significant problem during enilconazole treatment. Nutritional management of dogs with pneumonia, upper airway disease and inappetence is a major challenge. It is important to emphasize that any attempt to force- or syringe-feed a dog with upper airway dysfunction, such as laryngeal paralysis, should be avoided because of the high risk of aspiration pneumonia. This also extends to the forced administration of oral medications. It is far better to give these parenterally, if they are not willingly taken by mouth. The use of appetite stimulants in dogs with ongoing disease, especially those being treated with medications that affect appetite, often prove ineffective. In fact, there is little evidence demonstrating the efficacy of appetite stimulants in general in dogs. Acupuncture may stimulate appetite (see below).

Aspiration of food following laryngeal tie-back surgery is a common complication. Some advise withdrawal of food until the day after surgery to ensure pharyngeal function has returned fully after anaesthesia prior to feeding. Feeding balls of food of a sausagemeat consistency and avoidance of powdery foods, milk and gravy are also recommended to try to avoid aspiration.

An additional challenge in this dog is ensuring adequate feeding if the dog is sedated daily for tube flushes. It is advisable NOT to sedate dogs for tube flushing, and in most dogs this is not necessary, but a few become very distressed and require light sedation. Adequate daily food intake in spite of starvation for sedation may be achieved by feeding the dog in the evenings after recovery from sedation and then starving again for 12 hours prior to the next flush. There is more of a challenge if this dog is tube-fed, because the volumes given by tube need to be small (see below). Great care must therefore be taken in calculating the timing and calorie intake at each meal to ensure that the dog takes in enough calories daily in spite of the flushes.

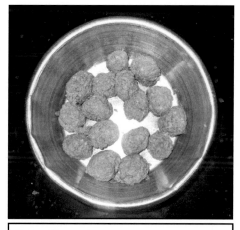

Balls of food of a sausagemeat consistency. (Courtesy of Rachel Lumbis)

Monitoring food intake and tube feeding

Good records should be kept of the dog's daily food intake; if this is less than about 85% of the daily RER (see Chapter 5) for 3 days, nutritional support should be implemented. It is very likely that this dog will NOT eat willingly. In this case, the most effective means for providing nutritional support would be to place an oesophagostomy tube or a percutaneous gastrostomy tube (see Chapter 5). This would allow for the continued treatment of the aspergillosis and pneumonia, and provide a means for effective nutritional support.

> **WARNING**
> A naso-oesophageal tube is contraindicated because of the ongoing nasal disease.

Diets typically used for tube feeding are usually energy-dense, high in protein and easily digestible. Initial feeding calculations should be designed to meet the dog's RER but could be adjusted upon reassessment of his body condition and appetite status.

There is a real risk of aspiration if the stomach is over-filled and food refluxes up the oesophagus. Therefore, feeding via either form of tube should be instituted slowly and carefully, with frequent small volumes. The tube should be aspirated before each feed to check for excessive gastric retention of the last meal; if this occurs feeding should be delayed. Prokinetics could be administered to aid gastric emptying and usually work within 30–60 minutes of administration; the tube can then be re-aspirated 1–2 hours later with a view to administering the next feed.

Physiotherapy

Physiotherapy is an important part of the treatment of aspiration pneumonia and should be applied from the time of diagnosis. It aids expulsion of airway secretions and encourages deep breathing. The protocol for chest physiotherapy should consist of nebulization and percussion (coupage). Nebulization with moist steam, using a hand-held nebulizer, should be performed prior to coupage to help break up airway secretions. Percussion should be carried out for periods of 30–60 seconds, followed by expiratory vibrations (4–6 expirations) and then a rest of one minute. This should be repeated several times and the protocol carried out up to every 4 hours.

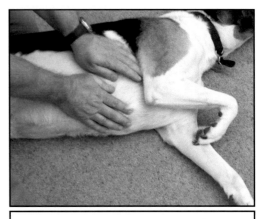

> **WARNING**
> If the dog is dyspnoeic, percussion should be removed from the protocol as it can cause breath-holding.

Expiratory vibrations: the hands are placed on the chest wall and, during expiration, a vibratory movement is applied in the direction of the normal movement of the ribs. (Courtesy of Brian Sharp)

Once the dog is able to walk, he should be allowed to do so for short periods to encourage deep breathing. Percussion/vibrations can continue to be applied.

Hydrotherapy

Hydrotherapy is not indicated for this patient.

Acupuncture

Analgesia
Acupuncture would not be of immediate consideration in this condition, but if other analgesics are not tolerated then acupuncture may have a role in relaxing the patient and providing some general analgesia. Care should be taken in needling over the thorax to avoid the interspaces, because of the risk of causing pneumothorax (well documented in humans). Paraspinal needling in multifidus muscles along the thoracic spine and on the sternum would be the treatment of choice based on the available evidence.

Appetite stimulation
Acupuncture may have an additional effect of stimulating the appetite, although the mechanism is unknown; but it will not improve the taste of enilconazole or the dog's sense of smell!

Other nursing and supportive care

Monitoring for neurological signs
This dog should be monitored for neurological signs, including seizures and central depression, both after surgery and during treatment. The integrity of the cribriform plate can be compromised in patients with aspergillosis, although in this dog the CT scan did not suggest this. The prognosis is poor if fitting occurs.

Fluid therapy
Intravenous fluid therapy with appropriate potassium supplementation is required to avoid dehydration caused by inappetence and increased fluid losses into the airway due to pneumonia. Serum electrolyte concentrations, packed cell volume and total protein should be checked at least twice daily while fluid therapy is required.

Monitoring oxygenation
Frequent monitoring of respiration and oxygenation status by pulse oximetry or arterial blood gas analysis would be recommended to ensure adequate ventilation and oxygenation in the face of pneumonia. Clinical assessment of respiration every 2 hours may be required in the first instance or during the period of ongoing oxygen requirement. Arterial blood gas analysis may be performed once to twice daily to assess the ongoing need for oxygen therapy and response to treatment.

Oxygen therapy should be instituted as required and could be provided via nasal prongs, nasal catheter or an oxygen cage.

Enilconazole treatment
Enilconazole treatment can be unpleasant, so it is important that the dog receives a lot of 'tender loving care'. Taking the dog for a walk after treatment may help to divert his attention.

Care of feeding tubes
If the dog has a PEG or oesophagostomy tube placed, this should be managed as outlined in Chapter 5.

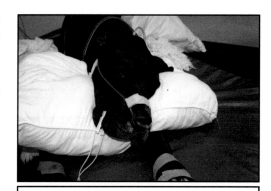

Administration of oxygen via nasal prongs in a Great Dane with aspiration pneumonia. A pulse oximeter has been placed on the lip to monitor oxygen saturation.

Owner advice and homecare recommendations

Homecare following laryngeal tie back
Homecare following laryngeal surgery should include rest for 6 weeks with short (5–10 minutes) lead walks, three or four times daily. A shoulder harness should be used long term instead of a neck collar.

Seroma formation is a common complication; the client should be advised that this will become firm and resolve over 1–2 weeks. Skin suture removal 10–14 days following surgery is recommended.

Feeding a diet of sausagemeat consistency for 6 weeks may help to avoid repeat aspiration. Sudden recurrence of inspiratory distress as seen prior to arytenoid lateralization may indicate failure of the lateralizing suture and the need for repeat surgery.

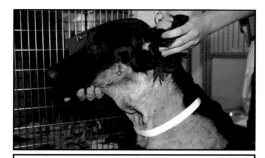

Focal seroma formation 2 days following left arytenoid lateralization.

Homecare for aspiration pneumonia
Homecare for aspiration pneumonia requires monitoring for deterioration. Signs to watch for include laboured breathing, purulent nasal discharge, inappetence and lethargy. The client needs to be advised of the importance of the completion of the courses of antibiotics prescribed. Revisit for repeat thoracic radiography at the end of the course of antibiotics will be required to confirm resolution of pneumonia.

Continued coupage at home may be useful, especially if the dog still has excessive airway secretions. Ongoing warm moist air therapy may also be useful to aid expulsion of airway secretions; the humid environment of a bathroom with the shower running can provide this.

Avoidance of powdery foods, milk and gravy may be recommended long term to decrease the risk and/or severity of aspiration pneumonia.

Homecare after enilconazole treatment
Homecare should include encouragement to return to a normal life, including encouragement to eat if this is still a problem.

The owner should be advised that the tube exit sites will heal by themselves; they should be monitored for increased redness, swelling or discharge suggestive of a secondary bacterial infection, but otherwise left alone. A serous nasal discharge may be present long term due to extensive turbinate destruction. A green mucoid nasal discharge and bleeding from the nose may indicate recurrence of the fungal infection.

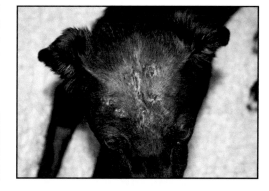

Temporal region of a dog one day after removal of four treatment tubes placed into the frontal sinuses for treatment of aspergillosis. The tube exit wounds were left to heal by second intention and have become sealed with eschars.

References

Sharp NJH, Sullivan M and Harvey CE (1993) Treatment of canine nasal aspergillosis with enilconazole. *Journal of Veterinary Internal Medicine* **7**, 40–43

Case 12.4
Pharyngeal stick injury in a dog

A 1-year-old female entire, boisterous Labrador was presented a few hours after running on to a stick with an open mouth. On lifting her head, a stick with a small amount of blood fell from her mouth. However, she continued to show signs of oral and neck pain and appeared anxious.

Clinical examination revealed anxiety, pain on palpation of the neck and reluctance to open her mouth. An emergency blood profile was unremarkable. Oral examination under anaesthesia revealed a 2 cm wound in the dorsal pharynx with a stick evident in the wound. Cervical and thoracic radiographs demonstrated free air within the soft tissues around the oesophagus and pneumomediastinum. Oesophagoscopy was unremarkable. Diagnosis of a pharyngeal stick injury was made.

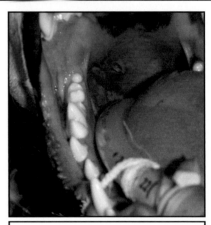

Oral examination, demonstrating a wound in the right side of the dorsal pharynx, containing a stick.

Agreed medical/surgical management

A 10 cm long piece of stick was retrieved from the pharyngeal wound, which was left to heal by second intention. Surgical exploration of the neck revealed a second stick of similar size dorsal to the oesophagus. This stick was removed and the remaining pocket lavaged with sterile saline. A swab was taken for bacterial culture after lavage. A Penrose drain was placed in the neck wound. The pharyngeal wound would be expected to take a few days to perhaps 2 weeks to heal. Repeat anaesthesia to assess the pharyngeal wound would be appropriate 3–7 days after initial surgery, especially if dysphagia were present, and would also permit assessment of laryngeal function if dysphonia, suggestive of injury to the larynx or recurrent laryngeal nerves, were present.

Bacterial culture of the swab from the neck wound revealed a scanty growth of *Pasteurella*, which was sensitive to all antibiotics tested. A 7-day course of amoxicillin was initiated at surgery, pending culture results, and then continued for a further 7 days.

A gastrostomy feeding tube was placed while the dog was under anaesthetic (see below).

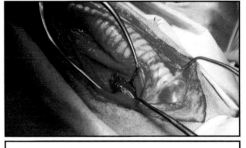

Intraoperative photo of a ventral midline exploration of the neck; a stick was found dorsal to the oesophagus.

Acute/chronic pain management

Perioperative
Methadone and an NSAID should be included in the premedication. Morphine is best avoided, as it can cause vomiting which is undesirable with pharyngeal trauma.

A local anaesthetic at the wound site can be helpful intraoperatively. Additional intraoperative analgesia may be needed and could be achieved with intermittent fentanyl boluses or a fentanyl CRI.

Postoperative
Opioids should be continued postoperatively; their use should be based on pain assessments, but will probably be necessary for 2–3 days.

The NSAID should be continued until the pharyngeal wound has healed. The drug can be given parenterally or via the PEG tube. For example, meloxicam liquid can be given easily via a PEG tube; or oral NSAID tablets can be crushed and administered with the food via the tube.

Chronic pain/analgesia on discharge

NSAIDs are the first analgesic of choice, although they should be administered with strict instructions to the owners to watch for signs of gastrointestinal toxicity, especially vomiting in this case. If NSAIDs are insufficient to control discomfort, tramadol can be added, starting at the lower end of the dose range to minimize the possibility of side effects (vomiting particularly, but also dullness and dysphoria, which may confuse the clinical assessment).

Chronic pain and sensitization around the wound site may be additionally treated with amitriptyline, amantadine or gabapentin (see Chapter 3).

Fear, stress, conflict concerns

This is an active dog, who will undoubtedly attempt to remove her drain. Her stress is likely to rise once she feels better in herself, when her activity levels will make management of wound and tube challenging. Distraction, gentle play and mental stimulation, including training exercises, may help in this regard. Sedation with a combination of acepromazine and opioid or with diazepam/alprazolam may be helpful if the dog is really boisterous after surgery.

Nutritional requirements

Resting the pharynx: tube feeding

Dogs with open pharyngeal wounds may or may not tolerate oral feeding. Oral discomfort and gagging may result in inappetence. In addition, a large pharyngeal wound may result in oral food entering the cervical tissues and exiting the body via the Penrose drain. In these circumstances the pharynx should be rested to allow healing and the dog should NOT be fed by mouth or by any type of tube that will pass through the affected area and delay healing; **i.e. neither a naso-oesophageal tube nor an oesophagostomy tube should be used.**

Provision of nutritional support in cases of extensive pharyngeal and/or oesophageal injury is best achieved via the placement of a gastrostomy tube, placed either surgically or endoscopically. Consideration should be given to surgical placement of this tube when the dog is anaesthetized for cervical exploration. Alternatively, a tube can be placed endoscopically while the dog is under anaesthetic for treatment of the stick injury. Feeding should be instituted as soon as possible after surgery and introduced gradually over a few days; the initial amount to feed should be calculated using the dog's RER (see Chapter 5).

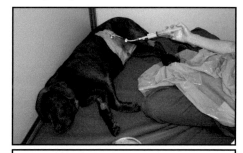

Feeding the patient via a PEG tube. In the absence of direct supervision, the dog would be wearing an Elizabethan collar.

Diet

There are no specific alterations to the nutritional requirements of the dog after surgery. Therefore, a maintenance diet can be modified by liquidizing a wet diet into a gruel with additional water. Alternatively, an energy-dense high-protein diet could be used.

Careful daily records should be kept of the dog's food intake, weight and body condition, and the amount of food adjusted to maintain body condition. After a few weeks, the dog can be transitioned to normal oral feeding.

Physiotherapy

Physiotherapy is not indicated for this patient.

Hydrotherapy

Hydrotherapy is not specifically indicated for this patient.

Acupuncture

Acupuncture is not applicable unless all other forms of analgesia are not tolerated.

Other nursing and supportive care

Care of the surgical wound

The surgical wound should be monitored for: exudates; erythema; haematoma; pain; odour; swelling; and wound breakdown.

Care of drains

Penrose drains should ideally be dressed with a non-adherent absorbent dressing and the dressing changed once or twice a day depending on the level of fluid production. Care must be taken to avoid tight cervical bandages as, in the face of ongoing pharyngeal/cervical inflammation, these can result in obstruction to venous drainage from the head and neck, and secondary oedema. Pharyngeal oedema could lead to airway obstruction. Cervical bandages should therefore be checked every 4 hours if placed. If oedema develops, it is better to leave the Penrose drain undressed and instead to barrier nurse the patient to avoid contamination of the Penrose drain and transfer of bacteria from the drain exudates to other patients.

Drainage from the Penrose drain should be monitored. The drain should be removed when fluid production falls to a steady low level and there is no evidence of ongoing infection. The latter can be checked by cytology of the draining fluid: the presence of intracellular bacteria and toxic or degenerate neutrophils would suggest ongoing active infection. Following removal of the drain, the exit wound should be left to heal by second intention.

Care of feeding tube

This patient will require an Elizabethan collar when left unattended, to avoid interference with her gastrostomy tube. Care must be taken to ensure that the collar does not interfere with the surgical wound.

The feeding tube will need careful monitoring: the majority of complications involve tube occlusion or localized irritation at the tube exit site. Serious complications such as infection, tube dislodgement and peritonitis should be watched for. The feeding tube is flushed with 5–10 ml of water after each feed to minimize clogging (see Chapter 5).

The dressings and bandages covering the feeding tube should be inspected daily for signs of infection and the site cleaned. Bodyweight should be monitored daily for patients receiving enteral nutritional support.

Fluid therapy

Oral food is withheld until the pharyngeal wound has closed. However, free access to water should be permitted. Fluid requirements should be dealt with by gastrostomy tube feeding, but intravenous fluid therapy may be required in the first 24 hours pending full initiation of gastrostomy tube feeding. Willingness to drink without difficulty would be an indication of a comfortable mouth.

Monitoring for postoperative complications

Possible postoperative complications include: dysphagia, pending healing of the pharyngeal wound; dysphonia, if laryngeal trauma occurred; cellulitis and infection of the cervical tissues; and late formation of a cervical abscess due to retention of a stick fragment within the cervical tissues.

Prior to complete healing the dog may demonstrate oral discomfort, retching or gagging when drinking water, a pharyngeal cough and blood-tinged saliva. Resolution of these signs would suggest appropriate healing of the pharyngeal wound.

Infection is one of the biggest concerns. Ongoing monitoring of body temperature, the Penrose drain and the surgical wound are required to detect uncontrolled infection.

Owner advice and homecare recommendations

Monitoring the wound site

The owner should be warned that a possible long-term complication is abscess or sinus formation if a fragment of stick remains within the neck. If the owner has any concerns, they should contact their veterinary surgery for advice. The client should be advised on how to monitor the wound, watching closely for signs of complications, such as drooling (possibly with blood-tinged saliva), dysphagia and facial/pharyngeal discomfort (pawing at the face).

The owner should be instructed to use a harness on the dog rather than a collar. In order to comply with UK law, an identity tag must be attached to the harness.

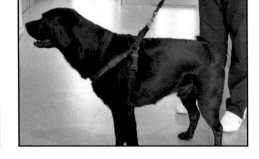

A harness should be used in place of a collar while the dog has a neck wound. (Courtesy of Samantha Lindley)

Feeding tube care

If the patient is going home with a feeding tube in place, the client must be fully competent in the provision of tube feeds and caring for the feeding tube.

Advice about play

The owner should be advised that **throwing sticks for dogs to catch is not recommended** for this or other dogs. Alternative safe playthings, such as balls of the correct size, should be suggested.

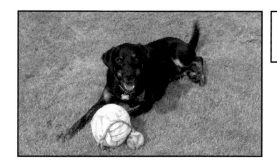

A ball is a much better 'fetch' toy than a stick. (Courtesy of Claire Corridan; reproduced from *BSAVA Manual of Canine and Feline Behavioural Medicine, 2nd edition*)

Follow-up and prognosis

The owners need to be aware of when they need to return for follow-up visits for skin suture/staple removal.

Prognosis is good, though failure to find a fragment of stick will result in a foreign body abscess after discontinuation of antibiotics. Chronic foreign bodies can be difficult to locate: CT or MRI would be recommended prior to repeat surgical exploration.

Case 12.5
Rectal adenocarcinoma in a dog

A 10-year-old neutered male Boxer dog was presented with straining on defecation. The dog was passing ribbon-like faeces, with some fresh blood. Rectal palpation revealed a rectal mass within the terminal colon. A proctoscopic biopsy confirmed adenocarcinoma. The owner was an elderly man and the dog was his only companion and very attached to him.

Right and left lateral thoracic radiographs revealed no obvious lung metastases. Pre-anaesthetic haematology and biochemistry blood screens were unremarkable.

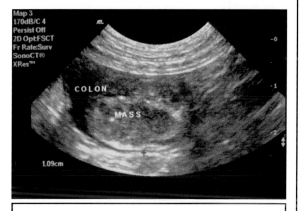

An ultrasound image of the descending colon, demonstrating an intraluminal soft tissue mass.

Agreed medical/surgical management

An exploratory laparotomy was performed. Prophylactic perioperative antibiosis was carried out with intravenous cefuroxime. In addition, oral metronidazole was administered for 3 days prior to and including the day of surgery. The dog was starved for 36 hours prior to surgery to reduce faecal volume within the colon. The presence of a mass lesion within the descending colon was confirmed at surgery, and several small nodules were noted in the liver.

Liver biopsy and surgical resection of the colonic mass were performed. Unfortunately, histopathology revealed extension of neoplastic adenocarcinoma cells up to the margins of the colonic resection, and metastatic spread to the liver. Meloxicam was prescribed to try to slow growth of the tumour.

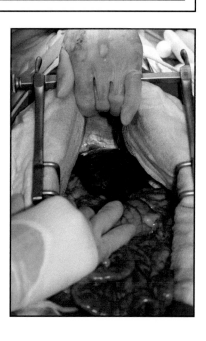

Exploration of the cranial abdomen revealed a nodular hepatic lesion with white discoloration.

Acute/chronic pain management

Perioperative

A full mu agonist, such as morphine, methadone or pethidine, should be used in premedication. Partial agonists, such as buprenorphine, should be avoided because they may interfere with the action of a full agonist if one is required later in the procedure (e.g. when using fentanyl). NSAIDs may also be included in premedication if there are no contraindications based on preoperative clinical signs and blood work-up (i.e. no gastrointestinal signs or renal/hepatic compromise).

Epidural analgesia with bupivacaine/morphine will provide ideal intraoperative analgesia. The morphine analgesia may last up to 24 hours postoperatively. Additional opioids may be necessary during surgery (e.g. fentanyl boluses) and will need continuing postoperatively (e.g. methadone) based on pain assessment.

Postoperative

Opioids may need continuing for 2–3 days postoperatively and the NSAIDs should be continued postoperatively until the wound has healed.

Chronic pain

There is some evidence that piroxicam (and therefore likely also the closely related meloxicam) may slow progression of the carcinoma postoperatively, so long-term use of NSAIDs may be indicated in this dog, provided there are no side effects. Tramadol can be added to the NSAIDs if necessary whilst the wound is healing. Pain assessments should be continued, to determine whether there are any other sources of pain and/or continuing sensitization of the surgical site. Although this dog has demonstrable hepatic metastases, these would rarely destroy enough liver to impair liver function. Therefore, provided there is no evidence of reduced hepatic function, gabapentin, amitriptyline, amantadine or paracetamol might be considered as alternative analgesics as necessary.

Fear, stress, conflict concerns

The dog and owner are very attached to each other. Therefore, the separation between them should be as little as possible, allowing visiting if appropriate. The previous experiences of the dog will influence the specific issues associated with this case. If the dog has had a very routine and predictable life with his elderly owner, then he may be particularly anxious about being in a novel environment with a different routine. Limiting the number of different carers, reducing disturbance, putting him in a quiet area, and keeping the routine as predictable as possible would help this patient.

Nutritional requirements

Importance of early postoperative feeding

Nutritional support of dogs following major surgery can be challenging. In the short term, it is important to ensure the dog eats while hospitalized. He should be fed as soon as possible after surgery (within 24 hours) to facilitate healing. Contrary to previous ideas, early feeding does not increase the risk of rectal suture breakdown and peritonitis. In fact, it is very much the reverse: intraluminal nutrition is needed to allow effective gut wall healing; and the 'giant migrating motility complexes' of the gut associated with fasting will be likely to put more strain on the sutures than the smaller postprandial peristaltic waves. However, in this dog it is important to choose a low-residue diet postoperatively to reduce the bulk of the faeces in the colon and rectum. The inclusion of some fermentable (soluble) fibre is wise to provide nutrition for the healing colonocytes. Lactulose is a suitable soluble fibre for postoperative use and will also make the faeces softer. It should be titrated to effect to produce two or three soft defecations a day – err on the conservative side to start with, as too much will result in diarrhoea. Ispaghula would be a suitable alternative.

Long-term dietary management

The major long-term dietary consideration in this case revolves around facilitating passage of stool and avoidance of the development of diarrhoea or tenesmus. For these reasons, a moderately fat-restricted, low-residue diet composed of highly digestible protein and carbohydrate and fermentable fibre may be ideal. There is a concern, however, that the fat and caloric content of such diets may not be appropriate for long-term use if the dog becomes debilitated from the metastatic carcinoma.

Once the rectum has completely healed, transition to a diet with a higher calorie content may be better in terms of supporting body condition, However this approach cannot fully reverse the catabolic effects of certain tumours. Therefore, it is important that the dog's bodyweight is measured regularly (ideally, every 2–3 weeks) and the diet and calorie intake adjusted accordingly.

Nutraceuticals

The precise nutritional requirements of small animals with neoplasia are unknown. Omega-3 fatty acids have been proposed to impact catabolic conditions favourably, by allowing animals to preserve lean body mass and even stimulating appetite. Furthermore, omega-3 fatty acids have been recommended for certain types of canine neoplasia (Ogilvie *et al.*, 2000). However, evidence of efficacy in prolonging disease-free state or length of remission is not convincing, and omega-3 fatty acids have not been properly evaluated in dogs with rectal carcinomas. Some veterinary diets contain omega-3 fatty acids already. If not, they can be supplemented in the form of fish oil capsules. Given that the 'ideal' dose of omega-3 fatty acids has not been ascertained, it is impossible to advise a dose rate or whether extra should be added to a diet already supplemented. Given the risk for developing diarrhoea when high doses of omega-3 fatty acids are introduced into the diet, supplementation should not be begin until the surgical site is fully healed.

Physiotherapy

Physiotherapy is not specifically indicated for this patient. The owner should be advised to increase exercise gradually following discharge. In cases where there is a strong bond between the pet and owner it can be helpful to teach the owner how to do gentle stroking massage (which can provide comfort to the dog and owner) and make the owner feel he is actively participating in the treatment process.

Hydrotherapy

Hydrotherapy is not specifically indicated for this patient.

Acupuncture

Acupuncture is unlikely to be appropriate. The only indication would be wound breakdown, which would need local needling close to the edge of the wound – this would probably not be well tolerated.

Other nursing and supportive care

Care of the surgical wound
The surgical wound should be monitored for: exudates; erythema; haematoma; pain; odour or swelling.

Feeding
Food should be offered as soon as possible following surgery (see Nutritional requirements, above). A stool softener may be added to the food for 2–3 weeks to facilitate passage of stools.

Patient comfort
As the dog is elderly, an especially soft and supportive bed should be provided. The patient should be prevented from lying on one side for long periods to prevent decubitus ulcer formation. Regular opportunities for the dog to go outside, for a short walk around the garden or yard, will promote mobility and encourage defecation.

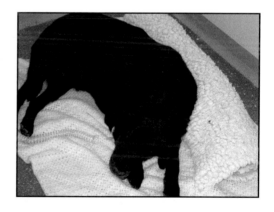

Supportive bedding is required for elderly patients and will aid in the prevention of decubitus ulcers. (Courtesy of Liz Mullineaux)

Monitoring for specific complications following colonic resection and anastomosis and liver biopsy
Complications of colonic resection and anastomosis include haematochezia, tenesmus, rectal prolapse, fecal incontinence, colonic stricture, colonic wound dehiscence and septic peritonitis, and surgical wound infection. Defecation and the perineal area need to monitored carefully postoperatively until return to normal. Haematochezia and tenesmus within the first week can be seen despite normal colonic wound healing and in isolation should not be a specific cause for concern. However, tenesmus can result in rectal prolapse, so oral laxatives may be beneficial. Faecal incontinence is unlikely following partial colonic resection and anastomosis; this complication is seen more frequently following large rectal resections.

Failure of colonic wound healing would result in septic peritonitis within the first 3–6 days after surgery and can occur in diseased intestines despite good surgical technique. Signs of septic peritonitis include ongoing inappetence, vomiting, abdominal pain, abdominal effusion, hypovolaemic shock and pyrexia. These findings should prompt complete clinical assessment and abdominocentesis: septic neutrophilic peritoneal inflammation would confirm suspicion of septic peritonitis. Exploratory laparotomy to repair colonic wound dehiscence and lavage of the peritoneal cavity, combined with intensive care support, would be required.

The major complication following liver biopsy is haemorrhage. Signs of hypovolaemic shock and pale mucous membranes, with or without abdominal distension, should prompt a check of blood haematocrit and abdominocentesis. Conservative management with fluid therapy, an abdominal bandage and blood transfusion, if required, is usually sufficient, but surgery to identify and ligate the bleeding vessel may be necessary if conservative management fails.

Owner advice and homecare recommendations

Rest
The client should be advised to rest the dog for 6 weeks following surgery, as required for healing of the abdominal wall and skin.

Wound care
The client should be advised to monitor the wound carefully and to contact the surgery if the wound develops any exudates, swelling, heat or erythema.

Follow-up and prognosis
The owners need to be aware of when they need to return for follow-up visits for skin suture/staple removal.

The owner should be informed carefully and sensitively of the dog's poor prognosis and the certainty that the tumour metastases will grow and spread in the long term, and eventually necessitate euthanasia. The owner should be informed of the signs to look out for (e.g. weight loss, vomiting, anorexia, return of dyschezia and haematochezia). The owner should monitor the dog's quality of life, reporting any changes in behaviour or deterioration in condition to the veterinary surgeon. Regular phone updates to the veterinary surgeon every 1–3 months are to be encouraged in this case to allow the owner to express any concerns and differentiate serious from non-serious clinical signs.

References

Ogilvie GK, Fettman MJ, Mallinchrodt CH *et al.* (2000) Effect of fish oil, arginine and doxorubicin chemotherapy on remission and survival time for dogs with lymphoma – a double blinded, randomized placebo-controlled trial. *Cancer* **88**, 1916–1928

Case 12.6
Bilateral thyroidectomy in a cat

> A 12-year-old neutered male DSH cat exhibited signs of weight loss, polyphagia and changed behaviour. A large bilateral goitre was palpable. The cat was easily stressed.
>
> Total T4 was markedly elevated (260 mmol/l; reference range 19–65) and biochemistry revealed mild to moderate elevations in alanine transferase and alkaline phosphatase, leading to a diagnosis of hyperthyroidism. The owner elected for surgical treatment.

Agreed medical/surgical management

The cat was treated with methimazole for 2 weeks prior to bilateral thyroidectomy. Surgery was performed using the modified extracapsular technique, whereby right and left external parathyroid glands were left *in situ*. Laryngeal function was checked prior to complete recovery from anaesthesia and found to be normal. Histopathology revealed bilateral thyroid hyperplasia and adenoma.

Acute/chronic pain management

Perioperative
This is relatively superficial surgery; buprenorphine may be sufficient for premedication, though the addition of acepromazine may also be useful. Untreated hyperthyroid cats have an increase in glomerular filtration rate which often masks pre-existing renal disease, so the use of NSAIDs is not advisable in these cases.

Local anaesthetic should be infiltrated into the skin before the incision is made. Buprenorphine should be continued for 1–2 days postoperatively, based on pain assessment. This may also relieve any short-term distress caused by the pain of swallowing.

Chronic pain would not be expected in this patient, but the possibility should always be borne in mind.

Fear, stress, conflict concerns

The cat appeared stressed in the clinic environment. This might have been related to his hyperthyroidism, which can be associated with a reduced threshold of response to changes in the environment. Peripheral signs of elevated T4, such as tachycardia, can have a positive feedback on emotional state, leading to increased anxiety. However, he might be poorly socialized to people, and/or responding to being in an unfamiliar and unpredictable environment. It would be helpful to ask the owner about the cat's behaviour in the past, before it became hyperthyroid, to try to differentiate.

In the veterinary clinic
- If the cat is anxious about people, minimal handling is important. As few people as possible should handle the cat and handling should be quiet and low-key. Attempting to stroke or pet the cat may not be perceived *by him* as positive, so should only be done if he responds with signs of a positive emotional state, such as purring, approaching and rubbing (purring alone may be a sign of pain or distress).
- Take time with the patient to help him relax before any intervention.
- In some cases pheromone therapy can be useful, but it is not a panacea, and appropriate handling and management is the main priority.
- Minimize exposure to potential stressors, such as dogs and other cats, noises and strong odours.
- Use the space in the cage to provide a hiding area (a cardboard box with a blanket or bedding will do) and use visual baffles (e.g. a towel over the cage door or hung to separate the cage) so the cat can choose to see and be seen, or to hide. In particular, visual access to unfamiliar cats should be blocked.
- Use minimal restraint during physical examination and the collection of blood for analysis. If possible, time blood sampling and other stressful procedures during sedation for imaging or other investigations. If the patient struggles and signs of respiratory distress appear, it is wise to postpone any handling and let the cat rest in a quiet and, ideally, oxygen-enriched environment. Any struggling will result in an increase in oxygen demand, leading to potentially fatal arrhythmias.

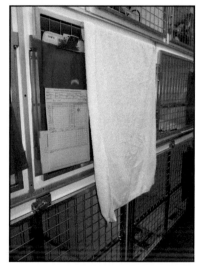

Blocking visual access to other cats can help with in-clinic anxiety. (Courtesy of Liz Mullineaux)

At home
Enhancing the core territory or environment will help the cat feel better. It is also necessary to make some adjustments so that an inactive and unwell patient can still exploit the improvements in the environment.

- **Food.** Increasing the number of feeding stations will increase a sense of security. The overall amount of food should not be increased, unless necessary for weight gain. Ensure the cat can easily reach the food; if he has previously fed at a height he may not feel like jumping, so adjust the position of the food, whilst making sure this does not make the cat anxious about it being available to competitors (the pet dog or a possible intruding cat if the food is placed near the cat flap, for example).
- **Water.** Cats generally prefer their water about a room's distance away from their food in a clear wide bowl, so provision of extra water bowls may be indicated.
- **Access inside and out.** Cats would normally have more than one access in and out of their core territory (usually the house). Consider providing a second access point or ensure that the cat can use the existing access points, i.e. that they are not too high or too difficult to negotiate when he feels unwell or uncomfortable. If he was previously allowed out and is now restricted, the owner will need to put more time into playing and interacting now he is inside all day – whether this is his choice, the owner's or the result of medical advice.
- **Scratching posts.** Are the scratching posts easily accessible and appropriate for this patient? If the cat tends to scratch on horizontal surfaces, then a horizontal scratch post should be provided. If the scratching post is an integral part of a piece of cat furniture, consider whether he can still reach it if he does not feel up to climbing.
- **Hiding areas.** Provide multiple safe and comfortable hiding areas at different levels, or make sure that there is a 'step' system to allow the cat to reach his old favourite places.

- **Bedding.** Provision of new beds such as radiator beds may improve comfort and wellbeing.
- **Play.** Modify games to very short bursts of gentle play, but continue to try gently to stimulate the cat.
- **Touch.** Use gentle touch, stroking and grooming in ways that the patient will not only tolerate but enjoy. This will improve the cat's feelings of wellbeing and also give the owner a sense of participating in their pet's treatment and nursing.

Nutritional requirements

Postoperative feeding

Initial postoperative nutritional support should centre on offering a highly palatable, easily digestible diet. It is important to feed the cat as soon as possible after surgery and to keep good records to ensure that he is in fact eating.

It is likely that appetite will be reduced as a result of the effects of surgery, analgesic drugs, and the removal of the 'drive' to eat associated with high circulating thyroid hormone. In addition, any transient postoperative hypocalcaemia will also interfere with appetite and the ability to eat, due to muscle fasciculations. If the cat does not eat its RER (see Chapter 5), attempts should be made to encourage eating (see Nursing care, below). Appetite stimulants could potentially be used, but only in the short term. If this fails to provide a significant proportion of the cat's daily calorie requirements, a naso-oesophageal tube may be placed and a suitable diet

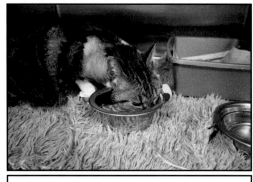

Three hours after a bilateral thyroidectomy, this cat has already started to eat.

administered until the cat recovers its appetite (see Chapter 5). This is the most appropriate form of tube feeding in this case because anorexia is likely to be short term, i.e. during the immediate preoperative period. Even so, early intervention is important, because even a thin cat is at risk of developing hepatic lipidosis when anorexic, if it has concurrent disease.

Long-term nutrition

In the longer term, because the cause for the catabolic state has been dealt with, nutritional support would normally centre simply on providing a good-quality, easily digestible diet. The use of omega-3 fish oils might be considered because they may help in the recovery of lean body tissue and may even help with appetite stimulation. However, the use of omega-3 fatty acids has not been evaluated in this clinical context.

Many cats with hyperthyroidism have mild to moderate elevations in liver enzymes, but this is *not* a reason to place them on proprietary feline liver diets. In most cases, these elevations are secondary to the hyperthyroidism and resolve as it is treated.

Diet if chronic renal insufficiency develops

Bilateral thyroidectomy often uncovers underlying renal insufficiency in cats, which can affect the choice of diet in the long term. If this is the case, the cat should, if at all possible, be moved on to a manufactured low-phosphate renal diet. These diets have been shown significantly to increase the life expectancy of cats with renal disease (see Chapter 5). The diet change should be gradual, but it is worth making the change early in the renal disease as the cat is more likely to accept a new diet at that stage than when it is very uraemic and sick.

Diet if long-term hypertrophic cardiomyopathy is present

The cat may have long-term hypertrophic cardiomyopathy as a result of his hyperthyroidism, although some resolution of cardiac hypertrophy should be expected after thyroidectomy. Dietary manipulation of patients with cardiac disease is controversial, but avoidance of high sodium content may be indicated in cats with a dilated left atrium or signs of volume overload. Restricting sodium, however, may be counterproductive in cats that become inappetent following surgery, as it may put them off their food; so, alterations to diet should be considered only after the appetite improves. Omega-3 fatty acids might be supplemented in these cases, as they are thought to reduce the risk of thromboembolism associated with hypertrophic cardiomyopathy in cats, although clear evidence for this is lacking.

Physiotherapy

This cat may benefit from regular calming and gentle massage (stroking techniques in particular are useful in this regard; see Chapter 9). These would be useful in both the hospital setting and at home, assuming the cat enjoys human contact. They are easy techniques to teach owners, allowing them to be involved in their pet's care.

Hydrotherapy

Hydrotherapy is not specifically indicated for this patient.

Acupuncture

Acupuncture is not indicated for this patient unless no other form of analgesia is tolerated.

Nursing and supportive care

Care of the surgical wound
Cats are poorly tolerant of dressings placed over the cervical region; therefore it may be best to leave the surgical wound undressed. The surgical wound should be monitored for: exudates; erythema; haematoma; pain; odour; swelling; and wound breakdown.

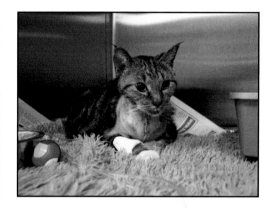

> A female DSH cat 3 hours after a bilateral thyroidectomy. She is comfortable following buprenorphine, administered as a premedicant. The ventral cervical wound was left uncovered to prevent undue irritation. Normothermia was restored within 1 hour after anaesthesia. Toys have been placed in the cage to enrich the environment. Intravenous fluid therapy was continued postoperatively via a left saphenous catheter.

Feeding
The cat should be offered food as soon as possible (see above). A highly palatable, easily digestible diet should be offered. If the cat is inappetent, eating may be encouraged by:

- Feeding small meals frequently
- Hand-feeding
- Providing fresh food
- Making sure the cat is offered its favourite food from home
- Warming the food to body temperature
- Adding flavour-enhancers (low sodium)
- Adding some chicken or other palatable foodstuff
- Not leaving large amounts of food in the cage if the patient is not interested in eating
- Providing privacy for eating (e.g. towel over cage door, see above).

Force-feeding should be avoided, as it could result in the development of food aversion.

Food intake and bodyweight must be monitored, and action taken quickly if the cat is not meeting its RER (see above).

Monitoring and management of specific complications of bilateral thyroidectomy
Reported early complications include hypocalcaemia and laryngeal paralysis. Horner's syndrome has also been reported (rarely) and is likely related to surgical trauma.

Hypocalcaemia is common after bilateral thyroidectomy because of both damage to the parathyroid glands or their blood supply and a sudden removal of the osteoclastic effects of elevated thyroid hormone. In this case hypocalcaemia would likely be temporary, as the external parathyroid glands were identified and left *in situ* at surgery. Hypocalcaemia can manifest up to 5 days after surgery, so cats should ideally be hospitalized for this period of time. Clinical signs of hypocalcaemia include muscle twitching, facial pruritus, inappetence, vocalization, irritability and seizures. These signs

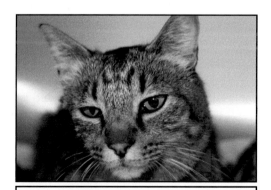

Horner's syndrome has also been reported following thyroidectomy.

should prompt blood sampling to check ionized calcium concentrations. Hypocalcaemia associated with clinical signs requires immediate calcium supplementation (initially intravenously), as it may be life-threatening. Once the cat is eating it can be sent home, with oral vitamin D ± oral calcium (as necessary) to maintain normocalcaemia. Ionized calcium levels should be rechecked 2 weeks after discharge from the hospital. If calcium concentrations are normal, vitamin D can be discontinued after 3–4 weeks and calcium concentrations rechecked 1–2 weeks later. (See *BSAVA Manual of Canine and Feline Endocrinology.*)

Laryngeal paralysis results from iatrogenic damage to the recurrent laryngeal nerves, which can be avoided by meticulous surgical technique. Clinical signs of upper airway obstruction and dysphonia may manifest immediately or weeks to months later. In this case laryngeal function was checked immediately after surgery and confirmed to be normal.

Owner advice and homecare recommendations

Rest
The cat should be confined to the house with a litter tray until the sutures have been removed, with all the considerations of care and core territory dealt with as outlined above.

Wound care
The client should be advised to monitor the wound carefully and to contact the surgery if the wound develops any exudates, swelling, heat or erythema.

Follow-up and prognosis
The owners need to be aware of when they need to return for follow-up visits for skin suture/staple removal.

Two weeks after surgery, blood and urine tests to check T4 concentrations and renal function are advised. High T4 concentrations may be due to ectopic or remnant thyroid tissue and are associated with persistence or recurrence of clinical signs of hyperthyroidism. Hyperthyroidism is associated with an increased glomerular filtration rate. Reduction of glomerular filtration rate with progression to euthyroidism may uncover pre-existing renal disease. Polyuria and polydipsia are clinical signs of both hyperthyroidism and renal disease, so may not be a useful indicator of renal disease in these cases.

Most cats do *not* become clinically hypothyroid after bilateral thyroidectomy; however, a few cases do, resulting in excessive weight gain and lethargy, and these cats may require thyroid supplementation.

Case 12.7
Surgical wound breakdown in a working dog

A 4-year-old neutered male Husky in ideal body condition, who was used for sled racing, was presented with wound breakdown over the medial aspect of the right stifle. Two weeks previously he had undergone wide surgical excision of an intermediate-grade cutaneous mast cell tumour. Histopathology had confirmed complete tumour excision. Debridement and resuturing of the wound had been unsuccessful in treating the complication.

Agreed medical/surgical management

On Day 1 the wound was lavaged and debrided and all suture material removed. A wet-to-dry dressing was tied into the wound. Culture of a swab from the wound prior to lavage revealed a scanty growth of a coagulase-negative *Staphylococcus*, sensitive to a range of antibiotics. Culture of the wound *after* lavage on Day 1 was negative. The wound was then lavaged, debrided and redressed daily for 7 days (under sedation with medetomidine and an opioid) until a healthy bed of granulation tissue was achieved. The dog was treated with oral amoxicillin/clavulanate initially, pending culture results. This treatment was discontinued when a healthy bed of granulation tissue was achieved.

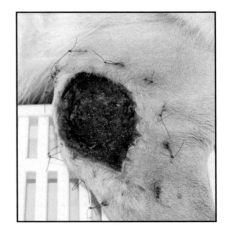

The wound contains some granulation tissue and some of the edges have begun to epithelialize and contract. Loose skin sutures have been placed around the wound to allow a wet-to-dry dressing to be tied into the wound.

On Day 8, the wound was closed with a 90-degree subdermal plexus transposition flap incorporating branches of the cutaneous genicular blood vessels. An active suction drain was placed local to the subdermal plexus transposition.

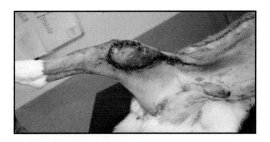

Reconstruction of the open wound using a 90-degree subdermal plexus transposition flap.

One day after flap placement the dog developed distal limb oedema, erythema of the flap and heat over the entire limb. These signs were not associated with infection but were believed to be secondary to decreased blood flow in the skin flap and alterations in blood flow in the distal limb. Oedema was therefore managed with gentle massage of the distal limb.

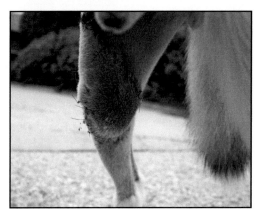

There is some swelling and erythema of the skin flap.

Acute/chronic pain management

Perioperative
Premedication should include a full mu agonist opioid (e.g. morphine, methadone, pethidine) and, because he is a fit young dog, medetomidine may also be a useful addition in view of its analgesic properties. Ketamine CRI can be very useful in these cases, after an initial loading dose. An NSAID licensed for perioperative use may also be included.

Postoperative
The dog should continue to be monitored for signs of pain and suffering postoperatively. NSAIDs are the first choice here, with the addition of tramadol if the dog appears to be really bothered by his wound. If there is sensitization of the area and resentment of its being touched, then gabapentin may be helpful. Amitriptyline may be used as an alternative to gabapentin, but the tramadol should be stopped if amitriptyline is used, since both increase serotonin and there is at least a theoretical risk of serotonin syndrome. Paracetamol ± codeine may provide additional analgesia when combined with other analgesics.

TENS and acupuncture may also be useful for pain relief (see below).

Fear, stress, conflict concerns

This Husky is likely to be a pack dog; as he is a racing dog it is likely that he is housed outside or, at least, with other Huskies. He may be distressed on being removed from the pack and this, and any problems when he returns to it, will need to be addressed as they arise. There is very little that can be done to limit potential problems, apart from limiting the time he is away. Separation may induce signs of anxiety and distress that are not alleviated, or only minimally so, by the attention of people. Inter-dog aggression is possible when he returns to the pack. Such problems would require a behavioural assessment and advice (see *BSAVA Manual of Canine and Feline Behavioural Medicine*).

Nutritional requirements

Feeding and daily sedation
Nutritional management of patients that require daily sedation for bandage changes and wound debridement presents particularly difficult challenges, as these patients often become catabolic and fail to maintain body condition. It is obviously not acceptable to starve this dog for the 7 days required for bandage changes and it is therefore necessary to time his feeding carefully to allow him to fulfill his caloric requirements, while avoiding eating too soon before sedation. This is best achieved by feeding him in the afternoon or evening, after recovery from sedation for bandage changes, and then starving him again overnight. It is important to allow adequate fluid intake, even when starved.

Because of the time restriction imposed, it is important to maximize food intake during the periods when the dog can eat. Diets should be highly palatable, energy-dense and high in protein. A very careful record should be kept next to the kennel of how much and when the dog eats so that early intervention can be instituted if he is not maintaining calorie intake. Initially, enough calories should be supplied to fulfil his RER (see Chapter 5). However, with frequent bandage changes and subsequent oedema, daily protein loss and thus protein and calorie requirements are likely to be high. It is important, therefore, to monitor his weight and body condition carefully and increase food intake if necessary.

Indications for feeding tubes

In many cases, unless the dog is eating well and willingly, it is preferable that a feeding tube is placed to facilitate feeding and ensure that an adequate amount of calories are provided each day. Relying on voluntary feeding in a catabolic dog with postoperative complications and restricted time for feeding often proves ineffective and results in significant weight loss and potentially longer recovery periods. Tube feeding with high-protein and energy-dense diets may help the dog maintain body condition and ensures an adequate supply of nutrients to support healing and recovery (see Chapter 5). A naso-oesophageal or oesophagostomy tube might be best for this dog.

Nutraceuticals

Supplementation of immune-enhancing nutrients, such as glutamine, arginine and antioxidants, have been recommended for human patients with severe illnesses, particularly those with surgical wounds. However, no data are available in dogs to support their use at this time.

Physiotherapy

Treating limb oedema

The most effective physiotherapy treatments for distal limb oedema are cold therapy, compression, effleurage massage and active exercise ('muscle pump'). Where there is generalized heat over the limb, cold therapy would again be the treatment of choice. Selection of the appropriate modalities to use would depend on the accessibility of the limb (bandaging, drains, etc.).

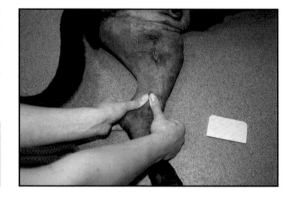

> Resolution of distal limb oedema is encouraged by effleurage massage: gentle stroking of the limb from distal to proximal. This dog had had an intramuscular lipoma removed from the medial thigh.

Pain relief

TENS may be useful for pain relief, with stimulation provided segmentally. It should be borne in mind, however, that electrode placement is not straightforward and that pain relief wears off quite quickly once the device is switched off, depending on the settings used.

Rehabilitation for return to work

If the long-term goal is to return this dog to sled racing it will be necessary to instigate an appropriate, progressive rehabilitation programme once the wound has healed. A sled dog must be able to pull a sled and driver (plus additional loads) over a variety of distances and terrains, so stamina and strength are the major functional requirements.

Because of the proximity of this dog's wounds to the stifle joint, loss of joint range is a real possibility and range of motion exercises (passive movements, stretches and active exercises) should be instigated at the earliest opportunity during the postoperative recovery period to offset this possibility. To some extent the practicalities of this will be dependent on the accessibility of the limb (bandaging, drains, etc.) but attempts should be made to maintain range as much as possible during this initial recovery period. Any remaining loss of range will need to be addressed during the subsequent rehabilitation programme.

To achieve a satisfactory return to work, a rehabilitation programme should also focus on aerobic conditioning and strengthening, especially as the dog will have been rested for long periods during his recovery. It may be more feasible to start aerobic and strength conditioning using hydrotherapy (water treadmill) and then land treadmill initially, but running within a 'team' environment must become predominant as rehabilitation progresses. Aerobic conditioning demands a steady increase in periods of running to develop improvements in aerobic capacity and endurance (cardiovascular and muscle). The repetitive nature of such training will also redevelop the specific motor skills required for the task, i.e. pulling a sled whilst running within a team. Strength and power will be developed through progressive overloading of weight being pulled during training periods.

Hydrotherapy

Hydrotherapy can be considered at the end of treatment once the wound has healed, to help to restore the dog's body condition, strength and stamina if he is going to be returned to sled racing.

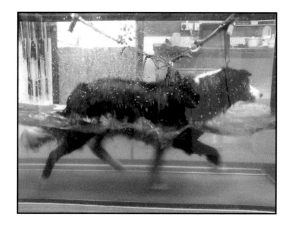

Aerobic and strength conditioning using a water treadmill may help return a working dog to full function. (© Linhay Veterinary Rehabilitation Centre)

Acupuncture

Wound healing
Acupuncture can be helpful for wound healing, through needling close to the edge of the wound in healthy tissue (see Chapter 11). **However, acupuncture should be used cautiously in oedema because of a theoretical increased risk of infection.**

Analgesia
For analgesia, 'mirror points' on the opposite leg can be used, or points further up the same leg (see Chapter 11).

Other nursing and supportive care

Kennelling
The dog should be cage-rested to decrease the tension on the surgical site, with careful lead walks outside to pass urine and faeces. As this dog is a working Husky, it is likely that he is used to spending long periods of time outdoors. He must therefore be monitored closely whilst hospitalized for signs of hyperthermia. Accommodation in a walk-in kennel should be considered, ensuring he has plenty of space; alternatively, a fan might be provided to prevent him from overheating.

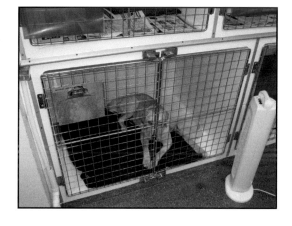

An electric fan can be used to keep a caged dog cool. (Courtesy of Liz Mullineaux)

Management of the drain
The dog must be prevented from interfering with the drain by placing an Elizabethan collar, and the drain must be protected from the dog's urine and faeces. The closed suction drain must be handled in an aseptic manner, monitoring and recording the fluid produced every 12 hours.

Drain removal is indicated when fluid production is <2 ml/kg per 24 hours, or when fluid production has reached a steady low level and cytology is not suggestive of ongoing bacterial infection. Once the drain has been removed, the stoma should be allowed to granulate over and must be kept clean at all times.

Feeding
Food intake must be monitored carefully (see above). Bodyweight should be recorded daily for patients receiving enteral nutritional support.

If a feeding tube has been placed, this should also be monitored carefully, as the majority of complications involve tube occlusion or localized irritation or infection at the tube exit site. The feeding tube is flushed with 5–10 ml of lukewarm water before and after each feed to minimize clogging (see Chapter 5).

The dressings and bandages covering the feeding tube and drain should be inspected daily for signs of infection. The tube exit site should be closely monitored and cleaned as necessary.

Food and water should continue to be offered *per os* even if a feeding tube is in place and the dog should be encouraged to eat voluntarily. It is best not to force-feed the dog as this could lead to development of food aversion.

Wound care

The surgical wound should be monitored for infection (redness, swelling, creamy discharge), wound breakdown or skin flap ischaemia (purplish skin discoloration). The dog should not be allowed to interfere with his wound. Specific cleaning of the wound should not be necessary if healing is uncomplicated.

Once the drain has been removed, the stoma should be allowed to heal naturally; special care is not usually required.

Exercise and return to work

The dog must be confined to a lead when out exercising *until all wounds have healed*. If he is usually housed with other dogs, the owner should consider moving him to a single kennel but must be observant for signs of distress relating to separation from the pack.

The dog should not recommence training until the wound has completely healed. If tension or wound breakdown is a problem postoperatively, healing could take 4–6 weeks or even longer.

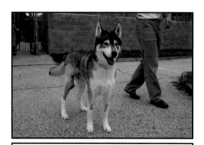

The Husky during a follow-up visit.

Follow-up

Suture removal should take place 10–14 days postoperatively. Further checks will be required until wound healing is complete.

Case 12.8
Splenic rupture in a dog

A 10-year-old entire male German Shepherd Dog was presented collapsed with tachycardia, weak pulses, pale mucous membranes, a peritoneal fluid thrill and a palpable mid-abdominal mass. His owners reported a 2-day history of progressive lethargy, depression, anorexia and weakness.

Blood tests showed a severe non-regenerative anaemia, thrombocytopenia, hypoproteinaemia and mildly prolonged partial thromboplastin and one-stage prothrombin times. Abdominocentesis results were consistent with intraperitoneal haemorrhage. Abdominal ultrasonography revealed a splenic mass but thoracic radiographs showed no evidence of metastatic disease.

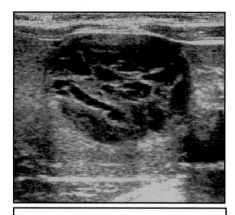

Ultrasound image of a spleen showing a rounded anechoic mass with hyperechoic strands, giving a septate appearance. (Courtesy of Frances Barr)

Initial fluid resuscitation was carried out with 90 ml/kg of intravenous lactated Ringer's solution. The anaemia and mild coagulopathy prompted a transfusion with 1 unit of DEA 1.1-positive fresh whole blood, which was initiated during induction to anaesthesia. (The dog was known to be DEA 1.1-positive and had no history of a previous blood transfusion, so cross-matching was deemed unnecessary.)

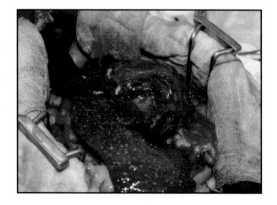

Intraoperative photo of the splenic mass. Bleeding has stimulated adhesion of the omentum to its surface.

Exploratory laparotomy confirmed a bleeding splenic mass. The abdominal organs were otherwise unremarkable. Total splenectomy was performed and histology revealed splenic haemangiosarcoma. The owner declined any palliative postoperative chemotherapy.

Acute/chronic pain management

Perioperative

Premedication should include a full mu agonist opioid (e.g. methadone, morphine or pethidine). An epidural with preservative-free morphine can provide up to 24 hours' analgesia postoperatively, but regular pain assessments are still essential; 'rescue' opioid analgesia can be given in addition to the epidural if required. A lidocaine CRI might also be useful in this case, not only because of its anti-arrhythmic effects, but also because it will provide additional analgesia (and reduce the amount of volatile anaesthetic agent needed).

Chronic pain

Postoperatively, this patient should continue to be monitored for signs of pain. Tramadol can be used once the perioperative period has passed. NSAIDs might be used, if the patient's progress is monitored well. It is important to check renal function in this older dog before using them and also to monitor carefully for any gastrointestinal side effects. Gabapentin may be helpful if the patient starts showing signs of progressive uncontrollable pain. It can be used alone or together with paracetamol ± codeine.

Fear, stress, conflict concerns

An older dog with pain and discomfort may display agitation and this should be taken into account when managing this case, both in the hospital and on return to his owners. The specific recommendations for this dog will depend on his perception of handling by unfamiliar people, and his response to being in a novel environment. The acute nature of the problem may mean that the dog has a limited awareness of his surroundings on admission, but subsequently shows signs of anxiety on recovery. Discussing with the owner what makes the dog anxious would be helpful, so that staff can be prepared. Discussion with owners should also explore their response to the dog's previous lethargy: misplaced anger or forcing him to go out may have precipitated some anxiety or avoidance responses, which would need addressing.

Nutritional requirements

Postoperative

Postoperatively the dog should be offered a highly palatable, easily digestible diet. There are no special dietary considerations for this patient.

Iron

Iron supplementation should be unnecessary, as any anaemia associated with intra-abdominal bleeding will not be associated with iron deficiency (the red cells will be recycled). If blood loss at surgery is marked, this is best treated with a blood transfusion. Absorption of iron from oral supplements is limited in dogs: most is excreted in the faeces unabsorbed. Absorption is significantly improved in humans by the concurrent administration of ascorbic acid (vitamin C) but the clinical usefulness of this in dogs is unknown. Oral iron also results in dark faeces and can cause constipation.

Monitoring food intake

It is important to monitor food intake while the dog is in the hospital, preferably via a record on the kennel, to ensure that he is eating. Stress of hospitalization, analgesic drugs and weakness associated with hypovolaemia and anaemia may all reduce his appetite. The amount fed should initially be calculated using his RER (see Chapter 5) and then the adequacy of this calorie intake assessed by monitoring bodyweight and body condition.

Nutraceuticals

There has been some suggestion that a diet high in omega-3 fatty acids could be useful in dogs with splenic haemangiosarcoma; however, there is no convincing evidence that such a strategy offers any advantage over their normal diet. Further studies are necessary to evaluate possible dietary approaches to dogs with this form of neoplasia.

Physiotherapy

Physiotherapy is not specifically indicated for this patient.

Hydrotherapy is not specifically indicated for this patient.

Acupuncture is not indicated for this patient.

Postoperative monitoring

The dog should be observed closely for the first 24 hours postoperatively for complications, which may include:

- Cardiac arrhythmias
- Haemorrhage or intra-abdominal bleeding
- Disseminated intravascular coagulation (DIC)
- Thrombosis
- Infections.

Vital signs and general condition are recorded. Heart rate and rhythm, concurrent pulse rate and quality, and mucous membrane colour should be regularly checked to assess for any evidence of haemorrhage and to ensure the dog remains normovolaemic in the postoperative period.

Frequent measurement of haematocrit (PCV) is *not* helpful in monitoring for acute haemorrhage of whole blood, since it takes several hours for fluid shifts to result in a drop in PCV; so frequent assessment for signs of hypovolaemia and hypotension is much more important. However, twice-daily monitoring of haematocrit and total protein is useful in this patient to assess the response to blood transfusion and will reflect ongoing blood loss. Blood pressure monitoring would also be useful. Any change in heart rate or rhythm should be checked with an ECG. Ventricular arrhythmias occur frequently in such patients but rarely require specific treatment due to maintenance of adequate cardiac output.

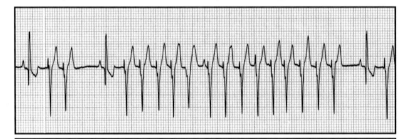

ECG showing a non-sustained, monomorphic ventricular tachycardia, with rate up to 230 bpm. A ventricular arrhythmia of this rate, if frequent or sustained, is likely to result in signs of haemodynamic compromise, often necessitating therapy. Lead II; paper speed 25 mm/s; gain 1 cm/mV. (Courtesy of Simon Dennis)

The dog must not interfere with the abdominal wound postoperatively. If necessary, an Elizabethan collar should be fitted.

Fluid therapy

Intravenous fluid therapy with isotonic crystalloids ± colloids – to maintain normovolaemia and normal blood pressure – should be continued until the dog is able to maintain his own hydration and any electrolyte and acid–base abnormalities have been corrected. Twice-daily checks of electrolytes, haematocrit and total solids should be continued until fluid therapy is discontinued.

Feeding

A highly palatable, easily digestible diet should be offerred as soon as possible postoperatively (see above). If the dog is inappetent, an attempt should be made to hand-feed him, since force-feeding could result in food aversion.

Comfort

As the dog is elderly, particular attention should be paid to the kind of bedding that will support him (see Case 12.5). He should also be prevented from lying on one side for long periods to limit the possibility of decubitus ulcer formation. Regular opportunities to go outside for a short walk should be provided; this will promote mobility and also help to limit understimulation during hospitalization.

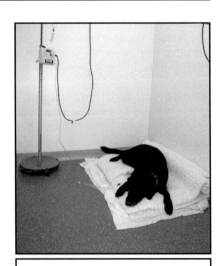

Fluid therapy to maintain normovolaemia. The dog is resting on comfortable bedding in a quiet area. (Courtesy of Liz Mullineaux)

Owner advice and homecare recommendations

Wound care

The owner must continue to ensure that there is no patient interference with the surgical wound. The dog should receive lead exercise only, until the wound is healed.

Prognosis and follow-up

The owners should be made aware of the poor long-term prognosis. They particularly need to be aware that recurrence of the tumour will likely result in a recurrent risk of intra-abdominal bleeding and they should be warned about the signs to look out for (e.g. weakness, lethargy, abdominal distension, collapse, pale mucous membranes). They should also be warned of the propensity for haemangiosarcomas to metastasize to the thorax and the signs to look out for (including coughing, laboured breathing and exercise intolerance). The veterinary surgeon and owner should reach an agreement as to how often (if at all) the dog will return for follow-up visits (after the initial mandatory visit for removal of sutures). As the client has declined chemotherapy, the client should be advised to give the dog a good quality of life and to treat him as usual, as long as he shows no signs of ill health.

13

Patients with neurological disorders

Edited by Natasha Olby

Introduction

Disorders of the nervous system include a wide range of conditions with very different needs in terms of rehabilitation, support and palliative care.

- Diseases of the forebrain, brainstem, cerebellum, spinal cord and peripheral nerves all have specific functional and behavioural consequences for the animal.
- Acute brain and spinal cord injuries are common and, while often self-limiting, the destruction of irreplaceable CNS tissue results in functional deficits that can be difficult to overcome.
- Many disorders, such as epilepsy, are chronic and require long-term drug therapy, leaving the owner and patient managing the consequences of both the primary disorder and the treatment.
- Others, such as many types of central nervous system (CNS) neoplasia, or multilevel spinal cord compressive disease, cannot be cured but require palliative care.

Principles of treating neurological cases

Diagnosis
The first general principle of treating these challenging cases is to attempt to establish an accurate diagnosis. The pathological effects of diseases of the nervous system manifest as syndromes specific to the *location* of the lesion. Thus, thoracolumbar disc herniation, degenerative myelopathy and neoplasia of the thoracolumbar spine will all result in similar clinical signs. While the history can be helpful in prioritizing a list of differential diagnoses, it is by no means diagnostic.

A full diagnostic work-up of a neurological problem often involves advanced imaging of the nervous system and cerebrospinal fluid (CSF) analysis. If these modalities are unavailable, or outside the financial means of an owner, there are still basic diagnostic tests that can and should be performed to rule out treatable diseases. Examples include: bile acid tolerance tests and blood pressure measurements in patients with signs of forebrain disease; and taking spinal radiographs of patients with signs that localize to the spine.

There is a tendency to omit these diagnostic steps if owners state they do not want a neurological work-up, but this can result in *inappropriate* palliative treatment of signs. For example, treatment of spinal pain with acupuncture, corticosteroids or other analgesic protocols will ultimately be ineffective, and is medically inappropriate if the cause of the pain is discospondylitis. This condition can be diagnosed with survey spinal radiographs (although sometimes the characteristic changes do not show up in the early stages of the disease) and the infectious agent involved identified from culture of a urine sample. Failure to treat with appropriate antibiotics may result in sepsis, pathological vertebral fractures and paralysis.

Quality of life
The second principle of managing neurological cases is to discuss with the owner, after the initial patient assessment, the implications of functional deficits for them and their pet. This discussion should be expanded to include a description of the possible course(s) of the disease and to define times at which an assessment of improvement or deterioration of the patient's and owner's quality of life will be repeated. This type of discussion helps the owner to understand what their pet might be experiencing and to understand what changes might constitute a clinical deterioration. It also ensures that the veterinary surgeon acknowledges the owner's role in caring for their pet and the need for the owner to be able to sustain a life outside their pet. Establishing timelines helps the owner to structure their approach to their pet's illness and ensures that pets are not lost to follow-up. Discussing and thinking about quality of life and potential endpoints ahead of time is very useful to the owner.

Nursing
The third principle is that the nursing team must be knowledgeable about the patient, because they will tend to have closer contact with the patient than will the veterinary surgeon. Whenever a new patient is hospitalized, a discussion should take place between the nursing team and the veterinary surgeon to ensure that all aspects of the patient's health problems are known by the whole team. There should be daily discussion between the nursing team and the clinicians, and treatment instructions for the day should be designed to allow all pertinent information (e.g. urination, appetite, pain score) to be recorded.

Managing recumbent dogs and cats
Patients with severe spinal or generalized lower motor neuron (LMN) disorders may be recumbent.

Recumbency can cause secondary problems associated with the respiratory system, bladder and bowel function, skin and musculoskeletal system, and can affect the patient's ability to eat and drink, and its demeanour. The principles of managing such patients include:

- Being aware of the range of complications associated with recumbency
- Assessing the patient carefully and regularly for these complications
- Taking appropriate steps to prevent the complications
- Early and aggressive treatment of developing complications.

Respiration

Any neurological condition severe enough to cause non-ambulatory tetraparesis or tetraplegia has the potential to cause hypoventilation. In addition, recumbency predisposes to atelectasis and aspiration pneumonia as secondary complications. Generalized LMN conditions, in particular, predispose to aspiration pneumonia due to the involvement of the laryngeal and pharyngeal musculature and oesophagus in the disease.

Assessment of any recumbent animal includes a careful assessment of the respiratory pattern (degree and direction of excursion of the thoracic and abdominal wall on inspiration) and rate. If there is a suspicion of hypoventilation or pneumonia, blood gas analysis should be performed to assess arterial carbon dioxide and oxygen levels. Respiratory rate and pattern should be recorded every 4–6 hours in patients that are severely affected, to facilitate early detection of problems. In stable patients, twice-daily assessments are adequate.

Respiratory complications (see also Chapter 17) can be prevented or limited by:

- Positioning the patient in as sternal a position as possible, using appropriate padding
- Turning the patient regularly (every 6 hours)
- Performing coupage at the time of turning, if the patient can tolerate it
- Only offering water and food when the patient is in a sternal position. Someone should sit with the patient whilst it is eating, and an upright position should be maintained for 30 minutes afterwards, to decrease the risk of regurgitation and aspiration.

More specialized care of animals with LMN disorders that cause regurgitation (such as myasthenia gravis, botulism, polyradiculoneuritis) may be necessary. In these cases, a naso-oesophageal tube may be placed for intermittent suction of the oesophagus, and a percutaneous endoscopic gastrostomy (PEG) tube may be placed for feeding (see Chapter 5).

Urination

As a general rule, paraplegic and tetraplegic animals cannot urinate voluntarily, while patients with motor function can do so. However, there are some exceptions; for example, patients with lesions of the sacral spinal cord or sacral nerves may be able to walk but not to urinate. In addition, some tetraparetic animals will choose not to urinate, even though they can, because they cannot adopt the appropriate posture. Neurogenic micturition disorders therefore cause a combination of urine retention and leakage. It is important to understand that whenever the intravesical pressure exceeds that of the urethra, urine leakage will occur; this can be incorrectly identified as voluntary urination. It is important to teach those caring for the patient how to palpate the bladder and to enable them to understand that paraplegic animals are unlikely to be able to urinate voluntarily.

Assessment of the bladder includes:

- Palpation to assess bladder size before and after urination
- Urinalysis on admission, with optional culture depending on results
- Recording of all urination in the medical record, noting whether voluntary, expressed manually or via a catheter
- Testing urine with a dipstick every 2–4 days for the presence of white blood cells and protein.

Appropriate management of the bladder in recumbent animals includes:

- Regular (at least three times a day) trips outside for the opportunity to urinate
- If unable to urinate, manual bladder expression 2–3 times a day (depending on bladder size)
- Where manual expression is not possible or is contraindicated (e.g. a victim of a road traffic accident with significant soft tissue injuries, where manual expression could be very painful or exacerbate injuries), intermittent catheterization should be performed, or an indwelling catheter placed
- Pharmacological therapy, where indicated. This involves the use of phenoxybenzamine and diazepam to relax the internal and external urethral sphincters. *Use of bethanecol to cause contraction of the detrusor muscle is contraindicated in any animal in which the bladder cannot be manually expressed,* to avoid causing detrusor contraction against high urethral sphincter tone.
- Suitable bedding that will allow liquid to wick away from the animal's skin
- Keeping the patient clean and dry at all times (see also Chapter 18).

Defecation

There is relatively little information in the literature about bowel function in animals with neurological problems. In general, because of the enteric neural plexuses, contractions of the gastrointestinal tract continue in the face of spinal cord disease. Therefore, the most significant issues faced by these patients are the lack of voluntary control over defecation, and severe soiling associated with sacral lesions that cause faecal incontinence. In cats with neurological problems, there is a tendency toward constipation and megacolon. It is important to monitor and record defecation, and to keep the patient clean and dry at all times. Dietary changes may be made to reduce the volume of stool (in cases of faecal incontinence) or to soften the stool (in cases of constipation) (see Chapter 5).

Skin care

Recumbent patients are at risk of developing decubital ulcers over pressure points and dermatitis secondary to urine scald or faecal soiling. In addition, repeated attempts to move, and dragging themselves over rough surfaces, can rapidly result in severe traumatic injuries to the skin and underlying soft tissues. When the patient is assessed, potential pressure points should be noted.

Complications can be prevented by:

- Appropriate soft bedding that will wick away moisture
- Decreasing pressure on pressure points by appropriate padding around the region
- Regular turning (every 6 hours) and massage of pressure points to increase local blood flow
- Clipping hair in the perineal region
- Prompt removal of soiled bedding
- Keeping the patient clean and dry
- Appropriate bladder management (see above).

Treatment of skin complications includes:

- Cleaning of dermatitis with a dilute chlorhexidine solution, followed by thorough drying and application of a barrier cream
- If decubital ulcers develop, care should be taken to ensure that pressure is no longer placed over the region.
- Debridement of dead tissue (may require surgery in severe cases)
- Elizabethan collars, if the patient is licking or chewing the region.

Muscle and joint problems

Spinal cord and peripheral nerve disorders resulting in paralysis cause muscle atrophy and contracture, and deterioration of joints and the associated soft tissues (Sherman and Olby, 2004; Olby *et al.*, 2005). Sometimes, particularly in LMN disorders, these consequences can be so severe that recovery of function is not possible, even with return of neurological function. In addition, many patients are in pain caused by their primary disease, surgical intervention or the secondary effects of recumbency and spasticity. Assessment of the musculoskeletal system includes a careful orthopaedic examination with consideration of muscle mass, joint range of motion (ROM) and pain. The level of pain should be assessed and recorded 2–4 times a day (dependent on the patient). Many clinics now use a pain scoring system to ensure consistency (see Chapters 2 and 3).

Management of these problems includes:

- Treatment of pain
- A rehabilitation plan, which should be made for each patient and instituted as early as possible. Exercises that the owner can perform at home can also be developed.

- Basic techniques, such as passive ROM exercises and massage, which may help to maintain joint mobility during recumbency. Passive ROM should be instituted as soon as possible
- A nutritional plan.

Details are given in relevant chapters and in the case studies below.

Changes in demeanour

Recumbency can cause patients to become frustrated, anxious or depressed. These emotions can be exacerbated by pain. Demeanour may be improved by:

- Ensuring the animal is comfortable, through the use of pain management and appropriate bedding. This includes tailoring the amount of contact with humans to the individual patient – some prefer to be quiet while many appear to do better if they can see and have regular interactions with people
- Arranging regular contact with the owner
- Taking the canine patient outside regularly. This is not appropriate for cats unless they are used to lead/harness walking; allowing a period for free exploration in a secure cat ward every day under supervision may be helpful for feline patients
- Placing a dog in a suitable sling to allow it to spend some time in a standing position every day; this also helps the pulmonary and musculoskeletal systems and skin
- Regular passive ROM exercises and massage.

References and further reading

Beal MW, Paglia DT, Griffin GM, Hughes D and King LG (2001) Ventilatory failure, ventilator management, and outcome in dogs with cervical spinal disorders: 14 cases (1991–1999). *Journal of the American Veterinary Medical Association* **218**, 1598–1602

O'Brien D (1988) Neurogenic disorders of micturition. *Veterinary Clinics of North America: Small Animal Practice* **18**, 529–544

Olby N, Halling KB and Glick TR (2005) Rehabilitation for the neurologic patient. *Veterinary Clinics of North America: Small Animal Practice* **35**, 1389–1409

Olby NJ (2005) Feline neurogenic micturition disorders. In: *Consultations in Feline Internal Medicine*, ed. JR August, pp.481–491. Elsevier, St. Louis

Sherman J and Olby NJ (2004) Physical rehabilitation of the neurological patient. In: *BSAVA Manual of Canine and Feline Neurology, 3rd edn*, ed. SR Platt and NJ Olby, pp. 394–407. BSAVA Publications, Gloucester

Clinical case studies

A variety of case scenarios in dogs and cats will now be presented to illustrate the considerations to be made and the options available within a specific clinical setting. Information relating to the rehabilitation and palliation of each condition has been contributed to each case by the authors in the first part of this Manual, plus notes on nursing and homecare from Rachel Lumbis RVN. The reader should refer back to the appropriate chapters for further details. Photographs used to illustrate the principles and techniques within the cases do not necessarily feature the original patient.

Case 13.1
Tail pull injury in a cat

A 5-year-old neutered male DSH cat had suffered a tail pull injury 2 days prior to initial presentation. General physical examination was unremarkable. The tail was limp and lacked nociception, but there was focal pain over the sacral region. He had good motor function but had slightly dropped hocks bilaterally. He was sent home with no treatment.

Two days later the cat was re-presented, leaking blood-tinged urine. He was walking well but had slightly reduced hock flexion when withdrawal reflex was tested. The tail was still analgesic and limp. Anal tone was reduced and there was no perineal reflex or perineal sensation. The owner reported that the cat had not defecated since the accident. Radiographs of the spine showed luxation of the first and second caudal vertebrae, but no evidence of fracture. An extremely large bladder was palpable, but attempts to express it manually were unsuccessful and produced a painful response.

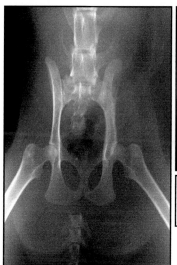
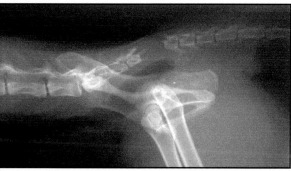

These radiographs show wide separation between the first two caudal vertebrae. (Courtesy of Sorrel Langley-Hobbs)

Agreed medical/surgical management

Urination

The cat was hospitalized to facilitate management of the bladder. A red rubber catheter was passed transurethrally into the bladder; the urine was removed and submitted for analysis, culture and sensitivity testing. Because the cat had severe haematuria, a red rubber catheter was used so that it could be left *in situ*; tomcat catheters, whilst easier to pass, cause significant trauma to the bladder mucosa and should never be left indwelling. The catheter was sutured in place and connected to a sterile urine collection system, with the aim of keeping the bladder empty for 48 hours to allow the detrusor muscle to recover from being overstretched, if possible.

The difficulty with manual bladder expression is caused by stimulation of the sympathetic innervation of the internal urethral sphincter by the hypogastric nerve. To address this, oral phenoxybenzamine can be started.

After 48 hours the catheter may be removed and the bladder expressed manually 3–4 times a day, with intermittent catheterization if manual expression is unsuccessful. If phenoxybenzamine does not aid bladder expression, prazosin can be tried.

In some cats, manual bladder expression is impossible, and in this instance a tube cystostomy should be placed. These can be managed effectively by owners and are tolerated well by cats. The cat will be able to urinate on its own with a tube cystostomy in place and so functional recovery will not be masked.

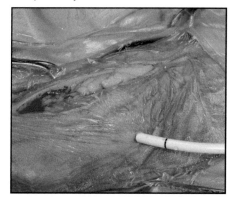

A cystostomy tube placed percutaneously at laparotomy to drain the bladder. The tube can be either connected to a closed collecting system, or emptied intermittently. (Courtesy of Stephen Baines)

Tail amputation

Because of the separation between the first and second caudal vertebrae and the lack of sensation, the tail is unlikely to recover motor or sensory function. In such cases amputation is indicated.

Acute/chronic pain management

Perioperative

Epidural morphine/bupivacaine would provide ideal intraoperative analgesia.

Pain before and after surgery can be treated with meloxicam (0.2 mg/kg orally once; then 0.1 mg/kg q24h for 3 days; then 0.025 mg/kg 2–3 times a week for 2 more weeks).

Chronic pain

It is possible that this cat will have continuing pain over the sacral area; this can be treated with longer-term use of meloxicam or with acupuncture (see below). If the pain is not controlled, or the cat shows signs of allodynia or hyperalgesia (see Chapter 3), then gabapentin or amitriptyline can be added to the meloxicam.

It is theoretically possible that this cat may suffer 'phantom' sensations, including pain, from the amputated tail, although this is arguably more likely to occur when there has been a chronic pain problem rather than a traumatic injury and subsequent amputation within a short period of time. Phantom pain would be inferred from the cat's behaviour: turning to look at the stump or beyond it; attacking the area where the tail should be; suddenly jumping or starting and running away. There is still controversy about the cause of such pain; whilst it is generally considered to be neuropathic (see Chapter 3), it is possible that soft tissue, especially muscle, pain around the stump or referred from the sacrum may generate this pain. (See also Case 14.1.)

Fear, stress, conflict concerns

It is appropriate to discuss quality of life for both the cat and the owner early in the course of managing this problem. This should include consideration of the extent to which the cat accepts handling and enjoys contact with people. Cats that are already anxious about handling may not be suitable for continuing treatment, as necessary treatment is likely to become progressively more stressful for cat and owner. Additionally, this cat may have ongoing balance and mobility problems. Optimizing his core territory will be helpful in restoring his confidence and helping him obtain necessary resources:

- **Food.** The cat must also be able to reach food easily, as he must not jump up for at least 6 weeks, and possibly as long as 3 months. Food should be repositioned if he has previously fed at height, making sure that this does not make him anxious about it being available to competitors (e.g. the pet dog or a possible intruding cat if the food is placed near the cat flap).
- **Water.** Cats generally prefer their water about a room's distance away from their food in a clear, wide bowl.
- **Access inside and out.** Cats normally have more than one access point into and out of their core territory (usually the house). Consider providing an additional access point, or ensure that he can use the existing access points (they are not too high or too difficult to negotiate when he feels unwell and uncomfortable).
- **Scratching posts.** Are these easily accessible and appropriate? A horizontal scratch post can be provided, so that the cat can still reach it if he does not feel up to climbing.
- **Hiding areas.** Provide multiple safe and comfortable hiding areas at different levels, or make sure that there is a 'step' system to allow the cat to reach his old favourite places.
- **Beds.** Provision of new beds, such as radiator beds, may improve the comfort and wellbeing of the patient.
- **Play.** Modify games to very short bursts of gentle play or try other ways to gently stimulate the cat.
- **Petting.** Use of gentle touch, stroking and grooming in ways that the patient will tolerate and enjoy will not only improve the patient's feelings of wellbeing but will also give the owner a sense of participating in their pet's treatment and nursing.

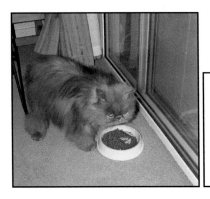

The cat will need to feed at ground level as he must not jump up for at least 6 weeks. (© Samantha Elmhurst)

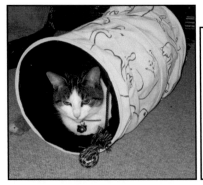

Safe and comfortable hiding areas should be provided. This cat also has some toys to hand for gentle play. (Courtesy of Lucy Hudson)

Nutritional requirements

With this type of injury the cat will not have voluntary control over defecation. This can lead to problems of faecal incontinence *or* constipation. The diet should address the over-riding problem for the individual cat: if it is becoming constipated, a stool softener can be used; if it is dropping large volumes of stool in the house, a low-residue diet is chosen. The use of a low-residue diet, containing moderate amounts of fermentable fibre, may be beneficial in modulating colonic water content, reducing faecal bulk and reducing risk of constipation.

Physiotherapy

If there are persisting balance and mobility issues that need addressing, exercises targeted at improving these (see Chapter 9) should be prescribed, if the cat will accept them.

Hydrotherapy

Hydrotherapy is not indicated for this patient.

Acupuncture

Acupuncture is often reported to be useful in urinary retention, but its effects will be determined by the type of injury/pathology causing the retention. If the cat is in too much pain to squat to urinate (e.g. following injury), then the immediate relaxation and analgesic effects of acupuncture may produce the desired effect.

If the problem is functional rather than pathological (i.e. the function is disturbed but there are no physical lesions preventing normal function), then acupuncture may have 'normalizing' effects on the bladder (as it appears to in irritative bladder syndrome in humans, for example; Kelleher *et al.*, 1994). In this cat, however, acupuncture is unlikely to have such a 'normalizing' effect, although it may be requested by the owner because of anecdotal reports of success in urinary retention in the veterinary literature (see Chapter 11).

Other nursing and supportive care

The cat should be given comfortable, soft bedding such as a covered foam mattress with fleecy bedding on top. Any bedding soiled with urine or faeces should be removed immediately.

Management of a urinary catheter
Whilst the cat is in the hospital, whether catheterized or not, urine should be monitored daily for changes in odour and colour. If there is an indwelling urinary catheter, it should be connected to a closed system and the amount of urine passed should be measured and recorded. When draining the bladder and emptying the urine bag, gloves should be worn and an aseptic technique employed.

It is best *not* to use *prophylactic* antibiotics in animals with indwelling urinary catheters because of the risk of resistant infections (see Chapter 18). However, the urine should be monitored carefully for evidence of infection (urine dipsticks can be used to check protein content and to detect blood). The urine should be cultured if an infection is suspected and antibiotics chosen on the basis of sensitivity testing. It is important to detect and treat any urinary tract infection in cases such as this one, as such patients are at increased risk of pyelonephritis: increased pressure in the bladder makes propulsion of bacteria up the ureters more likely.

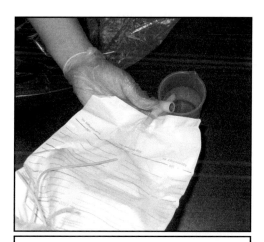

Gloves should be worn when emptying the urine bag. (Courtesy of Rachel Lumbis)

Owner advice and homecare recommendations

Urinary and faecal incontinence are extremely difficult for owners to manage in a pet that lives in the house, and urine retention can be a fatal complication for the pet.

Bladder management
Depending on whether the cat is discharged with a cystostomy tube or is to be managed using manual bladder expression, the owner needs instructions: either on tube management and emptying; or on how to express the

bladder. The latter is a skill that only some owners are confident to perform. It takes practice, so initially the owner should be encouraged to come into the clinic twice a day to express their cat's bladder with help of the veterinary staff.

If a cystotomy tube is placed, the owner should be advised regarding its long-term care. An Elizabethan collar will be fitted in the initial stages but can be removed after 24–48 hours, with the cat observed carefully to see if a collar is still required.

However the bladder is managed, it is very important to stress to the owners that persistent retention of a lot of urine will not only cause further detrusor muscle function loss, but can also result in acute renal failure. Therefore, it must be stressed that they should contact the veterinary surgery immediately if they have trouble emptying the cat's bladder.

Keeping the cat indoors

The owner should be advised that the cat will no longer be able to go outside without supervision, because he must have his bladder expressed at least twice a day. He should be confined to one room, with access to a litter tray when the owner is not at home, to limit the impact of faecal incontinence in the home environment and to allow the owner to monitor for evidence of urination and defecation. The owner should be counselled to provide appropriate toys so that the cat does not become understimulated.

Toys with food hidden inside can provide stimulatory play. (Courtesy of Lucy Hudson)

Prognosis

It is useful to establish timelines for the owner to feel that they have given their pet the chance to recover. One of the most important pieces of information for owners in this situation is to know at what point it will become apparent that recovery of function is *not* going to occur. If there is no recovery of perineal sensation by a month after the injury, it is extremely unlikely that voluntary urination and defecation will return.

References

Kelleher CJ, Filshie J, Burton G *et al.* (1994) Acupuncture and the treatment of irritative bladder symptoms. *Acupuncture in Medicine* **12**, 9–12

Case 13.2
Brain tumour in a dog

A 12-year-old male neutered Golden Retriever was presented with acute recent onset of generalized seizures, behavioural changes, and circling. Physical examination was unremarkable but neurological examination revealed lateralizing forebrain signs.

Routine blood work and thoracic radiographs were unremarkable. MRI of the brain showed a large, homogenously contrast-enhancing extra-axial mass in the left frontal/parietal lobe, most consistent with a meningioma. There was extensive peritumoral oedema.

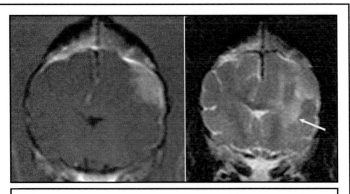

(left) T1-weighted post-contrast transverse image of the brain at the level of the thalamus. The extra-axial contrast-enhancing mass is clearly visible. **(right)** T2-weighted image, highlighting the oedema extending beyond the borders of the mass (arrowed).

Agreed medical/surgical management

Treatment with a combination of oral phenobarbital (2 mg/kg q12h) and prednisolone (0.5 mg/kg q12h for 5 days then tapered over the next 2 weeks) was initiated to address the seizures and the peritumoral oedema.

The meningioma was then removed surgically by a supratentorial approach. Since tumour-free margins were unlikely to be obtained, adjunctive radiation was recommended (but declined by the owner).

Acute/chronic pain management

Perioperative
A full mu agonist, such as morphine, methadone or pethidine, should be used in premedication. Partial agonists such as buprenorphine should be avoided because they may interfere with the action of a full agonist if one is required later in the procedure (e.g. when using fentanyl). Fentanyl continuous rate infusion (CRI) can be started during surgery and continued postoperatively. Immediate postoperative pain can be managed with a fentanyl CRI for 24 hours plus placement of a fentanyl patch. poss photo

Chronic pain
Chronic pain may be difficult to determine, given the behavioural changes that may occur with a brain tumour and its treatment; but it should always be borne in mind as a possibility and treated as required.

Fear, stress, conflict concerns

The behavioural effects of frontal lobe tumours include pacing, anxiety and changed interactions with the owner. These can be difficult for the veterinary surgeon to appreciate but can cause significant distress to the owner. In addition, the behavioural side effects of prednisolone and anti-epileptic drugs can be more pronounced in dogs with frontal lobe disease. All owners should be warned that they may see permanent behavioural changes of this kind.

Nutritional requirements

Phenobarbital and prednisolone both cause polyphagia, polyuria and polydipsia. These effects can be pronounced, particularly in dogs with frontal lobe disease, and the owners must be counselled to avoid feeding increased amounts.

If necessary, larger volumes of a low-calorie diet formulated for weight loss can be fed. Owners should also be counselled to try to increase the dog's exercise. It would *not* be appropriate to use the MTP inhibitor weight loss drugs in this context as they are not recommended for prophylactic use or with these other drugs (see Chapter 6). Some dogs can become so polyphagic that they eat inappropriate objects, with serious consequences. Phenobarbital has been chosen because of its established efficacy as an anti-epileptic drug and reasonable cost; however, owners should be informed of alternatives that will not cause polyphagia, such as levetiracetam, gabapentin and zonisamide (potassium bromide will also cause polyphagia).

Physiotherapy

Physiotherapy is not indicated for this patient.

Hydrotherapy

Hydrotherapy is not indicated for this patient.

Acupuncture

Acupuncture has been reported to control canine epilepsy in a few small case series (see Case 13.6). It would not be appropriate for this patient, but owners may request it because of reports of success in the literature.

Other nursing and supportive care

Assessment and first aid
On initial presentation and admission, the patient was assessed and first aid care provided, based on clinical signs. If the dog is seizuring or post-ictal, care should be provided as outlined in Case 13.6.

Perioperative care

The patient should be monitored for signs of pain and discomfort (see also Chapter 12). A recumbent patient needs to be turned regularly, at least every 2–4 hours. If the dog is ambulatory, assistance with walking may be required. Bladder size should be monitored; catheterization or manual expression may be required (see Chapter 18).

Avoiding increases in intracranial pressure

Increases in intracranial pressure could have serious consequences for the patient.

- Avoid placing intravenous catheters in the jugular vein.
- Minimize patient stress. For example, if a patient develops separation anxiety, time in the hospital prior to surgery should be minimal.

Owner advice and homecare recommendations

Behavioural changes or seizures

The owners should be educated about the behavioural changes that are likely to occur secondary to the medications, the location of the tumour and the surgery (see above). They should also be instructed in what to do if the dog suffers a seizure (see Case 13.6).

Medication

Phenobarbital

Phenobarbital levels will be measured 10–14 days after starting therapy to ensure that blood levels are within the therapeutic range, so the owners will need to bring the dog to the surgery for a re-check at this point. Owners should be warned about potential side effects, particularly polyphagia (see above), behavioural changes and sedation, and should report these at the re-visit. They must not stop the phenobarbital suddenly.

Prednisolone

Prednisolone is being dispensed at a tapering dose to control peritumoral oedema. The aim is to maintain the dog on the minimum dose possible and owners are instructed to follow the prescribed tapering dosing regimen. They should be warned about potential side effects, particularly when the dog is on the higher dose (polyphagia, PU/PD, sedation, behavioural changes).

- Owners should be advised that the side effects will decrease as the dose is reduced but to contact the surgery if the side effects are unacceptable (e.g. the dog starts to urinate in the house).
- *They must NOT stop the steroids suddenly.*
- If they notice a clinical deterioration (e.g. circling) after they have reduced the dose, they should inform the veterinary surgery and increase the dose back to the effective dose.
- No changes must be made to the dose of medication or frequency of administration without consultation.
- No additional medication should be administered.

Case 13.3
Cervical disc herniation in a dog

A 4-year-old castrated male Beagle had a 6-week history of severe neck pain, treated with fluctuating doses of oral prednisolone (from 2 mg/kg q12h to 0.5 mg/kg q24h). The owners reported a transient improvement when the prednisolone was first started, but the therapy no longer appeared effective. The dog had developed melaena in the last 2 days. His body condition score (BCS) was 6/9.

On examination, he had extreme cervical pain with a left-sided nerve root signature. There were no neurological deficits and no other abnormalities on physical examination. A blood cell count showed a stress leucogram consistent with steroid therapy, and mild regenerative anaemia likely due to the gastrointestinal (GI) bleeding. Serum biochemistry showed elevated alkaline phosphatase consistent with steroid therapy. Urinalysis showed decreased specific gravity (1.010) and the presence of bacteria and white blood cells. Urine culture revealed *Escherichia coli,* sensitive to most broad-spectrum antibiotics.

Cervical spinal radiographs and computed tomography revealed a disc herniation at C2/3.

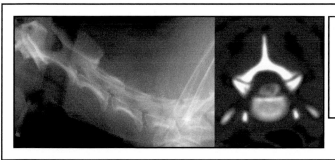

The lateral radiograph shows collapse of the C2/3 disc space, with a small amount of mineralized material visible in the canal. The nucleus of C3/4 is mineralized but there is no evidence of herniation at this site. The transverse CT scan at C2/3 shows a large mass of mineralized disc material on the floor of the canal.

Agreed medical/surgical management

The disc herniation was surgically decompressed via a ventral slot. The cervical pain also required aggressive management (see below).

The prednisolone therapy had resulted in gastrointestinal ulceration. This could be treated with sucralfate in combination with an acid secretory inhibitor, such as an H2 blocker (famotidine or cimetidine (whilst noting potential drug interactions) or ranitidine), or a proton pump inhibitor (omeprazole or pantoprazole) for 14–21 days. The oral prednisolone dose was tapered (current dose 0.5 mg/kg q24h) to 0.25 mg/kg q24h for 1 week, then 0.25 mg/kg q48h for 1 more week, then discontinued.

The urinary tract infection was treated with cefalexin.

Acute/chronic pain management

Perioperative

Given the severity and chronicity of the pain, and the current use of prednisolone, a fentanyl patch was placed preoperatively. Pain was managed immediately postoperatively with a fentanyl + lidocaine + ketamine CRI for 24 hours. As the dog was comfortable after 24 hours, the ketamine was withdrawn, followed by the lidocaine, and then the fentanyl.

If necessary, longer-acting opioids, such as morphine, methadone and, later, buprenorphine, can be used by other routes, at appropriate dosing intervals, in addition to the CRI. Oral tramadol is started when the dog is awake enough to eat. Oral diazepam can be added to the drug regimen if the dog is experiencing muscle spasms. Typically, the level of pain will improve dramatically within 48–72 hours of surgery and the problem should have resolved within 2 weeks. If severe pain does persist beyond 72 hours after surgery, a CT or MRI should be repeated to ensure that there is no residual disc material at the site.

Chronic pain

Given that the pain is severe and chronic, it may well continue after surgery. If pain is still present and significant 72 hours after surgery, and no residual disc material is seen on imaging, a further pain assessment should guide the clinician towards the use of further medication.

NSAIDs are contraindicated in this patient while there is evidence of gastrointestinal ulceration and while he is receiving concurrent steroids. If evidence of central sensitization or continuing severe pain is present at any stage after surgery (see Chapter 3), gabapentin or amantadine may help, or amitriptyline *(but do not use amitriptyline with tramadol)*. Specific adverse effects of gabapentin are ataxia and tripping/stumbling; the drug should be withdrawn or the dose reduced if these occur. Additional pain relief may be achieved by adding paracetamol: with codeine if tramadol is not used; but without codeine if tramadol is already being used.

Given the multiple medications and the complications already occurring, it would be wise to assess the dog carefully for signs of continuing pain or chronic pain syndrome (see Chapter 3), rather than just assuming he has it and using additional medication, any of which may cause sedation and/or gastrointestinal disturbance.

Fear, stress, conflict concerns

Many dogs that have suffered severe chronic pain are extremely anxious about being handled, in anticipation of the pain that might ensue. It is important to place the dog in a ground-level cage and approach him slowly, letting him step out of the cage himself. Leads should not be placed around the neck, but looped between the front legs or, preferably, a harness can be placed.

The dog is allowed to step out of a ground-level cage and approached gently.
(Courtesy of Rachel Lumbis and Catherine Kendall)

It may be necessary to desensitize this patient to handling by the owners and to the approach of strangers and other dogs, if his previous experiences have resulted in a learned anxiety about these encounters. Unpredictable reactions suggest continuing pain rather than learned associations, although the occurrence of responses should be investigated: owners may perceive responses to be 'unpredictable' when they are not. In the long term, replacement of favourite but inappropriate games such as jumping and twisting to catch things, with mentally stimulating games and varied walks will help to prevent frustration in this patient.

Nutritional requirements

Diet

In light of the gastrointestinal ulceration, the dog should be fed little and often on a low-fat digestible diet, such as one formulated for small intestinal disease. High-fat critical-care type diets are contraindicated because they delay gastric emptying and so may increase vomiting (see Chapter 5). *It is very important that the dog does eat*, because gastric ulcers will not heal effectively without products of intraluminal digestion for nutrition. It is completely inappropriate to try to 'treat' gastrointestinal ulceration with 'starvation'.

Monitoring food intake in the hospital

Although this dog is on steroid therapy, which would be expected to *increase* his appetite, the pain of his condition, the analgesics and the gastrointestinal ulceration may all *reduce* appetite. In view of the importance of feeding for gut healing, it is therefore vital to ensure that he eats in the hospital. Daily records should be kept and if he fails to meet his RER for 2–3 days, consideration should be given to some sort of tube feeding (see Chapter 5). The fact that he is slightly overweight at presentation does *not* mean that starvation in the hospital can be tolerated, as bodyweight lost in these circumstances will be predominantly lean body mass. An oesophagostomy or naso-oesophageal tube could be placed or, if the dog appears really averse to eating preoperatively, a gastrostomy tube could be placed at surgery. A gastrostomy tube has a wider bore and therefore allows use of a wider range of diets (including low-fat diets liquidized to gruel).

Long-term feeding

On discharge, consideration should be given to the dog's calorie intake, and methods of weight control should be discussed with the owners. This dog is already slightly overweight, is of a breed predisposed to obesity, and is likely to exercise less in the postoperative period. The owners should therefore be advised to reduce his calorie intake as soon as he goes home and monitor his bodyweight every 2 weeks. If the dog gains weight, they should contact the surgery for institution of a full weight management programme (see Chapter 6).

Physiotherapy

Gentle massage of, and warmth applied to, the cervical musculature two or three times a day may be helpful in the postoperative period but should be discontinued if it appears to cause pain. With a 6-week history of pain prior to surgery, muscle strength, joint range of motion, balance, joint stability, stamina and confidence in moving may all be reduced. An appropriate progressive rehabilitation programme should be devised. The owners should be involved, under the guidance of a veterinary physiotherapist.

Hydrotherapy

This patient has neck pain and no neurological deficits; swimming will cause him to extend his neck and has the potential to exacerbate the neck pain. Hydrotherapy would therefore *not* be recommended in this patient.

Acupuncture

If pain persists beyond 2 weeks after surgery, and repeat diagnostic work-up does not show evidence of a condition that needs intervention (e.g. surgical site infection, ongoing compression), acupuncture may be helpful. With these caveats in mind, acupuncture could be used adjunctively at any stage during this patient's recovery, although avoidance of the wound site is obviously preferable unless wound healing is a problem. Local needling would be most appropriate (see Chapter 11).

Other nursing and supportive care

Postoperative care

Postoperatively, the patient should be monitored closely for pain and discomfort (see Chapter 12 for full details of postoperative care). A padded bed should be provided and the dog turned regularly if he is recumbent. The bedding should have an incontinence sheet or absorbent bedding on top; this should be changed and the foam bed washed if the patient urinates or defecates on it. Urine and faecal scalding should be avoided by providing regular opportunities to urinate and defecate, and by changing any soiled bedding as soon as possible.

The patient should be fed in sternal recumbency to prevent aspiration pneumonia. The daily calorie intake should be recorded (see above) and antiemetics used as necessary if the gastrointestinal ulceration is making him vomit.

As soon as he is deemed comfortable, attempts should be made to move the dog out of the kennel and get him standing. The length of time is variable, depending on each individual case, but assisted standing is usually possible after 24 hours. A harness, together with a towel under the abdomen, will assist his mobility.

Heat and cold therapy

The incision should have cold packs applied for 5–10 minutes every 4–6 hours for the first 24–48 hours, i.e. during the initial acute phase after surgery; then hot packs should be applied for 5–15 minutes every 3–4 hours for the next week.

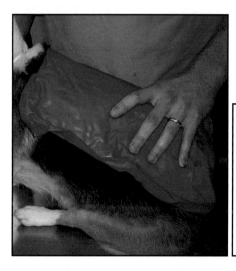

This dog's incision is being cooled using a custom-made pack that can be cleaned and disinfected and is kept in the freezer between uses. A pack of frozen peas can be used in a similar way.

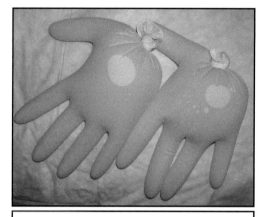

Hot packs can be made by filling disposable gloves with hot water.

Owner advice and homecare recommendations

Cage rest and exercise

The dog will be restricted to a crate for the first 2 weeks postoperatively.

Then a progressive walking schedule can be introduced:

- Initially, for the first 2 weeks following cage rest, he should be walked – on a harness – for 5 minutes, 3–4 times a day. Stairs should be avoided in this initial phase
- If the dog is improving then the walking can be increased gradually: e.g. in weeks 5 and 6 after surgery, 10 minutes 3–4 times daily; in weeks 7 and 8, 20 minutes 3–4 times daily.

It is better for the dog to exercise in a controlled fashion than to become frustrated from lack of exercise, but the restricted exercise must be enforced, even if improvement is marked. In the long term, the dog should *not* take part in vigorous exercise that involves twisting and jumping (e.g. playing Frisbee).

Owners should preferably play an active role in an appropriately devised rehabilitation programme that addresses all the dog's physical and mobility needs (see above). They should also reduce his calorie intake during the cage rest period to avoid further weight gain.

Follow-up

The patient should be re-checked and evaluated after 4 weeks. The owner should also observe the patient for signs of pain and discomfort.

Case 13.4
Cervical myelopathy in a dog

A 2-year-old spayed female Great Dane in ideal body condition (BCS 4/9) was presented for non-ambulatory tetraparesis, localizing to cervical spinal cord segments 1–5.

A diagnosis of cervical stenotic myelopathy was made, based on MRI of the cervical spine. There were three dorsal compressive lesions, at C4/5, C5/6 and C6/7. The dog was otherwise normal.

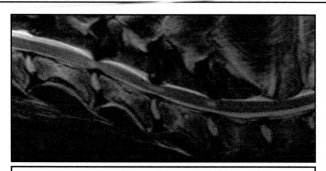

Severe dorsal compression of the spinal cord is evident at C4/5 and C5/6 on this sagittal T2-weighted MRI. There is less severe compression at C6/7, but all sites of compression are associated with increased signal within the underlying spinal cord.

Agreed medical/surgical management

In light of the severity of neurological signs and compression, surgical decompression by a multilevel dorsal laminectomy was performed.

Acute/chronic pain management

Perioperative

A full mu agonist, such as morphine, methadone or pethidine, should be used in premedication, along with an NSAID licensed for perioperative use such as carprofen. Partial agonists, such as buprenorphine, should be avoided, because they may interfere with the action of a full agonist if one is required later in the procedure (e.g. when using fentanyl).

Intraoperative analgesia can be provided with a CRI of fentanyl + ketamine, and these can be continued postoperatively. There is increased interest in the use of lidocaine by CRI, both intra- and postoperatively (see Chapter 2).

Immediate postoperative pain can be managed with a combination of carprofen (a single dose of 4 mg/kg s.c. given about 30 minutes before the end of surgery, followed by 2 mg/kg orally q12h for 10–14 days postoperatively) and opiates. A fentanyl patch can be placed postoperatively; hydromorphone is used in the first 24 hours after surgery until the fentanyl patch is working effectively.

Chronic pain

The patient should be monitored for continuing pain after the period of healing. If persistent pain occurs, changing the NSAID for another may be appropriate. Tramadol and/or gabapentin, depending on signs, or amitriptyline (without tramadol) or amantadine may be considered. Paracetamol ± codeine may help alongside other analgesics.

Fear, stress, conflict concerns

Although unable to move, and hence unable to display anxiety behaviour effectively, the patient is likely to have been very distressed by the tetraparesis. Care should be taken that she does not associate this anxiety, or postsurgical pain, with human interaction or handling.

During the recovery period, she will need continued and varied attention to prevent her becoming frustrated and understimulated. As well as nursing care from the practice team and her owners, they should use touch, grooming, talking, gentle play (as it becomes possible – may be only the agitation of a toy close to the mouth for her to try to grab, ensuring that she succeeds in the end) and different food delivery methods (as she becomes more capable of feeding safely).

Nutritional requirements

Postoperative nutritional requirements have not been demonstrated to differ from those in normal dogs, and alterations to diet may not therefore be necessary. However, it is important that the patient eats well postoperatively to allow effective healing. A digestible high-quality diet would be ideal; a low-residue diet should be used to limit the volume of stool produced and aid nursing care. If the pain and analgesic drugs reduce appetite, however, she may be most likely to eat her usual diet, which is acceptable. The dog should be placed in a sternal position for feeding and maintained in that position for 20–30 minutes after feeding to avoid regurgitation and aspiration.

Good records should be kept of daily food intake while in the hospital to ensure that she eats to fulfil her calculated daily resting energy requirement (RER; see Chapter 5). If she fails to do this, the effectiveness of analgesia should be re-assessed and methods of encouragement used. Consideration could be given to some sort of tube feeding, but this can be difficult in a large recumbent dog and carries an increased risk of aspiration pneumonia. Appetite stimulants are very rarely effective in large-breed dogs.

Physiotherapy

Physiotherapy needs to start immediately after surgery with passive range of motion (ROM) in *all four legs*, every 4–6 hours. Ideally, the dog will be transferred to a dedicated rehabilitation unit 48–72 hours after surgery, once postoperative pain is under control with oral drugs only.

A specific course of physiotherapy will be devised for her, based on her postoperative neurological status. It is important that the rehabilitation programme includes therapy to improve strength, ROM, balance, proprioception, joint stability, gait and confidence in walking. This should involve a variety of approaches including postural management and control of abnormal muscle tone, NMES to stimulate appropriate muscle activity, and a progressive exercise programme focussed on function and appropriate at every stage to the dog's current physical ability. Initially, she will require assistance to move, but it is hoped that this would gradually reduce as function returns.

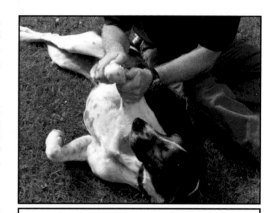

Passive movements to the carpus. (Courtesy of Brian Sharp.)

Once the dog can support her own weight, the owners will be able to manage her at home. The amount of time it might take for the patient to recover weightbearing ability is extremely variable. Most patients are worse immediately after surgery but are ambulatory within 2–4 weeks. A small proportion of patients will have a protracted recovery over 3–6 months.

Hydrotherapy

Hydrotherapy in the form of underwater treadmill training will form an important part of the rehabilitation. The water will help to support the dog's weight as she is recovering, and facilitate early treadmill use. Hydrotherapy should be started when the dog has some voluntary motor function. The surgical incision should be covered with sterile petroleum jelly if hydrotherapy is started in the first 10 days after surgery.

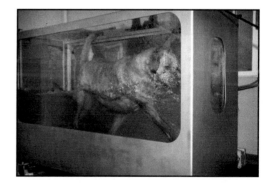

A dog using an underwater treadmill with the water at shoulder height; this gives buoyancy initially and increased resistance at later stages of recovery. (© Janet Van Dyke)

Acupuncture

There is experimental evidence that acupuncture at the time of acute disc prolapse reduces the short-term cord damage in rats, although the practical application of this to canine patients would be challenging (even if effective) given everything else that is required around the time of diagnosis, hospitalization and treatment. This dog has a chronic compressive condition; although acupuncture is often reported to be used in such conditions, it is not an alternative to surgery where that is indicated. If pain is uncontrollable postoperatively, then acupuncture should be considered, particularly the use of electroacupuncture (see Chapter 11).

Other nursing and supportive care

Monitoring

The dog should be monitored carefully for pain, preferably using a pain scoring system (see Chapters 2 and 3), and analgesics given as necessary. Fluid and food intake should also be carefully monitored.

Bedding

The dog must be kept on soft dry bedding and turned every 6 hours if she can't maintain sternal recumbency. If she can stay in a sternal position, her pelvis should be turned every 6 hours so that the pressure is shifted from one hindleg to the other. She must be placed in a sternal position for feeding (see above).

Prevention of decubitus ulcer formation is important and can be achieved by:

- Providing soft padded bedding that is kept clean and dry
- Turning the patient regularly
- Regular massage over the points of pressure to promote circulation; from a practical perspective this can be done each time she is turned
- Elevation of 'at risk' pressure points using 'doughnut' bandages.

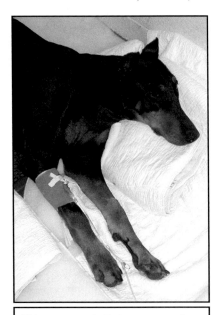

This tetraparetic Dobermann prefers to lie in lateral recumbency. Padding has been placed under her left shoulder and head, to maintain a more upright but still comfortable posture.

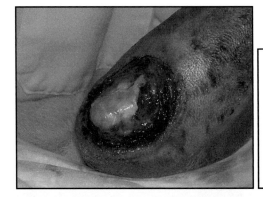

Large decubital ulcer over the elbow of a tetraparetic dog that was kennelled in a cage with no padding. His repeated abortive attempts to stand had caused severe injury to the soft tissues of both elbows.

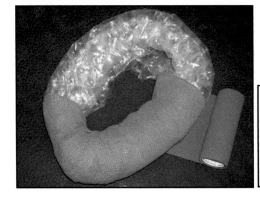

'Doughnuts' can be made using bubble wrap and adhesive bandage. They are placed to lift pressure points away from the ground.

Urination and defecation

If the dog maintains some motor control after surgery, she should have voluntary control of urination and defecation. She should be taken outside on a cart 3–4 times a day and supported while she urinates or while the bladder is manually expressed. If the patient is unable or unwilling to urinate, or cannot be taken outside (e.g. due to limited personnel, or pain associated with moving), an indwelling urinary catheter should be placed for up to 3 days. The risk of iatrogenic urinary tract infection increases with every additional 24 hours the catheter is left in place. If this were a male dog, intermittent catheterization could be performed.

If the patient defecates in her cage, she should be carefully cleaned as soon as possible.

Exercise

The dog should be confined for 4 weeks (2 weeks strict confinement and then, if doing well, 2 weeks of increasing controlled exercise). She should then be gradually reintroduced to normal activity, but *jarring of the head and neck must be avoided*.

Owner advice and homecare recommendations

Reduced mobility

The biggest concern in this case is preparing the owners for the potential for protracted recovery and the intensity of postoperative care needed. Targets for recovery that should be discussed include the expectation that their dog is likely to be weaker immediately postoperatively but that typically there is significant improvement over the 4 weeks after surgery. It is very difficult for a giant-breed dog that cannot walk to be managed at home. The owners are strongly recommended to place her in an appropriate rehabilitation facility until weightbearing is achieved.

Rehabilitation

Once the dog is adequately mobile and able to return home, it is vital that the owners continue rehabilitation themselves (or with the help of a local veterinary nurse or physiotherapist) to ensure optimal outcome. A demonstration of how to fit a chest harness should be given and the owner must be instructed *not* to fit a traditional neck collar. The owner should be advised to return to normal activity levels according to their pet's individual progress. The dog should be taken out into the garden up to three times a day.

Advice on suitable bedding and prevention of urine scalding, hypostatic pneumonia and decubitus ulcer formation must be given if mobility is still limited.

Case 13.5
Discospondylitis in a dog

A 2-year-old intact female English Mastiff was presented with a 1-month history of back pain and paraparesis. She had initially responded to dexamethasone and amoxicillin but had been para-plegic for the last week and managed at home due to financial limitations.

On physical examination, she had a BCS of 3/9. There was severe exudative superficial pyoderma over the ventral abdomen and inguinal region, and a severe flea infestation. Urine scalding was present in the perineal region, and extremely malodorous urine was expressed whenever she moved. Whipworms were found on faecal examination. She had autoamputated the nail and last phalanx of the third and fourth digits of her right hindfoot and constantly licked at abrasions on the dorsal aspect of the metatarsals.

Neurological examination revealed paraplegia, with reduced pain sensation in both pelvic limbs. Neurological signs were localized to the thoracolumbar (TL) junction, based on spinal reflexes (patellar, withdrawal and cutaneous trunci). Focal pain was elicited at the TL junction. A diagnosis of discospondylitis was made from spinal radiographs.

There was a profuse growth of *Escherichia coli* on urine culture, which was resistant to most broad-spectrum antibiotics but sensitive to ciprofloxacin, amikacin and imipenum.

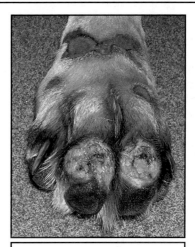

The dog had mutilated the third and fourth digits of her hindfeet, removing the nails and a part of the third phalanx. There were also severe decubital ulcers on the dorsal aspect of the tarsus.

Agreed medical/surgical management

Discospondylitis and the urinary tract infection (UTI) were assumed to be caused by the same organism, as this is usually the case. Treatment was commenced with oral ciprofloxacin for an in initial period of 4 weeks. It would be wise *not* to use imipenem for treatment of this dog, as use of this antibiotic is restricted in humans to avoid build-up of resistance. If progress is satisfactory, an additional 8 weeks of antibiotic will be required, with the caveat that longer-term therapy will be needed. As the dog has urinary incontinence, she requires manual help with bladder expression.

The mutilated digits were treated by application of sugar (manuka honey would be an alternative) and a light bandage once a day until a healthy bed of granulation tissue developed. An Elizabethan collar was fitted to prevent further mutilation.

The wounds were treated by the application of sugar, and a bandage that was changed twice daily to generate a healthy bed of granulation tissue.

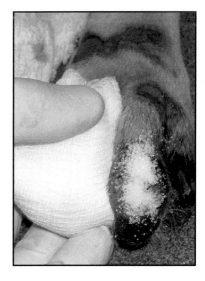

The pyoderma was treated by cleaning with a dilute chlorhexidine shampoo. Application of a suitable topical antibiotic cream to the lesions could also be considered, but care should be taken to avoid any cream that contains steroids; significant cutaneous absorption can occur, and this dog has a multiresistant infection and therefore should not be immunosuppressed.

A topical ectoparasiticide and an endoparasiticide should be used for the flea and worm infestations.

Acute/chronic pain management

Acute pain
The acute spinal pain was managed with carprofen and a fentanyl patch. It is important to monitor renal function in this dog because the UTI may also involve the kidneys (this is difficult to confirm); NSAIDs should be avoided if renal function appears to be compromised.

Chronic pain
If pain continues after acute management, an alternative NSAID could be considered (but monitor renal function). Tramadol could also be used, together with NSAIDs if necessary. The dog may be sensitized around the areas where she has amputated part of her digits; if so, gabapentin or amitriptyline or amantadine may help this. Amitriptyline may provide additional benefit via its antihistaminic and sedation effects. Secondary muscle pain in the spine might be treated with acupuncture.

Fear, stress, conflict concerns

As well as being caused by understimulation or frustration, persistent licking and self-mutilation may be a displacement activity precipitated by anxiety or emotional conflict in response to external factors, or a consequence of pain. The situation in which the behaviour occurs should be carefully investigated to distinguish these causes. Meanwhile, it would sensible to move the dog to an area in the hospital where she has a lot of human contact during the day. She may also be walked several times a day, with sling support.

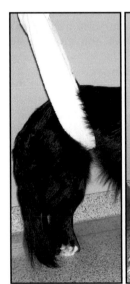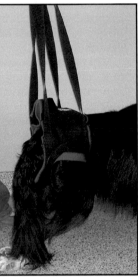

Paraplegic or paraparetic animals can be walked with sling support, using something as readily available as a towel (left). A custom-made sling (right) has the advantage of supporting the dog's entire pelvis and is more comfortable, so the dog is more likely to try to walk.

Nutritional requirements

Feeding in the hospital
The dog is in poor body condition and also has a serious inflammatory disease and significant skin disease. All of these are likely to increase her protein and calorie requirements, so it is important to feed her a digestible high-calorie diet with a good protein content. The ideal diet would be one formulated for small animal critical care use. These diets also tend to be relatively low-residue and so will help reduce faecal volume and thereby help nursing.

Initially, the dog's energy requirements are calculated (RER; see Chapter 5). Her bodyweight should be monitored on a daily basis and calorie intake increased if she is losing weight. Daily food intake should be carefully recorded. If she fails to meet her RER for 2–3 days, some form of assisted (tube) feeding should be considered. In this dog, the need for tube feeding is likely only to be short term, while the effects of pain and analgesic drugs wear off; a naso-oesophageal or oesophagostomy tube would therefore be most appropriate (see Chapter 5).

Feeding at home
The dog is likely to take several months to regain normal body condition, so feeding of a high-quality high-calorie diet should be continued at home. As there are financial considerations, it is unlikely that the owners will be able to afford to feed her on a critical care diet for months. However, they should be encouraged to feed the highest quality diet they can afford. They might even consider feeding a diet formulated for large-breed puppy growth, as long as it does not give her diarrhoea through its relatively high fat content.

Nutraceuticals

Cranberry juice capsules might be beneficial in helping to control the dog's UTI. There is some evidence that cranberry juice protects against infectious cystitis in humans (Jepson and Craig, 2008), although evidence of its effectiveness in dogs is currently only anecdotal.

Physiotherapy

Financial constraints limit the amount of physical therapy that can be performed on this patient. Initially passive range of motion (ROM) exercises can be performed on both hindlimbs 4 times a day for 5 minutes per leg. The hindlimbs should be massaged for 5 minutes twice a day. The dog can be walked outside 4 times a day using a sling or cart, with booties to protect her hindfeet.

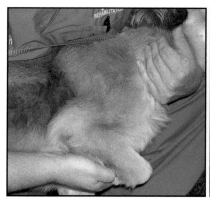 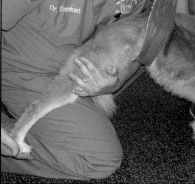 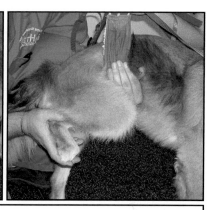

Passive range of motion of the pelvic limbs. (Reproduced from *BSAVA Manual of Canine and Feline Neurology, 3rd edition*)

Additional therapy in the early stages could include assisted standing (using physiotherapy rolls or harnesses), assisted 'sit-to-stands', and assisted walking (with foot placement). Standing exercises should be coupled with balance work to improve core stability, as well as improving speed and effectiveness of reaction. Balance exercises should be introduced into both walking and standing activities to improve dynamic and static balance. NMES (applied to appropriate muscle groups) can also be a useful therapy to help maintain muscle activity and provide valuable sensory stimulation.

Land treadmills can be effective in rehabilitation (to aid gait patterning and increasing strength) when the dog is walking better; but in the early stages the danger of knuckling and damaging paws remains and, for large dogs, hydrotherapy would be preferable (see below).

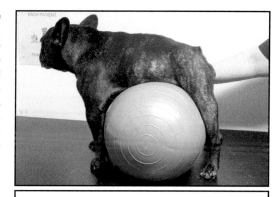

Animals with marked weakness may require assistance to stand and walk, using physiotherapy rolls. (Courtesy of Brian Sharp)

Hydrotherapy

It might not be possible to perform hydrotherapy in this particular case – initially, because of the UTI and pyoderma; and subsequently, because of financial constraints on the owners. However, in patients with fewer complicating factors, hydrotherapy (underwater treadmill or pool) should be used 1–2 times a day once some strength has returned to the hindlimbs. This is preferable to a land treadmill because of the dog's size. Hydrotherapy may allow more freedom of movement, improve coordination, provide more confidence in limb usage, and provide more effective strengthening of weakened muscles.

Acupuncture

Acupuncture is unlikely to be useful in the early stages but may be considered if the dog does not respond to other forms of analgesia or has unacceptable side effects from them. Areas of infected skin should be avoided, as should areas without sensation. The most painful areas should be targeted locally (see Chapter 11).

Other nursing and supportive care

- The digital lesions should be cleaned, dressed and bandaged (see above).
- Prevention of decubitus ulcer formation should be practised.
- Daily sling-supported walking to promote recovery of a normal gait, maintain interest, prevent understimulation and provide an opportunity for urination and defecation will be helpful. Protective boots should be fitted to protect the dorsal aspect of the metatarsals when she is taken outside.
- To help improve the dog's mental status, regular contact with her owner is essential; visits are to be encouraged unless the dog becomes very upset after the owner leaves. It is also beneficial for the owner so that they can learn how to care for their pet.

> **WARNING**
> This dog has a multiresistant *E. coli* infection. This could be a concern for any immunosuppressed in-contact persons or dogs. Precautions must be taken to prevent infection transmission. PPE (personal protective equipment) must be worn when handling and nursing the patient.

Monitoring
The dog should be assessed for pain regularly (preferably using some type of scoring system) and analgesia administered as necessary. Neurological signs should be regularly reassessed. Fluid and food intake should be recorded.

Incontinence
The dog is incontinent and requires manual bladder expression several times a day. It is important to remember that patients who are unable to urinate voluntarily or effectively are at risk of: developing UTI; damaging their bladder wall as a result of overdistension; or developing pyelonephritis.

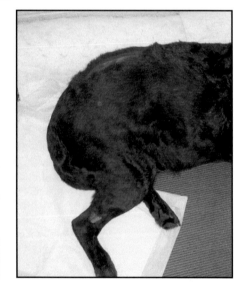

In a dog with urine scalding, the use of a urinary catheter with a closed collection system might be considered. This would assist with monitoring fluid balance, help to keep the animal comfortable and reduce the need for manual expression of the bladder. However, because this dog has a multiresistant *E. coli* infection, use of a urinary catheter would be unwise. A catheter could increase the risk of persistent infection and of ascension into the kidneys. Therefore, every effort should be taken to manage this dog effectively without a catheter.

The perineal and inguinal regions should be clipped and the urinary scalds treated. 'Nappy rash' cream can help to soothe affected areas. A waterproof barrier should be applied to clean dry skin to protect it from further urine scalding. Absorbent disposable pads can be placed under the dog's hind end and disposed of whenever she urinates or defecates.

> This dog is lying on a thick rubber mat with easily removable absorbent pads underneath its hind end.

Feeding
As discussed above, sufficient food intake is important. If the dog is inappetent, it is important to encourage food intake using measures such as:

- Feeding small meals frequently
- Adding moist food if the dog is eating a primarily dry food
- Warming the food to body temperature
- Adding some chicken or other palatable foodstuff
- Finding out what the dog's favourite food is at home, and feeding that.

Owner advice and homecare recommendations

Teaching the owner how to treat the dog
Because of the size of the dog and the need for regular bladder expression and skin/wound care, this dog will remain in the hospital until she can walk with sling support and can urinate on her own.

The owner may visit to learn how to perform ROM exercises and how to treat the skin wounds.

In addition to basic passive movements, the owner should be taught a range of appropriate exercises to help return the dog to optimal function (best prescribed, taught and monitored by a veterinary physiotherapist).

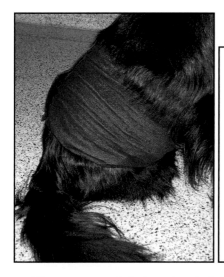

The owners of this chronically paralysed dog express their pet's bladder regularly. To prevent small 'accidents' in the house, the dog wears this velcroed waist band on a daily basis. An absorbent pad is placed in the waistband over this dog's penis and is changed regularly.

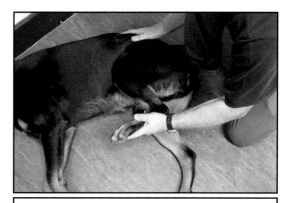

Hindlimb moved in a bicycling motion to simulate normal gait patterning; a useful technique for patients with neurological disease that are unable to walk.

- The owner needs to be educated about monitoring for ongoing self-mutilation and the patient should be discharged with an Elizabethan collar to be used if needed. The collar should be placed if the owner has to leave the dog for protracted periods.
- The owner should be educated about the importance of long-term flea and worm control.

Follow-up
- The patient should be reassessed at 2 and 4 weeks after presentation:
  o If there is no improvement by 2 weeks, urine culture and spinal radiographs should be repeated
  o If the dog is improving, the ciprofloxacin should be prescribed for an additional 8 weeks and urine culture then repeated to ensure that the therapy is being effective.
- The patient should be reassessed at 12 weeks and spinal radiographs repeated.
  o If the patient is doing well clinically, and there is no evidence of additional lesions radiographically, antibiotics can be discontinued.
  o A urine culture is repeated 2 weeks later to confirm resolution of infection.

References

Jepson RG and Craig C (2008) A systematic review of the evidence for cranberries and blueberries in UTI prevention. *Molecular Nutrition and Food Research* **51**, 738–745

Case 13.6
Refractory epilepsy in a dog

A 7-year-old castrated male German Shepherd Dog was presented with refractory epilepsy, currently treated with a combination of phenobarbital and potassium bromide. He had had clusters of 3–5 seizures every 8–12 weeks since he was 3 years old, but recently these had increased in frequency to every 4–6 weeks. He also had a history of degenerative joint disease (DJD) in both hips, and the owners reported hindlimb weakness and ataxia since a recent increase in potassium bromide dose.

A complete blood cell count was normal, but serum biochemistry showed downward trends in cholesterol and albumin (although both were within normal limits). There was no evidence of proteinuria on urinalysis and no history of gastrointestinal disease. A bile acid stimulation test was unremarkable.

Serum phenobarbital and potassium bromide levels were, respectively, 28 µg/ml (desired range 15–45 µg/ml) and 1.8 mg/ml (desired range 1–2 mg/ml).

Agreed medical/surgical management

The goals of treatment are to decrease seizure frequency while limiting side effects. Side effects of concern for this dog are hindlimb weakness and ataxia, and possible impairment of liver function.

The initial treatment plan was to reduce seizure frequency by adding in a third anti-epileptic drug with a different side-effect profile (e.g. zonisamide, gabapentin, levetiracetam) without changing the phenobarbital and bromide doses. The decision was made to add in a third drug, rather than increase phenobarbital or potassium bromide, because the most recent increase in bromide dose had caused worsening of hindlimb weakness.

The long-term aim is to reduce the dose of phenobarbital to avoid hepatotoxicity and to reduce signs of weakness. This dose reduction would be tried after at least 12 weeks have elapsed without a seizure, and would be done cautiously: typically, only a 10–20% reduction in dose every 3 months, as long as seizure frequency remains under control.

Acute/chronic pain management

Chronic pain
Chronic pain is associated with the hip DJD, which may also exacerbate hindlimb weakness. Management of pain in DJD is described in Chapter 14.

Fear, stress, conflict concerns

Owners should be informed that repeated seizures can result in behavioural changes. Aggression, or other, sometimes bizarre, behaviours are not unusual in the post-ictal phase, so the owner must be warned of these and informed that they are not signs that can be modified by behavioural intervention.

Behavioural changes may also occur in association with the DJD, where the dog learns that particular events precipitate pain, and develops an avoidance response (see Chapters 4 and 14).

Nutritional requirements

Diet
There are no special dietary requirements and this dog can stay on his usual diet. However, it is important to avoid changes in salt content, e.g. avoid intermittent feeding of high-salt tit-bits. Dietary salt concentrations appear to affect bromide elimination by the kidneys, with more bromide being eliminated on high-salt diets. If changes in diet that involve changes in salt intake become necessary in the future (e.g. moving to renal or cardiac diets – although even in these diets, sodium restriction is of questionable benefit (see Chapter 5)), the serum bromide level should be rechecked 2–4 weeks after the dietary change and the dose adjusted if necessary.

Phenobarbital and prednisolone both cause polyphagia, polyuria and polydipsia. These effects can be pronounced, particularly in dogs with frontal lobe disease, and the owners must be counselled to avoid feeding increased amounts.

Nutraceuticals
Nutraceuticals may have a role to play in hepatoprotection against phenobarbital toxicity. S-Adenosylmethionine (SAMe) is a potent antioxidant and glutathione precursor, which has been shown to offer some protection against paracetamol toxicity in small animals (Wallace et al., 2002) and should also help with phenobarbital toxicity (although no specific studies have been done). SAMe could be used alone, or in combination with silibylin (the active ingredient of milk thistle); silibylin has been shown to protect the liver against acute toadstool toxicity in dogs, though its use for phenobarbital toxicity has not been studied.

There is increasing interest in the potential for omega-3 fatty acid supplementation to reduce seizure activity in humans, so this dog could also have a trial treatment with omega-3 supplements. There is a single rather unconvincing but promising case report in a dog (Scorza et al., 2009) but generally it is unknown whether this has any effect in dogs and the ideal dose is unknown. Seizure activity should be carefully monitored during supplementation, since there is the potential for omega-3 supplementation to increase, as well as decrease, seizure frequency, at least in rats (Gilby et al., 2009).

Nutraceuticals might also be helpful for the DJD, especially in this case where NSAIDs might be avoided (see Chapter 14).

Physiotherapy

Physiotherapy is not specifically indicated in cases of epilepsy. It does have a very important role in the treatment of DJD (see Chapter 14). If the hindlimb weakness and ataxia in this case has a neurological cause, physiotherapy has an important role to maintain strength, joint stability, balance and proprioception through the prescription of appropriate exercise programmes (see Chapter 9).

Hydrotherapy

Although hydrotherapy may be useful for the DJD, it should be used with caution in patients with epilepsy. It would be wise to examine the triggers for seizures, if known, and then to avoid such therapy in dogs with these triggers; otherwise the therapist should always have physical contact with the patient, ready to withdraw them from the water at the first sign of any seizure. Although the dog would be under close supervision, both the therapist and the owner may decide the procedure is not worth the anxiety.

Acupuncture

Acupuncture has been reported to control canine epilepsy in a few small case series (e.g. Klide *et al.,* 1987; Panzer and Chrisman, 1994) and anecdotally. More recently, a controlled trial examining the clinical effects of gold wire inserted at acupuncture points in 15 dogs claimed no difference in EEG recordings between control and treatment groups, but there was a reduction in frequency and intensity of seizures in the treatment group (Goiz-Marquez *et al.,* 2009). These studies related to primary epilepsy, but the evidence is not very convincing. Acupuncture would not be appropriate in this case, but owners may request it because of reports of success in the literature.

Other nursing and supportive care

Care of the seizuring patient

1. Note the time.
2. Ensure that the airway is patent. Do not put anything in the patient's mouth.
3. Try to ensure that the patient does not harm himself.
4. Call for assistance from colleagues.
5. Diazepam may need to be administered (usually intravenous if a catheter is *in situ,* or via the rectal or nasal route). It should never be drawn up in advance as it will adhere to the syringe plastic within about 15 minutes.

- Monitor body temperature and cool if hyperthermic.
- Maintain a quiet and calm environment.

Post-seizure care

> **WARNING**
> The patient is likely to be disoriented and care should be taken when handling him.

- Ensure patent intravenous access, placing an intravenous catheter if there is not one already *in situ.*
- Observe closely for signs of further seizure activity.
- Monitor cardiovascular and respiratory effort.
- In the immediate recovery period, reduce stimuli such as light and sound.
- The patient should be accommodated in a padded kennel to prevent injury in the event of further seizures.

Owner advice and homecare recommendations

Seizures

Owners should be educated about seizure recognition (generalized, partial, and status epilepticus).

The owner should also be educated about what to do in the event of their dog suffering an epileptic seizure:

1. Make sure that the dog cannot injure itself.
2. If there are other dogs in the household, move them away (other dogs may attack a dog during or after a seizure).
3. Do not attempt to touch, move or restrain the dog during a seizure. (There is no need to pull the tongue out of the mouth, as owners often think they have to.)
4. Reduce noise and darken the room, then step back and observe.
5. Being able to describe the episode accurately is important; make notes and time the event.
6. Following the seizure, the dog may be disorientated and irritable. Some dogs become aggressive immediately following a seizure; therefore, take care when approaching the dog.

Owners often find seizuring dogs very distressing; they need reassuring that a brief seizure is neither dangerous nor distressing to the dog.

Owners should be advised to maintain an accurate seizure log. They should also record the severity of any side effects as new drugs are introduced and, in the longer term, when adjustments are made to drug doses.

Expectations for seizure control are that the dog will have fewer than one seizure a month; if the frequency is higher than this, the owners should inform their veterinary surgery. They should also contact the veterinary surgery immediately if a seizure is prolonged – they should be warned about the very real possibility of permanent brain damage in status epilepticus if they do not do this.

Date	Seizures (number, duration)	Comments (on seizures and drug side effects)	Treatment given	An example of a seizure log. Owners are asked to note seizures and any additional treatment that is given. They are also asked to make notes on the severity of side effects. This helps the clinician balance seizure control and the impact of unwanted drug effects.
4th July	2 seizures, lasted about 3 minutes	Seizures were 2 hours apart. The additional phenobarbital seems to have prevented a full cluster	One full dose of phenobarbital	

Owners should be informed when to bring the dog back to the surgery for reassessment of blood concentrations of drugs and liver enzymes: every 6 months, or if the seizure pattern changes or side effects worsen. No changes must be made to the dose of medication or frequency of administration without consulting the vet. Similarly, no additional medication should be administered and they should ensure that dietary sodium concentration is consistent (see above).

Exercise
As this dog has DJD of both hips, exercise should be within the dog's capabilities – provide short amounts of regular exercise. The owners should be shown how to perform manual therapy in the form of massage passive movements/stretches.

References

Gilby KL, Jans J and McIntyre DC (2009) Chronic omega-3 supplementation in seizure-prone versus seizure-resistant rat strains: a cautionary tale. *Neuroscience* **163**, 750–758

Goiz-Marquez G, Caballero S, Solis H, Rodriguez C and Sumano H (2009) Electroencephalographic evaluation of gold wire implants inserted in acupuncture points in dogs with epileptic seizures. *Research in Veterinary Science* **86**, 152–161

Klide AM, Farnbach GC and Gallagher SM (1987) Acupuncture therapy for the treatment of intractable, idiopathic epilepsy in five dogs. *Acupuncture Electrotherapy Research* **12**, 71–74

Panzer RB and Chrisman CL (1994) An auricular acupuncture treatment for idiopathic canine epilepsy: a preliminary report. *American Journal of Chinese Medicine* **22**, 11–17

Scorza FA, Cavalheiro EA, Arida RM *et al.* (2009) Positive impact of omega-3 fatty acid supplementation in a dog with drug-resistant epilepsy: a case study. *Epilepsy and Behaviour* **15**, 527–528

Wallace KP, Center SA, Hickford FH, Warner KL and Smith S (2002) S-Adenosyl-L-methionine (SAMe) for the treatment of acetaminophen toxicity in a dog. *Journal of the American Animal Hospital Association* **38**, 246–254

Case 13.7
Thoracolumbar disc protrusion in a dog

A 14-year-old neutered male Labrador Retriever was presented with a history of chronic, progressive hindlimb weakness, ataxia and pain. The owners reported these changes as happening over the last 18 months, but with a recent significant deterioration. The dog was overweight (BCS 7/9).

On examination, the dog was lame in both hindlimbs in addition to being paraparetic and ataxic. He had reduced range of motion (ROM) of both stifles and hips, and had thickening of the joints with medial buttresses on both stifles (indicating joint instability). He resented palpation of the thoracolumbar and lumbosacral spine. His patellar reflexes were normal to increased, and he had reduced hock flexion on testing his withdrawal reflexes.

Routine blood work was unremarkable as were thoracic radiographs. Magnetic resonance imaging of his spine revealed type II disc protrusions at T12/13, T13/L1, L1/2 and the lumbosacral junction, with milder protrusions at the remaining lumbar discs. The disc protrusions at T12/13, T13/L1, and L1/2 were causing spinal cord compression.

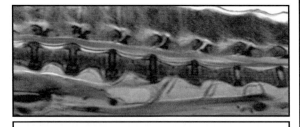

TL type II disc: A sagittal T2-weighted MRI of the lumbar spine shows protrusions of all the intervertebral discs. These are causing significant spinal cord compression at T12/13 (not shown), T13/L1 and L1/2.

Agreed medical/surgical management

Surgical decompression of the spinal cord and cauda equina was not recommended for this patient because of: the presence of multiple sites of compression; the lack of certainty about outcome with surgery; the presence of significant orthopaedic disease; and the age of the dog. As a general rule, removal of chronically protruded disc material is more technically challenging than removal of acutely herniated material. The disc material is fibrous and has to be sharply dissected to remove it from the canal. The potential to damage the spinal cord is greater than that encountered when decompressing an acute disc herniation. In addition, the chronicity of the compression has already caused significant, irreversible spinal cord damage. As a result, the potential for improvement is more limited than when treating an acute compressive disorder.

A short test course of anti-inflammatory doses of prednisolone was prescribed (0.5 mg/kg orally q12h for 3–5 days, then q24h for 7 days; then 0.25 mg/kg q24h for 7 days, then q48h for 7 days). The aim of this therapy was to treat the vasogenic oedema associated with chronic disc protrusions, and inflammation associated with degenerative joint disease (DJD). If the prednisolone does not produce an improvement, it will be discontinued. If it does improve the dog's ability to walk, tapering of the dose will help to identify the minimum dose that will control the signs.

Acute/chronic pain management

Pain was initially controlled using tramadol. Additional drugs may be added, depending on the response to tramadol. If the dog remains on a corticosteroid, NSAIDs should be avoided; otherwise an NSAID can be prescribed after allowing a suitable 'wash-out' period of several days after stopping the steroids. Additional drugs that may be added include gabapentin and amantidine; the choice will depend on the nature and intensity of the pain. The NSAID paracetamol can be used in conjunction with any of these medications, although its preparation with codeine may be best avoided with tramadol, in case the dog is particularly sensitive to the opiate effects of both.

Hydrotherapy and acupuncture may also be helpful to control pain (see below).

Fear, stress, conflict concerns

Chronic pain may result in signs of anxiety that are mistaken for behavioural problems (e.g. sound sensitivity, reluctance to get in the car, agitation when the car is moving, separation problems) or even for cognitive dysfunction in older dogs (e.g. pacing and panting at night). It is important that these behavioural signs of pain are not overlooked or misdiagnosed. In addition, the dog may learn to show an avoidance response, or aggression, to avoid specific events that predict a painful outcome (see Chapters 3 and 4).

This dog is overweight and may now need a weight reduction diet on top of other treatments; he may see this as a loss of an important resource. Delivery of the food in divided portions in a food ball, or plastic bottle with holes punched in it, will make him feel that he is being fed more rather than less. Once he gets the idea of this way of feeding then the ball can be hidden in increasingly challenging areas and the dog can hunt for it, his reward being the food itself. It is important that he still gets some food in a bowl at regular meal times and that the food ball is delivered at random times and not when the dog is asking or demanding it, since this can then become a new stressor for the dog and a nuisance for the owner.

Nutritional requirements

Weight management
Given that the dog is overweight, has a reduced ability to exercise and will be on steroids, a weight loss programme should be considered. This will provide great benefit in terms of improving current mobility and quality of life. Nonetheless, given the age of the dog, it is unlikely to provide much in the way of other benefits (reduction in risk of other diseases, improved longevity). Given that the natural lifespan of the dog is not known, nor is it know what additional medical problems may arise, the aim of the weight plan should be more to enable modest reductions in bodyweight, in the short term, rather than insisting that an ideal weight must be achieved. Subtle reductions in bodyweight many improve mobility and quality of life, even if the dog remains overweight. It would be sensible to consider a systemic health check prior to weight loss (including haematology, clinical biochemistry and urinalysis), to ensure that it is safe to start a weight management programme and to rule out any concurrent diseases predisposing to weight gain in this dog, such as hypothyroidism. It would be feasible to use either a conventional weight management regime (see Chapter 6) or drug therapy (e.g. dirlotapide or mitratipide) in this case.

In addition to dietary management (or drugs), the owners should be encouraged to instigate a daily exercise plan, tailored to their dog's abilities (see Physiotherapy, Hydrotherapy). This will help to promote weight loss, and preserve lean muscle mass during the programme.

The dog should be brought to the clinic on a 2-weekly basis initially, so that his progress can be monitored. The same set of electronic scales should be used on each occasion, so that any changes are known to be genuine rather than due to discrepancies between scales. Most dogs will lose 0.5–1.5% of their starting bodyweight per week; however, this dog may progress more slowly, and this could be acceptable while his mobility is restored. Once he has reached target weight, a maintenance regime should be instigated. The transition should be made gradually: the dog should continue to be weighed every 2 weeks, whilst energy intake is increased incrementally by 10% at a time. Once his bodyweight has stabilized, the interval between weight checks can be gradually extended (i.e. monthly, 3-monthly, 6-monthly) but weight monitoring should not be stopped altogether.

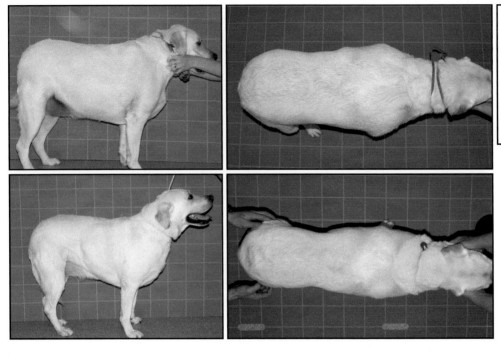

A Labrador Retriever before **(top)** and after a weight loss programme. (Courtesy of The Royal Canin Weight Management Clinic, University of Liverpool)

Nutraceuticals

The use of nutraceuticals for the treatment of chronic inflammation has been recommended for various conditions. Omega-3 fatty acids have been recommended for the management of inflammation associated with chronic degenerative orthopaedic conditions with mixed results (see Chapter 7). The rationale for their use includes reduction of inflammation and pain. Their use in chronic degenerative neurological conditions such as spinal cord compression has not been evaluated, although there may be parallels with osteoarthritis that may merit consideration.

Physiotherapy

Muscle strength is best improved by activities such as slowly progressive walking (5 minutes, 3–4 times a day), 'transfers' (e.g. sit-to-stand exercises) and hydrotherapy (underwater treadmill). Specific exercises should also be introduced to improve static and dynamic balance. NMES may also be useful to help improve muscle activity as well as providing valuable sensory stimulation.

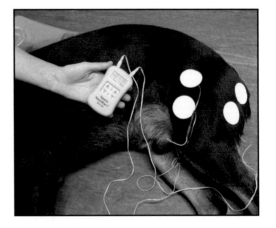

Application of NMES – shown here to the quadriceps and hamstrings – with the aim of achieving co-contraction of the two muscle groups. (Courtesy of Brian Sharp)

Weight loss can be helped by using a land treadmill, but the underwater treadmill or pool are likely to be much more effective as well as providing support to the joints. Joint mobility/range is best achieved via passive movements, massage and stretching, together with the use of heat to improve soft tissue extensibility.

Hydrotherapy

The aims of hydrotherapy for this patient are to support him as he returns to exercise, potentially retrain his gait, maintain cardiovascular fitness and contribute to weight loss. The warmth and buoyancy of the water may also help with pain relief. Initially an underwater treadmill may be safer than swimming; it is less strenuous for the animal but still provides support (see Chapter 10). An underwater treadmill is also easier to enter and exit. The dog may progress to gentle swimming exercise if this can be provided in a controlled environment with the equipment necessary (hoist) to get him in and out of the water in a controlled fashion. Additionally, an experienced therapist should be in the pool with this patient.

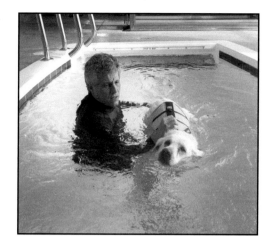

A therapist should assist the dog while he swims in the pool.
(© Steven Steinberg; http://veterinaryneuron.blogspot.com)

Acupuncture

Acupuncture may be helpful for the continuing pain experienced by this patient. It will usually give a response within the first 4 weeks; if there is no response, then electroacupuncture would be recommended (see Chapter 11).

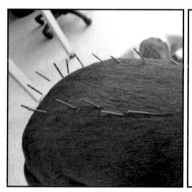

Manual needling would include targeting the gluteals and longissimus muscles, depending on the patient's distribution of pain.

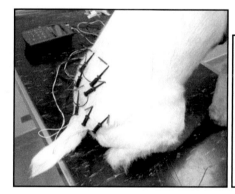

Electro-acupuncture is recommended if there is no response to manual acupuncture, or if a more potent or longer-lasting effect is needed.

Other nursing and supportive care

Whilst the patient is in the hospital for investigations, the use of a harness/abdominal sling may be useful to aid mobility. Suitable padded bedding should be provided and the patient should be monitored for deterioration and pain.

Owner advice and homecare recommendations

As dogs become ataxic they often scuff their nails and toes, and so the owners should be warned to look for this complication, to walk the dog on soft surfaces, and to try protective boots if scuffing does occur. Fitting a harness and using an abdominal sling should be demonstrated if necessary. Following appropriate tuition, the owners have a very important role in performing the physiotherapy techniques prescribed, and ensuring exercise is carried out as prescribed (see above).

Follow-up

The owner will need to return the dog to the surgery every couple of weeks to assess his weight and overall progress (see above).

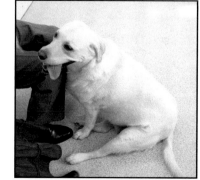

Weight management clinics also offer the opportunity for the owner to discuss any other care-related issues. (Courtesy of The Royal Canin Weight Management Clinic, University of Liverpool)

14

Patients with orthopaedic disease

Edited by Sorrel Langley-Hobbs

Introduction

Orthopaedic conditions are common in both dogs and cats, and there are two main scenarios where rehabilitation and palliative care are appropriate:

- Acute cases, including fractures, dislocation and ligament ruptures or sprains
- Chronic conditions, such as degenerative joint disease.

The most important considerations for supportive care are: to alleviate pain; and to maintain function or improve mobility of the patient. Multimodal management is usually most appropriate, with a plan designed around the patient and modified according to response. Consideration should be given to: pain assessment and analgesia; treatment of the underlying disease or condition; bodyweight; nutritional supplements; exercise; physiotherapy; and general factors.

Treatment of the underlying disease

It is important to try to obtain a specific diagnosis for lameness or mobility problems, so that treatment can be specific and patient-oriented. Animals should be investigated in a routine fashion, with a physical and orthopaedic examination to localize the problem. Ancillary diagnostic aids, such as radiography, MRI, CT and arthroscopy, may then be necessary to confirm suspicions or identify a cause (see *BSAVA Manual of Canine and Feline Musculoskeletal Disorders*). Symptomatic treatment of, for example, most fractures, incomplete ossification of the humeral condyle in Springer Spaniels, meniscal tears and cranial cruciate ligament ruptures in large-breed dogs, and shoulder osteochondrosis, would be inappropriate.

Recognizing pain

There are situations where it can safely be assumed that a dog or cat is experiencing pain when there are obvious injuries or after some surgical procedures. In other instances, the veterinary surgeon and owners have to be more observant and look for subtle signs of pain (see Chapters 2 and 3). It is very common for an owner to think that their dog or cat is not in any pain because the animal does not vocalize. However, if there is pain on manipulation or movement of a joint then it is fairly safe to assume this is real. Instead of using vocalization as a measure of pain in their pet, owners should be informed that reluctance to climb stairs or jump out of a vehicle, refusal to exercise, or a change in behaviour – such as reacting negatively to being picked up – can all be subtle signs of pain. Indeed, a change in behaviour may be the only clue that a dog or cat is in pain.

Analgesia

Pain relief for orthopaedic conditions will be required on a short-term basis for acute conditions such as fractures, dislocations or sprains, and on a more long-term basis for chronic conditions such as osteoarthritis. In the former situation, pain relief is usually provided by using a combination of drugs, such as opioids and non-steroidal anti-inflammatory drugs (NSAIDs), and external support. Often the most effective form of pain relief is stabilizing the fracture or reducing the dislocation, but this cannot always be done immediately, and there will usually be some residual periarticular soft tissue pain after corrective surgery that will need continued attention.

There are many analgesics available for use in osteoarthritis, ranging from NSAIDs to the potentially more potent, but unauthorized, drugs such as tramadol and amitriptyline (see Chapter 3).

Nutritional supplements

Supplements that contain ingredients such as glucosamine sulphate, chondroitin sulphate, methylsulfonylmethane (MSM), DL-phenylalanine (DLPA), fish oil, green lipped mussel and avocado/soybean unsaponifiables (ASU) may all have some beneficial effects for dogs with osteoarthritis (see Chapter 5).

Bodyweight

A reduction in bodyweight in an obese animal has been shown to reduce the need for analgesia and to decrease lameness scores in dogs with hip osteoarthritis (Impellizeri *et al.*, 2000). A long-term study comparing two groups of matched Labradors monitored osteoarthritis development in the presence of obesity. This study showed that the Labradors that were fed *ad libitum* became obese and their osteoarthritis progressed significantly faster and to a more severe degree than Labradors fed on a lower plane of nutrition (Smith *et al.*, 2006).

Anaesthesia

If surgical stabilization is required, the animal will need a general anaesthetic. Adequate perioperative analgesia is essential to limit the development of chronic pain problems and facilitate rapid rehabilitation (see Chapters 2, 3 and 11).

Radiography may require animals to be positioned in such a way that it contributes to the pain. For example, obtaining a ventrodorsal radiograph of the coxofemoral joints of a dog with severe coxofemoral osteoarthritis will require extending the hips, which will be uncomfortable and probably resisted. It should be anticipated that the patient may show a worsening of clinical signs after this procedure. With careful planning and the use of analgesia, this pain or anticipated deterioration can be alleviated or minimized.

Heat and cold application

Immediately postoperatively, and after an acute soft tissue injury such as a sprain, the application of cold (cryotherapy) to an area to decrease swelling and inflammation is often beneficial. A protocol of holding a wrapped cold pack on the affected limb or joint immediately postoperatively for 15 minutes and then for 20 minutes three or four times daily for 2–3 days, or until swelling has subsided, is recommended (see Chapter 9).

Once the initial acute phase of inflammation has passed, the application of heat to a damaged area may be substituted. The aims in using a hot pack are to loosen up the soft tissues, relax the muscles and improve blood supply. However, such packs should be wrapped in a towel to protect the tissues. Heat application is useful prior to physiotherapy or massage of an area but tends to reach only superficial areas. Therapeutic ultrasound can be used for warming deeper tissues (see Chapter 9).

Physiotherapy

The use of physiotherapy after cranial cruciate ligament surgery (tibial plateau leveling osteotomy) has been compared to leash walks in a small number of dogs (Monk *et al.*, 2006). The results of this survey concluded that early physiotherapeutic intervention should be considered as part of the postoperative management to prevent muscle atrophy, build muscle mass and strength, and increase stifle joint flexion and extension range of motion (Chapter 9).

Complementary therapies

There is some evidence that acupuncture, body manipulation, chiropractic and massage can noticeably decrease discomfort and improve function in many dogs and, to a lesser extent in terms of evidence, cats. Many veterinary surgeons and allied health professionals are gaining training and qualifications in such techniques, which are usually used as an adjunct to conventional veterinary medicine. However, the evidence is still limited and these are not recommended as alternatives to a specific conventional treatment.

Exercise

Exercise enhances return to function and is essential following orthopaedic surgery and in the long-term management of osteoarthritis. Therapeutic exercise is the core of most rehabilitation plans. Exercise can improve periarticular muscle strength to help protect a joint, and improve mobility in a stiff joint. Combined with weight loss, regular exercise helps promote loss of fat rather than muscle, and helps prevent a decrease in metabolic rate that can occur with calorie restriction.

Homecare

There are many general factors to consider in the rehabilitation and palliation of the orthopaedic patient. For example:

- Ramps can provide easy access into the back of the car for an elderly dog with coxofemoral osteoarthritis
- A low-sided litter tray for a cat with elbow arthritis can help prevent inappropriate urination and soiling
- Comfortable padded bedding and avoiding placing a bed in a draughty place in the kitchen may help ensure the dog and cat (and owner) all get a good night's sleep.

References and further reading

Houlton JEF, Cook JL, Innes JF and Langley-Hobbs SJ (2006) *BSAVA Manual of Canine and Feline Musculoskeletal Disorders*. BSAVA Publications, Gloucester

Impellizeri JA, Tetrick MA and Muir P (2000) Effect of weight reduction on clinical signs of lameness in dogs with hip osteoarthritis. *Journal of the American Veterinary Medical Association* **216**, 1089–1091

Lascelles BDX, Hansen BD, Roe S *et al.* (2007) Evaluation of client specific outcome measures and activity monitoring to measure pain relief in cats with osteoarthritis. *Journal of Veterinary Internal Medicine* **21**, 410–416

Monk ML, Preston CA and McGowan CM (2006) Effects of early intensive postoperative physiotherapy on limb function after tibial plateau leveling osteotomy in dogs with deficiency of the cranial cruciate ligament. *American Journal of Veterinary Research* **67**, 529–536

Montavon PM, Voss K and Langley-Hobbs SJ (2009) *Feline Orthopedic Surgery and Musculoskeletal Disease*. Elsevier, Edinburgh

Pead MJ and Langley-Hobbs SJ (2007) Acute management of orthopaedic and external soft tissue injuries. In: *BSAVA Manual of Canine and Feline Emergency and Critical Care, 2nd edn*, ed. LC King and A Boag, pp.251–268. BSAVA Publications, Gloucester

Robertson S and Lascelles BDX (2010) Long term pain in cats: how much do we know about this important welfare issue? *Journal of Feline Medicine and Surgery* **12**, 188–199

Smith GK, Paster ER, Powers MY *et al.* (2006) Lifelong diet restriction and radiographic evidence of osteoarthritis of the hip joint in dogs. *Journal of the American Veterinary Medical Association* **229**, 690–693

Clinical case studies

A variety of case scenarios in dogs and cats will now be presented to illustrate the considerations to be made and the options available within a specific clinical setting. Information relating to the rehabilitation and palliation of each condition has been contributed to each case by the authors in the first part of this Manual, plus notes on nursing and homecare from Rachel Lumbis RVN. The reader should refer back to the appropriate chapters for further details. Photographs used to illustrate the principles and techniques within the cases do not necessarily feature the original patient.

Case 14.1
Leg amputation in a cat

A **15-month-old female neutered cat** was initially presented after a road traffic accident that had resulted in pelvic fractures and neurological deficits. The pelvic fractures were repaired.

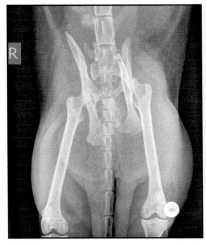

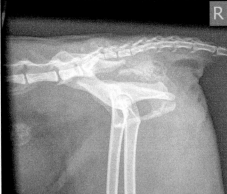

Following the accident, pelvic radiographs revealed a right sacroiliac luxation, a long oblique left iliac body fracture and pubic fractures.

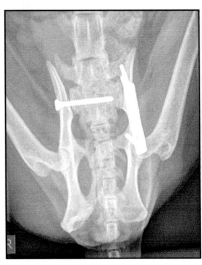

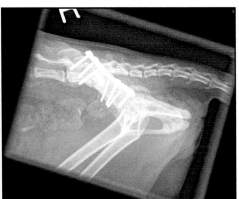

The pelvic fractures were repaired with a 2.7 mm lag screw across the sacroiliac joint and a dorsally applied 2.0 mm bone plate.

The cat made a good recovery but was re-presented with persistent neurological deficits in one pelvic limb, with knuckling over of the foot. She also licked constantly at the leg and had caused a small area of excoriation on the caudal aspect of the thigh.

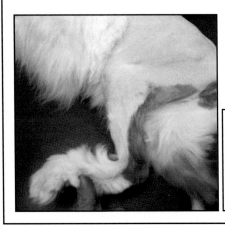

Contraction of digital flexor tendons leads to knuckling of the paw when hindlimb joints are flexed.

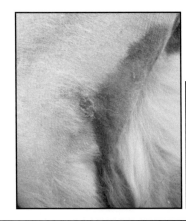

The cat's excessive licking had caused a small lesion on the caudolateral aspect of the thigh.

After discussion with the owners regarding the prognosis, it was decided to amputate the leg.

Neuropathic pain

Trauma may result in a neuropathic pain problem but also referral of pain from traumatized muscle. The more intense and long lasting the muscle pain, the more widespread the referral pattern tends to be.

Licking of an area may indicate:

- A displacement activity – conflict (such as pain elsewhere, or restriction of activity, or anxiety) resulting in a behaviour that is not relevant to that situation but which fills a behavioural 'vacuum'
- A compulsive behaviour – resulting from continued conflict and neurotransmitter changes
- Local pain, dysthesia (an abnormal unpleasant sensation) or paraesthesia (a morbid or perverted abnormal sensation, e.g. 'pins and needles')
- Referred pain or dysthesia – this can arise from nerve damage or muscle damage
- Neuroma/direct nerve damage – neuropathic pain is described by human subjects as 'sharp, burning, lancinating pain' and it is inferred from this that the reaction to such pain is a sudden starting or jumping movements, followed by running away or attacking the area.

Steady licking of the area could therefore arise from any of these sources (see Chapter 3).

Genuine neuropathic pain generally responds well to either gabapentin or amitriptyline (Cashmore *et al.*, 2009), but prior to starting either of these meloxicam would be worth trying, along with acupuncture (see below), which appears to be one of the better treatments for muscle pain.

Tramadol, although a potential source of analgesia for the cat, has been associated with seizures at the dose rates recommended for dogs and should be used with care in cats, even at lower doses (see Chapter 3).

Perioperative pain

When amputation is planned, very aggressive multimodal analgesia is necessary to provide complete blockade well before, and especially during, the surgery. This would include local anaesthesia and opioids, plus various chronic pain treatments (e.g. gabapentin, amitriptyline) preoperatively. Buprenorphine can be added to this both pre- and postoperatively at 10–30 (or even 40) micrograms/kg transmucosally 2–3 times per day (O'Hagan, 2006).

Intraoperative epidural analgesia may not be possible if the anatomy of the pelvic region has been distorted by the fractures. If there is no distortion, then both long-acting local anaesthetics (e.g. bupivacaine) and morphine may be used. Ketamine CRI should also be considered, especially if epidural analgesia is not possible. This may be continued postoperatively at a lower dose, provided dysphoria is not a problem.

Local anaesthetic should be applied around nerves at the site of transection before they are cut (taking care not to give a toxic dose).

'Phantom limb' pain

Pain arising from the original injury, especially if neuropathic in origin, may not resolve quickly, even following amputation, and the issue of phantom limb pain may need consideration. Because of the lack of conclusive evidence for the benefit of any one treatment for phantom limb pain, an interdisciplinary approach is worth considering.

- There have been good reports for the use of transcutaneous electrical nerve stimulation (TENS) to reduce phantom limb pain in humans. However, placement of the electrodes on the stump itself has generally been found to be unreliable, and often uncomfortable.
- Targeting the segmental innervation would be worth considering if the cat were amenable to this form of treatment. Good results have been found when the electrodes have been positioned on the remaining aspects of the amputated limb (not relevant for this case) and, especially, on the contralateral limb.

There are a number of anxiety issues to be dealt with:

- The cat may have lost confidence in going outside generally or in her surroundings generally, which will probably depend on how aware she was of what had happened to her (i.e. did she make a direct association with a car or just that something painful and frightening happened when she was outside?). She may not want to go outside or may behave differently from before when outside, and may perform displacement activities such as overgrooming, licking or inappropriate toileting

- Continuing pain will cause ongoing anxiety/fear
- The loss of one limb will cause physical difficulties such as balance, but also psychological difficulties such as feeling more vulnerable.

Improving and enhancing the cat's core territory should help her deal with any or all of these issues, although effective pain relief must be a priority. The following should help the cat feel more secure:

- **Food.** Increase the number of feeding stations. The cat must also be able to reach food easily; if she has previously fed at a height she may not feel like jumping, so adjust the position of the food, whilst making sure this does not make her anxious about it being available to competitors (e.g. the pet dog or a possible intruding cat if the food is placed near the cat flap).
- **Water.** Cats generally prefer their water about a room's distance away from their food in a clear, wide bowl.
- **Access inside and out.** Cats normally have more than one access point into and out of their core territory (usually the house). Consider providing an additional access point, or ensure that she can use the existing access points (they are not too high or too difficult to negotiate when she feels unwell and uncomfortable).
- **Scratching posts.** Are these easily accessible and appropriate? A horizontal scratch post can be provided, so that the cat can still reach it if she does not feel up to climbing. The preference for horizontal *versus* vertical scratching may change with the loss of a limb.
- **Hiding areas.** Provide multiple safe and comfortable hiding areas at different levels, or make sure that there is a 'step' system to allow the cat to reach her old favourite places.
- **Beds.** Provision of new beds, such as radiator beds, may improve the comfort and wellbeing of the patient.
- **Play.** Modify games to very short bursts of gentle play, but continue to try to stimulate the cat.
- **Petting.** Use of gentle touch, stroking and grooming in ways that the patient will tolerate and enjoy will not only improve the patient's feelings of wellbeing but will also give the owner a sense of participating in their pet's treatment and nursing.

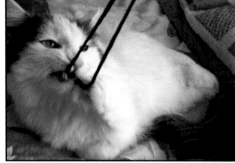

During recovery from surgery the cat was keen to play with a piece of string, biting and pawing at it.

Pheromones (see Chapter 4) may help reduce anxiety and promote feelings of comfort and wellbeing if the cat is continuing to show signs of anxiety despite all the above measures.

Nutritional requirements

Feeding in the hospital
Nutritional requirements after surgery may be increased (see Chapter 5). Common strategies for nutritional support of postoperative patients include the use of palatable, easily digestible diets.

It is most important that the cat eats, because if she becomes anorexic when presented with unfamiliar food there is always a risk of hepatic lipidosis, even in a lean cat. Therefore, feeding her normal diet to encourage eating is acceptable. Good records should be kept of daily food intake while in the hospital to ensure she eats to fulfil her calculated daily resting energy requirement (RER; see Chapter 5). If she does not eat enough to satisfy her RER, serious consideration should be given to special nutritional support such as short-term naso-oesophageal or oesophagostomy tube feeding.

Long-term feeding
It will be important thereafter that the cat does not put on weight as, with only three legs, she may exercise less after surgery. It will also be important for future joint health that she does not become overweight. Long-term management should focus on maintaining lean bodyweight. Body condition should be assessed frequently to ensure an appropriate feeding regimen; neutered cats tend not to regulate bodyweight when fed *ad libitum*.

Physiotherapy

Physiotherapy and rehabilitation are important aspects of postoperative care following amputation, to ensure an optimal functional outcome; however, with cats, success is very dependent on the cat's willingness to be handled and guided to perform certain activities. There may also be physical problems related to the original injury (such as reduction in joint range and muscle strength in the remaining limbs) that must be considered alongside the amputation requirements, and it is recommended that a veterinary physiotherapist should be involved in the planning of the programme to ensure the most appropriate treatments/rehabilitation regimes are applied. In particular, an assessment needs to be made of the remaining three limbs to assess joint range and muscle strength and whether any secondary muscle or joint pains are occurring as a result of compensatory postures/gaits. If present, these should be treated appropriately, and may involve the use of various joint and soft tissue treatments and electrotherapy. The use of TENS for phantom limb pain is addressed above.

An appropriate rehabilitation programme should be devised to improve strength, joint and muscle range, balance, proprioception, joint stability and stamina. In particular, the inclusion of balance and proprioception exercises to improve core stability and speed of reaction will enable the cat to cope more effectively with the enforced changes in weight distribution caused through the amputation. Basic standing and walking exercises should be made increasingly more challenging, but all exercises should be progressed in line with the cat's recovery and increasing functional abilities. With cats, exercise is best instigated through the use of short play sessions, using toys and other items of interest, such as beams of light flickered across the floor and on walls.

Hydrotherapy

In a small number of cases, cats can be introduced to water quite successfully, and in those cases, it can form a valuable part of the physiotherapy management programme. Hydrotherapy can improve strength and stamina and allows freedom of joint movement. The warmth of the water would help reduce pain and may permit more effective passive movements and stretches to be carried out if required to improve joint range of motion.

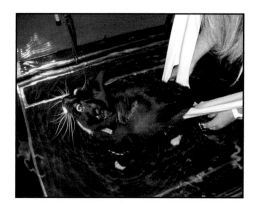

Hydrotherapy can be used successfully in some cats. (© Linhay Veterinary Rehabilitation Centre)

Acupuncture

Acupuncture may well be helpful in treating secondary muscle pain, trigger points secondary to trauma and pain around the stump. It would also be worth trying prior to amputation, in case the licking is secondary to referred muscle pain rather than neuropathic pain. Segmental needling (see Chapter 11) should be performed around the sacrum and gluteals. Mirror points (i.e. the points that would have been used in the absent leg) in the contralateral leg and myofascial trigger points would be the needling targets of choice.

Other nursing and supportive care

- Soft comfortable bedding and a low-sided litter tray should be provided.
- Vital signs should be monitored.
- Any signs of pain and discomfort should be recorded, using a pain scoring system (see Chapter 2) to ensure a standardized approach.

Postoperative care
- The surgical wound should be kept clean and dry. The incision site should be kept covered by a self-adhesive dressing, which is checked and changed regularly. Patient interference should be avoided by fitting an Elizabethan collar.
- The surgical site should be monitored for swelling, redness and/or discharge. The application of a cold pack to the surgical site after surgery can help reduce swelling and pain in the area. This should be continued for 2–3 days.
- There can be considerable blood loss from cut muscle ends if diathermy is unavailable; therefore intravenous fluids may be required to assist with a rapid recovery.
- Postoperative complications that can occur, and should be monitored for, include:
  o Seroma – a common postoperative complication; accumulation of fluid in the area can be painful. Seromas will usually resolve when treated conservatively but removal of fluid by intermittent drainage using a needle and syringe or by placing a closed suction draining system or bandage should be considered if the seroma is very large
  o Bleeding
  o Infection
  o Suture line dehiscence.
- Cage rest is required but the cat will need help to adjust to walking on three legs. Slippery floors should be avoided; rubber mats help prevent the patient from slipping. Limb use and mobility should be observed.

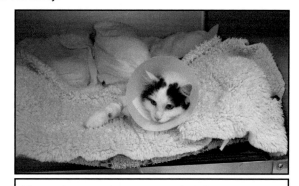

The cat is recovering postoperatively in a cage with plenty of bedding. She is on a ketamine CRI for pain relief. She is wearing an Elizabethan collar to prevent interference with the surgical incision.

Owner advice and homecare recommendations

Welfare and home environment

The owner should be advised to:

- Keep the cat indoors until the sutures have been removed; then she can be allowed to return to normal activities
- Assist the cat in adjusting to getting about on three legs – avoiding slippery floors or laying down rubber mats
- Prevent the cat interfering with the wound.

Suggestions for improving the cat's core territory are given in 'Fear, stress, conflict concerns', above.

Follow-up and prognosis

The cat made a full and rapid recovery. The owners felt that she had a better quality of life after surgery and that the right hindlimb had been causing her constant and chronic pain.

References and further reading

Cashmore RG, Harcourt-Brown TR, Freeman PM, Jeffery ND and Granger N (2009) Clinical diagnosis and treatment of suspected neuropathic pain in three dogs. *Australian Veterinary Journal* **87**, 45–51
O'Hagan BJ (2006) Neuropathic pain in a cat post-amputation. *Australian Veterinary Journal* **84**, 83–86

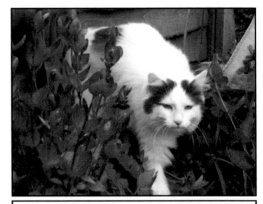

The cat enjoying a stroll through the garden 14 days after surgery.

Case 14.2
Total hip replacement in a dog

A 7-year-old male neutered 40 kg German Shepherd Dog was presented with a history of 18 months' progressive stiffness and exercise intolerance. He had difficulty rising in the morning and after sleeping following exercise. His signs were worse when it was cold outside. He was still keen to go for walks but slowed down after the initial excitement of being outside wore off. When he ran, he 'bunny hopped', using both back legs together.

On general examination, he was healthy with no evidence of pre-existing infection such as skin disease, dental disease or perianal furunculosis. On orthopaedic examination, the dog had bilateral pelvic limb lameness with adduction and a shortened stride length. On hip manipulation, there was a marked decrease in the range of motion, particularly in extension, with the right worse than the left.

Radiographs were taken of the coxofemoral joints and the dog was diagnosed with coxofemoral osteoarthritis, likely to be secondary to hip dysplasia as a puppy.

The condition had been managed non-surgically and the owner felt that some improvement had occurred, but the dog was still stiff and unable to exercise as much as the owner would have liked.

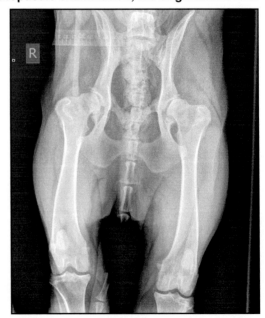

This ventrodorsal extended pelvic radiograph shows bilateral coxofemoral osteoarthritis, worse on the right side.

Agreed medical/surgical management

Total hip replacement surgery was discussed, with the potential risks and benefits described, and the owner opted for this approach. Although non-surgical management had not worked satisfactorily in this dog, it should be noted that it would be appropriate for many dogs.

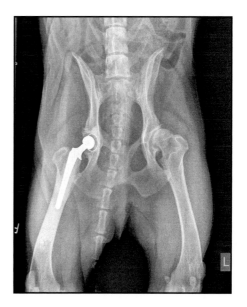

A right total hip replacement has been performed.

Acute/chronic pain management

Perioperative

Epidural morphine can be used but is not sufficient on its own to blunt the autonomic response to surgical trauma. The use of fentanyl/ketamine CRI intra- and postoperatively or, alternatively, morphine + lidocaine + ketamine infusion, also continued postoperatively, should be considered.

Another alternative is to place a fentanyl patch 24 hours preoperatively to provide postoperative analgesia. The use of a long-acting local analgesic into the epidural space should be avoided, as this can cause postoperative ataxia or paresis, which might predispose to postoperative luxation of the total hip replacement.

Postoperative analgesia should be continued until no longer required (see Chapter 2 for assessment).

Fear, stress, conflict concerns

Anxiety can be addressed by presurgical assessment of the patient, determining which resources are important in the dog's life. If he is very attached to his owners, separation should be minimized and may be partly helped by a lot of attention from the veterinary practice team (see Chapter 4). Some effort should be made to discover whether the patient is better off in a part of the hospital where he can see what is going on or whether he is better in a quiet, darker place where he can settle. Touch and massage can reduce blood pressure and release positive mood neurotransmitters (see Chapter 8).

Pheromone diffusers may help, but their overall efficacy is unclear. The pre-emptive use of alpha-casozepine prior to and after surgery may help in some cases where anxiety and agitation are anticipated, but there is currently no scientific evidence to support its use in this regard.

The use of acepromazine may not be ideal as, quite aside from its potentially negative cardiovascular effects, it may disguise the expression of pain; diazepam or alprazolam may be preferable, although it is important to be aware of potential disinhibition of aggression with any behaviour-modifying drugs and especially diazepam. These drugs should therefore be reserved for animals that will damage themselves by being agitated.

Nutritional requirements

Postoperative

Postoperative nutritional requirements have not been demonstrated to differ from those of normal dogs and therefore alterations to diet may not be necessary. However, it is important that the dog eats well postoperatively to allow effective healing. A digestible, high-quality diet would be ideal. If stress and analgesic drugs reduce appetite, the dog may be most likely to eat his usual diet, which is acceptable. Accurate records should be kept of daily food intake while in the hospital to ensure that he eats to fulfil his calculated daily RER (see Chapter 5).

Feeding long term

Long-term management of dogs with chronic degenerative orthopaedic disorders mainly centres on prevention of obesity. Feeding a balanced diet to maintain stable bodyweight, split into two meals a day, and avoiding high calorie tit-bits would be the best way to achieve this (see Chapter 6).

Nutritional supplements

Other long-term strategies proposed for the management of osteoarthritis have included the use of nutraceutical agents such as chrondroitin sulphate and glucosamine. However, there are limited data supporting their use (see Chapter 7). Other, more recent, strategies include supplementation of omega-3 fatty acids, which may reduce joint inflammation and thus reduce requirements for NSAID therapy. Further work is required to confirm the benefits of omega-3 fatty acid supplementation in dogs with osteoarthritis. These nutraceuticals can either be supplemented separately or formulated within a diet designed for joint disease.

Physiotherapy

Surgical management should always involve carefully planned postoperative physiotherapy and rehabilitation. A protocol should be designed for each dog individually, considering both hindlimbs and any concurrent joint and muscle problems.

Preoperative

It would be beneficial to place this dog on a preoperative physiotherapy programme, to optimise his physical condition and maintain the optimal condition of the other limb, and with the aim of achieving improved outcomes following surgery. This should include an individually designed exercise programme addressing strength, stamina, flexibility, balance and proprioception (see Chapter 9); a preoperative programme would provide the dog and owners with an opportunity to become accustomed to the exercise programme *before* surgery.

Postoperative

In the immediate postoperative period (week 1) the protocol should comprise: cold therapy; effleurage; and passive movements (to help with pain relief, keep swelling under control and maintain joint range). TENS may also be beneficial to help with pain relief and can be applied locally or segmentally.

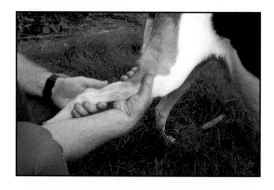

Effleurage of the hindlimb forms part of immediate postoperative physiotherapy. (Courtesy of Brian Sharp)

Passive movements should be carried out on all joints of the operated limb, but ensuring that movements of the hip are restricted to pure flexion and extension, being careful not to take the joint beyond its normal limits. These should be continued until normal range is achieved. Abduction, adduction and rotation movements of the hip should be avoided to prevent dislocation. It would also be advisable to maintain range of motion and comfort in the joints of the other hindlimb, through regular massage, passive movements and stretches. Treatments such as joint mobilizations, various soft tissue techniques and electrotherapy can also be usefully provided.

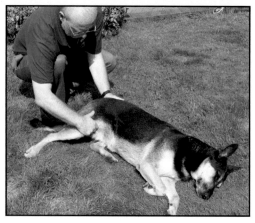

Passive movements should include hip extension, taking care not to take the joint beyond its normal limits. (Courtesy of Brian Sharp)

Once the acute heat and swelling is under control (normally from day 4 or 5 postoperatively), *cold* therapy can be replaced by *heat* therapy. The heat, along with other massage techniques (e.g. kneading, picking-up, wringing; see Chapter 9) will help relax muscles, improve circulation to healing tissues, and also provide pain relief.

During the first 2 weeks, walking should be limited to three or four short (5 minutes) slow walks each day, with a belly band or abdominal sling support provided as required to prevent slipping or abduction of the pelvic limbs.

During the later postoperative period (after 2 weeks) until the radiographic check at 6–8 weeks, the dog should continue to be managed carefully, with passive movements, massage and slowly progressive walking permitted. Each walk should be increased by 5 minutes every 2 weeks. Passive movements can now include gentle bicycling movements of the limbs. Gentle weight-shifting exercises, together with flexor reflex stimulation and neuromuscular electrical stimulation (NMES; see Chapter 9) can also be introduced at this stage. Appropriate treatments should also continue on the other limb until the dog is mobilizing normally; and if there are secondary problems (such as back pain) these should also be addressed.

After week 8, the emphasis in the rehabilitation programme should primarily be on muscle strengthening and re-educating the dog's gait, as well as improving the dog's balance and proprioceptive mechanisms.

Controlled progressive walking should be continued, and start to include steps and slopes. Balance and proprioception exercises should also be gradually increased in difficulty.

Weeks 12–16 should see a gradual return to normal activity with continued physiotherapy.

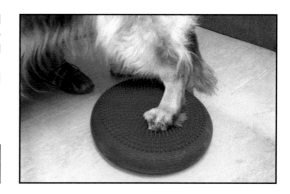

Balance exercise using an air cushion. (Courtesy of David Prydie)

Hydrotherapy

If hydrotherapy is planned as part of postoperative rehabilitation, introduction to the pool prior to surgery would help with muscle strengthening and help the dog become accustomed to the water, procedures and staff, thus providing a less stressful introduction after surgery.

Postoperative hydrotherapy can be introduced as soon as sutures are removed in a calm dog that is used to swimming. However, if the dog is liable to panic and kick or thrash around in the water, and has not been introduced to the water preoperatively, hydrotherapy is best delayed until after the first postoperative check at 6 weeks. There is a danger of luxation of the new implant if the dog struggles or slips in the pool. Therefore, an underwater treadmill would be preferable and more useful than swimming for gait re-education.

Acupuncture

Acupuncture may be indicated for continuing secondary muscle pain, if present, or for pain in the other hip if that does not yet require surgery.

WARNING
Implants and prostheses should not be needled directly because of the increased risk of infection.

Other nursing and supportive care

- Vital signs should be monitored.
- Any signs of pain and discomfort should be recorded, using a pain scoring system (see Chapter 2) to ensure a standardized approach.

Postoperative care
A light adhesive dressing should be applied over the surgical incision immediately postoperatively and this should remain in place until a fibrin seal has formed; otherwise, no external support is used on the limb. The incision site should be monitored carefully for signs of infection (swelling, redness, heat, discharge). The application of a cold pack to the surgical site after surgery can help reduce swelling and pain in the area. This should be continued for 2–3 days. The surgical wound should be kept clean and dry (see Case 14.1 and Chapter 12).

A sling, bellyband or hoist should be used to aid mobility and prevent falls or slipping in the hospital. Limb use and mobility should be observed, using a bellyband under the dog's abdomen when he is walked outside.

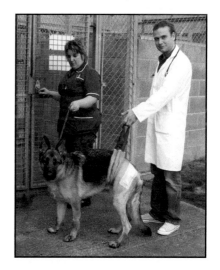

Use of a sling under the abdomen helps to support a dog's weight and prevent slipping when walking outside and on smooth or wet surfaces.

Owner advice and homecare recommendations

Welfare and home environment
The dog must be kept confined, with only limited lead exercise for the first month postoperatively. The owner should be advised to avoid potential frustration by spending time with him. Touch, grooming, massage, gentle mental stimulation and imaginative delivery of food may help to keep him calm and content. The use of

ramps (e.g. to get into cars), comfortable beds and sensible play (e.g. toys to chew but no throwing games) should be considered.

Follow-up and prognosis

The owner should bring the dog back to the surgery for a re-check and suture removal after 10 days and again at 6 weeks to evaluate gait, assess range of motion of the hip, look for evidence of pain and for radiography. Owners should be made aware of what to expect in terms of postoperative limb use: most dogs are weightbearing within 2 days of surgery and continue to improve after this time.

The owner should be advised of potential postoperative complications, including dislocation, infection, femoral fracture, acetabular fracture and implant loosening. Dislocation is the most likely complication to occur in the short term (up to 4 weeks after surgery). With all complications the owners should be advised to look for a change in leg position or carriage and an acute or deteriorating lameness.

Lameness should be imperceptible by the 6-week recheck. If functionally sound, and postoperative radiographs are normal, the animal is then likely to be allowed an increase in lead exercise over the following 6 weeks, with off-lead exercise introduced at the end of this period. The owner should be informed that it can take as long as 6 months for muscle atrophy to resolve and for maximal function to return.

The owner should be advised that prophylactic antibiotics are recommended prior to ear cleaning or removal of dental calculus, and any infections should always be treated promptly after a dog has had a total hip replacement.

Case 14.3
Hip dysplasia in a puppy – conservative management

A 7-month-old male entire Labrador puppy, weighing 30 kg, was brought into the practice because the owners were concerned that he was not keen to exercise, he 'bunny hopped' and he had a strange 'wiggly' pelvic limb gait. The puppy preferred to sit, but when he did walk it was with bilateral pelvic limb adduction, a short stride and a pronounced lateral sway. The puppy was overweight (BCS 8/9).

On manipulation there was bilateral hip subluxation, palpable because there was dorsocranial displacement of the greater tubercles. The puppy resented hip extension. There was marked gluteal muscle atrophy. Hip dysplasia was suspected. Radiography confirmed bilateral hip dysplasia with marked hip subluxation. Laxity tests confirm marked laxity, with loss of the dorsal acetabular rim.

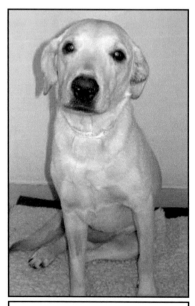

A Labrador puppy with hip dysplasia prefers to sit rather than stand.

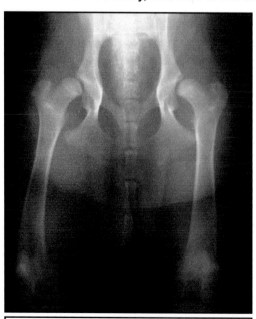

Ventrodorsal extended hip radiograph showing bilateral severe hip subluxation.

Agreed medical/surgical management

The hip dysplasia was too severe to be considered for corrective osteotomies, so the puppy was treated conservatively. Failure to respond to non-surgical management, however, would prompt future consideration of salvage surgery (total hip replacement or femoral head and neck excisions).

A 5–10% reduction in weight could have a significant effect on this patient but dieting should be approached very carefully in a dog that is still maturing (see below). The puppy should be assessed for potential complications of therapy, but also of exercise restriction: how can a 7-month-old puppy's normal exercise be replaced with mental stimulation? Also, restriction of food could be a major source of conflict for this breed (and the owner), but it will depend on how this is approached.

Chronic pain management

The puppy was placed on the maximum dose of NSAIDs for the first 7 days, with the dose halved for a further 2 weeks. He was then re-examined to evaluate the response and the need for further drugs.

Further chronic pain management could include:

- The use of two or three different NSAIDs in succession, with a washout period of 24–48 hours between them. During the washout period, tramadol or paracetamol + codeine may be necessary to maintain analgesia. Each NSAID should be used for a period of time sufficient to allow evaluation of the response (4–6 weeks). Owners should be given strict instructions to watch for signs of gastrointestinal toxicity and nausea. Regular blood testing should be carried out to monitor, as far as possible, for hepatic and renal toxicity
- The addition of further pain relief such as tramadol if the dog is clearly struggling with pain and the NSAIDs alone are inadequate
- The addition of gabapentin or amantadine if the patient develops chronic pain syndrome/central sensitization (see Chapter 3) or if a combination of NSAIDs and tramadol is not providing sufficient analgesia
- Acupuncture (see below)
- Dietary and weight management (see below). Bodyweight is a major priority for this patient: reduction in weight may reduce, or preclude, the need for surgery or even analgesia over time.

Fear, stress, conflict concerns

Conflict and frustration may arise as a result of dieting this puppy and restricting his exercise. Novel ways of delivering food, such as playing hide and seek or using food balls, or hiding dry food under objects or within boxes of shredded paper, will give gentle exercise, mental stimulation and the sensation of acquiring more food without acquiring more calories.

The puppy is in pain; since pain, fear and anxiety are linked, analgesia is a priority to reduce anxiety and inappropriate associations (with people, other dogs, noises, traffic, etc.), which might result in the development of aversive behaviour towards those objects associated with pain (see Chapters 3 and 4).

Nutritional requirements

Nutritional management of young dogs with developmental orthopaedic disease centres on: decreasing their rate of growth whilst meeting nutrient requirements for growing dogs; and preventing or correcting weight gain. Given that this puppy is obese (BCS 8/9) and has concurrent orthopaedic disease, a weight loss programme should be considered. However, he is still within his growth phase, so the timing of this regime is critical. In this respect, it is perhaps not advisable to instigate caloric restriction or drug therapy to reduce bodyweight at this stage. Instead, it would be preferable to continue with a diet appropriate to the lifestage to allow slow continued growth and prevent further adipose tissue gain.

A growth diet designed for large-breed dogs might be ideal for this patient. These diets meet the protein and mineral requirements of growing dogs, but have a relatively low caloric density and are intended to slow rate of growth and decrease the risk of developing obesity. By providing energy requirements for only a slow rate of growth (approximately 1.2–1.6 times maintenance), the majority of tissue gain should be lean muscle and skeletal tissue. Therefore, body condition may gradually begin to normalize, even without caloric restriction.

Advice on cutting out high-calorie tit-bits would certainly be worthwhile at this stage. The weight and body condition should be recorded on a monthly basis to ensure that the rate of growth is acceptable.

Weight control

Once the dog has reached adult size (which should be by 18 months) his weight and body condition should be reviewed and, if appropriate, a weight management regime should then be instigated. Details of weight loss regimens are given in Chapter 6.

In addition to dietary management (or drugs), the owners should be encouraged to follow a daily exercise plan, tailored to their dog's abilities. This should take into account the current orthopaedic disease. It may be that novel exercise techniques, such as hydrotherapy (see below) will prove beneficial in stimulating activity and encouraging weight loss, although weight loss may be limited depending on the amount of hydrotherapy.

Given that hip dysplasia will predispose to osteoarthritis in the future, and obesity will contribute to the pain experienced, it is critical to ensure that the dog remains in optimal (even lean, e.g. BCS 4/9) body condition throughout life. To achieve this, he should be weighed and his condition scored every 6 months throughout his life.

Nutritional supplements

Although the use of nutraceutical agents such as chondroitin sulphate and glucosamine has been advocated in degenerative joint disease, there is limited evidence to support their use in severely affected cases (see Chapter 7). More recent approaches have included the supplementation of omega-3 fatty acids to reduce inflammation in affected joints. There is currently limited clinical evidence demonstrating the efficacy of this approach. However, there may be individual animals that respond positively. These nutraceuticals can either be supplemented separately or formulated within a diet designed for joint disease.

Physiotherapy

An appropriate programme of exercise should be designed to:

- Strengthen the periarticular hip musculature
- Improve speed of muscle activation (via balance and proprioception exercises) to protect the unstable joints
- Maintain adequate hip range of motion (especially extension and rotation)
- Prevent compensatory postures and gaits.

A selection of land-based exercises would be appropriate to achieve these aims, in conjunction with a hydrotherapy programme (see below).

The use of neuromuscular electrical stimulation (NMES; see Chapter 9) may be appropriate to improve strength in particularly weak muscles (such as the gluteals). Massage, hot or cold therapy, laser or ultrasound may be useful in conjunction with medications. Electrotherapy should always be performed by a trained operator. Certain modalities of electrotherapy would not be advisable at such a young age but may be beneficial as the dog matures.

All activities (walking or prescribed exercise) must be controlled, paced (within the tolerance of the puppy) and carried out on a regular (little and often) basis. This will prevent undue stress being placed on the unstable hip joints; though to achieve improvements in strength and stability the difficulty of the activities must be progressively increased.

Hydrotherapy

Hydrotherapy should form an important component of a thorough physiotherapy management programme. It may also help with weight loss (although that cannot be relied upon) and relieve frustration from reduced exercise. It would be easy, however, to over-exercise the puppy in the pool, especially if he is having fun and seems comfortable. Over-exercise will lead to increased pain and discomfort after the swim, later that evening or the next morning, so it is important not to over-swim young keen dogs.

Acupuncture

Acupuncture may be helpful in non-surgical management of hip dysplasia (and osteoarthritis), especially as part of a multimodal analgesic programme. Acupuncture is not, as far as is understood, directly anti-inflammatory, and is therefore not an alternative to NSAIDs, but it may be a helpful adjunct if these are not sufficiently helpful in relieving pain or are contraindicated. Acupuncture is safe to use concurrently with NSAIDs, tramadol and any of the osteoarthritis drugs. Electroacupuncture, a more potent form of stimulus, should be tried before it can be said that acupuncture is not working for an individual patient. Treatment is with local (segmental) needling (see Chapter 11).

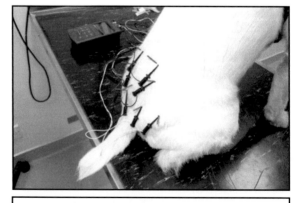

Electroacupuncture applied to the hip region of a small dog. (Courtesy of Samantha Lindley)

Other nursing and supportive care

Nurses can and should play an active role in the management of hip dysplasia and develop nurses' clinics to provide clients with information and support, as well as an opportunity to monitor a patient's progress formally.

Patient monitoring

Range of movement of the hip joint can be measured with a goniometer. Signs of pain, discomfort and inflammation should be watched for, using a pain scoring system to ensure a standardized approach (see Chapters 2 and 3).

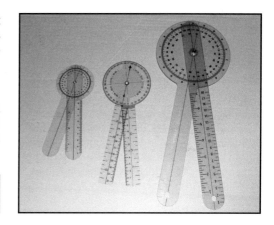

Goniometers can be used to measure angles of joint extension and flexion (see Chapter 9). (Courtesy of Brian Sharp)

Owner advice and homecare recommendations

Welfare and home environment

A comfortable bed will be required, and the patient's preferences should be considered (e.g. support, softness, room to stretch out). The addition of an insulated heat source may help soothe the dog's stiff joints, making them more comfortable and promoting rest. However, some dogs seek cool areas when in pain and may avoid such heat sources.

A daily exercise regime should be instigated: regular periods of low-intensity exercise based on the puppy's ability. It is important to maintain optimal or slightly lean body condition. Novel exercise, such as hydrotherapy, should be encouraged; Labradors usually love the water and as this patient is so young it should not be difficult to introduce him to swimming. The exercise and diet regime may need to change as the dog gets older.

Arthritis care

It is important to recognize the integral role of the owner in assessing and adjusting therapies and lifestyles to suit the individual dog's needs and the importance of the veterinary team and owner working together long term for the dog's benefit (see Case 14.8).

Case 14.4
Cruciate ligament repair in a dog

A 6-year-old male neutered crossbred dog was presented with acute-onset right pelvic limb lameness after playing with another dog on the beach. On examination he was 7/10ths lame, with swelling and pain around the stifle.

Radiographs showed a joint effusion and periarticular osteophytosis. Cranial drawer and tibial thrust tests were positive. A ruptured cranial cruciate ligament (CCL) was diagnosed.

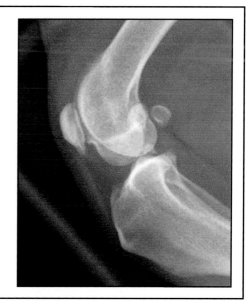

Mediolateral radiograph of the stifle, showing a joint effusion and periarticular osteophytosis; these changes are commonly seen with cranial cruciate ligament disease.

Agreed medical/surgical therapy

Agreed medical/surgical therapy

A right stifle arthrotomy was planned to debride the ruptured CCL and check for meniscal tears, followed by stabilization with a lateral suture (tibial–fabella suture).

Acute/chronic pain management

Acute pain

If surgery is delayed, for example because the owner is going on holiday, the dog should be kept comfortable on NSAIDs. The addition of opioids (ideally oral buprenorphine, because other opioids are too short-acting) or tramadol, to make sure the dog does not become sensitized to the pain, might be helpful, depending upon how much the patient is judged to be suffering (see Chapter 3).

Cold therapy (together with elevation, compression and effleurage) may help to reduce the post-injury swelling in preparation for the surgery, and may also help to reduce pain and discomfort (see Chapter 9).

Perioperative

This is an ideal case for epidural analgesia using a combination of bupivacaine (or ropivacaine, which may cause less motor block postoperatively) and morphine. If this is not possible, femoral and sciatic nerve blocks can be performed; these are much more likely to be effective if located accurately with a peripheral nerve stimulator (see *BSAVA Manual of Canine and Feline Anaesthesia and Analgesia*).

Postoperative

Opiates and NSAIDs should be used immediately postoperatively. The dog should go home with NSAIDs and tramadol, as appropriate.

Fear, stress, conflict concerns

The restriction of exercise in this dog may be a problem if he has a high drive to exercise and if the stifle is not causing him so much pain that he does not want to exercise. Mental stimulation in terms of training, attention, games with food, meeting (but not playing with) his canine and human 'friends', can all help to alleviate this frustration.

Changes in exercise after surgery may also be considered, i.e. looking at the kinds of games he routinely plays and how these can be altered to minimize the stress on the operated leg and the chances of the other cruciate tearing (as far as this is possible) but to avoid him being frustrated. Since the injury occurred whilst playing with other dogs, the possibility that the dog has associated the close proximity of other dogs with an aversive consequence should be investigated. Where signs of anxiety, withdrawal or aggression towards other dogs is apparent, a controlled programme of desensitization and counter-conditioning should be instigated (see *BSAVA Manual of Canine and Feline Behavioural Medicine*).

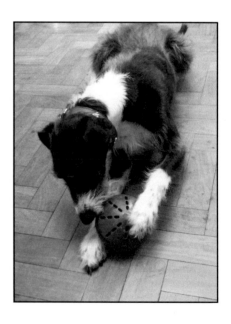

Hiding food within toys can provide mental stimulation for a dog that is exercise-restricted.

Nutritional requirements

Postoperative

Postoperative nutritional requirements have not been demonstrated to differ from those of normal dogs and therefore alterations to diet may not be necessary. A high-quality easily digestible diet would be most appropriate. However, if the stress and analgesic drugs make the dog anorexic, encouraging him to eat with his 'usual' diet might be most successful. Good records should be kept of daily food intake while in the hospital, to ensure he eats to fulfil his calculated daily RER.

Feeding long term

Long-term management of dogs with chronic degenerative orthopaedic disorders mainly centres on prevention of obesity. It is important that the owner recognizes that there may be a reduced energy requirement in this dog, associated with reduced exercise postoperatively (i.e. that it will not necessarily be appropriate to feed the 'usual' amount of food). The owner should be encouraged to weigh the dog regularly after surgery (every month or so) and to feed him to maintain a stable bodyweight.

Nutritional supplements
There has been a recent interest in the use of omega-3 fatty acids in animals with inflammatory orthopaedic disorders (see Chapter 7). This approach has not been applied to acute types of injury and further work is required to confirm the benefits of omega-3 fatty acid supplementation in this context.

Physiotherapy

Preoperative
During the 2 weeks *before* surgery, there is no reason to delay the rehabilitation process as long as pain relief is effective.

Even at this stage physiotherapy is important for pain relief, control of swelling, maintenance of joint range and muscle strength, and gait re-education (as much as is practical during this short period). Appropriate techniques would include cold therapy with compression, limb elevation, and effleurage massage for pain relief and control of swelling. Passive movements (within the tolerance of the patient) will help maintain/restore range. A gentle exercise programme should include: walking (slow, short periods) to encourage limb use; balance exercises to improve core stability; and exercises to encourage hamstring activity (such as stepping over low poles).

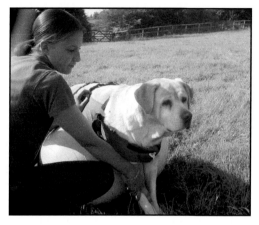

Improving balance and core body strength in a dog, using a 'physio ball'. (Courtesy of David Prydie)

An effective preoperative rehabilitation period should prepare the dog much better for the impending surgery, and (as is the case with human cruciate surgery) may result in better (and quicker) functional outcomes following surgery (see Chapter 9).

Postoperative
During the immediate postoperative period (first 2–3 days minimum), physiotherapy should comprise cold therapy, elevation of the limb, effleurage and passive movements (within the tolerance of the patient) to help with pain relief, keep swelling under control and maintain joint range. Passive movements should be carried out on all joints of the operated limb and continued until normal range is achieved. It is often beneficial for the veterinary physiotherapist to perform mobilization of the patella to ensure mobility is maintained and stifle range is not being restricted.

Once the acute heat and swelling are under control (normally from day 4 or 5), cold therapy can be replaced by heat. The heat, along with massage techniques (such as kneading, picking-up and wringing) will help relax muscles, improve circulation to healing tissues and may provide pain relief.

During the first 2 weeks postoperatively, walking should be limited to three or four short slow walks; once the dog can bear weight on the operated limb, gentle weight-shifting exercises can be started. Stimulation of the flexor reflex and use of NMES can also be introduced during this period to improve muscle strength and reflex hamstring activity. If the dog is not bearing weight particularly well by the end of week 2, exercises to encourage this should be started, such as baiting and low step-overs.

Weeks 2 to 3 can see an introduction to more functional exercises, such as sit-to-stands and step-overs. Exercises can be steadily progressed from week 4 onwards, with an emphasis on muscle strengthening, restoration of full joint range, joint stability, and balance and proprioception. In particular, hamstrings require specific rehabilitation to achieve adequate strength and improve reaction time. Weeks 9–12 (see Homecare) should see a gradual return to normal activities, including running.

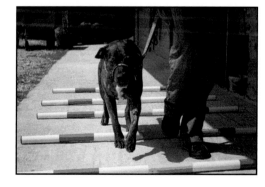

A dog undergoing proprioceptive retraining using Cavalletti poles. (Courtesy of David Prydie)

Hydrotherapy

Once the initial acute phase is over, the dog may benefit from short periods in the hydrotherapy pool (or preferably on an underwater treadmill) to accustom him to the water and begin the process of muscle strengthening and usage of the limb (see below) prior to surgery.

Swimming can be commenced slowly from week 2 postoperatively, and gradually progressed and continued up to 12 weeks. If the dog still has an abnormal gait following hydrotherapy, the use of an underwater treadmill for gait re-education may be beneficial to avoid postural changes that may lead to more pain.

Acupuncture

Acupuncture may be useful for analgesia prior to surgery if NSAIDs are not sufficient or are contraindicated.

Other nursing and supportive care

- Vital signs should be monitored.
- Any signs of pain and discomfort should be recorded, using a pain scoring system (see Chapter 2) to ensure a standardized approach.

Postoperative care

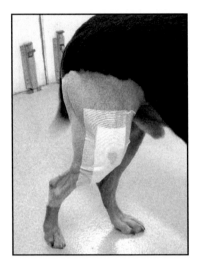

The surgical wound should be kept clean and dry and watched for postoperative complications (see Case 14.1 and Chapter 12).

A sling, bellyband or hoist should be used to aid mobility and prevent falls or slipping in the hospital. Limb use and mobility should be observed, using a bellyband under the dog's abdomen when he is walked outside (see Case 14.8). When taking the dog outside, he should be walked *slowly* to encourage him to weightbear on all limbs.

An adhesive dressing prevents contamination of the surgical site from the environment in the immediate postoperative period.

Owner advice and homecare recommendations

Welfare and home environment

- The owner should be advised to use a sling or hoist (such as a bath towel) to aid the dog's mobility as necessary, and to place mats on slippery floors.
- The dog's feeding regime will need to be adapted to maintain a stable bodyweight (see above).

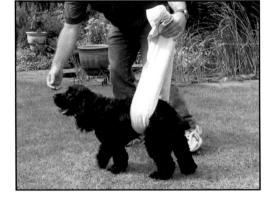

A towel can be used to support a dog's weight and aid mobility. (Courtesy of Brian Sharp)

Exercise

The owner should be provided with a progressive exercise programme covering the 12-week postoperative period, taught how to perform the exercises, and encouraged to continue them at home. The programme should ideally be monitored at intervals by a veterinary physiotherapist who can make appropriate adjustments to the programme as necessary. Exercise is limited to specific physical rehabilitation exercises and lead walking for several weeks, followed by a gradual return to normal activity. When lead-exercising the dog, he should be walked *slowly*, encouraging him to weightbear on all his limbs. The prospect for a return to function for patients that have undergone a reconstructive procedure is usually good in the long term.

Case 14.5
Tibial fracture repair in a cat

A 9-month-old neutered male DSH cat, who had been missing for 5 days, returned home 8–9/10ths lame on his right pelvic limb. On presentation he was bright and alert, with slightly pale mucous membranes. He appeared mildly dehydrated and in poor body condition.

On examination the cat had a palpably unstable right tibial fracture. Nerve function to this limb was normal. Haematological and biochemical blood analyses confirmed mild dehydration and anaemia (PCV 23%, total protein 60 g/dl). Thoracic radiographs did not show any abnormalities. Radiographs of the tibia showed a transverse, mid-diaphyseal tibial fracture.

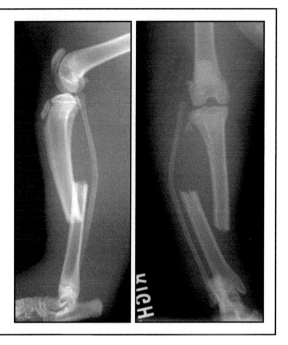

There is a mid-diaphyseal simple transverse tibial fracture and a proximal fibular physeal fracture with bending of the mid-diaphyseal fibula.

Agreed medical/surgical management

Because of his poor body condition and mild dehydration, the cat was given intravenous fluids at twice maintenance levels and offered food, which he ate ravenously.

A plan was made to reduce the fracture and stabilize the tibia with an intramedullary pin and unilateral external skeletal fixation. External fixators can usually be removed once sufficient callus is visible radiographically; this takes about 4–8 weeks.

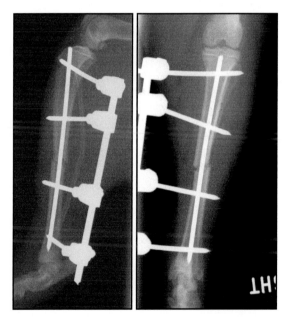

The fracture was stabilized with an intramedullary pin and a 4-pin unilateral external skeletal fixator.

Acute/chronic pain management

This cat will need appropriate premedication, intraoperative pain relief during anaesthesia, and postoperative analgesia. The use of NSAIDs should be considered carefully because of their potential to cause renal compromise with the dehydrated state of the patient preoperatively. Ideally, their use should be delayed until the patient is properly rehydrated.

Intraoperative

Epidural administration of bupivacaine/morphine would provide ideal intraoperative analgesia (see Chapter 2). If this is not possible, ketamine CRI is also very useful and can be continued postoperatively if there is no dysphoria caused by the ketamine.

Postoperative

It is likely in this case that fracture reduction will be difficult and will result in increased postoperative pain because of the muscle contracture that needs to be overcome during surgery. A fentanyl patch placed on the dorsal neck area may be useful for additional postoperative analgesia.

Physiotherapy and acupuncture may also help with pain relief in the immediate postoperative period (see below).

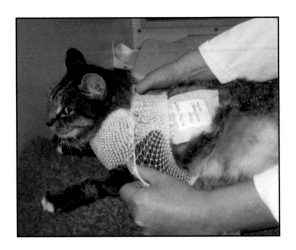

> A fentanyl patch can be placed on clipped skin and covered with a flexible dressing to prevent the edges curling and excessive interference from the cat. It takes several hours to provide peak plasma fentanyl concentrations so it should be placed well in advance of surgery, and additional analgesia provided for the first few hours. (Courtesy of Polly Taylor)

Chronic pain

The cat should be monitored for signs of postsurgical chronic pain, through careful physical examination and by questioning the owners as to changes in behaviour since the trauma. Careful interpretation of the information is required, since the cat may have been psychologically traumatized by the incident itself (rather than the pain), but this should not be assumed. Chronic postoperative pain would be managed in the first instance with NSAIDs (meloxicam is the only NSAID authorized for use in chronic musculoskeletal pain in cats) and acupuncture (see below).

Fear, stress, conflict concerns

It is likely that this cat will be anxious after surgery. Post-anaesthesia excitement can be anticipated, and small doses of acepromazine and/or medetomidine can be given as necessary to control this.

There are two major considerations: treatment and handling at the veterinary clinic; and the patient's home environment.

At the veterinary clinic

- The extent to which the cat will find human contact positive will depend on his perception of people. Members of the veterinary team should be aware of the signals that may indicate that a cat does not find attention positive: as well as active withdrawal or aggression, cats may respond passively when anxious.
  - o Where cats find attention aversive, handling should be minimized.
  - o Where cats find attention positive, stroking and rubbing around the chin, grooming with a massaging groomer or gentle stroking of the chest can be used to increase relaxation.
- Minimize exposure to potential stressors, such as dogs and other cats, noises and strong odours.
- Use the space in the cage to provide a hiding area and visual baffles (a towel over the cage door or hung to separate the cage so the cat can choose to see and be seen or to hide). It is particularly important to block visual access to unfamiliar cats.
- In some cases pheromone therapy may be helpful. However, overall efficacy remains unclear, and this type of intervention should not be used instead of minimizing external stressors. Maintaining the scent environment within the cage, by, for example, not removing all bedding each day, has been demonstrated to aid adaptation to a cattery environment.
- Take time with the patient to help them relax before any intervention.
- Use minimal restraint during procedures where possible.

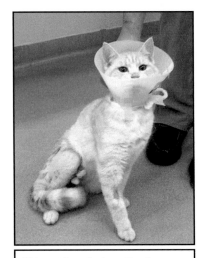

This cat is enjoying attention. He has been allowed out of his cage for some controlled exercise and stroking.

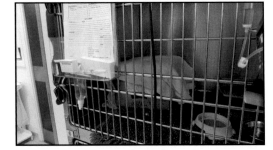

> A cardboard box with a blanket over it will make a hiding area for an anxious cat.

At home

The cat may have some postoperative or chronic pain and may be feeling insecure and vulnerable after the incident that resulted in the fracture. Enhancing the core territory will help him feel better and cope with his discomfort more easily:

- **Confinement.** The cat will be confined to a cage for the initial weeks following surgery and will not be allowed outside until the external skeletal fixator has been removed. The cage environment can be improved by providing sufficient room for a litter tray, food and water bowls, and even some grass.
- **Petting.** Using gentle touch, stroking and grooming in ways that the patient will not only tolerate but enjoy will improve its feelings of wellbeing and will also give the owner a sense of participating in their pet's treatment and nursing.

Pheromone diffusers may help reduce anxiety and promote feelings of comfort and wellbeing. Alpha-casozepine may be helpful if the cat continues to display signs of anxiety.

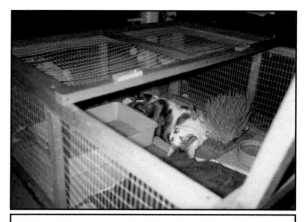

This cat, that presented with ipsilateral humeral and femoral fractures, has an enriched cage environment with a bed, litter tray, food and water bowls, and some fresh grass. The cage is also of a low height which prevents jumping and the mesh is small to prevent the clamps of the external skeletal fixator becoming entangled in the wire. The cage was modified from an outside rabbit run.

It is important to rule out chronic pain, as far as possible, before assuming that inappropriate behaviours such as spraying, over-grooming or inappropriate toileting are due to anxiety *per se.*

Nutritional requirements

The loss of body condition indicates a *catabolic state*, which should be addressed with some urgency because of its potential negative effects on healing and immunity (see Chapter 5). Cats deemed to be in catabolic state may require higher levels of protein and calories than normal and may also have a risk of development of hepatic lipidosis if adequate food intake is not restored. Nutritional support usually entails providing highly palatable and easily digestible, high-protein diets formulated for hospitalized cats. It would be wise to allow the cat a day or two of adequate feeding prior to surgery, although this may not be ideal if the fracture is very painful or unstable.

As the cat is eating voluntarily, further nutritional interventions are not required at this stage. However, it is important to keep an adequate daily record of his food intake, particularly after surgery when stress and analgesic drugs may reduce his appetite. The cat's daily intake should be compared to the calculated resting energy requirement (RER); if it falls well below this for 2 or 3 days, more aggressive nutritional support should be initiated. In this case, a naso-oesophageal tube would be the most appropriate means of achieving this, because the anorexia is likely to be short term. The use of pharmacological appetite stimulators in these circumstances is of limited usefulness and not encouraged (see Chapter 5).

Physiotherapy

Gentle physiotherapy of the operated limb is recommended, particularly addressing any decrease in flexion of the stifle and hock. Treatment can begin once the area is accessible (and bandaging has been removed), but should nevertheless start within the first few days after surgery. Stroking massage may help to reduce stress and anxiety at all stages of recovery, assuming the cat enjoys being handled. Success of physiotherapy will very much depend on the willingness of the cat to be handled.

Pain control

This can be aided through the use of TENS, cold or heat therapy, and massage.

- TENS may be applied locally (if appropriate) or via segmental innervation and can be particularly effective for acute pain, bearing in mind that the effects may wear off quickly once the device is removed depending on the settings.
- Cold therapy should be applied in the immediate postoperative period (first 3–5 days) and would probably be best applied via cold flannels, especially with superficial metalwork present (cold packs should not be applied directly over metalwork).
- Heat can be used once the immediate acute inflammatory phase is over and can be useful to relax any muscles in spasm that may be restricting movement of the joints (see Chapter 9).

Controlling swelling

This would be best aided through the use of cold therapy and compression (if possible in the presence of the external fixator), with effleurage massage performed every 3–4 hours. Cold therapy should be applied in the immediate postoperative period (first 3–5 days) followed by heat therapy after this time.

Minimizing loss of joint and muscle range

The aim is to minimize such loss by the application of gentle flexion and extension passive movements (within the tolerance of the cat) to the hip and stifle, and all other joints of the affected limb. Passive movements should be performed after cold application, or, in later stages, after heat application. Effective pain relief (see above) together with appropriate analgesia is essential in the early stages of healing to allow effective passive movements to be performed (and range to be restored).

Joint mobilizations (see Chapter 9) can also be applied to retain/restore the natural accessory movements of the joints. Although all joints of the limb should be considered, this form of treatment should only be carried out *once the repair is sufficiently stable*. In addition to passive movements, the hindlimb joints should also be mobilized via active exercises – allowing the cat short periods of (controlled) walking and simple standing/balance exercises.

If joint and muscle range are still restricted at 2 weeks, stretches should be applied; these should be preceded by massage, heat or therapeutic ultrasound. Stretches must be continued for at least a month (often more) to counteract contracture.

Active exercises should be progressed further from 4 weeks. The use of obstacles encouraging the cat to step over, walk around and crawl under should be discouraged in the presence of the external skeletal fixator to avoid the pain from entanglement.

Minimizing loss of muscle strength

Gentle massage techniques, such as kneading, can be usefully applied in the early postoperative stages to help reduce local muscle spasm and mobilize the soft tissues. This can be particularly important when external fixators are *in situ*, and muscles are not being adequately used. Neuromuscular electrical stimulation (NMES) may be effectively used to maintain muscle activity during the initial period of relative inactivity, and can be used even with external fixators in place.

The cat should receive short, slow periods of exercise that should be gradually progressed. In cats, exercise is best instigated through the use of short play sessions. Once the external fixator is removed, hydrotherapy (see below) may also be considered, though it is often not well tolerated by cats.

Minimizing loss of balance and proprioception

Sensory input to stimulate mechanoreceptors can help restore the 'body awareness' of the limb. This can be achieved through massage, passive movements, NMES and joint mobilizations. Basic balance exercises should be introduced by the end of week 1 after surgery, even if the cat is still mobilizing on three legs; but they will be especially useful once weightbearing through the operated limb is achieved. As with all exercises these should be gradually progressed as the fracture heals.

Minimizing compensatory postures and gaits

An assessment should be carried out to identify secondary problems, such as muscle and joint pains, arising as a result of compensatory postures and gaits. Appropriate treatment plans may include various joint and soft tissue treatments as well as electrotherapy.

Hydrotherapy

In a small number of cases, cats can be introduced to water quite successfully, and in those cases, it can form a valuable part of the physiotherapy management programme (see Case 14.1). For this patient, hydrotherapy would be best started following natural sealing of the external fixator pin tracts.

Acupuncture

Postoperative pain

Cats often tolerate acupuncture surprisingly well and appear to be very responsive to it, probably because, as a species, they are highly reactive to any stimulus. Local (segmental) needling would not be indicated here, because avoidance of the surgical site immediately postoperatively would be advisable. Points over the sacrum would be helpful, as might so-called mirror points in the opposite leg (see Chapter 11).

WARNING
Implants and prostheses should not be needled directly because of the increased risk of infection.

- Adequate dry bedding should be provided and patient warmth and comfort maintained.
- The cat should be encouraged to move around the cage.

Patient monitoring
The cat should be observed for signs of pain, using a pain scoring system to ensure a standardized approach to monitoring and pain management (see Chapter 3). If the cat is recumbent, it is important to monitor him for decubital ulcer formation. Food and fluid intake should be recorded (see Chapter 5).

Postoperative care
Postoperative complications should be anticipated, to allow early detection and treatment. For example: there may be postoperative swelling, which will particularly affect the distal part of the limb. A bandage can be placed around the leg, including the distal foot, for 3–5 days. After this time the leg and fixator pins should be left unbandaged to reduce the chance of pin tract infections and bandage-related sores. The surgical site and pin tracts should be monitored daily for signs of postoperative infection.

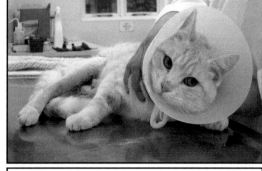

The cat has some swelling of the crus and paw.

External fixator care:

- The site where the pins exit the skin will not completely heal while the pin is in place, but a viable and functional seal usually forms.
- Dried discharge from the area can be cleaned using cotton buds or similar. **Only clean if there is a lot of discharge**; otherwise it is best to leave alone, in order to allow a seal to form around the tract.
- Cover the cut ends of the transosseous pins with cohesive tape, to prevent sharp edges from catching on furniture or the opposite limb.

Fracture patient care
Requirements for postoperative care of fracture surgery patients must be explained clearly to owners and commented on in case notes. Written instructions should be provided where possible.

- The cat should be kept confined to an area where he cannot jump or climb, and where there is nothing that can catch on the fixator.
- Instruct the owner in a few simple flexion–extension exercises, if appropriate.
- External fixator management will include daily pin care as needed (see above).
- Provide an appropriate exercise programme designed specifically to cater for all of this cat's needs.

Follow-up and prognosis
The owner should be aware that the cat will need to return to the clinic for the fracture healing to be assessed physically and radiographically at regular intervals, usually monthly or bimonthly.

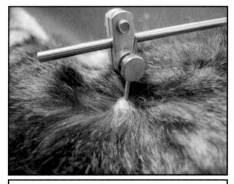

The skin–pin interface of a cat where the ESF was left on for 18 months due to the owner failing to return for its removal at 10 weeks post-application. A functional seal has formed.

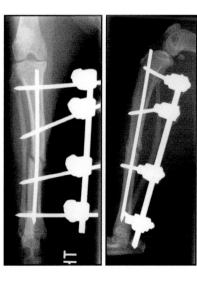

Radiographs taken 4 weeks postoperatively show early callus formation at the tibial fracture site. Further radiographs were scheduled to be taken in another 4 weeks; no change to the external skeletal fixator was made at this stage.

Case 14.6
Patellar luxation in a dog

A 2-year-old aggressive, entire male Jack Russell Terrier was presented with a history of intermittent right pelvic limb lameness for 2 months. He was intermittently non-weightbearing on the leg. The owner was able to muzzle the dog to allow veterinary examination in a standing position and it was possible to luxate both patellae. The luxations were graded as II (right) and II/I (left) (see *BSAVA Manual of Canine and Feline Musculoskeletal Disorders*).

Agreed medical/surgical management

Surgical *versus* continuing conservative management for the right patellar luxation was discussed with the owners and they opted to try non-surgical management initially. The dog was discharged home on NSAIDs for 2 weeks, with another appointment made at the end of this time to check on progress. At the recheck appointment the owner reported that there had been no change in the frequency of patellar luxation, with the same number of periods of non-weightbearing lameness, although they thought that the dog may have been a bit more keen to exercise. The details of surgical therapy were discussed with the owners, including possible complications. Radiographs were taken to check alignment and rule out concurrent problems.

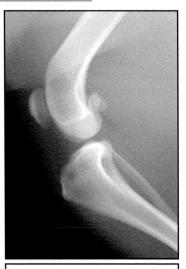

Mediolateral radiograph of the right stifle, showing no evidence of concurrent problems.

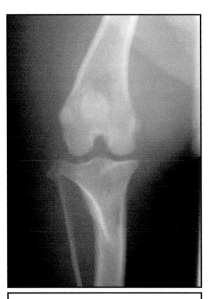

Craniocaudal view, showing no evidence of concurrent problems.

The owners decided to opt for surgical correction of the right patellar luxation. Given the dog's temperament, the owner muzzled and restrained him for injection of the premedication. A wedge recession trochleoplasty was performed. Unusually, no tibial tuberosity transposition was necessary. Closure, with overlap of the joint capsule and fascia lata, was routine. Postoperative radiographs were taken to confirm correct patellar position.

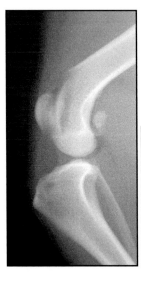

Mediolateral radiograph of the right stifle after surgery, showing better and deeper seating of the patella in the trochlear groove.

Acute/chronic pain management

Premedication

A full mu agonist, such as morphine, methadone or pethidine, should be used in premedication. Partial agonists, such as buprenorphine, should be avoided because they may interfere with the action of a full agonist if one is required later in the procedure (e.g. when using fentanyl; see Chapter 2).

Intraoperative

Epidural administration of bupivacaine/morphine will provide ideal intraoperative analgesia. If epidural injection is not possible, intermittent fentanyl boluses, fentanyl CRI or ketamine CRI should be considered to provide properly balanced anaesthesia.

Postoperative

The use of opioids for longer than usual after acute surgical pain is recommended in this patient, because of the chronic nature of the existing pain. This chronic pain may now be an issue because the condition has been present for 2 months. The pain may be local to the stifle, but may also be present further up the leg and in the muscles of the other hindleg, the back and even the forelimbs (because of transferring weight forwards). Chronic pain should be considered as a cause of this dog's aggression; an assessment of when the aggression started and toward whom it is directed would help in determining this. Whatever the cause, pain and a feeling of vulnerability will certainly make the aggression worse.

NSAIDs prior to and after surgery would be the first line of treatment, being aware of outcome measures other than use of the leg (e.g. keenness to exercise, playfulness, interaction with the family). Tramadol may be helpful in relieving suffering, although there is a possibility that it could make aggression worse (presumably via disinhibition, although this response has by no means been proven). Paracetamol ± codeine may be a useful adjunct.

Fear, stress, conflict concerns

The dog's aggression should be discussed with the owners in terms of their management of him in the postsurgical phase. If he is aggressive to them, this may well be worse after surgery and some basic behavioural advice about approaching him (or not) may help them to deal with him more successfully.

In the longer term, the reason for the aggression should be investigated further and treated with appropriate behaviour therapy. In addition, the dog is likely to benefit from a programme of desensitization and counter-conditioning to attending the veterinary practice, as any pre-existing anxiety will have become worse after associating the clinic with handling and pain (see *BSAVA Manual of Canine and Feline Behavioural Medicine*).

Nutritional requirements

Postoperative

Postoperative nutritional requirements have not been demonstrated to differ from those of normal dogs and therefore alterations to diet may not be necessary. See Case 14.2.

Feeding long term

Long-term management of dogs with chronic degenerative orthopaedic disorders mainly centre on prevention of obesity. See Case 14.4.

Nutritional supplements

There has been a recent interest in the use of omega-3 fatty acids in animals with inflammatory orthopaedic disorders (see Chapter 7). This approach has not been applied to acute types of injury and further work is required to confirm the benefits of omega-3 fatty acid supplementation in this context.

Physiotherapy

Given the dog's temperament, it was not possible to perform hands-on physiotherapy on this particular patient. Postoperatively, he was walked at a slow pace to encourage weightbearing on the operated limb.

Where owners cannot handle a patient, a 'hands-off' exercise approach can be used. This would include a variety of exercises to promote stifle stability, in particular to improve proprioception and quadriceps activity. The type of muscle activity to concentrate on would depend on the type of luxation and the type of surgery. Exercises prescribed in this way will also be of benefit for the remaining hindlimb which, in this case, would still have a luxating patella.

The following should be considered for more amenable patients.

Preoperative

Physiotherapy as part of conservative management of patellar luxation may help with lower grade luxations. Preoperative physiotherapy may also improve muscle activity, which may be beneficial to postoperative outcome. Appropriate exercises are likely to be more effective in conjunction with NSAID treatment, as the patient will be more likely (and willing) to perform them correctly. Where the patient can be handled, some manual therapies and electrotherapies may also be possible before and after surgery.

Postoperative

During the immediate postoperative period (first 2–3 days minimum), physiotherapy should comprise cold therapy, effleurage and passive movements (within the tolerance of the patient) to help with pain relief, keep swelling under control and maintain joint range. Passive movements (flexion and extension) should be carried out on all joints of the operated limb and continued until normal range is achieved. These techniques will be dependent on the availability of the limb to be handled (i.e. taking into account bandaging, etc.) and the willingness of the dog to be handled (by staff or owners). TENS may be useful to help with pain relief, bearing in mind that analgesic effects are often short lived once the device is turned off (depending on the settings used).

Once the acute heat and swelling are under control (normally from around day 4 or 5), the cold therapy can be replaced by heat. The heat, along with massage techniques (such as kneading, picking-up and wringing; see Chapter 9) will help relax muscles, improve circulation to healing tissues and provide pain relief.

During the first 2 weeks postoperatively, walking should be limited to three or four short slow walks; once the dog can weightbear on the operated limb, gentle weight-shifting exercises can be started. Stimulation of the flexor reflex and use of the NMES can also be introduced during this period to improve muscle strength and activity. Lead walks should be carried out slowly, but in a gradually progressive way. If the dog is reluctant to use the limb, exercises such as gentle standing/balance exercises, low step-overs, shaking hands/paws (while standing) and baiting may be effective.

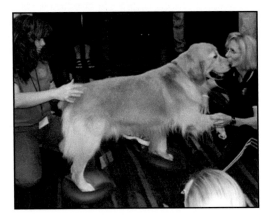

Working on body awareness, balance and core strength. This Golden Retriever is standing on two legs on balance disks.
(© Janet Van Dyke)

Weeks 2 to 3 can see an introduction to more functional exercises, such as sit-to-stands and step-overs. Exercises can be steadily progressed from week 4 onwards, with an emphasis on muscle strengthening, restoration of full joint range, joint stability, and balance and proprioception. Weeks 9–12 should see a gradual return to normal activities, including running, with continuing physiotherapy.

Hydrotherapy

After a re-examination at 3 weeks postoperatively, to check that the patella is still reduced and stable, hydrotherapy can be started. (Tibial tuberosity transpositions may require a radiograph at 6 weeks before hydrotherapy is started.) Hydrotherapy may be beneficial to build muscle mass and strength, which will also help to support the stifle joint and aid in keeping the patella reduced. Hydrotherapy can be a particularly effective way of encouraging greater limb use and should be continued (and progressed) throughout the whole rehabilitation period.

Hydrotherapy may prove more difficult in this case, due to the dog's temperament, but involving the owners and any favourite treats or toys may help. It may mean that the first couple of sessions are used to allow the dog to become familiar and relaxed with the people, environment and the water. The use of the underwater treadmill may be more useful than swimming, given that joints undergo full flexion *and* extension with treadmill walking.

Acupuncture

Aggression is not necessarily a contraindication for acupuncture. Although results appear to be better if the animal is relaxed, some aggressive or very anxious animals come to accept the treatment well and, although one is always cautious, it should never be ruled out if analgesia is not being achieved by other means.

Other nursing and supportive care

Pain

The patient must be monitored closely for signs of pain and discomfort, using a pain scoring system to ensure a standardized approach. Postoperative pain may seriously inhibit attempts to use the limb.

Postoperative care

The incision site should be kept covered by a self-adhesive dressing. With severer grade luxations (grade III/IV), where more soft tissue dissection is necessary, a postoperative bandage is usually applied for 3 days. The application of a cold pack to the surgical site after surgery can help reduce swelling and pain in the area. This should be continued for 2–3 days. The surgical wound should be kept clean and dry and watched for postoperative complications (see Case 14.1 and Chapter 12).

A sling, bellyband or hoist should be used to aid mobility and prevent falls or slipping in the hospital.

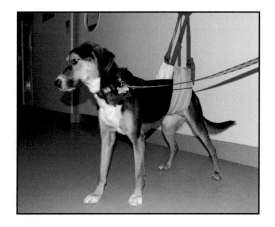

A bellyband is being used to facility this dog's mobility within the hospital. (Courtesy of Rachel Lumbis and Catherine Kendall)

Owner advice and homecare recommendations

Exercise and mobility
The owner should be advised to use a sling (such as a bath towel) to aid mobility, if necessary and to place mats on slippery floors. Exercise should be restricted to specific rehabilitation exercises and lead exercise only for 6 weeks. The dog should then be gradually returned to unsupervised activity over a further 6-week period.

Follow-up and prognosis
The owner should be advised to return the dog to the surgery: after 10 days for suture removal; at 3 weeks for assessment that the patella is still correctly reduced; and then at 4–6 weeks (depending on the surgical approach) for radiography to evaluate healing.

Case 14.7
Humeral fracture in a dog

A 4-year-old male neutered Springer Spaniel was rushed into the clinic after stumbling while jumping a ditch. He yelped and was immediately unable to walk on his left thoracic limb. The owner had carried him back to the car and brought him straight in.

On examination the dog had pale mucous membranes and an elevated heart rate. When placed on the surgery floor he was able to walk on three legs but not on the left thoracic limb, which was visually unstable with marked swelling around the distal humerus and elbow joint. After administering analgesia (opioids) the results of examination were suggestive of fracture. Radiographs confirmed the suspicion that the dog had sustained a combined intracondylar and supracondylar fracture of the left humerus ('Y' fracture).

As surgery was delayed until the next day, a body bandage (spica splint) was applied to minimize movement of the left elbow.

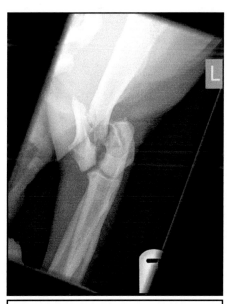

A 'Y' fracture of the distal humerus.

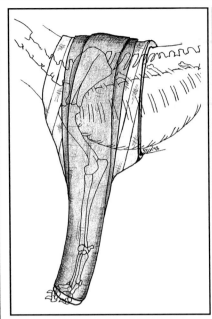
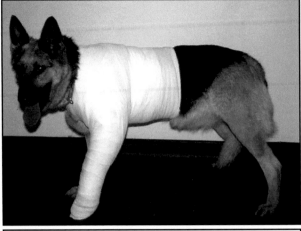

A spica splint stabilizes the elbow and humerus. The flat lateral splint is held in place with adhesive tape over a Robert Jones dressing and a body bandage around the thorax. Reproduced from *BSAVA Manual of Canine and Feline Emergency and Critical Care.*

Agreed medical/surgical management

The fracture needed fairly immediate surgical repair. A medial surgical approach was made, reducing the medial aspect of the humeral condyle to the humeral diaphysis with a 3.5 mm bone plate and screws. The dog was then repositioned in right lateral recumbency and a lateral approach made to the humeral condyle to reduce the articular component of the fracture and stabilize this fragment with an intracondylar lag screw and a 2.7 mm bone plate up the lateral epicondyle. A padded bandage was applied postoperatively and left on for 3 days.

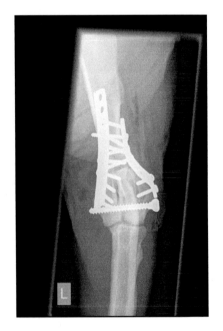

The Y fracture was stabilized with a medial bone plate, lateral bone plate and a transcondylar bone screw. Fracture reduction is good but there is a small gap in the condyle, which may indicate that the dog was suffering from incomplete ossification of the humeral condyle prior to acute complete fracture.

Acute/chronic pain management

Acute/preoperative
Preoperatively, pain was managed with NSAIDs and opiates.

Intraoperative
Brachial plexus blocks are not always effective for surgery at, or proximal to, the elbow. Such surgery is likely to be very painful, so an opioid in the premedication may not be sufficient. Fentanyl by intermittent bolus or CRI, and/or ketamine CRI should be considered. An alternative is morphine/lidocaine/ketamine CRI. All CRIs can be continued postoperatively. If no facilities for CRI are available, full mu-agonist opioids, such as morphine, methadone or pethidine, can be given by intravenous or intramuscular injection, based on pain assessment.

Postoperative pain management
A lumbosacral morphine epidural injection may provide some analgesia in the forelimb. A fentanyl patch placed up to 24 hours before surgery may also be useful for postoperative analgesia, although these cases

should not be unduly delayed as ultimately surgical stabilization will give the best analgesia. NSAIDs should be continued postoperatively.

Physiotherapy (see below) may help with pain relief in the immediate postoperative period.

Chronic pain

Chronic pain should not be an issue after the immediate postoperative phase, but, in case of complications or continued manifestations of anxiety, it should be considered and monitored for. If postarticular fracture osteoarthritis develops and causes lameness, NSAIDs are the treatment of first choice. If these do not appear to be sufficient, tramadol may be added to help reduce suffering. Paracetamol ± codeine, and gabapentin in the event of central sensitization occurring (with hyperalgesia and allodynia), may be indicated, depending on the progress of the pain and the individual's response to it.

Fear, stress, conflict concerns

If the stress is primarily pain-related, this should be addressed as a priority (see above).

Sedation

The patient is a nervous spaniel who is under stress pre- and postoperatively. There are two main options for sedation of an anxious or agitated animal. Clearly the clinical condition will have some bearing on this choice, as well as the route of administration.

- Benzodiazepines: diazepam or alprazolam tablets can be used to effect, but one should beware of possible disinhibition of excitement/aggression.
- Acepromazine (ACP) combined with opioids can a useful alternative. ACP has a variable effect, depending on the individual.

For additional sedation, butorphanol is preferable. If analgesia is required as well as sedation, one of the mu receptor agonists is better and the choice depends upon the required duration. Pethidine has the shortest duration of action at 30 minutes; methadone and morphine are longer lasting but beware of vomiting with morphine; buprenorphine is the longest lasting. An additional consideration is the amnesic effect of benzodiazepines, which will help prevent the dog from associating the clinic with painful handling.

At the veterinary clinic

Simple measures such as addressing comfort, reducing noise and discussing with the owners the individual needs of this dog (What does he like? What does he dislike? What is he afraid of?) can help the practice team to develop a plan that will best accommodate him. The following should be considered:

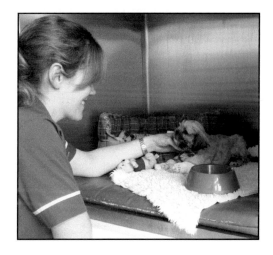

- Calm, quiet handling to minimize pain and maximize the pleasant aspects of physical interactions
- Ensuring that the dog is in the quietest possible place in the ward, but talked to and interacted with as much as possible
- A pheromone spray or a diffuser nearby may be helpful for some dogs, although overall efficacy is unclear.

Gentle interaction with a patient in a quiet area of the ward can help address anxiety.

Exercise restriction

This dog is going to have his exercise curtailed and the owners will be worried about him fracturing his other leg as he is suspected of having incomplete ossification of the humeral condyle(s). There is, therefore, the danger that this dog will be so restricted as to cause behavioural difficulties. Training, division of feeding and novel food delivery systems will help to maintain mental stimulation. A progressive (and written) exercise plan will enable the owners to see, and be reassured by, the progress they are allowed to make in increasing the dog's exercise and should mitigate against their being overprotective.

Nutritional requirements

Postoperative

Postoperative nutritional requirements have not been demonstrated to differ from those of normal dogs and therefore alterations to diet may not be necessary (see Case 14.2).

Feeding long term

Long-term management of dogs with chronic degenerative orthopaedic disorders mainly centres on prevention of obesity. While this is not usually as much of a problem in Springer Spaniels as in some other breeds, the owner should be warned that the dog's calorie requirement may be reduced while exercise is limited and should be encouraged to weigh the dog regularly (monthly) and feed to maintain stable bodyweight.

Nutritional supplements

There has been a recent interest in the use of omega-3 fatty acids in animals with inflammatory orthopaedic disorders (see Chapter 7). This approach has not been applied to acute types of injury and further work is required to confirm the benefits of omega-3 fatty acid supplementation in this context.

Physiotherapy

Physiotherapy of the operated thoracic limb can be started with gentle range of motion exercises within 3–4 days of surgery. Full flexion of the elbow is often lost after this sort of fracture, so particular attention should be paid to maintaining this. Stroking massage may help to reduce stress and anxiety at all stages of recovery.

Pain control

This can be aided through the use of TENS, cold or heat therapy, and massage (see Case 14.5). If post-articular fracture arthritis develops, heat, massage, cold therapy, electrotherapy, joint mobilizations and soft tissue treatments may be helpful.

Controlling swelling

As for Case 14.5.

Minimizing loss of joint and muscle range

As for Case 14.5.

- If surgical repair permits, supination and pronation passive movements to the forearm should also be included from an early stage.
- In addition to passive movements, the elbow should also be mobilized via active exercises – initially, short slow lead walks and simple standing/balance exercises.
- Range of movement exercises should be progressed further from 4 weeks, and should include such exercises as step-overs and 'shaking hands'.

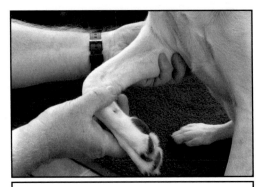

Passive supination of the forearm. (Courtesy of Brian Sharp)

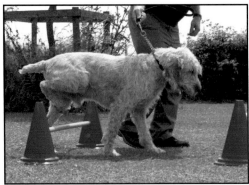

Step-over exercise. (Courtesy of Brian Sharp)

Minimizing loss of muscle strength

As for Case 14.5. Once the dog is permitted to walk, it should receive short, slow periods of exercise that should be gradually progressed.

Minimizing loss of balance and proprioception

As for Case 14.5.

Minimizing compensatory postures and gaits

As for Case 14.5.

Hydrotherapy

Hydrotherapy is recommended after suture removal if the dog is progressing well postoperatively. This may help maintain and regain muscle bulk and joint range of motion. This patient may also benefit from the physical and mental stimulation of hydrotherapy sessions. Care must be taken if he is excited by swimming, as he may injure his healing leg by slipping, running, or while getting in or out of the pool.

Acupuncture

Acupuncture should not be necessary unless there is uncontrolled postoperative pain or post-articular fracture osteoarthritis develops and causes lameness. Usually, local (segmental) needling would be indicated but in this case it is probably not possible because of all the implants.

> **WARNING**
> Implants and prostheses should not be needled directly because of the increased risk of infection.

Other nursing and supportive care

Patient monitoring
- Signs of pain should be watched for pre- and postoperatively, using a pain scoring system to ensure a standardized approach.
- Food and fluid intake should be recorded.

Postoperative care
- Postoperatively the leg is bandaged immediately with a medium-sized bandage for 3–5 days, to minimize postoperative swelling and increase patient comfort. Correct bandage care is important:
  - o Do not allow the bandage to become soiled or wet
  - o Check that the bandage is not slipping or causing discomfort
  - o Check for irritation of adjacent skin
  - o Monitor for signs of infection, such as odour
  - o Protect the bandage (e.g. cover with a non-porous bag if the dog goes outside; remove the bag immediately once back inside)
  - o Prevent patient interference with the bandage and wound by applying an Elizabethan collar.
- The dog should be encouraged to move around his cage.
- A sling or hoist should be used to aid mobility and prevent falls or slipping.

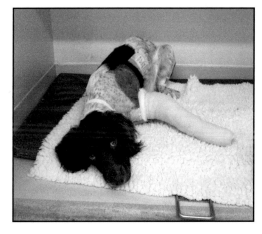

> A bandage ending as proximally as possible in the axilla will help reduce perifracture swelling and increase patient comfort. A body bandage could also be used after surgery, and this would provide more support of the limb.

Owner advice and homecare recommendations

The owners should be advised that the implants are generally left *in situ*.

Welfare and home environment
The owner will need advice on how to look after the bandage (see above). They should also lay down rubber mats on slippery floors.

Exercise and physiotherapy
The owners should be given strict, preferably written, instructions. They should restrict activity to lead walking and physical rehabilitation until the fracture has healed. Physical rehabilitation thereafter will encourage controlled limb use and proximal limb function (see above).

Follow-up and prognosis
The dog should be weightbearing tentatively on the operated limb after bandage removal, and use of the limb should gradually improve thereafter. If lameness occurs, veterinary attention should be sought. The owner will be required to bring the dog back into the surgery after 4 weeks for radiography and analysis of fracture repair.

Case 14.8
Osteoarthritis in a dog

A 10-year-old male Rottweiler was presented with a chronic 6-week history of right thoracic limb lameness and a 3-month history of generalized stiffness and exercise intolerance. He had a history of cruciate surgery – on one leg 7 years ago, and on the other 5 years ago. He was not overweight (BCS 4/9).

On examination, he had enlarged elbows, stifles, metacarpophalangeal and metatarsophalangeal joints. These joints all had reduced range of motion and crepitus on manipulation. Radiography revealed bilateral elbow, hip, stifle and metacarpophalangeal osteoarthritis, with fragmentation of sesamoids.

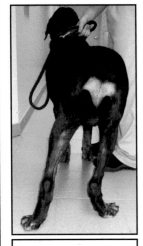

The Rottweiler, showing an abnormal stance due to multiple joints affected by osteoarthritis.

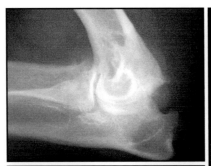

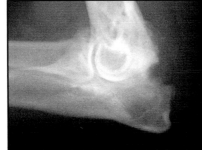

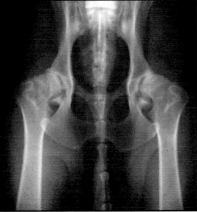

Mediolateral elbow and pelvic radiographs showing well established osteoarthritis.

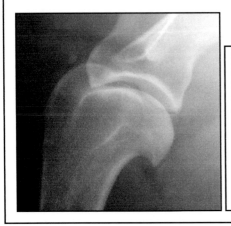

Mediolateral shoulder radiograph, showing very mild osteophytic changes on the caudal glenoid and humeral head and an area of mineralization in the supraspinatus muscle.

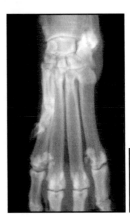

Dorsopalmar view of the forefoot, showing fragmentation of sesamoids II and VII.

Agreed medical/surgical management

The dog was treated non-surgically. In some situations, arthroscopic evaluation and flushing may be suitable for elbow osteoarthritis, but in this case the osteoarthritis was very well established, so this option was thought not to be appropriate.

A full general examination, haematological and biochemical analysis of blood, and urinalysis were performed because of the age of the dog and the likelihood of prescribing drugs metabolized via the kidney or liver. As no abnormalities were detected, he was placed on NSAIDs at the maximum dose for the first 7 days, with the dose halved for a further 2 weeks. He was then re-examined to evaluate the response and the need for further drugs.

Chronic pain management

A chronic pain assessment (see Chapter 3) will determine outcome measures for this patient and guide the practice as to how much medication/intervention he needs.

NSAIDs are the first-line treatment in osteoarthritis. Non-response to the first NSAID used indicates trying one or two others in succession, with suitable washout periods between them and strict instructions to the owners of what to look for in case of gastrointestinal toxicity. Pentosan polysulphate is effective in some patients, but needs to be given during a short break from NSAIDs. If the patient is not responding sufficiently to NSAIDs, the addition of tramadol is the next option; care should be taken to monitor the patient for dysphoria, dullness, nausea and excessive sedation.

Continued pain, as the condition progresses, would indicate the need for the addition of gabapentin, watching for sedation, gastrointestinal signs and, specifically, stumbling or tripping. Amantadine is an alternative to gabapentin but may also be associated with gastrointestinal signs. Paracetamol ± codeine may be beneficial.

Such multimodal analgesia will result in a better overall result, with a possible reduction in individual medications.

Physiotherapy and acupuncture (see below) are also likely to be of value in helping this patient's pain.

Fear, stress, conflict concerns

The occurrence of chronic pain may lead to sensitization to external stimuli. Because the pain causes emotional arousal, there is an increased chance that external events will lead to anxiety. For example, it is not uncommon for dogs experiencing pain to become fearful of specific noises, anxious around other dogs, or very dependent on owner attention. This general sensitizing effect will also decrease the threshold for the display of aggression. In addition, dogs will often learn that specific events result in the sensation of a bout of acute pain. For example, a dog may learn that when owners get out a towel to dry their feet, the associated joint flexion causes pain, and may either show aggression or withdraw to avoid this negative outcome.

The problem with older dogs that have osteoarthritis is that the restriction of exercise usually means that they are walked short distances, on concrete, on the same route. This is concussive to the joints and mentally unstimulating for the dog. An effort should be made to take him to interesting places and let him walk on grass, interact with other dogs and people (if appropriate), and to continue to have access (albeit in a reduced way) to resources.

Nutritional requirements

Long-term management of dogs with chronic degenerative orthopaedic disorders mainly centres on prevention of obesity (see Case 14.4). The owner should be advised that the dog's energy requirement will have probably decreased since he was a young adult because of the reduced exercise associated with joint disease.

Nutritional supplements

Supplementation of omega-3 fatty acids may reduce joint inflammation and thus reduce requirements for non-steroidal therapy. Further work is required to confirm the benefits of omega-3 fatty acid supplementation in dogs with osteoarthritis (see Chapter 7). Nutraceuticals can either be supplemented separately or formulated within a diet designed for joint disease.

Physiotherapy

Management of osteoarthritis should preferably involve an interdisciplinary approach including weight control, medication and physiotherapy.

Pain relief

Heat, massage, passive movements and stretches can be beneficial in improving comfort and mobility (especially in the mornings and prior to exercise).

Restoring function

Osteoarthritis is progressively detrimental to an animal's strength, joint and muscle range, balance, proprioception, joint stability, stamina and overall function. To counter these effects an appropriate exercise programme should be designed which is low-impact and addresses all of these elements (see Chapter 9). A controlled low-impact exercise programme alone has been shown to improve pain and overall function scores in geriatric dogs with osteoarthritis (Hudson and Hulse, 2004). All exercises (including walking) should be paced (within the tolerance of the patient) yet provided regularly (little and often). This approach should be continued throughout the dog's life.

All activities should be markedly reduced during flare-ups of the osteoarthritis, and steadily returned to normal as the flare-up subsides. If the osteoarthritis remains under control, the exercise programme should be gradually progressed.

Other interventions that can be beneficial for patients with osteoarthritis include joint mobilizations (to improve joint range and reduce pain) and soft tissue techniques (such as myofascial release and trigger pointing) (see Chapters 9 and 11).

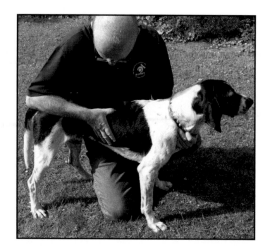

Spinal mobilizations may be performed by a veterinary physiotherapist. (Courtesy of Brian Sharp)

Hydrotherapy

Underwater treadmill exercise may be potentially beneficial for this patient (with the usual considerations of slow, graduated, paced exercise), but with progression to swimming as he becomes stronger. Swimming generally allows more freedom of movement and can be more 'fun' for dogs that have limited land exercise.

Acupuncture

Acupuncture is likely to be of some benefit in generalized OA, depending on the responsiveness of the patient. The targets would be:

- To reduce pain from the joint
- To reduce pain from the soft tissues, especially secondary muscle pain caused by joint dysfunction
- To reduce secondary muscle strain due to postural change
- To reduce central sensitization.

Acupuncture can be added to the multimodal analgesia plan at any stage.

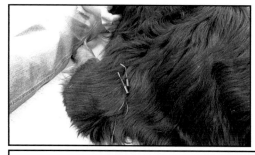

Acupuncture applied to the infraspinatus muscle to treat the pain of elbow arthritis. (Courtesy of Samantha Lindley)

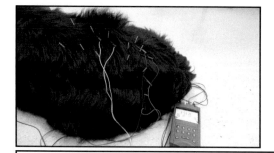

Electroacupuncture applied to hip and back points for the treatment of pain secondary to hip arthritis. (Courtesy of Samantha Lindley)

Other nursing and supportive care

Nurses can and should play an active role in the management of osteoarthritis and develop nurses' clinics that can provide clients with information and support, as well as an opportunity to monitor a patient's progress formally.

Comfort

Placing the dog in a walk-in kennel or crate will help to promote activity and prevent long periods of recumbency. He should be taken outside for frequent short walks to allow urination/defecation and to prevent him from becoming stiff and uncomfortable. Deep, comfortable bedding should be provided. The addition of an insulated heat source may help soothe stiff joints, making them more comfortable and promoting rest, although some dogs seek cool areas when in pain and may avoid such heat sources.

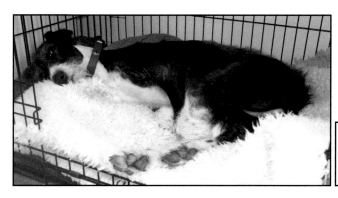

A crate with deep comfortable bedding would be most suitable.

Patient monitoring

Range of movement of joints can be measured with a goniometer (see Case 14.3). Signs of pain, discomfort and inflammation should be watched for, using a pain scoring system to ensure a standardized approach (see Chapters 2 and 3). Food and fluid intake should be recorded.

Owner advice and homecare recommendations

Osteoarthritis management is a lifelong commitment. This must be explained to the owner. It is important to recognize the integral role of the owner in assessing and adjusting therapies and lifestyles to suit the individual dog's needs and the importance of the veterinary team and owner working together long term for the dog's benefit. Clients must be well informed regarding the disease process and the need for ongoing re-evaluation. The management of osteoarthritis is dynamic and responsive to the individual patient's needs. Owners should not think that what they are doing now will be what they will always be doing to manage the condition. During periods of acute exacerbation of clinical signs, analgesia should be administered and exercise adjusted according to the dog's capabilities. NSAIDs may be able to be given by the owner on an 'as necessary' basis, provided the owner can judge when they are necessary and not allow breakthrough pain to become a problem; early indications of pain and suffering should be agreed. Attendance at nurse-led clinics may be helpful.

Welfare and home environment
- The use of heat, massage, passive movements and stretches may be beneficial in improving comfort and mobility (especially in the mornings before walks, and during those months when the dog is particularly stiff and uncomfortable).
- Owners should also be provided with an appropriate exercise programme designed specifically to cater for this dog's needs, and an explanation should be given regarding the pacing of all activities:
  o The dog should be given regular frequent periods of low-intensity exercise
  o The owners should avoid taking the dog for excessively long walks or vigorous exercise such as chasing or playing.
- Environmental modification:
  o A ramp will aid the dog to get into the car
  o A slightly raised bed placed away from drafts and with plenty of soft bedding may be helpful
  o Avoid slippery floor surfaces – provide a non-slip carpeted runner across the floor to the exit doors if necessary.

Follow-up and prognosis
- The need for ongoing evaluation and regular attendance at nurse clinics should be emphasized.
- Exercise and diet regimes may need to change as the condition progresses. The dog's weight and body condition score should be checked carefully on each visit to make sure she is not gaining weight.
- The dog will also be monitored for side effects from chronic use of NSAIDs; blood samples every 3–6 months are recommended.

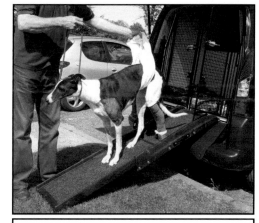

Ramps can help dogs with limited mobility get in and out of cars.

References

Hudson S and Hulse D (2004) Benefit of rehabilitation for treatment of osteoarthritis in senior dogs. *Proceedings, 3rd International Symposium on Rehabilitation and Physical Therapy in Veterinary Medicine, Raleigh (NC)* p.235

Case 14.9
Elbow arthritis in an elderly cat

A 15-year-old male neutered overweight (BCS 8/9) cat was presented with stiffness and inappropriate urination outside his litter tray.

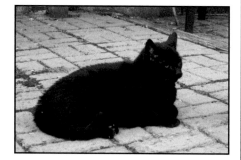

An overweight cat that is reluctant to exercise unless it is feeding time.

On examination he had bilateral hip pain, reduced elbow flexion and extension, and a stiff gait with lameness in all four legs. Radiographs confirmed bilateral hip and elbow osteoarthritis with several 'joint mice' (synovial osteochondromatosis) around the elbow joint.

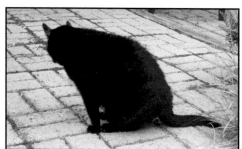

The cat is stiff and has difficulty rising from sitting or lying.

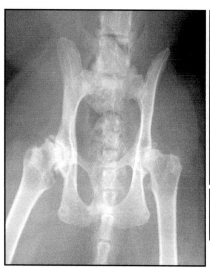

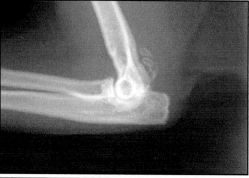

The hip radiograph shows coxofemoral and intervertebral osteophytosis. The elbow radiograph shows multiple 'joint mice'.

The stiffness was considered to be related to the osteoarthritis. It is possible that the inappropriate urination may be related to a reluctance to climb into the litter tray which was found, on questioning the owners, to have high sides.

Agreed medical/surgical management

Non-surgical management was planned. A full general examination, haematological and biochemical analysis of blood, and urinalysis were performed. There was a mild elevation in urea but no elevation in creatinine. Urinalysis was normal. Given the cat's age and the mild azotaemia, it is critical to have accurate knowledge of renal function. This is important in light of the need for pain management (use of NSAIDs) and weight management (use of a high-protein diet). Given that in cats urine specific gravity (SG) can remain well within the hypersthenuric range, even in the face of renal insufficiency, it may be sensible to determine glomerular filtration rates (GFR) more accurately, e.g. exogenous creatinine clearance. No abnormalities were detected in SG or GFR, so the cat was placed on NSAIDs at a high dose for the first 7 days, moving to a lower dose for a further 2 weeks. The cat was then re-examined to evaluate the response and the need for further drugs (see below).

This cat was to be treated non-surgically initially. In some circumstances surgery may be appropriate, e.g. femoral head and neck excision for hip osteoarthritis, and elbow arthroscopy for debridement and lavage.

Chronic pain management

NSAIDs can be given, judiciously monitoring the cat regularly for side effects and regularly checking blood levels of urea and creatinine in particular. Very few NSAIDs are authorized for use in the cat. Meloxicam is authorized in the UK for long-term use in musculoskeletal pain. NSAIDs should be discontinued if vomiting, diarrhoea or loss of appetite occurs. They should be used under very careful veterinary supervision if there is any suggestion of blood disorder, kidney, liver or heart disease, or gastrointestinal ulceration. Drug interactions can occur (e.g. with steroids).

In addition to NSAIDs, gabapentin may helpful if the cat is showing signs of central sensitization (hyperalgesia and allodynia). Tramadol is used in cats but has been reported to trigger seizures in the doses that are recommended (off licence) for dogs, so may be better avoided. Amitriptyline appears to work well for pain in cats, but requires competent renal and hepatic function and normal heart rhythm for safe administration. It also tastes bitter and is therefore difficult to administer. Short-term oral transmucosal buprenorphine may be useful for acute flare-ups, as it is well absorbed transmucosally in cats.

Given the safety issues of using unauthorized analgesics in cats, acupuncture (see below) should be considered as a realistic option early in the management of pain in this species. Optimizing the cat's core territory (see below and Case 14.1) may help the cat cope with its pain and may be a real contributor to a decrease in suffering from that pain.

Polysulphated glycosaminoglycans (PSGAGs) have anti-inflammatory activity and may help modulate cartilage and synovial membrane metabolism. They are usually given as weekly injections for a month and then every few months. This product is not authorized for use in cats in the UK.

Fear, stress, conflict concerns

Urination outside the litter tray

This cat may:

- Have physical difficulty getting into his litter tray because of his arthritis
- Have unpleasant associations with attempting to squat in his litter tray because of pain
- Be expressing the fact that the pain is a source of stress and conflict.

The current litter tray should be replaced with one that is identical in all respects – except that it has lower sides. Seed trays (from garden centres) will sometimes be acceptable, and allow entry at the low end and the use of deep litter at the high-sided end. Once the right litter tray is found, a number of these should be made available in different locations (easily accessed but not in busy thoroughfares) to see if the cat can use an alternative tray (or the one in the original position).

It should also be considered that the change in elimination site may be unrelated to the arthritis, and other possible causes of this change should be explored (see *BSAVA Manual of Canine and Feline Behavioural Medicine*).

Environmental changes

Improving and enhancing the core territory or environment (see Case 14.1) will help the cat feel better and help him cope with his discomfort more easily.

Pheromone diffusers may help reduce anxiety and promote feelings of comfort and wellbeing; and alpha-casozepine may be helpful if the cat continues to display signs of anxiety. However, neither product has proven efficacy in such situations.

It is important to rule out chronic pain, as far as possible, before assuming that inappropriate behaviours such as spraying, over-grooming or inappropriate toileting are due to anxiety *per se*).

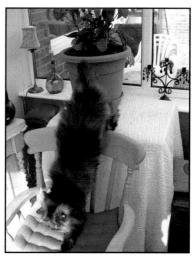

Stepped access to and from favourite areas may help a cat with limited mobility. (© Samantha Elmhurst)

Nutritional requirements

Prevention of obesity *versus* dietary treatment of kidney disease

Long-term management of cats with chronic degenerative orthopaedic disorders mainly centres on prevention of obesity. However, the age of this cat and potential concerns over early chronic kidney disease (CKD) should be taken into account.

As the cat is already 15 years old it is unlikely that longevity will be improved by weight management. Further, if CKD exists, bodyweight and condition is usually gradually lost, even when appropriate dietary management is provided. Moreover, the choice of diet would need to be carefully considered; it is usually preferable to increase protein relative to dietary energy for weight loss in cats, so that lean tissue is preserved during weight loss. However, increasing protein content may not be sensible in the face of early CKD. Instead, a diet with only a modest increase in protein may be preferable, coupled with modest energy restriction to enable a slow rate of weight loss. Regular monitoring of haematological and serum biochemical parameters would also be essential, and the diet strategy should be changed if azotaemia worsens.

Weight management

The degree of current adiposity (BCS 8/9) means a long-term plan would be necessary (12–18 months). Given that the natural lifespan of this cat is not known, nor is it known what additional medical problems may arise, the aim of the weight plan should be more to enable modest reductions in bodyweight, in the short term, rather than insisting that an ideal weight must be achieved. Even subtle reductions in bodyweight many improve mobility, decrease pain and improve quality of life.

Weight control will require calorie restriction and frequent monitoring of body condition to guide further alterations to the feeding regimen. Implementation of meal-feeding strategies are more effective than *ad libitum* feeding.

Prior to starting the weight management regime, the cat should be weighed. This, and his body condition score, will enable the degree of excess weight to be estimated, and a target bodyweight to be set. The main aim of this calculation is to estimate the correct energy intake for weight loss, rather than expecting the cat to achieve this final weight. Thereafter, a purpose-formulated diet, designed for feeding during weight management, can be commenced (see Chapter 6).

In addition to dietary management, the owners should be encouraged to increase activity levels; the level and type of exercise should be tailored to suit the needs of the cat, given its orthopaedic disease. The owners should start by instigating play sessions (see Homecare, below). Since overweight cats are likely to be unfit, only two sessions of 2–3 minutes may be a sensible starting point. The type of toy should be varied; usually, those that create rapid unpredictable movements are best, and the cat should be allowed to catch the object periodically to avoid frustration. As weight loss progresses, and fitness improves, the amount of daily play can be increased. Since cats are used to exercising in short frenetic bursts, it may be sensible to increase the number of play sessions, rather than their duration.

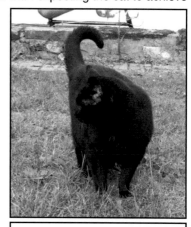

An outdoor cat may spontaneously increase activity.

Activity can also be increased in other ways; for instance, if a dry food is used, a feeding toy can be used to increase activity at meal times. Some dry food (part of the ration) can be fed in different places to encourage the cat to move around. Finally, outdoor cats may spontaneously increase activity, and should be encouraged to do so.

Measuring progress

The cat should be brought back to the clinic on a fortnightly basis, initially, so that progress with weight loss can be monitored. Most cats will lose between 0.5 and 1.0% of their starting bodyweight per week. Dietary caloric intake may need to be modified if weight loss slows.

If the cat reaches his target weight, a maintenance regime should be instigated. The transition should be made gradually; he should continue to be weighed every 2 weeks, whilst energy intake is increased incrementally by 10% at a time. Once weight has stabilized, the interval between weight checks can be gradually extended (e.g. monthly, 3-monthly, 6-monthly) but weighing should not be stopped altogether.

It is vital throughout that the cat's weight loss is *gradual*. If any diet change actually stops him eating, then it is important to revert to the previous, acceptable diet to avoid the very real risk of hepatic lipidosis developing in this patient.

Nutritional supplements

Other strategies proposed for cats with orthopaedic disorders have included the use of nutraceutical agents such as chrondroitin sulphate and glucosamine, but there are limited data supporting their use, especially in cats. Other more recent strategies include the supplementation of omega-3 fatty acids, which may reduce joint inflammation and thus reduce requirements for non-steroidal therapy (see Chapter 7). Further work is required to confirm the benefits of omega-3 fatty acid supplementation in cats with osteoarthritis.

Physiotherapy

Management of osteoarthritis in cats should preferably involve an interdisciplinary approach including weight control, medication and physiotherapy. Physiotherapy has an important role in the provision of pain relief and maintenance of function, but, with cats, is very dependent on the cat's willingness to be handled and guided to perform certain activities.

Pain relief
As for Case 14.8.

Restoring function
See Case 14.8. With cats, exercise is best instigated through the use of short play sessions, using toys and other items of interest. If the osteoarthritis remains under control, the exercise programme should be gradually progressed to improve body condition and help with weight loss.

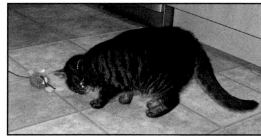

Short play sessions can be used to provide exercise for cats. (Courtesy of Brian Sharp)

Hydrotherapy

In a small number of cases, cats can be introduced to water quite successfully. The warmth of the water would help reduce pain and may permit more effective passive movements and stretches to be carried out if required to improve joint range.

Acupuncture

Acupuncture appears to be very useful in the treatment of pain in cats, especially nociceptive pain such as that of osteoarthritis. Ideally, it would be used as an adjunct to other medication as part of a multimodal analgesia plan, but for all of the reasons discussed in 'Chronic pain', above, is often used as a sole modality. Cats tolerate acupuncture surprisingly well in most cases and appear to be sensitive to its effects, probably because, as a species, they are highly reactive to many stimuli.

Other nursing and supportive care

Nurses can and should play an active role in the management of OA and in weight control and develop nurses' clinics to provide clients with information and support, as well as an opportunity to monitor a patient's progress formally.

Comfort
A litter tray with low sides should be provided.

Patient monitoring
- Cats generally resent extension of the joints, so the use of a goniometer to measure range of movement is not so helpful here.
- The patient should be observed for signs of pain, discomfort and inflammation (e.g. crepitus, heat).
  NB: Cats often show none of these signs and yet may have significant pathology.
- A pain scoring system should be used to ensure a standardized approach to monitoring and pain management, bearing in mind that *there are no validated scoring systems for cats.*
- Customized plans for cats are useful. For example, the return of the ability to jump up on to a favourite sofa would be a good indication that treatment is being effective.

Owner advice and homecare recommendations

OA management is a life-long commitment. This must be explained to the owner (see Case 14.8).

Welfare and home environment
- The use of heat, massage, passive movements and stretches may be beneficial in improving comfort and mobility. All these techniques can be applied by the owners, following appropriate instruction.
- Owners should be provided with advice regarding exercise for the cat, and an explanation should be given regarding the pacing of all activities. The owners should be made aware of the flooring within the house, and encouraged to do exercises on non-slip surfaces or outside.
- Core territory improvements that will help the cat cope with its pain and disability are outlined in Case 14.1. A litter tray with low sides should also be provided.

15

Patients with neoplastic disease

Edited by Gerry Polton

Introduction

The field of oncology covers myriad presentations with ever increasing numbers of strategies for management. Important distinctions can be made between cancer that is managed by curative surgery and that which is managed by palliative therapy (including non-curative surgery, chemotherapy, radiotherapy or a combination of these).

Surgical management, even if curative, can sometimes result in conformational change that incurs a change in function or appearance. In general, owners and veterinary surgeons are more prepared to accept or inflict a functional or conformational change if the patient makes a substantial gain in quality or length of life in return.

Palliative management strategies, by definition, are not expected to result in a cure, although lengthy periods of complete remission can sometimes be achieved. Palliative therapy may also induce functional or conformational consequences with which both owner and pet have to cope (see below).

Systemic medication is frequently used in cancer therapy in general veterinary practice and this does expose the patient to a risk of treatment-induced adverse events. In addition, the veterinary surgeon and owner may expose themselves to the potential risks of handling cytotoxic drugs. Owners and veterinary surgeons must be fully aware of the risks associated with any procedures they choose to pursue to ensure that appropriate measures are taken to prevent, identify and manage any potential adverse events that may arise.

Owner considerations

It is easy to overlook the social consequences of the diagnosis and treatment of cancer. Many owners will have encountered cancer in their own lives, either as a sufferer themselves or because an immediate family member or close friend has been affected, or because another of their pets has had cancer. For many, a cancer diagnosis is synonymous with a death sentence. The prevailing expectation is that cancer induces significant suffering and that its treatment is worse. For many owners this point of view can not be challenged and the veterinary team must be sympathetic to this. For others, there is a need for gentle but honest examination of their anxieties and an explanation of the implications and risks as far as their pet is concerned.

Curative excision of a tumour or palliative excision, for example in cases of primary bone tumours, may result in alterations in appearance and/or function. Owners need to be adequately informed about the impact of the functional consequences for their pet. It is often hard for owners of patients that might be well managed by limb amputation to believe that their pet will be able to enjoy an acceptable quality of life subsequently. Sometimes the simplest way of answering their questions is by allowing them to make contact with another owner who has been confronted with the same problem. It is also important to attempt to inform owners fully about the possible impact on them, and the people around them, of a change in the physical appearance of their pet, although this is usually less important from a veterinary perspective than it is in human medicine. It can be emotionally very disturbing for owners to find that their usual circle of pet-owning friends express controversial opinions about the wisdom of an intervention once performed.

The practice of chemotherapy in pets carries certain negative connotations, and understandably so. Many individuals have had direct or indirect experience of chemotherapy. It is not unreasonable for owners to assume that chemotherapy in pets induces severe and protracted quality of life issues. It is vital, therefore, that owners are fully informed about the risks associated with therapy, not only to their pet but also to other individuals and the environment, as well as the potential benefits of treatment. Owners need to be given a realistic appraisal of the probability of a successful outcome, how such a successful outcome is defined and what they can expect in terms of adverse consequences *en route*. They must be fully informed about recognition and management of the most likely side effects of chemotherapy, such that they feel confident that they could act appropriately should an undesirable event arise.

Intercurrent disease

Cancer typically arises in patients of relatively advanced age. This patient group is also likely to have other age-related medical conditions. It is easy for the diagnosis of cancer to assume greatest importance, but this is not always appropriate. Many cancers can be cured by minimalistic surgery, or are sufficiently indolent that their treatment poses a greater risk to the patient than the decision not to treat. The philosophy of palliative care is to examine the patient *in toto* and to address all concerns appropriately. Patients are frequently presented for management of an oncological complaint that poses no immediate threat to their quality of life, while at the same time their owner has overlooked an intercurrent disease state, such as significant osteoarthritis, that is causing the patient to suffer *now*.

The consideration of intercurrent disease is also important on prognostic grounds. A decision to perform radical surgery might be considered inappropriate if a patient has a separate disease process that is expected to impose a limit on their life expectancy independent of the cancer.

In addition, the metabolic consequences of intercurrent disease can affect a patient's ability to detoxify and eliminate cytotoxic drugs or to tolerate and recover from anaesthesia and surgery. Renal and hepatic insufficiency both predispose to chemotherapy-induced toxicity, frequently inducing further perpetuation of the renal or hepatic problem.

Risks associated with cancer surgery

Cancer surgery carries the generic risks associated with surgical procedures of any kind, i.e. haemorrhage, infection and wound breakdown (see Chapter 12). It is also an established fact that dogs with advanced cancer are at increased risk of coagulopathy (Kristensen *et al.,* 2008). These clotting problems are not always identified by routine assays such as activated partial thromboplastin time and one-stage prothrombin time. Coagulopathy is particularly prevalent in patients with haemangiosarcoma and metastatic cancer of any type.

An additional risk associated with cancer surgery is failure to achieve the surgical objective, which is often complete eradication of the tumour.

Administration of systemic chemotherapy

- Oral chemotherapeutic agents should be supplied in clearly labelled containers. In addition to the usual labelling requirements, the label must also read 'CYTOTOXIC DRUGS' and 'WEAR GLOVES TO HANDLE' or words to that effect.
- Loose tablets and capsules must be dispensed in child-proof containers if these can be opened by the owner. Treatments that are supplied in blister packs must be dispensed in their packaging.
- Tablets or capsules must *never* be crushed or split. They must be dispensed in whole tablet or capsule amounts only.
- If tablets or capsules need to be reformulated for safe and accurate dosing, this must be performed by a licensed pharmacist.

Intravenous chemotherapy should always be administered via an intravenous cannula (see Case 15.2). The consequences of perivascular injection range from loss of local skin and soft tissues in less severe cases (e.g. following vincristine extravasation) to severe, extensive, protracted necrotic changes usually necessitating amputation (e.g. following extravasation of doxorubicin and related compounds).

Health and safety considerations

Based upon animal studies, cytotoxic agents are considered to be mutagenic, teratogenic, abortigenic and carcinogenic. These are just four of the reasons why these agents should be treated with caution and only prescribed in appropriate circumstances. Over the last decade it has become recognized that chemotherapy is most definitely associated with an increase in the incidence of second malignancies in human patients. Even tamoxifen, lauded for its lack of classic cytotoxic effects, has been shown to result in a 5.5% increase in endometrial cancer risk after only 5 years of use. Risk of second malignancy is a probability function. Thus, while the risk of developing acute myeloid leukaemia after receiving >1 g of platinum chemotherapeutic agents is 7.6 times higher than if the person had not received platinum chemotherapy, a single exposure still carries a tangible risk of causing malignant transformation.

The question of increased risk of genotoxic effects if patients are exposed *in utero* is frequently posed. Data are largely derived from individual case reports, as clinical trials on such questions could never be performed. Doxorubicin is teratogenic in chicks and rats, but not in mice or rabbits. There are several cases described of pregnant women receiving doxorubicin (at therapeutic doses) and no malformations being detected in their offspring. Other anthracyclines and platinum drugs have been given to women in the second and third trimesters and the only reported adverse effect for the infant was leucopenia in one case. Vincristine has been shown to be teratogenic in all species and associated with chromosomal abnormalities and myelosuppression in mid and late pregnancy. Hydroxyurea is shown to be teratogenic in all animal species tested but women have taken it throughout pregnancy on many occasions and only one case of stillbirth has been described (that this author [GP] knows about). In short, the effects are often less severe than expected but it cannot be assumed that individuals are not at risk.

- Chemotherapy should be administered in accordance with Local Rules as required under the Health and Safety at Work etc. Act 1974.
- All staff who may be involved in handling and administration of cytotoxic substances should be appropriately trained.

Ideally, totally enclosed systems should be used for the preparation and administration of cytotoxic substances to limit risk of accidental spillage or leakage (see photos in Case 15.1). Where this is not possible or practical, substances should be handled in areas with adequate ventilation, with low human traffic levels and where eating, drinking and smoking are prohibited. Administration of chemotherapy should be carried out in an area away from disturbances and away from food or drink items. A chemotherapy 'spill kit' should be considered a mandatory requirement before handling cytotoxic liquids.

If risk of exposure cannot be adequately prevented or controlled by the means stated above, protective clothing should be provided for *all* staff who may be at risk of exposure. This should include some or all of the following:

- Protective gloves:
  o Natural rubber is not impermeable to some chemotherapy agents
  o Latex gloves will protect the wearer from accidental splashes but tend not to be a snug fit and will therefore reduce dexterity
  o Nitrile rubber gloves are recommended
  o There is no protective glove that will be completely chemical-proof for extended periods. Glove type is irrelevant if chemical exposure arises by contact via the cuff
- Respiratory protective equipment:
  o In the absence of a suitable safety cabinet, pharmaceutical isolator or other device, suitable respiratory protective equipment should be provided and used.
  o Surgical facemasks do *not* protect against the inhalation of aerosols
- Goggles
- Protective gown or apron:
  o Gowns and aprons can help protect against accidental spillage
  o Liquid can seep through cloth gowns and therefore these are less protective than some operators assume
  o Conversely, impermeable materials lead to discomfort with prolonged wear and this must also be a consideration when constructing a protocol for use.

Staff and owners must be aware that urine and faeces from patients receiving chemotherapy can contain active metabolites or unchanged chemotherapeutic agents, and suitable protective equipment should be worn and handling measures taken. Chemotherapy residues have been recorded in the urine of canine patients as much as 11 days after administration. Separate containers for cytotoxic waste should be available and clearly labelled (see photos in Case 15.2). Contaminated sharps and syringes must be disposed of as 'cytotoxic sharps'. Waste should not be allowed to accumulate.

Risks of systemic chemotherapy to the patient

All chemotherapeutic drugs carry risks of inducing side effects. The principal effects potentially shared by all cytotoxic drugs are gastrointestinal and myelosuppressive. Essentially, cytotoxic drugs work by interfering with the process of cell multiplication. Therefore, any normal cells undergoing multiplication at the time of chemotherapy exposure are also potentially at risk. This includes the crypt epithelial cells of the stomach and intestine, and the proliferating cells in the bone marrow.

Gastrointestinal signs

The clinical signs of gastrointestinal side effects resemble those of enteric disorders generally, and include the whole spectrum of responses from mild nausea or inappetence through to severe haemorrhagic gastroenteritis. Therapy for these should be the same as for any gastrointestinal disorder in the *absence* of chemotherapy or a diagnosis of cancer. Gastrointestinal side effects are typically seen within 72 hours of chemotherapy administration. The incidence of significant gastrointestinal side effects varies with the chemotherapy strategy employed, but is between 10% and 20% of cases.

Myelosuppression

Myelosuppression manifests primarily as a susceptibility to bacterial infection secondary to chemotherapy-induced neutropenia. This typically presents 7–10 days after chemotherapy is administered. A neutropenic patient can develop bacterial sepsis that would be fatal if left untreated. The cardinal signs of sepsis include depression, lethargy, inappetence and listlessness, in association with a marked pyrexia (>40°C). Some owners are able to measure their pet's temperature. Identification of pyrexia within the timescale described should prompt administration of intravenous, followed by oral, bactericidal antibiotics; treatment needs to be administered relatively urgently, and certainly within 12 hours of identification of the problem. In extremely unusual instances, the septicaemia is due to the presence of antibiotic-resistant bacteria and, despite prompt intervention, this can be fatal. The incidence of neutropenic sepsis varies with the chemotherapy strategy employed, but is between 2% and 10% of cases. Periodic haematological analyses are recommended, according to the risk involved, to monitor white cell and platelet parameters. In the event that a significant neutropenia is noted, treatment should be delayed until normal haematological values have been demonstrated.

Myelosuppression can also arise with chronic chemotherapy. It is normal to note a slowly declining packed cell volume, but frank bone marrow failure can also arise. For this reason, it is advised that no patient on long-term chemotherapy goes for more than 3 months without a full haematological profile being performed.

Haemorrhagic cystitis

Haemorrhagic cystitis following cyclophosphamide administration is often too severe by the time that the patient is overtly symptomatic for it to recover spontaneously. There is therefore great merit in training owners to perform urine dipstick analyses periodically; weekly evaluation is recommended. Any dipstick evidence of blood in the urine can then be reported, and cyclophosphamide treatment stopped before clinical signs manifest.

Thrombocytopenia

Thrombocytopenia is unusual, but it can be fatal if it is not identified and is allowed to progress. It arises as a manifestation of myelosuppression, particularly in association with the platinum chemotherapy agents. Regular haematology analyses are performed during the course of such treatments and this monitoring allows identification of potential problems before it is too late. Chemotherapy administration must be delayed or stopped altogether if thrombocytopenia develops.

Risks associated with radiotherapy

Ionizing radiation can be cytotoxic. The cytotoxic effects can be prompt, or they may be delayed for a prolonged period. The application of radiation to cancer takes advantage of a differential sensitivity to radiation between normal and neoplastic tissues, to achieve a therapeutic benefit. Radiotherapy is generally administered on a 'some is good, more is better' premise, with the last four decades of radiotherapy research being largely directed at how to administer greater total doses of radiation to the target tissues without encountering intolerable side effects. The simplest strategy that has been defined for maximization of radiation dose is fractionation, i.e the administration of multiple divided doses in (often daily) succession. In veterinary radiotherapy, fractionation regimes are governed by practical, financial and toxicity issues. An increased number of fractions imposes a need for serial anaesthetic events. Increasing the number of treatments increases the cost arithmetically, as the cost of delivering one big dose would be indistinguishable from the cost of delivering one small dose. Delivery of multiple small fractions allows administration of a higher total dose, but incurs a significant risk of acute inflammatory consequences in the treatment field.

Acute side effects are typically superficial, and range from erythematous skin changes through to extensive moist desquamation. The incidence and severity of acute side effects are proportional to the total dose of radiation delivered and they are therefore seen most frequently with more highly fractionated regimes.

Late-onset side effects occur months to years after radiation administration. Superficial effects include persistent, non-healing ulcer formation. Deeper effects include second malignancy formation, spontaneous fracture and spontaneous tendon rupture. The incidence and severity of late effects are proportional to the radiation delivered per dose.

Radiotherapy is frequently used in the management of brain tumours in cats and dogs. There are undoubtedly cognitive consequences of this treatment, but this area of veterinary oncology remains poorly explored.

Nutrition

Advanced or systemic cancer is recognized to place a significant metabolic burden on patients. Cancer can also disengage mitochondrial energy transduction pathways, leading to cachexia. While there are scientific reports of investigations into the impact of gross calorie intake and of the role of specific nutrients in cancer management, nutrition is an exceptionally difficult field to investigate objectively in spontaneous cancer-bearing cases. As a general principle, cancer sufferers, like other veterinary patients, require a balanced and adequate diet. Energy and nutrient demands must be met but over-supplementation can cause unwanted medical consequences, including obesity in some patients.

Analgesia

'Is my pet in pain?' This is always of paramount concern to the owner of a pet recently diagnosed with cancer. Often there is an assumption that there will be suffering due to pain, and a natural concern that this pain will elude detection. While cancer certainly can cause pain, for the most part cancer pain occurs due to invasion into bony structures (as in osteosarcoma) or due to cancer-associated inflammation (e.g. with some squamous cell carcinomas, particularly of the head and neck region). Appropriate use of anti-inflammatory and analgesic medication is advised. As long as the owner and veterinary surgeon are aware of the potential hazards, there is rarely a significant contraindication for a trial course of non-steroidal anti-inflammatory or opioid therapy if there is a concern that a patient may be experiencing significant discomfort.

In many cases in which there is pain associated with cancer, optimal management of this pain requires treatment of the underlying cause. This can present something of a dilemma, as interventions carry a risk of failure or complication, and uncertainty prevails as to the likelihood of achieving the desired analgesic or therapeutic response.

Some mention must be made of the current interest in the use of piroxicam specifically, and cyclooxygenase (COX) inhibitors generally, in the management of cancer. Over the last 15 years there has been a rapidly increasing body of evidence indicating that certain tumours can demonstrate clinical responses to the administration of piroxicam. Initial assumptions were that this agent mediated its anti-cancer effect through inhibition of COX-2, and so rational extrapolations have been made and alternative COX-2 inhibitors have also been used. Anecdotal data abound, but we are still unclear about the true mechanism of action of piroxicam and, therefore, about the potential role for other related compounds. This is a rapidly changing field of veterinary oncology and so up-to-date advice should be sought from a veterinary oncologist. For the time being, this author [GP] recommends that if COX inhibition therapy is considered appropriate for anti-neoplastic reasons, piroxicam is used. If COX inhibition is required for other reasons, then authorized alternatives should be used according to the veterinary surgeon's expertise and preference.

Waxing and waning course of disease

One final consideration, that is not unique to oncology but that must be acknowledged to offer the best palliative care, is the fact that many neoplastic conditions have a waxing and waning course. These normal variations can mislead the unwary clinician and can be deeply distressing to the owner. For best management, owners should be informed of the range of changes that they might expect to see, and this will help them to determine when unscheduled appointments should be made. For the owner to be optimally informed, the veterinary surgeon needs to understand the nature of the disease process and to have experience in its management. Often this experience takes time to acquire and it therefore pays to manage these cases together with your clinical team, sharing experiences and expectations, and seeking advice readily when unfamiliar situations present themselves. Far too many oncology patients undergo euthanasia due to uncertainty about disease progression, rather than development of a significant or life-threatening progression.

References and further reading

Arnon J, Meirow D, Lewis-Roness H and Ornoy A (2001) Genetic and teratogenic effects of cancer treatments on gametes and embryos. *Human Reproduction Update* **7**, 394–403

Nind F and Mosedale P (2009) *BSAVA Guide to the Use of Veterinary Medicines*. (www.bsava.com)

Dobson JM and Lascelles BDXL (2010) *BSAVA Manual of Canine and Feline Oncology, 3rd edn*. BSAVA Publications, Gloucester

Health and Safety Executive (2003) *Safe Handling of Cytotoxic Drugs*. (http://www.hse.gov.uk/pubns/misc615.pdf)

Kristensen AT, Wiinberg B, Jessen LR, Andreasen E and Jensen AL (2008) Evaluation of human recombinant tissue factor-activated thromboelastography in 49 dogs with neoplasia. *Journal of Veterinary Internal Medicine* **22**, 140–147

Clinical case studies

A variety of case scenarios in dogs and cats will now be presented to illustrate the considerations to be made and the options available within a specific clinical setting. Information relating to the rehabilitation and palliation of each condition has been contributed to each case by the authors in the first part of this Manual, plus notes on nursing and homecare from Rachel Lumbis RVN. The reader should refer back to the appropriate chapters for further details. Photographs used to illustrate the principles and techniques within the cases do not necessarily feature the original patient.

Case 15.1
Osteosarcoma in a dog

A 6-year-old neutered female Rottweiler was presented with severe right forelimb lameness, associated with heat and swelling over the right proximal humerus. The dog had pre-existing osteoarthritis due to bilateral cruciate ligament rupture and was overweight (48 kg; BCS 6/9).

A radiograph of the limb raised strong suspicions of neoplasia. Core biopsy confirmed proximal humeral osteosarcoma. Right and left lateral thoracic radiographs showed no evidence of gross metastases.

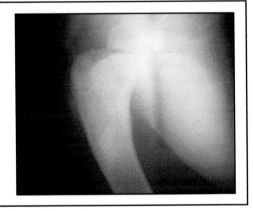

Radiograph showing a lytic lesion affecting the proximal humerus, consistent with osteosarcoma.

Agreed medical/surgical management

The treatment plan for this dog was amputation, followed by carboplatin chemotherapy to slow down growth of micrometastases.

Chemotherapy administration was delayed until wound healing was proceeding uneventfully. The most frequent adverse event associated with carboplatin is myelosuppression; if significant neutropenia were to coincide with development of a fulminant surgical wound infection, septicaemia would likely result.

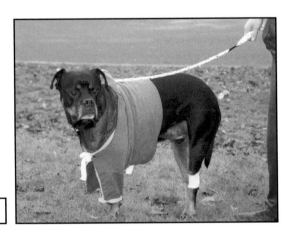

The patient one day after amputation of her right forelimb.

Acute/chronic pain management

Perioperative

A full mu agonist, such as morphine, methadone or pethidine, should be used in premedication. Partial agonists, such as buprenorphine, should be avoided because they may interfere with the action of a full agonist if one is required later in the procedure (e.g. when using fentanyl). An NSAID can be added to the premedication as long as there is no contraindication. It would be wise to assess renal function with blood and urine samples in this dog before using NSAIDs.

Intraoperative analgesia should be achieved with fentanyl (bolus or CRI) and ketamine CRI. Alternatively, a morphine + lidocaine + ketamine CRI could be used. These CRIs can be continued postoperatively. During surgery, bupivacaine should be applied to the nerve roots before sectioning, but the nerve should not be injected.

A fentanyl patch could be considered for postoperative analgesia, but this would need to be put in place 24 hours prior to surgery. If no CRI or fentanyl patch is used, full mu agonist opioids can be given, based on pain assessment.

NSAIDs should be continued postoperatively.

Chronic pain

Overall, removing the limb affected by the osteosarcoma should result in significant pain relief. However, after perioperative pain has been dealt with, the dog should be re-assessed to find out how she is coping with the osteoarthritis (OA) in the stifles (given that it is not always painful), bearing in mind that the strain on the remaining limbs (because there will be a tendency for the dog to throw its weight backwards) may cause a joint in a chronic silent phase of OA to flare up into a chronic active state. All joints (and muscles) and the limb stump should be assessed for pain.

The first line of treatment for the pain of OA is NSAIDs, and the NSAID treatment that was started perioperatively should be continued. Renal function should be monitored in this patient (blood and urine samples every 3 weeks) because of the potential renal toxicity of carboplatin. NSAIDs should not be used if there is evidence of renal failure. If NSAIDs are contraindicated or are not dealing with the pain, tramadol may be used. Central sensitization and/or continuing hyperalgesia/allodynia at the stump or at the site of OA may require the addition of gabapentin, starting daily in two or three divided doses. Both gabapentin and tramadol require renal clearance, so lower dosages should be considered if renal function is compromised. Amantidine added to NSAIDs has been reported to improve analgesia in arthritic joints. Paracetamol ± codeine may be helpful and can be used safely in dogs with reduced renal function, provided there is no evidence of hepatic dysfunction. Acupuncture may be helpful (see below).

'Phantom limb' pain

Phantom limb pain or at least sensations and apparent 'movements' of the absent limb have been reported anecdotally in dogs and cats (see also Case 14.1). Phantom limb pain is generally considered to be neuropathic, although there is some controversy about this classification. Signs to look for would include excessive licking or nibbling around the stump (which may just be stump pain) or hyperalgesia/allodynia at and around the surgical site. It is important to differentiate nociception due to central sensitization from local inflammation, as the latter may simply indicate infection or a sterile suture reaction for which management would be different. Stump movement is normal. Attempts to carry out normal behaviours (such as phantom scratching of the ears) may imply sensation, but on their own do not imply pain. In a case of phantom limb pain, the patient should display distress towards and about the absent limb. Gabapentin is probably the first-choice treatment for such a case. Amitriptyline (a tricyclic antidepressant) is commonly used in human patients with phantom limb pain. Care should be taken with both of these medications in patients with compromised hepatic and renal function and/or receiving concurrent medications requiring detoxification and clearance by the liver or kidneys. Acupuncture may be helpful for phantom limb pain (see below).

Fear, stress, conflict concerns

The main concern with this patient will be how she copes with the loss of a limb, but before she has to deal with this, she needs to cope with the potentially frightening experience of hospitalization, pain and numerous interventions by veterinary staff; these may be minimized by some of the techniques described in Case 15.2.

Most dogs appear to cope well with three legs in terms of their social interaction with other dogs. Similarly, other dogs do not appear to react differently to three-legged dogs. Communication depends on many behavioural and physical cues, but not, as far as we understand, on the number of limbs. However, this is a large dog who may feel unsteady at first. In addition, she may still have pain from the surgical site and her osteoarthritis, so may feel more vulnerable than she used to when she meets other dogs. Therefore, reintroduction to other dogs (assuming she was previously friendly with dogs) should be undertaken with care. It is best to start with calm dogs that she knows and a loose lead, but with the ability to achieve adequate control if necessary. The owner is far more likely to be concerned with potential, rather than real, problems and may be overprotective towards the dog, thereby interrupting important body language by pulling her away abruptly or petting her when she is trying to communicate with another dog. This could trigger aggression from either dog. The owner should display a positive attitude towards the patient rather than over-sympathizing or constantly reassuring her.

Nutritional requirements

Food intake during hospitalization

The dog's food intake should be carefully monitored during the perioperative period. Pain and the effect of analgesic drugs may reduce her appetite. Although she is overweight, perioperative anorexia is not helpful as it will result in an loss of lean body mass and may prolong recovery (see Chapter 5). A high-quality digestible diet is indicated.

It has been suggested that dogs with neoplasia should be fed high-fat diets, because fat is not well metabolized by poorly oxygenated neoplastic tissues. However, there is very little hard evidence in support of high-fat diets in canine neoplasia (see Case 15.2). Other complications may arise, including diarrhoea in dogs with gastrointestinal fat intolerance, so high-fat diets should be used with caution in susceptible animals. Additionally, a high-fat diet would not be sensible in this already overweight dog with concurrent OA.

Weight management

A weight loss programme should be considered but it is important to acknowledge that the potential health benefits of a strict programme would not be realized in the limited time before surgery. Deliberate induction of a negative energy balance prior to surgery and chemotherapy are more likely to cause problems than benefits.

Osteosarcoma is the most pressing complaint and will likely be the reason for ultimate euthanasia prior to the end of the dog's natural lifespan. Weight management may not extend her lifespan significantly but, because weight loss reduces pain in osteoarthritis, it may be expected to improve the *quality* of life in those dogs that go on to enjoy a prolonged survival. For those that fail to respond to chemotherapy and those that develop gastrointestinal complications of chemotherapy, an active weight loss programme would be counter-productive. Cancer cachexia does occur in veterinary oncology patients but it is an end-stage presentation and therefore plays a small role in general management.

Therefore, on balance, weight management is recommended but, rather than insisting on reaching an actual target weight, the main outcome would be to produce sufficient weight loss to improve mobility. Usually, even modest amounts of weight loss (5–10%) will produce significant benefits in terms of mobility. The exact endpoint can be difficult to predict for a particular case, and will need to be tailored as weight loss and the treatment of other diseases progresses. The weight loss regime may need to be halted periodically, depending on the outcome of other therapies that are used; for example, chemotherapy may cause gastrointestinal side effects, including anorexia, vomiting and diarrhoea. It may be more appropriate to feed a highly digestible diet rather than a weight loss diet while the dog is having chemotherapy, or possibly to tempt her with palatable foods in addition to her calorie-restricted diet so that appetite is regained. The weight loss regime should therefore only proceed as and when the dog is otherwise fit and well.

The choice of strategy for weight loss could feasibly involve either a conventional plan, using diet and exercise exclusively, or a plan involving drug therapy (see Chapter 6). Given the potential for gastrointestinal side effects (and anorexia) with chemotherapy, it may be preferable to avoid drug therapy as this can also cause anorexia and, in some cases, vomiting. However, the preference should depend upon the wishes of the owner and clinician involved in the case and the response of the dog.

Prior to starting the weight management regime, the dog should be weighed and her body condition score determined (see Chapter 6). This will enable the degree of excess weight to be estimated, and an ideal bodyweight set. *This is mainly of benefit for calculating her caloric requirements, and not necessarily for setting the endpoint of the diet.*

Most dogs will lose between 0.5 and 1.5% of starting bodyweight per week; however, this dog may progress more slowly. The most important outcome is not necessarily the amount of weight lost. If the rate of weight loss is slow, a reduction in dietary energy intake (again typically 5%) should be considered. However, as mentioned above, other therapeutic needs must also be taken into account.

Once the dog has reached a target weight with which both clinician and owner are happy, a maintenance regime should be instigated. It may be preferable for the dog to remain on the purpose-formulated weight loss diet, since this will contain supplemental protein and micronutrients and help to maintain lean tissue mass. If the diet is changed, the transition should be made gradually, e.g. the dog should continue to be weighed every 2 weeks, whilst the energy intake is increased incrementally by 10% at a time. Once weight has stabilized, the interval between weight checks can be gradually extended (e.g. monthly, 3-monthly, 6-monthly) but they should not be stopped altogether.

Nutraceuticals

Nutritional supplements have been proposed to aid in the management of patients with neoplasia. However, there have been no specific nutritional recommendations for osteosarcoma. In general, as chemotherapeutic agents often lead to the generation of oxygen free radicals, supplementation with antioxidants, such as vitamins C and E and selenium, would seem logical to minimize oxidative injury to non-neoplastic tissue. However, the effectiveness of these supplements has not been properly evaluated in animals and the effects of antioxidants in animals with various neoplasms are not always positive, e.g. antioxidants have been shown to diminish the effects of radiation and cytotoxic drugs (Palozza *et al.*, 2008). Given the lack of any evidence demonstrating benefits of antioxidant supplementation to animals with neoplasia or those being treated with chemotherapeutic agents, no recommendation for supplementation can be justified at the present time.

For a discussion of the use of nutritional supplements in osteoarthritis see Chapter 7 and Case 14.8.

Physiotherapy

Physiotherapy would be involved in several aspects of the treatment of this case: management of the pre-existing osteoarthritis (see Case 14.8); rehabilitation following amputation to achieve an optimal outcome; and weight loss exercise programmes.

A veterinary physiotherapist should be involved in planning to ensure that the most appropriate treatments are applied, especially in cases such as this where several different types of treatment need to be coordinated into a single management plan.

Postoperative rehabilitation

Physiotherapy can help with pain relief and return to function. An appropriate rehabilitation programme should be devised, taking into account the limitations of the pre-existing OA, and all exercises should be carried out in a paced manner (within the tolerance of the dog). The programme should address all aspects of the dog's physical abilities, in particular to improve strength, joint and muscle range, balance, proprioception, joint stability and stamina. Many of the exercises utilized for the OA (see Case 14.8) will be valuable for this purpose as well. Balance and proprioception exercises to improve core stability and speed of reaction will enable the dog to cope more effectively with the enforced changes in weight distribution caused by the amputation. Gait re-education and functional exercises are also likely to be required to ensure that she uses her remaining limbs optimally.

Exercise as an aid to weight loss

A progressive exercise regime should be instigated in conjunction with dietary management (see above). Hydrotherapy may be a useful component of this programme (see below). Consideration of the patient's pre-existing OA and postoperative status will dictate the starting level of exercise and the speed of the programme's progression.

Hydrotherapy

Hydrotherapy may be useful, once the surgical site has healed, to maintain cardiovascular fitness and provide non-concussive exercise. Swimming would be preferable but the dog will need correctly positioned floats to compensate for the missing limb and will need extra help getting into and out of the pool.

Acupuncture

Chronic pain relief

Acupuncture may provide additional pain relief for the osteoarthritic stifles and any secondary muscle pain arising from this joint dysfunction and the postural changes that will have already occurred. If one or both stifles have chronically active arthritis, there will be: pain in and around the joints; and also pain and trigger points in the upper quadriceps muscles, the gluteals and the longissimus muscles of the lumbar spine (and beyond if the pain and abnormal gait has been present for some time). In some patients, the pain and postural strain will extend to the forelimb muscles and even the neck.

An additional complication in this patient is the fact that she has had a painful tumour in the forelimb. This pain may have already set up active painful trigger points in the remaining forelimb muscles and in the muscles of the opposite limb as it has had to take the strain of weightbearing (see Chapters 3 and 11). Pain and lameness in the forelimb (and now its absence) will also cause the patient to shift her weight backwards, often causing pain at two pivotal points – the thoracolumbar and the lumbosacral junctions, as well as increasing the strain on the hindlimbs.

Therefore, depending on the duration of the condition before amputation, the state of the arthritic joints and the potency of concurrent analgesia, this patient may have extensive areas of pain to be potentially treated by acupuncture.

With regard to phantom limb pain, targeting trigger points around the stump, pain on the stump itself and needling of so called 'mirror points' on the opposite limb have been reported to be effective in human patients.

Reducing side effects of chemotherapy

There is convincing evidence in human patients that acupuncture works well in reducing post-chemotherapeutic nausea and vomiting, but the needling needs to be performed at the time of the emetic stimulus (i.e. when the patient is starting to feel ill, not necessarily when the chemotherapy is administered) and needs to be fairly robust to compete with the feelings of nausea. The correct timing of the treatment in dogs can be problematic, therefore, unless one takes the approximate timing of previous events as a guide. An additional difficulty with nausea in dogs is recognizing the sensation, since a nauseous dog does not always vomit (and a vomiting dog need not always be feeling nauseous). In the case of carboplatin, this drug induces nausea promptly if at all. Pharmacological anti-emesis is best achieved by administration of antiemetic approximately 30 minutes before chemotherapy is administered, but acupuncture would probably be best performed (if practical and if needed) immediately after the administration of carboplatin.

The 'famous' and much tested acupuncture point for nausea is PC6 in humans, on the medial aspect of the forearm above the median nerve. It is unlikely, however, that there is only one specific point for nausea in any species, and treatment for analgesia in this patient may also effectively treat any nausea.

Safety concerns

The primary concern in this case is linked to the likely immunosuppression caused by carboplatin. Severe immunosuppression increases the risk of introducing infection with needle penetration. This risk should be discussed with the owner and any acupuncture treatment structured around predictable changes in immune function. Carboplatin can be extremely immunosuppressive in a minority of cases; haematological analyses should be performed prior to every chemotherapy treatment to ensure that the patient has recovered fully from any myelosuppression. If acupuncture is to be performed, it would also be advisable to take blood samples at 4, 7, 10 and 14 days after the first chemotherapy treatment to define the timing and extent of the neutrophil nadir, so that an acupuncture programme can be designed that avoids treatment during times of significant concern. The likelihood of a neutropenia developing that would permit bacterial infection secondary to acupuncture needle placement is very low. Aseptic preparation of needle points and confirmation of satisfactory neutrophil numbers ($>2.0 \times 10^9$/l) would render this risk almost negligible.

Other nursing and supportive care

Preparing chemotherapy

General principles and health and safety considerations are discussed in the Introduction to this chapter.

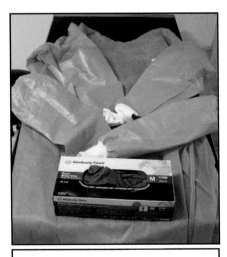

A chemo-proof long-sleeved gown or chemo-proof sleeves can be worn with suitable nitrile latex gloves, depending on the perceived risk of exposure.

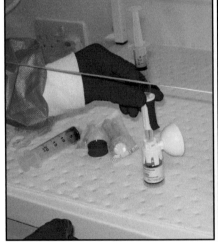
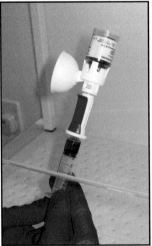

Preparation of a chemotherapy agent (in this case doxorubicin) in a biological safety cabinet. A full-length gown is not necessary for this, so chemo-proof sleeves are more appropriate.

Monitoring

Vital signs should be monitored perioperatively and during the hospital stay. Nutritional intake should be recorded and the patient observed for anorexia and other signs of pain and depression. A pain scoring system (see Chapter 3) will ensure a standardized approach to monitoring and pain management.

Mobility

The patient's limb use should be observed. She should be assisted in adapting to walking on three legs. The use of a sling or towel under the abdomen when exercising may help her feel more secure and stable for the first few days after surgery. It is also important to avoid slippery floors or lay down rubber mats to prevent slipping.

Wound care

The wound should be monitored daily until sutures are removed. Signs of acute inflammation include heat, redness, swelling and pain. The wound should also be observed for signs of a discharge.

Amputation induces a significant amount of surgical trauma and seroma formation is likely; this provides a perfect medium for the adverse progression of bacterial contamination and can retard healing. Every effort should be made to limit patient interference with the healing wound as that can result in wound complications, though it is important to note that most patients would not interfere with a wound that is bacteriologically clean and is not under tension.

Owner advice and homecare recommendations

Health and safety considerations of chemotherapy are discussed in the Introduction to this chapter.

Mobility

While the dog is adapting to walking on three legs, it will be important to avoid slippery floors or lay down rubber mats to prevent the dog slipping. Reintroduction to other dogs (assuming she was previously friendly with dogs) should be undertaken with care (see Fear, stress, above).

Weight management

The owner will require close support in order to succeed with such a regime. The dog should return to the clinic on a 2-weekly basis, initially, so that progress with weight loss can be monitored. The same set of electronic scales should be used when weighing the dog, so that any changes are known to be due to genuine changes in bodyweight rather than inaccuracies between scales.

The initial target to aim for could perhaps be 5–10% below current bodyweight. It would be helpful to set a different target for the owner, in addition to loss of bodyweight, on which to gauge success, such as improved mobility or decreased joint pain.

The owners should be encouraged to instigate a daily exercise plan, tailored to their dog's abilities. This should take into account the current disease and the effects of the surgery. Novel exercise techniques (e.g. hydrotherapy, see above) may prove beneficial in stimulating activity. Given that the dog's ability to exercise will be reduced, there will be a greater reliance on dietary caloric restriction or drug therapy.

References

Palozza P, Simone R and Mele MC (2008) Interplay of carotenoids with cigarette smoking: implications in lung cancer. *Current Medicinal Chemistry* 15, 844–854

Case 15.2
Lymphoma in a dog

A 6-year-old neutered female Golden Retriever was presented with enlarged, firm peripheral lymph nodes but no other clinical signs. Her BCS was 4/9.

Fine needle aspiration of the lymph nodes confirmed a diagnosis of multicentric lymphoma. Haematology and biochemistry blood screens were unremarkable, with no evidence of immunosuppression, circulating neoplastic cells or elevated ionized calcium.

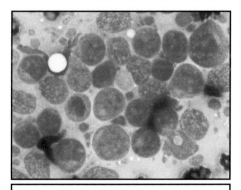

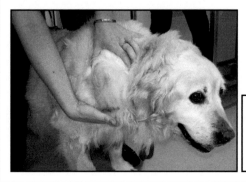

Golden Retriever with peripheral lymphadenopathy due to multicentric lymphoma.

Fine needle aspirate from the enlarged right prescapular lymph node, showing a population of atypical large lymphoid cells. Cellular pleomorphism, open chromatin, multiple nucleoli, bare nuclei and lymphoglandular bodies led to a diagnosis of lymphoma. Modified Wright's stain; original magnification X1000.

The dog was treated with a 6-month CHOP protocol (vincristine, cyclophosphamide, doxorubicin and prednisolone). Median life expectancy with this treatment is 12 months.

Week	Dates treatment due	Drug	Dose (mg/m²)	Instructions	Dates for blood tests
1	01-Jan-10	V	0.75	Intravenous via cannula	
		P	30	1 x 25 mg tablet once daily	06-Jan-10
2	08-Jan-10	C	200	4 x 50 mg tablets **once only**	
		P	20	4 x 5 mg tablets once daily	13-Jan-10
3	15-Jan-10	V	0.7	Intravenous via cannula	
		P	10	2 x 5 mg tablets once daily	20-Jan-10
4	22-Jan-10	D	30	Intravenous by slow infusion	
		P	5	1 x 5 mg tablet once daily	27-Jan-10
5	29-Jan-10	V	0.7	Intravenous via cannula	
6	05-Feb-10	C	200	4 x 50 mg tablets once only	
7	12-Feb-10	V	0.7	Intravenous via cannula	17-Feb-10
8	19-Feb-10	D	30	Intravenous by slow infusion	24-Feb-10
9	26-Feb-10	V	0.7	Intravenous via cannula	
10	05-Mar-10	C	200	4 x 50 mg tablets once only	
11	12-Mar-10	V	0.7	Intravenous via cannula	17-Mar-10
12	19-Mar-10	D	30	Intravenous by slow infusion	31-Mar-10
14	02-Apr-10	V	0.7	Intravenous via cannula	
16	16-Apr-10	C	200	4 x 50 mg tablets once only	
18	30-Apr-10	V	0.7	Intravenous via cannula	12-May-10
20	14-May-10	D	30	Intravenous by slow infusion	26-May-10
22	28-May-10	V	0.7	Intravenous via cannula	
24	11-Jun-10	C	200	4 x 50 mg tablets once only	
26	25-Jun-10	V	0.7	Intravenous via cannula	07-Jul-10
28	09-Jul-10	D	30	Intravenous by slow infusion	

A 6-month CHOP protocol for canine lymphoma. A diary format aids understanding and planning for the owner. C = cyclophosphamide; D = doxorubicin; P = prednisolone; V = vincristine.

An alternative treatment strategy is the COP protocol, which uses cyclophosphamide, vincristine and prednisolone. The author's [GP] preferred COP protocol is shown below. In the COP protocol a greater cumulative dose of cyclophosphamide is administered. Once prednisolone is no longer given daily, timing of administration should coincide with that of cyclophosphamide to enhance water excretion and reduce the risk of development of sterile haemorrhagic cystitis.

Drugs	Weeks 1–8	Weeks 9–24 (provided patient is in complete remission)	Weeks 25+ (provided patient remains in complete remission)
Vincristine	0.7 mg/m² i.v. q7d	0.7 mg/m² i.v. q14d	0.7 mg/m² i.v. q28d
Cyclophosphamide **NB Do not divide tablets**	150 mg/m² orally per week, spread over each 7 days	150 mg/m² orally per 14 days, spread over **one** week	150 mg/m² orally per 28 days, spread over **one** week
Prednisolone	20 mg/m² orally q24h for the first 7 days, then 20 mg/m² on alternate days	No further prednisolone therapy	No further prednisolone therapy

The author's preferred COP protocol. After 12 months of 'Week 25+' treatment, the protocol can be stopped. The patient should be monitored every month for evidence of relapse. On identification of relapse at any time, the protocol is recommenced from the start, or rescue chemotherapy may be considered. Note: Blood is taken for haematological analysis prior to institution of therapy and then prior to every second vincristine treatment.

Blood testing is performed regularly to monitor for the development of significant myelosuppression secondary to chemotherapy administration. The objective of testing is to identify patients that would be at risk of clinical signs associated with myelosuppression *if further chemotherapy were given*. Therefore, chemotherapy should be withheld until the results of blood testing are known. Neutropenia of 2.5 x 10^9/l and thrombocytopenia of 100 x 10^9/l do not pose a significant risk of bacterial sepsis or spontaneous haemorrhage, respectively, if no further therapy is given at that time. Treatment delay of 3–7 days is indicated until further haematological evaluations have proved that the bone marrow has recovered. Subsequent chemotherapy doses might be given at a reduced dose. Exact recommendations for dose reduction cannot be prescribed; however, in most instances a 5–10% dose reduction is appropriate for an asymptomatic episode of myelosuppression.

Not all fully informed owners would choose to pursue a course of chemotherapy for canine lymphoma; such decisions should be respected.

Acute/chronic pain management

Although lymphoma is usually not a painful condition, the possibility of pain should be borne in mind and a plan formulated to be used if required. Traditional NSAIDs are contraindicated because prednisolone forms part of the chemotherapy protocol. Alternatives would be tramadol (probably first choice in this case), gabapentin (bearing in mind partial liver metabolism in the dog), amantadine or paracetamol + codeine (although paracetamol should be avoided with liver dysfunction).

It can be challenging to differentiate loss of vitality due to chronic pain from loss of vitality for other reasons such as cancer- or chemotherapy-induced nausea or, simply, cancer progression. Patients can experience pain from gastritis, which typically responds best to antacid and sucralfate therapy. Some chemotherapeutic agents can induce gastrointestinal ileus, most notably the vinca alkaloids. Patients so affected can be almost paralysed by abdominal discomfort due to bowel distension for 12–24 hours; this would not be expected to respond to conventional analgesics and would be better managed using prokinetics.

Cyclophosphamide induces sterile haemorrhagic cystitis in a proportion of canine cases. The discomfort associated with this is so debilitating that some dogs undergo euthanasia due to the cystitis, despite being in complete remission from the lymphoma. This pain is exceptionally difficult to manage successfully. Options for management include: efforts to increase water turnover such as the use of prednisolone or furosemide, and analgesic medication. These could include steroids (or NSAIDs if prednisolone has been withdrawn), tramadol, amitriptyline, ketamine, gabapentin, amantadine. The sheer number of options reinforces the notion that none is truly effective. This may be something that is best managed by a veterinary oncologist should it develop. The best treatment is prevention (see Nursing and Homecare sections, below).

Fear, stress, conflict concerns

It is important that the dog copes well with the frequent visits to, and interventions by, the veterinary team. Owners may not persist with treatment if their pets become increasingly distressed with each visit. It is therefore vital that the whole veterinary team work to make the visits as pleasant as possible for both dog and owner.

- Application of local anaesthetic cream prior to venepuncture reduces pain and therefore reduces the likelihood of aversion developing.
- Touch is a powerful stimulus and targeting touch to trigger relaxation can be useful in some individuals (see Chapter 8).
- The use of pheromone sprays, collars and diffusers may also help individual patients to make positive associations with the visit and intervention, although the response appears to vary considerably between patients, and overall efficacy is unclear (see Chapter 4).
- High-value food rewards, where appropriate, will help food-oriented dogs to make positive associations.
- Teaching the owner not to over-sympathize with their anxious-looking animal will stop them reinforcing the patient's anxiety. The usual advice is to ignore the dog, but it is difficult to completely ignore a pet in such circumstances. So adopting a bright, positive approach and/or giving the dog a series of commands to distract it (and the owners) will help both owner and dog.

Nutritional requirements

Nutrition for lymphoma

Nutritional strategies have been proposed – and marketed – to prolong disease-free intervals and remission rates for dogs with lymphoma but there is limited evidence demonstrating efficacy. The strategy entails altering the composition of the diet to limit carbohydrate content and increase fat, in particular omega-3 fatty acid content (Ogilvie *et al.*, 2000). This approach was intended to support non-neoplastic cells preferentially whilst 'starving' neoplastic cells, since fat metabolism requires oxygen and neoplastic cells tend to have a poor blood supply. However, studies have not corroborated the benefits of such an approach, and many have questioned the benefit of dietary manipulation in the context of lymphoid neoplasia, where blood supply is less relevant. In addition, further studies have shown that carbohydrate metabolism remains disrupted even after lymphoma goes into remission (Ogilvie *et al.*, 1992). Supplementation of omega-3 fatty acids is unlikely to do harm in this case.

Antioxidants

See Case 15.1 for the cautions and caveats involved in using antioxidants in neoplastic conditions. On balance it would be better to avoid these.

Bodyweight

It would be wise to monitor this dog's bodyweight and BCS regularly throughout treatment. Her bodyweight could go up or down and early intervention to normalize it would be wise. It is not uncommon for dogs to *gain* weight during chemotherapy, likely partly because of the effects of steroids and also potentially because of increased feeding of high-calorie tit-bits by a sympathetic owner. It is also possible that the dog could *lose* weight, particularly if the chemotherapy makes her anorexic. All chemotherapeutic agents have been associated with altered taste sensation (dysgeusia) in human patients. The same can be inferred from the behaviour of those veterinary patients that appear to be hungry but lose interest in their food once they approach or taste it. The primary objective should be that patients ingest sufficient calories to sustain them and to meet their increased energy demands. Excessive weight gain should be avoided. Since chemotherapy requires that patients' weights are assessed extremely frequently for dose modification, it is easy to make this a focus for discussion in the serial visits that follow.

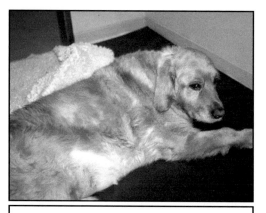

This Golden Retriever with lymphoma was overweight and required dieting while on chemotherapy. Significant weight loss was achieved simply by cutting out tit-bits. (Courtesy of Penny Watson)

Physiotherapy

Physiotherapy is not indicated for this patient.

Hydrotherapy

Hydrotherapy is not indicated for this patient.

Acupuncture

There is no evidence from a neurophysiological perspective that acupuncture could influence progress of lymphoma *one way or the other*. Acupuncture is mainly indicated for the treatment of any concurrent pain where NSAIDs are contraindicated during chemotherapy. It has also been advocated for alleviating side effects of chemotherapy (see Case 15.1). There is a theoretical risk that needling directly into a tumour could spread the condition via the needle track; thus, this should be avoided.

Other nursing and supportive care

Monitoring

Vital signs should be monitored while the dog is in the clinic. In the early stages she may appear well but the cancer can have a profound effect, causing weakness, poor appetite, loss of weight and general poor health. Any signs of pain and discomfort should be watched for and discussed with the owner. An objective pain scoring system (see Chapters 2 and 3) should enable a standardized approach. The dog's nutritional intake should also be recorded.

Reducing risk of infection

Some patients with lymphoma are susceptible to infection. This is of particular importance in those with alimentary lymphoma or bone marrow infiltration or who are otherwise systemically unwell. Furthermore, chemotherapy induces myelosuppression in a proportion of cases, which can result in a temporary period of susceptibility to infection. Such infection would be most likely to arise secondary to translocation of intestinal bacteria into the circulation.

Nursing care should address the perceived risk:

• Barrier nursing may be indicated in some cases
• Careful aseptic practice with intravenous catheters or indwelling urinary catheters is of significant importance
• Any evidence of catheter-based infection should prompt removal of the catheter, which should be submitted for bacteriology
• Urine culture is indicated on removal of an indwelling urinary catheter, as lower urinary tract infection will often be subclinical in those lymphoma patients that are receiving chemotherapy and also have an indwelling urinary catheter.

Administering chemotherapy

Full details about safe preparation and delivery of chemotherapeutic agents are given in the Introduction to this chapter. Intravenous chemotherapy must always be administered via a catheter to prevent perivascular injection. Both vincristine and doxorubicin can induce severe necrotic reactions should extravasation occur. With vincristine extravasation, the patient is likely to slough a 1–2 cm length of tissue, including the vein and the surrounding soft tissues. With doxorubicin extravasation, severe and progressive necrosis will ensue and limb amputation is often the ultimate outcome.

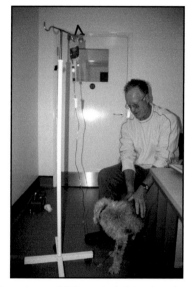

This Bedlington Terrier is receiving doxorubicin chemotherapy for multicentric lymphoma. The chemotherapy is being given through a Luer locking secure closed system, so there is no risk of exposure to the dog's owner. Chemotherapy can be administered in this way in the presence of staff and owners, so long as the preparation of the dose is performed in a suitable biological safety cabinet (see Case 15.1). The presence of the owner frequently diminishes anxiety for the patient, leading to a better overall veterinary experience.

All intravenous agents are capable of inducing an anaphylactic response but this is described more frequently with doxorubicin. Rapid infusion of doxorubicin can induce cardiac arrhythmia and death. Chronic, cumulative doxorubicin administration is associated with progressive cardiomyopathy. Objective data are lacking but it is believed that most cases are at very low risk of cardiomyopathy if they only receive a total cumulative dose of doxorubicin of 150–180 mg/m^2.

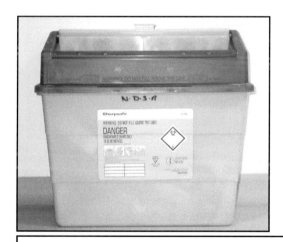

Contaminated sharps and syringes are disposed of as 'cytotoxic sharps' without separation prior to disposal.

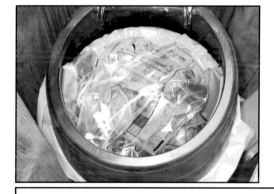

Non-sharp cytotoxic waste from preparing and administering chemotherapy is kept separately. In this case all individual waste packages are in separate sealed bags within the separate waste bin, which is in a separate outbuilding.

Owner advice and homecare recommendations

Urine monitoring

The owner must be aware of potential toxic effects. Of particular concern in the context of *oral* agents, which are often administered at home, is the risk of sterile haemorrhagic cystitis associated with chronic administration of cyclophosphamide to dogs. Sterile haemorrhagic cystitis can be catastrophic in dogs, sometimes necessitating euthanasia in a case that was otherwise in complete remission. Owners should be supplied with urine dipsticks and coached to perform urine dipstick analysis. They should be instructed to do this once a week for all patients receiving chronic cyclophosphamide treatment. Identification of haematuria should prompt veterinary attention and withdrawal of the cyclophosphamide treatment should be considered. (It is helpful to know that there is no evidence of haematuria before treatment commences.)

Health and safety considerations

- Owners who are administering oral chemotherapeutic drugs should wear disposable gloves to handle the treatment and should return empty vials to the veterinary practice for proper disposal.
- The owner must be provided with clear instructions about drug handling and administration. All owners are different but for many it helps to present the treatment plan in a diary format.

Opinions differ regarding the length of time that owners should avoid direct contact with body waste from a patient receiving chemotherapy. The author's [GP] preferred advice is that all direct contact with urine, faeces and vomit is undesirable. The owner should be advised to treat urine, faeces and vomit from their pet as though they are contaminated by cytotoxic drugs for the duration of their pet's chemotherapy protocol. Faeces should ideally be recovered from wherever they were deposited and disposed of down the toilet. Sites of defecation and urination, whether at home or in the local environment, should be irrigated to dilute or even wash away any potential cytotoxic contamination.

References

Ogilvie GK, Fettman MJ, Mallinchrodt CH *et al.* (2000) Effect of fish oil, arginine and doxorubicin chemotherapy on remission and survival time for dogs with lymphoma – a double blinded, randomized placebo-controlled trial. *Cancer* **88**, 1916–1928

Ogilvie GK, Vail DM, Wheeler SL *et al.* (1992) Effects of chemotherapy and remission on carbohydrate metabolism in dogs with lymphoma. *Cancer* **69**, 233–238

Case 15.3
Oral tumour in a dog

A 4-year-old neutered male Labrador Retriever was presented with a rapidly growing mandibular mass, which was beginning to interfere with his ability to eat. He had a bouncy vivacious temperament and was in normal body condition (bodyweight 34 kg).

An incisional biopsy was performed under general anaesthetic and a fibrosarcoma was confirmed. The clinical stage of the disease is defined by its local and systemic extent. Local disease extent can be determined, to an acceptable degree, by local radiography or CT examination. Local regional lymph node status is best defined by cytological or histological evaluation of fine needle aspirates or biopsy samples from lymph nodes, though the nodes are not always enlarged (or even detectable in some cases). A pragmatic approach is to perform fine needle

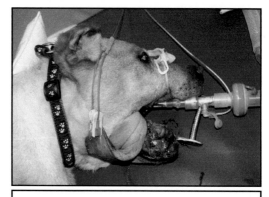

Labrador Retriever with a large mass affecting the right hemimandible.

aspiration on local lymph nodes where there are detectable changes in size or consistency. If CT examination of the primary tumour is performed, the local regional lymph nodes can also be evaluated. Distant metastases from oral tumours can develop anywhere; the thorax should be checked for pulmonary metastases by radiography or CT.

It is prudent for patients that might be candidates for invasive, complex or expensive management to undergo other peripheral organ evaluations to ensure that their general health is understood. Therefore, routine haematological and biochemical evaluations and urine analysis are advised. In this case, no other problems were identified.

Agreed medical/surgical management

After clinical stage determinations indicated that this was a locally invasive but non-metastatic tumour, a plan was made to perform a unilateral rostral mandibulectomy. The surgery was hoped to be curative. However, as fibrosarcoma in this location can be a remarkably invasive disease, consideration should be given beforehand to the action that might be taken in the event that incomplete excision is reported by the histopathologist.

Fibrosarcomas in this location are not expected to respond to chemotherapy or radiotherapy. In principle, however, adjuvant radiotherapy would be considered if excision proved incomplete.

Following unilateral mandibulectomy, patients can develop persistent drooling, palatal ulceration and possibly, in the long term, arthritis of the temporomandibular joint (TMJ). Drooling can arise due to loss of normal lip conformation and failure to retain the tongue and/or saliva within the oral cavity.

Palatal ulceration arises if the unadulterated hemimandible drifts towards midline without its contralateral counterpart to prevent this. The remaining canine tooth can impinge on the palatal mucosa and cause ulceration. This may require further work to shorten the length of the offending canine tooth crown, with the associated risks and costs.

If the remaining hemimandible is sufficiently unstable, TMJ inflammation can arise. Identification of the behavioural indicators of suffering (see Chapter 3) should be discussed *prior to surgery* to help the owner and the veterinary team to identify problems postoperatively or at a later date, e.g. the development of TMJ arthritis.

Acute/chronic pain management

Perioperative

For rostral mandibulectomy, a full mu agonist opioid should be included in the premedication, with an NSAID if not contraindicated by preoperative clinical examination and blood work-up (i.e. no evidence of significant gastrointestinal or renal compromise). In addition, a bilateral mandibular nerve block with bupivacaine should be administered before surgery.

Fentanyl can be used as required during surgery (as an intermittent bolus), but if the nerve block is successful then this should not be necessary.

Opioids can be continued postoperatively, based on pain assessment, along with an NSAID until the wound is healed.

Chronic pain

After dealing with perioperative pain, the dog should be assessed for continuing pain. A pain assessment (see Chapter 3) will be more difficult than usual as there may be many behavioural indications of suffering that may not necessarily be pain-related, e.g. physical difficulty in carrying toys rather than not doing so because of pain. Continuing pain after surgery can be managed with NSAIDs, with the addition of tramadol if NSAIDs are not sufficient. Care should be taken to watch for dysphoria and/or dullness with tramadol; this will make assessment of the patient's demeanour difficult. Persistent pain in spite of NSAID and tramadol treatment would indicate the addition of paracetamol (avoiding adding the paracetamol/codeine combination to tramadol as the opiate effects may cause excessive sedation or dysphoria.) Gabapentin can be added to any combination of NSAIDs, tramadol and paracetamol. Amantadine similarly can be added to this combination. Amitriptyline can be used, but not with tramadol.

Electrotherapy (ultrasound, laser) can be helpful for pain relief (see Physiotherapy). Acupuncture could also be used both postoperatively and for continuing pain (see below).

Fear, stress, conflict concerns

As a Labrador Retriever, the dog is said to be 'soft-mouthed' and may be less likely to play rough tugging games than other breeds, such as terriers and bull breeds. However, even carrying and fetching using the mouth may be a problem in the short term following surgery. Alternative mental stimulation would include: new training repertoires, rewards (touch) for finding and signalling items rather than picking them up; and chase and stay by the item, for which the dog is rewarded. If he can take high-value food rewards then this may partially substitute for the oral satisfaction of carrying objects.

Drooling may cause the owners some irritation, and it is important that they understand the importance of consistency in their own behaviour. Greeting the dog and making a fuss of him when they are not worried about the drool, but pushing him away or shouting at him when they are wearing their best clothes will only result in confusion and anxiety in the dog. To prevent this, the owners may be best advised to teach him a particular greeting (e.g. sitting) which avoids his drooling on them.

Nutritional requirements

Ensuring adequate food intake

Nutritional support of animals with oropharyngeal tumours can be particularly challenging. The dog's food intake should be carefully recorded both before and after surgery. If he fails to eat his calculated resting energy requirement (RER; see Chapter 5) for more than 2–3 days, some form of tube feeding may be necessary. If this is likely to be for only a few days, a naso-oesophageal tube may be used. In some cases it may be necessary to bypass the oropharyngeal area with oesophageal or gastrostomy tubes in order to allow the dog to be fed. Careful consideration should be given to placing such tubes at the time of the original surgery for rostral mandibulectomy to avoid a second general anaesthetic.

Support may be required for only a short period of time, as many dogs with partial mandibulectomies are able to adjust well and eat normally in a few days – perhaps surprisingly so, given the extent and location of surgery.

Diet

In terms of the composition of the diet there are no specific requirements. It may be supposed that soft food would be easier for these patients to eat but, in practice, many of them seem to cope better with dry food.

Diets used for tube feeding are typically made into a gruel and are usually relatively high in calories, protein and fat. This allows a reduction in both the volume and frequency of tube feeding. Diets for naso-oesophageal tube feeding should be very liquid to avoid tube blockage.

There are no specific recommendations for nutraceuticals or dietary ingredients to treat this dog's neoplasia as most, if not all, of the tumour mass will have been removed by surgery and no specific dietary interventions have been shown to have any impact on tumour metastasis or recurrence.

Physiotherapy

Electrotherapy (ultrasound, laser) may be helpful for pain relief, although it should not be applied to areas of active neoplasia or recent irradiation. Through careful placement of electrodes, TENS may provide effective pain relief (albeit short lived once the device is turned off, depending on the stimulation used) through segmental stimulation.

If TMJ arthritis develops, this dog may benefit from physiotherapy to help with function and pain relief. The application of warmth and gentle massage to the jaw muscles may help with pain and relaxation of muscles, although this will be dependent on the dog's tolerance to being handled around this area. Trigger points in associated muscles (see Acupuncture, below) can be treated manually and this may be tolerated better by the patient than acupuncture (although sometimes the converse is true). Heat is best applied via warm flannels to the jaw area for approximately 10–15 minutes. Alternatively, cold therapy can be applied (using cold flannels) to help with pain relief and control of inflammation. These are simple methods that owners can provide several times daily. To improve jaw function (and secondarily aid pain relief) mobilizations to the TMJ can be provided by veterinary physiotherapists.

Hydrotherapy

Hydrotherapy is not indicated for this patient.

Acupuncture

Postoperatively, acupuncture may help to reduce the amount of opiate analgesia required and give a clearer picture of the patient's demeanour if he seems dull or dysphoric. The principles of point selection in this case would be partly driven by the patient's tolerance of handling around the head following surgery and would avoid direct needling of the surgical site. Temporalis and masseter muscles should be examined for trigger points, which can be needled if tolerated. If the patient cannot tolerate needling on the side of the surgery then mirror points on the other side can be used. Needling in the neck muscles close to the back of the head may achieve segmental analgesia. Electroacupuncture may be necessary to provide effective relief of postoperative pain if opiates are not tolerated. General points such as ST36 (in tibialis cranialis) and SI11 (in infraspinatus) may be better candidates for providing heterosegmental relief at every spinal segment since these will generally be easier to stimulate more strongly and provide a more potent 'competition' for the pain.

If arthritis develops in the TMJ then acupuncture can be helpful for the pain associated with this. Again, trigger points in associated muscles (temporalis and masseter but also cleidobrachialis and cranial trapezius if the dog has been holding his head abnormally) should be looked for and treated. If tolerated, points in the head such as GV20, Yintang and GV17 can act as local acupuncture points.

Other nursing and supportive care

Perioperative care

One concern for the veterinary staff may be coping with the dog's bouncy nature during his stay for surgery. However, perioperative analgesia will probably cause a degree of sedation and he should only be in the clinic for 2–3 days postoperatively. Patient warmth, comfort and quality of life should be maintained.

The patient should be watched closely, especially in the immediate postoperative period, for signs of pain or discomfort. To this end, a pain scoring system may ensure a standardized approach (see Chapters 2 and 3). Postoperative problems associated with partial mandibulectomy include wound dehiscence, infection, injury to salivary ducts, subcutaneous emphysema, mandibular instability, abnormal salivation with secondary cheilitis/dermatitis, pain and discomfort, lingual dysfunction, and prehension difficulties and anorexia. Monitoring for the presence of mucoceles, seromas or haematomas is also required. An Elizabethan collar or neck brace should be fitted if necessary to stop him interfering with the operative site.

Assistance with feeding
Most patients resume eating immediately on recovery from surgery, but delays in feeding may occur as a consequence of inadequate postoperative analgesia or the development of surgical complications (see above). The dog may need help to eat – it may take several days for him to learn an efficient method of prehension.

If a feeding tube has been placed, this should be monitored carefully as the majority of complications involve tube occlusion or localized irritation at the tube exit site. (See Chapter 5 for a full discussion of feeding and tube care.) Bodyweight should be monitored daily for patients receiving enteral nutritional support.

Owner advice and homecare recommendations

Cosmetic considerations
There may be lateral deviation of the remaining hemimandible toward the resected side. In young patients, this laxity may be considerably greater than in older patients. The owner should be warned about potential management considerations such as persistent drooling (see Fear, stress, above) and protrusion of the tongue.

Play
Postoperative instructions are to avoid 'mouthing' and carrying games for 6 weeks. A veterinary evaluation is recommended prior to permitting unlimited mouthing activities once again. Alternatives to regular 'fetch and carry' games can be devised (see Fear, stress, above).

Case 15.4
Anal sac gland carcinoma and hypercalcaemia in a dog

A 13-year-old neutered male Cocker Spaniel was presented with depression and polydipsia. On presentation he was dull and lethargic. He had been straining to defecate and was passing only small stools; these were formed and not flattened. The owner reported that the dog was drinking excessively but that no change had been noted in his urination. His BCS was 7/9 and he weighed 14.5 kg.

Blood sampling revealed normal sodium, potassium, phosphate, total protein and albumin levels, but mild elevations in urea (12.7 mmol/l; reference range 2.5–9.6) and creatinine (162 µmol/l; reference range 44.0–159.0). Total serum calcium was 4.03 mmol/l (reference range 1.98–3.0); serum ionized calcium was 1.92 mmol/l (reference range 1.25–1.50). Haematology was unremarkable.

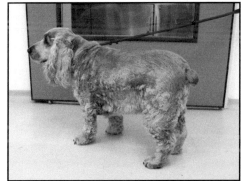

This overweight Cocker Spaniel was diagnosed with anal sac gland carcinoma and hypercalcaemia.

Careful examination revealed a small mass in the right anal sac and radiography showed marked enlargement of the sublumbar lymph nodes but no visible lung metastases. A diagnosis of anal sac carcinoma was made on cytological evaluation of fine needle aspirates from the anal sac mass.

The increased abdominal effort on defecation and the production of small faecoliths may indicate weakness of the smooth muscle of the colon and rectum.

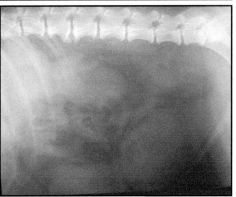

Radiography showed sublumbar lymph node enlargement. This was due to metastasis from the primary anal sac gland carcinoma.

Agreed medical/surgical management

Hypercalcaemia induces renal water loss by inhibiting the action of antidiuretic hormone. The patient would therefore be expected to be dehydrated at the time of presentation and pre-renal azotaemia would be expected. There was some indication of dehydration and a mild azotaemia. Initial management therefore required correction of fluid deficits. An estimation of the degree of dehydration was made and fluid replaced, using 0.9% saline for infusion. In patients that maintain good urinary output, further intravenous fluid therapy can be given at rates of up to 6 ml/kg/h. A high sodium load such as this can act as a calciuretic, making a modest contribution to control of serum calcium concentration. Additional calciuresis can be achieved with furosemide; care must be taken not to use loop diuretics in cases that are hypovolaemic, so the patient must be rehydrated first.

The primary medical problem affecting this dog's quality of life was the hypercalcaemia. In some cases this can be managed by tackling the underlying disease process. In this patient, the substantial sublumbar lymphadenopathy was not amenable to surgical management. A plan was made to manage the hypercalcaemia using bisphosphonate therapy. There are a number of agents available for use, all without veterinary authorization. Oral bisphosphonates are associated with a risk of gastritis but are otherwise considered to be reasonably safe. Some agents have a low bioavailability, which means that the oral dose can be very high compared to human patients; it can also mean that significant plasma concentrations of drug are never attained and that the agent fails to achieve the desired outcome. Intravenous agents that have been clinically evaluated in dogs include pamidronate and zoledronate. These are regarded to be considerably superior to the oral bisphosphonates in their capacity to restrict osteoclasis. Side effects include sudden death; this occurs with rapid administration and for this reason it is recommended that infusions are given over 1–2 hours. Experience with these agents is limited so undoubtedly further, less common side effects will come to light with increased usage. The author [GP] recommends initial re-evaluations after 1 and 4 weeks for plasma ionized calcium concentration determination. A decision can then be made about the efficacy of therapy. Some patients can be extremely well controlled on oral or injectable bisphosphonates; others may remain hypercalcaemic. Oral treatment continues in the long term. The objective of therapy is to restore normal vitality so persistent mild hypercalcaemia need not be a major concern if clinical signs have abated. With injectable bisphosphonates the clinician needs to identify the optimal interdose interval. This will be defined by careful history taking and blood test results.

Persistent hypercalcaemia may respond to more definitive therapy for the lymph node metastases such as chemotherapy or radiotherapy. The risks associated with these treatments must be fully discussed beforehand.

Acute/chronic pain management

Chronic pain

It is extremely rare for this tumour to cause pain. Patients that do demonstrate discomfort usually do so because of infection in the tumour or lymph node. This patient should be evaluated regularly for chronic pain but it should not be expected.

Renal compromise must be expected secondary to the hypercalcaemia, even if it has not registered on serum biochemistry and urinalysis. Therefore, any potentially nephrotoxic analgesic agents should be prescribed with extreme caution.

If pain becomes evident, tramadol can be used for immediate analgesia and the patient evaluated for evidence of infection. It may be simplest to prescribe broad-spectrum antibiotics in such an instance. This patient is being managed for a terminal condition; the need for lengthy or invasive investigations, or the presence of persistent chronic pain, should prompt a discussion about euthanasia.

Fear, stress, conflict concerns

If the dog needs frequent visits to the vet, for example to test blood calcium levels, it is important that he copes well (see Case 15.1 for details on how to reduce anxiety at repeat visits).

Nutritional requirements

There are limited nutritional implications for dogs with terminal forms of neoplasia.

Nutritional support in hypercalcaemia

Hypercalcaemia is likely to induce renal, gastrointestinal and neurological signs, which will likely suppress appetite. The most important consideration may therefore be to offer palatable food. Although the dog is overweight, anorexia is not advisable – a dog with concurrent neoplasia will lose a considerable proportion of lean, as well as fat, body mass and the owner is likely to elect for euthanasia earlier if the dog becomes inappetent. Continued nutritional support in cases such as these may rely upon the use of long-term feeding tubes, such as oesophagostomy or gastrostomy feeding tubes, although the decision to place these must be preceded by a discussion about the dog's long-term prognosis and quality of life.

Use of supplements
Other nutritional supplements such as antioxidants and omega-3 fatty acids have been proposed for other forms of canine cancer, but there are no studies supporting their use in anal sac carcinoma.

Weight loss?
Although this dog is overweight, a weight loss programme is not the first priority. The dog has a poor long-term prognosis and quality of life is more important at this stage than weight loss. However, some gentle advice to the owners to avoid high-calorie tit-bits and replacing them with low-calorie alternatives if possible would be wise.

Physiotherapy

Physiotherapy is not indicated for this patient.

Hydrotherapy

Hydrotherapy is not indicated for this patient.

Acupuncture

If analgesia is not sufficient when treated with the drugs listed above and/or some/all or those are contraindicated or not tolerated by the patient, then acupuncture may provide analgesia for the pain of carcinoma. Segmental needling rather than direct local needling would be recommended.

Other nursing and supportive care

Monitoring
While the dog is in hospital for investigations and fluid therapy, comfort and warmth should be maintained. Signs of pain and discomfort should be watched for; using a pain scoring system will ensure a standardized approach.

Fluid therapy
Most patients can tolerate fluid administration rates of 4–6 ml/kg/h but the clinician must be aware of the risk of interstitial kidney damage leading to a reduced ability to excrete free water and volume overload. Careful monitoring is required to ensure that the fluid therapy is given at the appropriate rate.

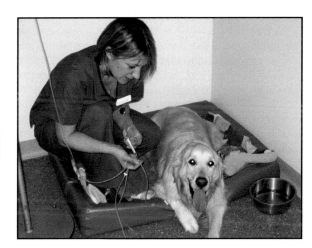

This Golden Retriever is receiving intravenous fluid support and nursing care. (Courtesy of Liz Mullineaux)

Feeding
Food intake should be monitored while the dog is in hospital. If a feeding tube is placed this should be monitored carefully as the majority of complications involve tube occlusion or localized irritation at the tube exit site. (See Chapter 5 for details on feeding and tube care.) Bodyweight should be monitored daily for patients receiving nutritional support.

Owner advice and homecare recommendations

The owners should monitor the dog for signs associated with kidney failure (as a result of hypercalcaemia): lethargy; loss of appetite; vomiting; increased drinking; increased urination.

They should also look for signs of relapse of the hypercalcaemia. These signs will usually be familiar as they were present prior to therapy. In many cases the recovery of vitality is quite marked with normalization of plasma calcium concentration, so a return of lethargy is frequently the first sign reported on relapse. A return of polydipsia is also frequently noted.

Other signs to look for relate to progression of the cancer. It is likely that the dog will develop obstipation, due to further enlargement of the metastatic sublumbar lymph nodes. At this time stool consistency can be modified with appropriate stool softeners, or more definitive therapy can be applied such as chemotherapy or radiotherapy. It is likely that the hypercalcaemia will be refractory to treatment by this time. The prognosis at such a time is going to be very poor and it is probable that the combination of refractory hypercalcaemia and advanced cancer would indicate to most pet owners that consideration of euthanasia would be appropriate.

Hypocalcaemia due to bisphosphonate therapy is exceptionally unusual. It can occur, however, in cases that undergo definitive management of the neoplastic complaint and concurrent treatment directed at the hypercalcaemia. Under those circumstances, which would not apply in this case, clinical signs of hypocalcaemia would include weakness, hyper-reflexia, tremors and collapse. Owners should be warned about this possibility and prompt veterinary attention should be sought in such cases.

Case 15.5
Insulinoma in a dog

A 7-year-old neutered male Boxer was presented with episodes of collapse and loss of consciousness. His BCS was 4/9 and he weighed 26 kg. He used to exercise three times a day.

Blood samples revealed low blood glucose levels and an inappropriately high concurrent serum insulin concentration. Otherwise, results of biochemistry and haematology were largely unremarkable. A diagnosis of insulinoma was presumed on the basis of history and elevated serum insulin concentration.

Abdominal ultrasonography revealed a mass 1 cm in diameter and of uniform echogenicity in the left limb of the pancreas. Administration of ultrasonographic contrast medium highlighted the lesion, indicating a significant vascular supply consistent with insulinoma. There was no evidence of hepatic or regional lymph node abnormalities.

Agreed medical/surgical management

Resection of the mass was uncomplicated. Detailed visual assessment of the liver and regional lymph nodes at surgery was unremarkable, consistent with the ultrasonographic findings. Histological examination of the resected pancreatic mass confirmed insulinoma.

Euglycaemia was recorded 26 hours postoperatively. Recovery from surgery was uneventful.

Partial pancreatectomy is associated with a high mortality rate (10%). Complications of surgery include acute pancreatitis and diabetes mellitus. Complications specific to insulinoma are associated with the neurological effects of withdrawal of excessive insulin from patients that have adjusted to this altered internal environment. Neurological complications include seizures and changes consistent with distal denervation.

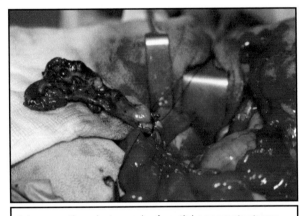
Intraoperative photograph of partial pancreatectomy.

This patient remained normoglycaemic for 14 months before clinical signs consistent with insulinoma returned. At this time ultrasonographic examination of the abdomen revealed a large (5 cm diameter) and non-resectable gastric lymph node. Medical management for hyperinsulinism was implemented.

Management of cases of persistent hyperinsulinaemia comprises changes in feeding and exercise (see below) and medical therapy. Options for medical therapy include prednisolone, diazoxide and streptozotocin. Of these, only prednisolone has consistently achieved durable periods of remission without significant, sometimes fatal, adverse effects. Prednisolone should initially be given at a dose of 1 mg/kg once daily and the dose can then be modified to the lowest daily dose that is required to maintain satisfactory glycaemic control.

Acute/chronic pain management

Perioperative
A full mu agonist opioid, such as morphine, methadone or pethidine, should be included in premedication for the partial pancreatectomy, along with an NSAID if this is not contraindicated on preoperative work-up.

Epidural morphine will provide analgesia into the postoperative period (up to 24 hours). During surgery, fentanyl can be given by intermittent bolus or CRI. Lidocaine CRI can also be considered.

The opioid and NSAID can be continued postoperatively. Opioid continuation should be based on regular pain assessments (see Chapter 2).

If the dog suffers from acute pancreatitis after surgery, it may be refractory to opioids or NSAIDs and the pain can be very difficult to treat (see Case 19.3).

Fear, stress, conflict concerns

Avoiding stress and hypoglycaemia

It is important for owners to be aware that fluctuations in blood glucose can have direct effects on behaviour. Hypoglycaemia, for example, has been associated with a lowered threshold to display aggression. For this reason, situations in which the dog currently displays signs of anxiety or emotional conflict should be addressed, to ensure that an aggressive response to these contexts does not develop. A consistent predictable routine will help maintain stable glucose levels and will also reduce the risk of aggression occurring during periods of hypoglycaemia.

Regulating exercise

Exercise reduces serum glucose, so individual episodes of exercise should be limited and, ideally, timed to coincide with peak serum glucose concentrations. This is likely to be 30–90 minutes after a meal.

Enforced changes in exercise can lead to frustration. The change in routine can be managed to minimize this by:

- Identification of the motivation for exercise for the patient
- Identification of his favourite games
- Identification of the time constraints on the owner
- Identification of the amount of unregulated exercise the dog was previously used to. For example: Did he chase about with other dogs he met when on a walk? Did he run off-lead or chase birds/rabbits? Did the children play with him (lots of exercise when the weather is good and there is no homework, very little when circumstances change)?
- Alteration of the management accordingly so that the dog has a routine to which the owner can keep
- Regulation of exercise so that the owner can estimate the amount of off-lead exercise the dog has had in one bout and then restrict it by putting him back on the lead, for example.

Frustration can be minimized by:

- Rewarding being put back on the lead with food, praise, or brief play
- Substituting short fun training exercises for wild games
- Using mentally challenging games such as hide and seek, 'track back' and 'treasure hunt'
- Taking the dog, where possible, to different exercise areas.

Clicker training may have a role in increasing mental stimulation and rewarding desired behaviours.

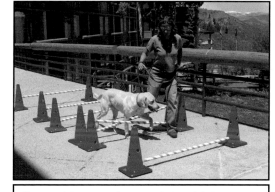

Short training exercises can help minimize frustration for dogs that cannot exercise freely. (© Janet Van Dyke)

Nutritional requirements

Perioperative

Careful attention and consideration should be given to how long the dog is starved prior to surgery. The period should be minimized and the dog's blood glucose checked frequently during this period, as hypoglycaemia is a real risk during perioperative starvation before the bulk of the tumour is removed. A dextrose infusion may be necessary, but must be given with caution as it can also stimulate insulin release.

Postoperative pancreatitis is a real risk after insulinoma surgery: manipulation of the pancreas may disrupt its blood supply. If this occurs, the dietary management during the bout should be the same as in Case 19.3.

Acute management of hypoglycaemia

If the dog shows signs of hypoglycaemia during hospitalization and in the immediate perioperative period, it should be fed immediately and preferably given foods low in simple sugars. These should not be the types of oral preparations usually used for human diabetic hypoglycaemic attacks. Something like some dried dog kibble or a piece of cheese, or even a biscuit, is preferable to sugar or honey, as the latter are more potent stimuli for more insulin release from the tumour, which may result in a rapid rebound hypoglycaemia.

Long-term nutrition to control blood glucose

The aim in long-term feeding of dogs with insulinoma is to minimize hypoglycaemia by feeding a highly digestible diet that has limited quantities of simple carbohydrates. The bulk of calories are derived from protein and fats and also some complex carbohydrates. This avoids the sudden release of insulin from the tumour that can be stimulated by simple carbohydrates and also allows a more prolonged absorption of sugars to counteract the hypoglycaemic effect of the tumour. Lower glycaemic index components such as dietary fibre may also have a role.

Dogs with hyperinsulinaemia can be fed a variety of high-quality digestible diets which at least partly fulfil these nutritional goals; a clinical diet is often unnecessary. High-fat, high-protein, low-carbohydrate diets have been formulated for cats but not for dogs. These diets have been designed for the management of diabetes and obesity in cats, although there are no data on efficacy or applicability of such an approach in dogs with insulinoma. There is a commercial diet formulated for the management of dogs with neoplasia, which is low in simple carbohydrates and relatively high in fat (mainly omega-3 fatty acids) and protein. It would be logical to use a diet like this in these cases, although there are no data to support its use in dogs with insulinoma.

For a variable period after debulking surgery, dietary management may be less important as the hyperinsulinaemia is temporarily controlled. However, with time, hyperinsulinism usually recurs due to the development of regional lymph node or hepatic metastases; control of clinical signs can then often be achieved for a prolonged period with a combination of dietary manipulations and drug therapy. *The most important thing in dogs with insulinoma and symptomatic hyperinsulinaemia is to feed multiple small meals a day and not leave prolonged periods between meals.* This can be difficult for owners who work or are away from the dog for long periods and they may have to make arrangements to have the dog fed during those times.

Weight management

This dog is not overweight. However, dogs with insulinomas can present significantly overweight because of the effect of chronic hyperinsulinaemia increasing the lay-down of fat. During the initial bout of illness the dog should be fed to maintain bodyweight and not for weight loss. Once the dog is stable postoperatively, it is appropriate to try to gently normalize its bodyweight. Where the dog is underweight, like this dog, a gradual increase in bodyweight to normal should be aimed at; where a dog is overweight, a gentle weight loss programme can be instituted for the dog's quality of life. In cases where the long-term prognosis from the tumour is poor, this weight loss programme should be 'gentle' and advisory only and should not put undue pressure on dog or owner.

Details of weight loss programmes are given in Chapter 6. In line with feeding recommendations for dogs with insulinoma, the chosen diet should be high in protein and contain reduced levels of simple carbohydrates. The food ration should be fed over a number of small meals (ideally at least 5–6 a day). In addition to dietary management, the owners should be encouraged to instigate a daily exercise plan, tailored to their dog's abilities. The owner may be rightly concerned about hypoglycaemic attacks on exercise, so this should never be too vigorous and they should always bring some food with them to give in the case of such an attack.

Physiotherapy

The risk of hypoglycaemia imposes a limit on the amount of exercise this dog can take. However, a variety of other exercises can be used, including: functional-type exercises (e.g. sit-to-stand, lie-to-sit) to help improve overall strength and function (and obedience); and balance exercises (to improve core stability, joint stability and speed of reaction to alterations in posture and gait).

Hydrotherapy

Hydrotherapy is not indicated for this patient.

Acupuncture

Acupuncture is not indicated unless the dog has postoperative pancreatitis, when acupuncture might be considered as an adjunct to analgesia (see Case 19.3).

Other nursing and supportive care

Avoiding hypoglycaemia

Serum glucose concentration should be determined prior to surgery and the patient should receive a glucose infusion during surgery. An infusion of 5% glucose in crystalloid solution is advised at an administration rate of 10 ml/kg/h during the surgical procedure.

The patient should be monitored closely postoperatively for complications such as:

- Hyperglycaemia
- Persistent hypoglycaemia
- Pancreatitis.

In the immediate postoperative period, blood glucose should be monitored every hour for the first 4–6 hours and then every 2–4 hours, with the administration of dextrose boluses or dextrose infusions as necessary. Note: Some dogs may be normoglycaemic or hyperglycaemic following surgery and will not require dextrose-containing fluids.

Owner advice and homecare recommendations

Dealing with hypoglycaemia
The owners should be educated about the signs associated with hypoglycaemia, including lethargy, weakness, incoordination, seizures, nervousness, tremors and hunger. In severe cases the dog may become unconscious.

Feeding advice
Frequent feeding of small high-protein, low-carbohydrate meals in addition to exercise modification may control hypoglycaemia. However, if the dog has a poor appetite, it must be emphasized that *starvation is more hazardous than consumption of non-ideal foodstuffs*. In such cases the owner should encourage the dog to eat by offering palatable warm aromatic foods and by hand-feeding him.

Exercise
To maintain interest in walks on-lead (for owner and dog) activities such as stepping over obstacles, changes of direction, incorporating slopes/steps/different surfaces and transitions (e.g. walk-stop-walk, slow-fast-slow) can all be included and progressed according to ability. Owners should carry a source of complex carbohydrate, such as a biscuit, with them whenever they exercise the dog, for use in a hypoglycaemic attack.

Follow-up
In a patient in which euglycaemia has been achieved following partial pancreatectomy, relapse of insulinoma is exceptionally unlikely in the immediate short term; median remission duration for dogs achieving normoglycaemia following partial pancreatectomy is 496 days.

The client should be advised to bring the dog into the clinic if any signs of lethargy, listlessness or inappetence develop in the 2 weeks following surgery. Pancreatitis and diabetes mellitus can develop many days after surgery. The client should present the dog for serum glucose evaluation should they become concerned that he is showing signs of relapse, particularly during exercise.

In a patient with persistent hyperinsulinaemia, serial blood glucose determinations are advised, initially once every 2 weeks until the clinician is comfortable that the medication and management routine has resulted in satisfactory glycaemic control. The purpose of blood testing is to ensure that severe and persistent hypoglycaemia is not present. Satisfactory glycaemic control in these cases is defined most by clinical signs, not by a drive to achieve ideal blood glucose concentrations. Despite failure to maintain normal serum insulin concentrations, dogs can enjoy a surprisingly long period of remission from clinical signs of hypoglycaemia on a combination of strategic husbandry and prednisolone therapy; median remission duration in one study was approximately 15 months.

Median survival time for patients undergoing partial pancreatectomy for insulinoma is 785 days.

Case 15.6
Leukaemia in a cat

A 7-year-old male neutered DSH cat was presented with a 3-week history of inappetence, weight loss and increased thirst. His BCS was 3/9. He was an indoor/outdoor cat.

Examination revealed abdominal organomegaly and dehydration.

Haematological evaluation demonstrated a moderate anaemia (PCV 16%) and a marked (95%) lymphocytosis (WBC 51.3 x 10^9/l; reference range 6.0–15.0). His neutrophil count was at the low end of normal and his platelet count slightly below normal (107 x 10^9/l; reference range 150–550). There was some variability in the size of the lymphocytes; the enlarged forms had irregular nuclei with fine granular chromatin and increased cytoplasm.

Blood biochemistry was unremarkable apart from mild elevations in urea (11.35 mmol/l; reference range 5.0–10.0) and creatinine (158 µmol/l; reference range 40.0–150.0) and an elevated total bilirubin (13 µmol/l; reference range 0–10 µmol/l). Blood tests for FeLV and FIV were negative.

Abdominal ultrasonography revealed enlarged and uniformly echogenic liver and spleen and enlarged hypoechogenic mesenteric lymph nodes. Fine needle aspiration of the liver, spleen and bone marrow revealed a predominance of mature lymphocytes, resulting in a diagnosis of chronic lymphocytic leukaemia.

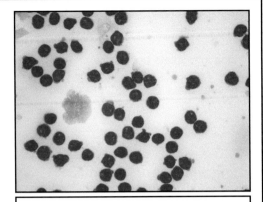

There is a predominance of mature lymphocytic cells in this peripheral blood sample from a cat with chronic lymphocytic leukaemia. Wright's stain; original magnification X400.

Agreed medical/surgical management

The patient was treated with vincristine, chlorambucil and prednisolone.

Drugs	Weeks 1–4	Weeks 5–12 (provided patient is in complete remission)	Weeks 13+ (provided patient is in complete remission)
Vincristine	0.5 mg/m² i.v. q7d	0.5 mg/m² i.v. q14d	0.5 mg/m² i.v. q28d
Chlorambucil	20 mg/m² orally q14d	20 mg/m² orally q14d	20 mg/m² orally q14d
Prednisolone	For the first 7 days: 5 mg/cat orally q24h Then: 5 mg/cat orally q48h	No further prednisolone therapy	No further prednisolone therapy

Treatment plan for feline chronic lymphocytic leukaemia. On identification of relapse, treatment is recommenced from the start but *without* prednisolone. Blood is taken for haematology prior to institution of therapy, then prior to every second vincristine treatment. (Source: Polton and Elwood, 2008)

The patient achieved a prompt complete remission, but this lasted only 90 days. After this time the cat experienced a period of waxing and waning disease that correlated with administration of cytotoxic therapy. During relapse the spleen was palpably grossly enlarged and this corresponded with episodes of listlessness and anorexia.

The patient was moderately to severely anaemic on initial presentation and this improved with initial therapy, with the PCV reaching 26% by Day 29 of treatment. This was sustained until Day 71 when the PCV was recorded at 23%. With continued treatment the cat developed a progressive non-regenerative anaemia with a PCV of 18% recorded.

Once relapse was detected, the objective of treatment in this case was palliation of clinical signs rather than attainment of another complete remission at all costs. In this situation it is appropriate to attempt to define the least chemotherapy that can be given to achieve the required goal. It is therefore not unusual to see a waxing and waning nature to the signs, as described here. Non-regenerative anaemia develops for a combination of reasons, including chronic disease, chronic myelosuppressive drug administration and intermittent inappetence. More aggressive management of the leukaemia would promote further deterioration in haematological parameters. Failure to treat the leukaemia in this case led to rapid deterioration in constitutional signs.

Non-regenerative anaemia can be treated with recombinant erythropoietin. Treatment is administered by subcutaneous injection two or three times a week until a satisfactory PCV is achieved. Further treatment can be given to maintain a stable PCV as indicated by PCV evaluations. Typically, six treatments given over 2 weeks will establish a stable PCV between 22 and 27%, and a single dose once every 2 weeks thereafter will sustain this. Erythropoietin administration has been associated with immunological reactions that result in failure of the exogenous product to elicit a beneficial effect. This is typically seen 8–10 weeks into treatment. There are reports of human patients who have received recombinant erythropoietin developing an immunological reaction not only to the exogenous drug but also to their own endogenous hormone, resulting in a considerable deterioration and, in rare cases, aplastic anaemia.

Acute/chronic pain management

Although this condition is not usually considered to be painful, pain assessment should be performed on a regular basis and a treatment plan formulated if necessary. NSAIDs are contraindicated because of prednisolone in the treatment protocol.

Fear, stress, conflict concerns

This patient sounds relatively easy to treat, but he may not stay that way with repeated interventions and when he feels unwell. Additional stress will not help either with the condition or with his general wellbeing. There are two major considerations: treatment and handling at the veterinary clinic; and the patient's home environment.

At the veterinary clinic

- Reward and reinforce any positive experiences and associations with the veterinary practice and its team. Use positive touch (stroking and rubbing around the chin, grooming with a massaging groomer, gentle stroking of the chest) to release mood neurotransmitters, drop the blood pressure and encourage bonding.
- Take time with the patient to help him relax before any intervention.
- Pheromone therapy may be helpful, although its efficacy in such situations is not clear.
- Minimize exposure to potential stressors such as dogs and other cats; noises and strong odours.
- Ideally this patient will remain in hospital for only minimal periods of time sufficient for appropriate evaluations and treatment to be administered. In the event that he needs to be admitted, use the space in the cage to provide a hiding area (a cardboard box will do with a blanket or bedding over it) and visual baffles (a towel over the cage door or hung to separate the cage so the cat can *choose* to see and be seen or to hide).
- Use minimal restraint during procedures where possible.

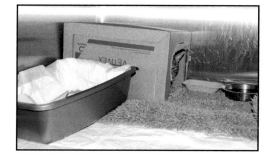

A cardboard box can be used to fashion a hiding place within a cat's cage. (Courtesy of Rachel Lumbis)

At home

The cat will feel unwell sometimes. Enhancing the environment will help him feel better (help him cope with his discomfort more easily), but it is also necessary to make some adjustments so that an inactive and unwell patient can still exploit these improvements.

- **Food.** This patient is inappetent and may need his appetite stimulating. Novel areas and food delivery may be helpful if an unpleasant association has been made with the routine feeding bowl/area. These should not be removed, however, but rather alternatives added elsewhere. Ensure the cat can easily reach the food (if he has previously fed at a height he may not feel like jumping), so adjust the position of the food, whilst making sure this does not make the cat anxious about it being available to competitors (the pet dog or a possible intruding cat if the food is placed near the cat flap, for example).
- **Water.** Cats generally prefer their water about a room's distance away from their food in a clear, wide bowl so provide extra water bowls.
- **Access inside and out.** Cats would normally have more than one access in and out of their core territory (usually the house). Consider providing a second access point or ensure that the cat can use the existing access points (they are not too high or too difficult to negotiate when the cat feels unwell and uncomfortable).
- **Scratching posts.** Are these easily accessible and appropriate for the patient? If the cat tends to scratch on horizontal surfaces, then a horizontal scratch post can be provided. If the post is an integral part of a piece of cat furniture then the patient must still be able to reach it if he does not feel up to climbing.
- **Hiding areas.** Provide multiple safe and comfortable hiding areas at different levels or make sure that there is a 'step' system to allow the cat to reach his old favourite places.
- **Beds.** Provision of new beds such as radiator beds may improve the comfort and wellbeing of patient.
- **Play.** Modify games to very short bursts of gentle play, but continue to try to gently stimulate the cat.
- **Touch.** Use gentle touch, stroking and grooming in ways that the patient will not only tolerate but enjoy, to improve feelings of wellbeing and also to give the owner a sense of participating in their pet's treatment and nursing.

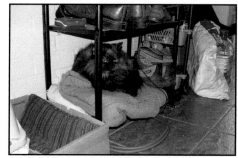

Hiding areas should be available at various levels, including at low level if the cat cannot climb. (© Samantha Elmhurst)

Encouraging and monitoring food intake

The cat is underweight and his food intake needs to be monitored closely. He is reported to be intermittently inappetent and is therefore going to require encouragement to feed. This might take the form of trying his usual favourite foods while in the hospital or warming the food or adding strongly smelling foods such as pilchards. Firm stroking sometimes encourages anorexic tractable cats to eat. On the other hand, some cats prefer to eat in privacy, so putting a towel over the front of the cage may help. In the short term, use of appetite stimulants may help to get the cat started with eating (see Chapter 5). However, if the cat is not easily eating his RER within 3 days, consideration should be given to placing a feeding tube, especially as he is debilitated and future treatments may also put him off his food.

Even though he is underweight, this cat would be at significant risk of hepatic lipidosis and other serious metabolic derangements if he suffered from prolonged anorexia in combination with the neoplasia and chemotherapy. It is therefore very important that, even if he is not tube-fed, his daily calorie intake is carefully monitored and action taken if this fails consistently to meet the RER.

Nutritional support

The waxing and waning nature of the disease and the insidious catabolic effect have resulted in a debilitated state. The various treatments can also have adverse effects on food intake and, therefore, unless encouragement to eat works rapidly and effectively, initiation of nutritional support via the placement of feeding tubes such as an oesophagostomy or gastrostomy tube is recommended (see Chapter 5). With a feeding tube in place the owner can supplement food when the cat has episodic bouts of inappetence and this will allow better maintenance of body condition.

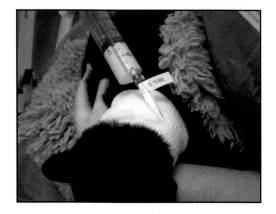

This cat is being fed via an oesophagostomy tube. (Courtesy of Rachel Lumbis)

Diet

It is most important that this cat eats some type of balanced diet for cats that he finds palatable. The type fed is of secondary consideration. Although nutritional strategies have been devised for *dogs* with lymphoid neoplasia, this has not been applied to *cats*. The approach in dogs (see Case 15.2) has included reducing the amount of simple carbohydrates in the diet and increasing protein and fat. Much of the fat content is derived from omega-3 fatty acids. The effectiveness of these diets in cats is unknown. A similar type of diet (with high fat and low carbohydrates, although without the specific increases in omega-3 fatty acids) might be achieved with some of the feline high-protein diabetic diets.

Nutraceuticals

Antioxidant supplementation has also been proposed in cases of neoplasia, especially in animals being treated with chemotherapeutic agents. However, currently there is no evidence supporting a beneficial role of antioxidants in this context and there is some evidence, at least in human patients, that antioxidants can actually have adverse effects in neoplasia (Palozza *et al.*, 2008), so at present their use cannot be recommended.

Physiotherapy is not indicated for this patient.

Hydrotherapy is not indicated for this patient.

There is no evidence that acupuncture can influence this disease one way or the other, but it may be helpful in palliation of some of the signs. Cats often tolerate acupuncture surprisingly well and it is worth considering in many cases; cats appear to respond to acupuncture overall better than dogs, probably because they are a very reactive species and acupuncture is, after all, an unusual stimulus.

Appetite stimulation

Anecdotally, acupuncture has been used to stimulate appetite in anorexic cats; this may be via its effects on feelings of nausea, or via some other mechanism (experimental work in rats demonstrates that needling at ST36, a point in tibialis cranialis, just below the stifle, significantly reduces the production of stomach acid, for example). Generalized humoral effects such as the release of endorphins and other neurotransmitters may improve general feelings of comfort and wellbeing.

Relieving side effects of chemotherapy

One specific indication for acupuncture in animals receiving chemotherapy is the relief of nausea and vomiting (see Case 15.1).

Safety concerns

The primary safety concern with the use of acupuncture in patients receiving chemotherapy for cancer is the increased risk of infection with needling if the patient is significantly immunosuppressed. This risk should be discussed with the owner and acupuncture treatment structured around favourable blood results.

Other nursing and supportive care

Care of feeding tube

If a feeding tube has been placed, this should be monitored carefully as the majority of complications involve tube occlusion or localized irritation at the tube exit site. Full details of feeding and tube care are given in Chapter 5. Bodyweight should be monitored daily for patients receiving enteral nutritional support.

Preparation and administration of chemotherapy

See also the Introduction to this chapter and the photos in Cases 15.1 and 15.2.

Owner advice and homecare recommendations

Paying attention to the cat's home environment, as noted above (see Fear, stress), may aid his recovery.

Care of feeding tube

If the cat is discharged with a feeding tube in place, the owner needs to be given clear instructions on tube care and how to administer food. A demonstration should be given on all aspects and the owner encouraged to demonstrate this back to check their understanding.

Once the feeding tube has been removed, the owner should be advised on how to care for the wound and how to encourage the cat to feed, e.g. offer highly palatable, aromatic, warm food, hand-fed if necessary.

References

Palozza P, Simone R and Mele MC (2008) Interplay of carotenoids with cigarette smoking: implications in lung cancer. *Current Medicinal Chemistry* **15**, 844–854

Polton G and Elwood CM (2008) Pulmonary oedema as a suspected adverse drug reaction following vincristine administration to a cat: a case report. *The Veterinary Journal* **177**, 130–133

Case 15.7
Sarcoma in a cat

An 8-year-old neutered male DSH cat was presented with an interscapular mass that the owner reported had appeared over a period of 8 days. The cat's BCS was 5/9. He was an indoor cat – with attitude!

General physical examination was otherwise unremarkable and thoracic radiography was normal. A biopsy confirmed that the mass was a sarcoma. Because of its rapid onset and position, it was deemed to be an 'injection site sarcoma'.

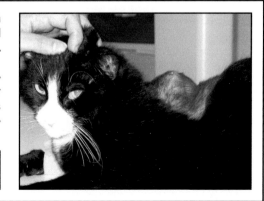

Large interscapular tumour diagnosed on incisional biopsy as an injection site sarcoma.

The cat was managed using a combination of surgery and epirubicin chemotherapy.

Planned treatment protocol

1. Epirubicin is administered by slow intravenous infusion once every 3 weeks for a total of three doses, provided there is evidence of a sustained beneficial effect. The tumour is measured using calipers to ensure objectivity.
2. Following completion of the first chemotherapy protocol, an MRI scan of the tumour and surrounding tissue is performed to delineate the precise anatomical location of the tumour for surgical planning. In some cases, MRI will indicate that definitive surgery is inappropriate because it would induce too much morbidity or because the probability of complete removal is too low.
3. Following surgery, the wound is managed with a closed active suction drain and intralesional administration of local analgesia (bupivacaine) using a wound diffusion catheter.
4. After adequate time for postoperative wound healing, typically 7–10 days, a further three chemotherapy treatments are given, as before, once every 3 weeks.

All chemotherapy treatments are preceded by haematological evaluation to ensure there is no evidence of myelosuppression that should result in a postponement of treatment. Renal parameters must also be assessed, as epirubicin is potentially nephrotoxic and anorexia causes dehydration which will promote nephrotoxic effects. Renal dysfunction induced by epirubicin can remain stable if further chemotherapy is not given, though there will undoubtedly be some negative impact on the patient's prognosis, whether due to tumour- or kidney-related events, and therefore consideration should be given to whether radical surgery remains indicated.

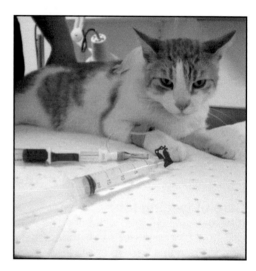

Cat receiving chemotherapy for an injection site sarcoma. Note the totally enclosed needle-free, Luer lock system. The larger syringe contains (colourless) physiological saline for dilution of the epirubicin and for flushing the catheter before and after administration of the drug. The total volume of fluid administered over 25 minutes is 25 ml.

Side effects

In this cat, chemotherapy-induced nausea developed following the first dose of epirubicin. Short-term care involved intravenous fluid support, antiemetic therapy (metoclopramide 1 mg/kg q24h CRI) and provision of warmed strongly smelling foods to tempt him to eat.

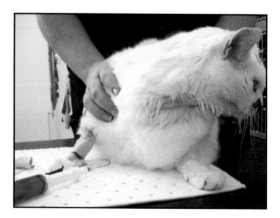

Anthracycline agents such as epirubicin, and other chemotherapeutics, are known to induce taste changes in humans and it is believed that they do the same in veterinary species. In the cat shown here, chemotherapy triggered marked ptyalism starting approximately 3 minutes into every treatment and finishing promptly once the infusion was complete. Other patients show a reduced appetite, which can last up to 5 days after chemotherapy administration.

The chemotherapy dose was reduced by 10% for the subsequent treatments and mild signs of nausea were noted for less than 12 hours after each treatment, so no specific therapy was administered to counter these effects.

In some patients undergoing radical surgical excision of large tumours, significant persistent pruritus develops. The true pathogenesis of this is unknown and it is extremely challenging to manage. The best treatment is prevention, which appears to be achieved satisfactorily by avoiding resection of large areas of skin and subcutis such that significant tension is then applied to the remaining skin edges when closure is achieved.

Perioperative

A full mu agonist opioid should be included in the premedication. Medetomidine may also be used if there is no underlying cardiovascular disease.

Ketamine CRI should be administered during the procedure. Ketamine is preferred here because of toxicity and efficacy concerns about the use of lidocaine CRI in cats. It is readily available in most practices.

Postoperatively, the cat will need good quality analgesia for several days; full mu agonist opioids can be continued initially, with a change to buprenorphine by the second postoperative day. The ketamine CRI can be continued for up to 48 hours postoperatively unless dysphoria is a problem. Intractable postoperative pain may necessitate either intermittent boluses or CRI of medetomidine.

A wound diffusion catheter could be placed during surgery to allow local perfusion of the wound bed with an appropriate analgesic; bupivacaine is the agent of choice and wound diffusion catheters are commercially available for this purpose. NSAID therapy could also be provided perioperatively unless there is evidence of renal dysfunction on previous blood tests.

Chronic pain

Once he is home, the cat should be assessed by monitoring any behavioural changes, by physical examination of the wound site and by watching for postural changes and restricted mobility (muscular pain from myofascial trigger points would be pertinent here, see Chapters 3 and 11). Ideally, the cat's general behaviour at home should have been assessed prior to surgery, so that changes after surgery can be quickly identified as being probably due to pain, although the contribution of potential psychological upset (see below) to altered behaviour postoperatively should also not be underestimated.

Wound pain and healing may be treated with acupuncture (see below) to attempt to reduce the drug burden for the patient. NSAIDs (those safely metabolized by the cat), if tolerated, would be the first-line treatment for pain. It is important to check renal function first, as NSAIDs are contraindicated in renal failure. Gabapentin or amitriptyline may be helpful if there are indications of allodynia or hyperalgesia. Amitriptyline may also help with pruritus; it requires competent renal and hepatic function for clearance, and should be used with caution in patients with existing cardiac arrhythmias. The pharmacokinetics of gabapentin in the cat are unknown but it would seem wise to assume some degree of renal and hepatic clearance/detoxification. Oral transmucosal buprenorphine may also be helpful (see Chapter 3).

Fear, stress, conflict concerns

Aggression

This cat is described as having 'attitude'. Aggression in cats is often misunderstood as being related to being deliberately difficult or associated with control of resources. In reality, aggression is shown either because the cat is anxious about interaction and has learnt that aggression is a successful strategy to avoid the perceived threat, or because of inappropriate learning about interaction with people during development. Since this cat is likely to have experienced pain, and aggression is associated with approach for handling, its 'attitude' is likely to be a defensive response. Minimizing stressful handling would be ideal, together with a desensitization and counter-conditioning programme, where the cat learns to approach people for a positive outcome, such as food. This type of programme can be started in the clinic with the owners encouraged to continue it after the cat is sent home (see *BSAVA Manual of Canine and Feline Behavioural Medicine*) .

Minimizing stress at the clinic

Measures that can be taken are outlined in Case 15.6. It should be noted, however, that feline facial pheromone fraction 4 is not indicated where cats are anxious or aggressive about the approach of hands: where the olfactory signal gives one message to the cat, and yet visual cues suggest an approaching threat, the resulting emotional conflict can cause a more extreme aggressive response.

Postoperative confinement

Being confined after surgery could have an impact on a cat that is used to having control of their territory and core territory. Enhancing the core territory or environment (see Case 15.6) will help such a cat to cope with frustration and/or discomfort more easily.

Pruritus

The use of plastic claw covers, on the hindpaws, may be helpful in reducing self-trauma due to pruritus. These covers should remain in place until the wound site is healed, but it should be borne in mind that the cat's climbing and defensive abilities will be reduced.

Nutritional requirements

Perioperative

It is important to monitor this cat's food intake while he is hospitalized, before and after surgery and during chemotherapy. The combined effects of the surgery, analgesic drugs and the cat's temperament may make him unwilling to eat in the hospital. If he eats significantly less than the calculated RER for more than 3 days, action should be taken to increase food intake. It is unlikely that an appetite stimulant or encouragement will be effective for this cat, and some type of tube feeding may be necessary (naso-oesophageal or oesophagostomy would be most appropriate in this case).

Longer-term nutrition

If nausea persists during the course of chemotherapy, this may negatively impact appetite and food intake. If antiemetic therapy such as maropitant is not effective at controlling nausea, nutritional support may require placement of an oesophagostomy feeding tube. There are no specific nutritional requirements for cases such as these. If a feeding tube is placed, gruel-type diets are typically used. These diets are typically high in protein and fat and can meet energy requirements with smaller volumes and fewer meals. It has been suggested that *dogs* with neoplasia should be fed diets higher in fat and lower in carbohydrates than normal (see earlier cases) although the evidence for the effectiveness of this in dogs is limited and in cats, there is no evidence. However, most cat 'critical care' diets fulfil these requirements.

Physiotherapy

There are several physiotherapeutic approaches that may be considered for this cat in respect of pain and reduced mobility, but these will obviously depend on his acceptance of treatment. Physiotherapy assessment would help identify the specific causes of the mobility problems, and treatments such as joint mobilizations and soft tissue therapies (e.g. massage, myofascial release, acupressure, trigger pointing) may be beneficial for both pain relief and mobility. Exercises to promote mobility and maintain strength, flexibility and balance/proprioception should be prescribed, and will generally offer a less hands-on approach if the cat is not amenable to handling.

The use of electrotherapy (ultrasound, laser) to help with wound healing and pain relief can be helpful, although should *not* be applied to areas of active neoplasia or recent irradiation. TENS (for pain relief) is not always easy to use in animals with 'attitude' because of the length of time it needs to be applied for, but if it can be used it is quite relaxing due to the release of endorphins. Through careful placement of electrodes TENS can be applied distant from the actual site of operation (i.e. on a more comfortable body area) yet still provide effective pain relief through pain gate activity and/or endogenous opioid release.

Hydrotherapy

Hydrotherapy is not indicated for this patient.

Acupuncture

It should not be assumed that cats with 'attitude' will not be amenable to acupuncture; it is well worth trying in cats of any character, since they may be sensitive and profoundly sedated by the treatment.

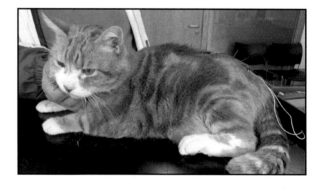

Electroacupuncture may produce sedation in cats.
(Courtesy of Samantha Lindley)

Chronic pain

Pain around the area of surgery and in the related muscles may be treated by local needling to the level of muscle in healthy tissue. The cat should be examined for secondary muscle pain and pain secondary to postural changes.

Wound healing

There is good experimental evidence in rats and clinical evidence in human patients for a role for acupuncture in promoting wound healing. This effect is mediated by the local release of neurotransmitters and vasodilation. Needles should be placed in healthy tissue as close as possible to the edge of the wound, about 2.5 cm apart, to the depth of tissue that requires healing (i.e. in this case, into muscle). The treatment should be repeated twice a week. Evidence suggests that this approach can be used as needed if the wound shows signs of poor healing.

Pruritus

Acupuncture *may* reduce pruritus, although the effects are by no means certain. It may be that it improves wound healing and reduces pain rather than affecting the pruritus *per se*. Local needling around the wound site is the preferred treatment of choice, although some 'strong' general points such as Li11 and ST36 may also be useful or necessary if local needling is not tolerated by the cat.

Relieving side effects of chemotherapy

See Case 15.1.

Safety concerns

The primary safety concern with using acupuncture in patients receiving chemotherapy for cancer is the increased risk of infection with needling if the patient is significantly immunosuppressed. This risk should be discussed with the owner and acupuncture treatment structured around favourable blood results.

Other nursing and supportive care

Postoperative wound care is described in Chapter 12. Use and care of feeding tubes are detailed in Chapter 5. Bodyweight should be monitored daily for patients receiving enteral nutritional support.

Handling a fractious cat

Scruffing the cat should be avoided. Restraint aids such as a cat bag, muzzle or towel may be used, if necessary, but taking into account the points made in 'Fear, stress' above.

Preparation and administration of chemotherapy

This is detailed in the Introduction to this chapter. Epirubicin carries some specific risks: severe and extensive tissue necrosis secondary to extravasation; and nephrotoxicity associated with cumulative dosing.

Owner advice and homecare recommendations

Waste disposal

The owner should be advised to treat urine, faeces and vomit from the cat as though it were contaminated by cytotoxic drugs for the duration of the chemotherapy protocol. While there are data that indicate that faeces remain contaminated for 3–5 days after treatment administration, this author [GP] advises that direct contact with urine and faeces is avoided for the entire duration of the protocol. Faeces should be recovered from wherever they were deposited and disposed of down the toilet. Owners should dilute any urine passed; this can be difficult if the cat has access to outdoors, so confining the cat indoors or to a small area of the garden for the first 3 days after drug administration will enable the owners to minimize the potential risks of environmental contamination.

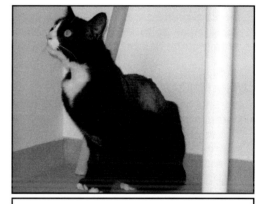

The cat one week after surgery, on the day of discharge.

Vaccination

There is no doubt that injection site sarcomas are induced by inflammatory reactions that are triggered by the act of injection. Most data implicate adjuvanted vaccines as the aetiological factors of greatest significance; but injection site sarcomas have been seen in cats that have never received a vaccination, so other injections must also be considered potential threats, including lufenuron and microchip implantation.

There are data to suggest that certain cats are predisposed. It is rational to assume that if this is the case, a cat that has already experienced an injection site sarcoma is likely to be one of them. For this reason, it is advised that cats that have previously suffered an injection site sarcoma NEVER receive an adjuvanted vaccination product again, by any route. Any other injections that are intended for subcutaneous or intramuscular administration should only be given subject to a risk/benefit analysis discussion with the client. This discussion will necessarily have to address the fact that the true risk of a further neoplastic event cannot be quantified, but there needs to be an awareness on both sides that a similar event could occur.

If there were to be a second tumour in a similar location, the overwhelming likelihood is that it would represent a relapse of the previous tumour rather than a new tumour induced by injection of a different product after the first tumour was managed. However, continued vaccination, particularly the practice of vaccination in an extremity, would conclusively prove whether a subsequent injection were guilty of inducing a subsequent tumour.

Many owners of cats that have experienced an injection site sarcoma have other cats and they are naturally exceptionally concerned that they receive the best advice in deciding how to manage these. The emotional distress of learning that a probably fatal condition will arise through following trusted veterinary advice to adhere to a vaccination protocol in the first place is hard to measure and the owners may be unwilling therefore to vaccinate their other cats. The importance of an annual health check should be emphasized and the risks of non-vaccination compared with the very low relative incidence of injection site sarcomas should be honestly appraised with the owner.

Vaccination is an act of veterinary medicine and as such should be subject to the same rigorous risk/benefit analysis that all veterinary procedures are subject to. Not all cats are exposed to the same risks of contracting infectious disease. Owners should be adequately informed to make an educated choice about vaccination for their cats based upon local factors, husbandry factors and their own attitude to risk. The owners should be advised that dogs are NOT predisposed to these tumours.

The reported prognosis for cats with this condition is remarkably variable. One of the most significant factors in determining prognosis is the quality of surgery performed. Median survival times quoted range from 2 months to 2 years. This author's [GP's] own observations (unpublished data) are that these cases can be cured but the likelihood of a cure is significantly adversely affected by incomplete early attempts to perform a biopsy or excise the mass.

Case 15.8
Pituitary tumour and acromegaly in a cat

A 12-year-old neutered female DSH cat was presented with poorly controlled diabetes mellitus (DM) requiring high doses of insulin. Prior to presentation the owners suspected that she had developed total blindness, as she had started walking into chair and table legs around the house and had shown a reduced enthusiasm for outdoor life. The DM had been identified 6 months earlier and had required steadily increasing doses of insulin to maintain some degree of glycaemic control. Serial blood glucose curves indicated that the cat had insulin resistance. On presentation the cat was of substantial build (BCS 8/9) with obviously large paws and interdental spacing evident on oral examination. The cat appeared to be very relaxed.

At the time of presentation the cat was receiving 28 IU lente insulin twice daily. Blood tests revealed mild elevations of urea (13.6 mmol/l; reference range 3–10) and alkaline phosphatase (52 IU/l; reference range 0–50) but routine biochemical and haematological evaluations were otherwise unremarkable, apart from a fasting hyperglycaemia. The mild elevation in urea was considered to be due to pre-renal causes.

Acromegaly was diagnosed on the basis of high serum insulin-like growth factor 1 (1488 ng/ml; reference range <1000). A pituitary mass, suspected to be a macroadenoma, was diagnosed on MRI.

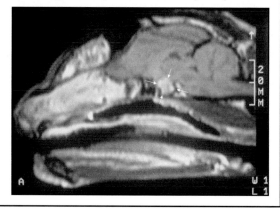

Sagittal MRI scan image of a cat with pituitary macroadenoma (T1W, post-gadolinium). (Reproduced from Littler *et al.*, 2006)

Agreed medical/surgical management

The cat was treated with radiotherapy, employing a once-weekly course of five fractions. Treatment was administered on an outpatient basis, with hospital stays lasting no more than 45 minutes at a time. Each treatment was performed under short-acting general anaesthetic with an endotracheal tube in place. Acromegaly can induce significant soft tissue proliferation, which can result in airway compromise under anaesthetic, though this was not the case in this patient.

Restoration of normal glycaemic control is unpredictable in patients undergoing radiotherapy for a functional pituitary macroadenoma. The cat's blood glucose concentration should be closely monitored, as hypoglycaemia can develop quickly without apparent warning; insulin doses will need to be changed over the following 6 months. The optimal method of blood glucose testing is home testing by the owners using an ear prick device (see Case 19.5). This can be performed daily or weekly or as the veterinary surgeon deems appropriate. Once radiotherapy has started, the owner should be aware of possible behavioural changes that might indicate a change in glycaemic control, such as altered appetite and thirst, reduced urination and altered energy levels. If owners are comfortable with home testing, weekly veterinary assessments are likely to be adequate for the first 6 weeks. If any behavioural changes are noted, additional blood glucose evaluations can be performed and the owners should be educated on how to react given different glycaemic situations.

In this cat, normoglycaemia returned quickly and all insulin was withdrawn within 10 weeks of commencing radiotherapy. Visual function returned before the third once-weekly treatment was performed and there was no return of neurological signs for the rest of the cat's life.

More than half of acromegalic diabetic cases treated in this way will experience complete remission of their DM but not their acromegaly. This interesting phenomenon is not clearly understood but it is important to note that progressive changes in other organs will develop associated with acromegaly. Terminal consequences are typically renal failure or cardiac failure due to hypertrophic cardiomyopathy. These potential consequences should be regularly screened for in patients that respond well to radiotherapy. In this cat, there was no evidence of renal insufficiency on blood evaluations performed later in the radiotherapy protocol but she did develop renal insufficiency 6 months after completion of the radiotherapy course, and this ultimately proved terminal.

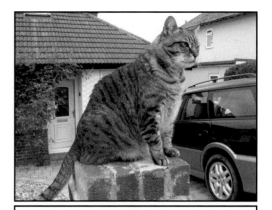

The cat 4 months after completion of the treatment course; enthusiasm for outdoor life has returned. (Reproduced from Littler *et al.*, 2006)

Acute/chronic pain management

The cat was regularly assessed for changes in behaviour that might indicate pain; none were recognized. Pain is rarely apparent in acromegalic cats. When pain is recognized it is usually in association with more marked neurological deficits and those patients rarely, if ever, respond adequately to radiotherapy.

Fear, stress, conflict concerns

Anecdotally, cats with acromegaly are often more 'laid back' than other cats. However, although the cat appears to be very relaxed it is important to look for subtle signs that might indicate anxiety about specific cues. Many cats appear superficially inactive or unresponsive to events, despite high physiological indicators of stress. Equally, behavioural inhibition may be a clinical sign (e.g. of pain) rather than the cat's natural response style. Signs of approach or positive reactions to people would be a better indication of a positive perception of handling than a passive response.

Furthermore, although the patient may be relatively easy to treat initially, she may not stay that way with repeated interventions or when she feels unwell. Additional stress will not help with her condition or general wellbeing and is best avoided (see Case 15.6).

Nutritional requirements

Nutritional management of diabetes mellitus
Acromegaly causes marked insulin resistance, so dietary therapy is unlikely to have a significant impact on diabetic control in this cat. Nevertheless, it is important to keep her daily calorie intake as stable as possible. She will have problems with fluctuating insulin requirements after radiotherapy and altering daily calorie intake would just add another, unwanted variable. Meal feeding is much less important in diabetic cats than in diabetic dogs (because the postprandial glucose peak is less significant in cats) and *ad libitum* feeding is tolerated as long as it is consistent from day to day.

Older feline diabetic diets included the use of dietary fibre (both soluble and non-soluble types) and components aimed at weight loss. More recently, an approach has been developed for type II DM in cats, which includes low-carbohydrate and high-protein diets. This can result in significant reduction in insulin requirements in some cats with type II DM and even reversion to a non-diabetic state. However, this approach has not been applied or evaluated in cats with acromegaly and DM. It is unclear whether such an approach would aid in this cat, as the marked insulin resistance induced by circulating growth hormone is likely to overwhelm any beneficial effect.

Weight management
This cat's BCS (8/9) indicates that she is obese. However, much of that bodyweight increase is likely to be a direct result of the acromegaly and may resolve on successful treatment. If obesity remains a problem, a careful weight loss programme should be considered (see Chapter 6), bearing in mind the concurrent requirements for DM control.

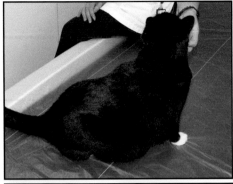
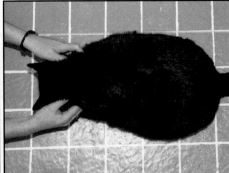
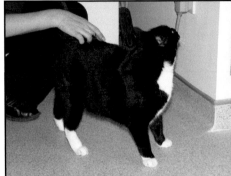
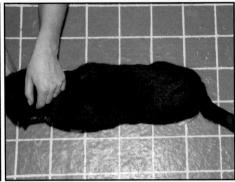

Photographs of a 7-year-old neutered male DSH cat, taken before **(top)** and after weight loss. Starting bodyweight was 10.30 kg (BCS 9/9), the final weight was 6.45 kg (BCS 5/9), and percentage weight loss was 37%. The weight loss programme took 490 days, and the mean rate of weight loss was 0.53% per week. (Courtesy of The Royal Canin Weight Management Clinic, University of Liverpool)

Physiotherapy

Physiotherapy is not indicated for this patient.

Hydrotherapy

Hydrotherapy is not indicated for this patient.

Acupuncture

Acupuncture is not indicated for this patient.

Other nursing and supportive care

Stabilization of diabetes mellitus

It should be noted that diabetic patients undergoing radiotherapy can experience an alteration in exogenous insulin requirement and subsequent unpredictability in the control of their diabetes. Blood glucose should be regularly monitored and insulin doses reduced as necessary when glucose concentrations fall.

Owner advice and homecare recommendations

Diabetes management and control

As this cat is already on insulin therapy, it is assumed that the owner has already been advised on correct storage, mixing, measuring and administration of insulin. The most important message for this cat's owners is that her insulin requirement can *change* precipitously as a result of the radiotherapy. For this reason, serial blood glucose monitoring is required. The technique that allows this with the least anxiety for the cat is optimal and a technique which can be applied at any time of concern is preferred. For this reason home testing is ideal. Owners should be trained to obtain blood using an ear-prick kit and trained to read and record blood glucose measurements accurately (see Case 19.1). A once-weekly blood glucose evaluation is a rational minimum but if the owner is comfortable and confident with the technique they can also perform impromptu checks at times when the cat's behaviour may indicate a possible hypoglycaemic episode. The owner should be educated to look for changes such as listlessness and alterations in urination and appetite. In the event of a diabetic complication or hypoglycaemic episode, food should be offered to the cat. Hypoglycaemia is harder to reverse quickly in cats than in dogs, so if the owners are worried they should ring the surgery urgently.

Disease progression

The owner should be informed about signs of disease progression, including degenerative arthropathies, congestive heart failure and renal failure. Pituitary tumours may cause local neurological damage resulting in stupor, somnolence, poor appetite, adipsia, temperature deregulation, circling, seizures, and changes in behaviour.

References

Littler RM, Polton GA and Brearley MJ (2006) Resolution of diabetes mellitus but not acromegaly in a cat with a pituitary macroadenoma treated with hypofractionated radiation. *Journal of Small Animal Practice* **47**, 392–395

16

Patients with cardiac disease

Edited by Ruth Willis

Introduction

Cardiac disease is commonly encountered in small animal practice and is usually an acquired condition in middle-aged and older dogs and cats. On detecting signs of cardiac disease, such as a cardiac murmur on auscultation, further investigation is indicated to determine the underlying cause and severity of the problem (see *BSAVA Manual of Canine and Feline Cardiorespiratory Medicine*). A proportion of patients with heart disease will show clinical signs related to congestive heart failure or arrhythmias (or a combination of both problems) and will require supportive care.

The palliative treatment of dogs and cats with heart disease is a challenging proposition for veterinary surgeons from both technical and emotional standpoints. However, this area also offers a unique opportunity to demonstrate the veterinary surgeon's overriding concern for animal welfare and understanding of the human–animal bond.

Supportive care for dogs with heart disease

Exercise

Provided that signs of acute heart failure are controlled, a regular exercise regime at a level that the dog can tolerate comfortably is appropriate and desirable for maintaining a routine and sustaining cardiovascular reserve. Shorter, more frequent walks during the cooler times of day may result in improved exercise tolerance, although owners should avoid exercising the dog to exhaustion. Although it is unlikely that exercise will cause a life-threatening event in cases with congestive heart failure secondary to degenerative atrioventricular valve disease, many owners will adjust where they walk the dog, avoiding remote areas without good vehicle access, and will carry a mobile phone to facilitate calling for help, especially if the dog is large and difficult to carry.

Managing respiratory distress

Management of acute respiratory distress is discussed in Chapter 17 and in the *BSAVA Manual of Canine and Feline Cardiorespiratory Medicine*.

Managing cachexia

Cachexia is common in congestive heart failure, particularly in dogs, and results from a combination of anorexia, in some dogs, and an increased breakdown of muscle mass associated with the increased energy demands in heart failure (see Chapter 5 for more details). Anorexia can be very frustrating for owners, particularly in patients that previously had a good appetite. Offering small, frequent, warm, odorous meals may be helpful, though owners will often report that foodstuffs eaten enthusiastically one day will be rejected the next.

Whilst a low-salt diet may be beneficial in enhancing the effects of diuretics, these diets sometimes appear to be poorly accepted and may result in aversion if introduced whilst the dog is unwell and hospitalized. Therefore, aiming to use these diets exclusively may not be beneficial if intake is minimal. For cases with advanced cardiac disease in particular, any calorie intake is better than no intake and therefore it may be acceptable to allow dogs to eat whatever they prefer, even if this may be nutritionally suboptimal.

There is some research suggesting that fish oil administration is useful in ameliorating the effects of the detrimental cytokines thought to be responsible for the cachexia seen in dogs with heart disease (Freeman *et al.,* 1998). However, if administration of fish oils appears to affect food palatability adversely, then their use should be discontinued.

Animals with cachexia often appear to age rapidly, sometimes in as little as a few weeks, and this may be a major factor in the decision to euthanase, even in cases where the other signs of congestive heart failure appear to be well controlled (Mallery *et al.,* 1999). Therefore, the impact of cachexia should not be overlooked and careful discussion with owners is required to facilitate consideration of how they are coping with this difficult issue.

Some drugs have appetite-stimulating effects; while they are not authorized for use for this application in small animals, they may be useful in some cases provided informed owner consent can be obtained.

Electrolyte balance

High doses of diuretics, as often used in congestive heart failure, have the potential to affect electrolyte balance adversely, particularly in anorexic patients that are at risk of hypokalaemia. Regular monitoring and, if required, diuretic dose adjustment may be required in anorexic patients; owners should be made aware of the need to contact their veterinary surgeon for advice if anorexia persists.

Monitoring

Regular monitoring is important to detect and pre-empt changes in the severity of heart disease. Owners often find it useful to be aware of 'intervention points' that may serve as rough guidelines on when it is necessary to contact the veterinary surgery for help. Some owners become adept at monitoring heart and respiratory rates at home, whereas others are better with more subjective criteria such as exercise tolerance and demeanour. Monitoring of clinical parameters, such as heart rate, respiratory rate and bodyweight, may be sufficient at some checks, but electrolyte balance and renal function should also be monitored regularly, particularly in anorexic patients.

If there is sudden worsening of respiratory distress, further tests may be required to establish the cause as this will dictate the most appropriate treatment. For example, dogs with congestive heart failure secondary to myxomatous atrioventricular valve disease may suddenly deteriorate due to worsening heart disease, resulting in further pulmonary oedema or a pleural effusion, development of a tachyarrhythmia (such as atrial fibrillation) or, less commonly, rupture of chordae tendinae or development of an atrial tear.

Providing support for owners

Regular contact with owners whose dogs have severe and terminal heart disease allows the veterinary surgeon to provide owners with emotional support from the objective standpoint of an experienced professional. Within a household there are often widely differing opinions regarding the severity of disease and the dog's quality of life. While these patients are unlikely to be in severe pain, owners are rightly concerned about the changes they see in their pet, which can progress at an alarming rate, especially in some large-breed dogs with dilated cardiomyopathy. The veterinary surgeon is expected to provide an objective assessment of the patient and to give information to guide the owners regarding disease progression.

Whilst, thankfully, the number of medical treatments available continues to increase, veterinary surgeons must ensure that the medication regimes recommended are practical for the owner:

- Medication that has to be given three times daily is awkward for owners working full time
- The timing of diuretic therapy should be adjusted to ensure that the dog is likely to urinate most at times convenient to the owner; this will help minimize 'inappropriate' urination in the house and nocturia, which are distressing for owners and pets
- Some clients find use of a pill box helpful to minimize the chances of administering the wrong medication; this is particularly important with anti-arrhythmic drugs, given the risks of toxicity and pro-arrhythmia.

Dealing with sudden death

Dogs with arrhythmias, particularly Boxers and Dobermanns, are at risk of collapse, which may be followed by sudden death. This presents a considerable emotional challenge for owners. Exercising the dog (see above) may become a stressful event instead of an enjoyable aspect of pet ownership and owners often describe the feeling of walking a 'time bomb'. Whilst minimizing exercise may not postpone this event, collapsing episodes at exercise may be embarrassing and stressful for owners, and guidelines need to be given about what to expect. Simple practical steps, such as ensuring that the airway is clear, can be advised to help owners feel they are doing something useful. Owners attempting cardiopulmonary–cerebral resuscitation in a rural environment are unlikely to be successful, and those who can accept a pragmatic approach of 'what will be will be' often cope best. However, this degree of detachment may be difficult to achieve for many normal owners.

Timing of euthanasia

Dogs with heart disease, even severe congestive heart failure, rarely die peacefully in their sleep. Owners are often understandably reluctant to ask about timing of euthanasia as, whilst they may find their pet's condition distressing, they do not wish to request euthanasia too late or too soon. Often there is no 'correct' time but, with careful discussion, owners can be provided with information that helps them to make an informed choice about the timing of euthanasia.

In cases where there is clearly a need for euthanasia but owners are reluctant because they feel that there is still 'some hope', setting objective criteria can sometimes be useful to help them to see that their pet is deteriorating. Using measures such as food intake, respiratory rate, clinicopathological data (particularly azotaemia) and heart rate can sometimes be more useful in providing objective evidence of decline, rather than relying on more subjective criteria such as level of activity.

Young dogs with heart disease

A considerable challenge for owners of puppies with heart disease, that are likely to have reduced life expectancy, is to treat these dogs as normally as possible with a normal routine and training to prevent or minimize behavioural problems and maximize quality of life. Euthanasia of young dogs with congenital heart disease is a particularly traumatic event for owners, even if the complications were anticipated, and extra support may be required.

Supportive care for cats with heart disease

The tenets mentioned above may be also applied to cats, bearing in mind a few, pertinent, species differences.

- Cats rarely cough and their tendency when diseased or in pain is to do very little except withdraw, so they may present with heart failure that is at a more advanced stage than when dogs are usually presented. At this time these cats are very fragile and measures should be taken to minimize stress and unnecessary diagnostic interventions until they are more stable.

- Anorexia may present a considerable challenge in cats and may be exacerbated by hypokalaemia in patients receiving furosemide. Appetite-stimulating drugs may be useful to ameliorate the general decline associated with this anorexia, although their efficacy is limited (see Chapter 5).
- Cats are often difficult to medicate and this may result in compromises in the medication regime. Such compromises may include the consideration of larger, less frequent doses of diuretics to minimize unpleasant cat–owner interactions at medication times. Diuretics may be given parenterally, or the whole day's medication placed in a single empty gelatin capsule and given as a single dose. Veterinary surgeons should be sensitive to, and understanding of, the difficulties owners experience when medicating cats and do their best to help owners to find a practical solution.

References and further reading

Freeman LM, Rush JE, Kehavias JJ *et al* (1998) Nutritional alterations and the effect of fish oil supplementation in dogs with heart failure. *Journal of Veterinary Internal Medicine* **12**, 440–448

Luis Fuentes V, Johnson L and Dennis S (2010) *BSAVA Manual of Canine and Feline Cardiorespiratory Medicine, 2nd edn.* BSAVA Publications, Gloucester

Mallery KF, Freeman LM, Harpster NK and Rush JE (1999) Factors contributing to the decision for euthanasia of dogs with congestive heart failure. *Journal of the American Veterinary Medical Association* **214**, 1201–1204

Clinical case studies

A variety of case scenarios in dogs and cats will now be presented to illustrate the considerations to be made and the options available within a specific clinical setting. Information relating to the rehabilitation and palliation of each condition has been contributed to each case by the authors in the first part of this Manual, plus notes on nursing and homecare from Rachel Lumbis RVN. The reader should refer back to the appropriate chapters for further details. Photographs used to illustrate the principles and techniques within the cases do not necessarily feature the original patient.

Case 16.1
Acute heart failure in a dog

A 4-year-old entire male Dobermann was presented with sudden-onset coughing and dyspnoea. He had marked dyspnoea and orthopnoea at rest and appeared anxious. His BCS was 4/9 and the owners reported that he was a fussy eater.

The dog had a respiratory rate of 60 breaths per minute and an irregular heart rate of 176 beats per minute. Femoral pulse quality was variable but generally weak with a pulse deficit. Mucous membranes were pale and extremities cool. There was a pink frothy bilateral nasal discharge. Cardiac auscultation revealed grade 3/6 systolic murmur, gallop sound and bilateral adventitious lung sounds.

The results of clinical examination suggested that the dog was showing signs of cardiogenic shock, with poor cardiac output. In view of his age and breed, dilated cardiomyopathy (DCM) resulting in congestive heart failure (CHF) was considered a likely diagnosis.

Agreed medical/surgical management

Emergency oxygen therapy was given; as a facemask resulted in stress, flow-by oxygen was used and the dog also placed in front of a fan. Opioids such as methadone can be useful for reducing anxiety levels, thereby facilitating slower, deeper breaths that result in more efficient ventilation.

Intravenous access was obtained and furosemide administered via this route. Blood samples were taken for baseline haematology and serum biochemistry. Percutaneous glyceryl trinitrate was applied to the underside of the pinna as a venodilator.

The dog was then moved to a kennel and made comfortable with adequate bedding, a cool room, access to fresh water and use of a fan. Once he had settled, an ECG was obtained. As minimizing stress is paramount, the trace may be recorded in whatever position the dog finds comfortable, rather than insisting that the patient lies in the conventional position (right lateral recumbency). The resulting trace showed atrial fibrillation with a ventricular rate of 180 beats per minute.

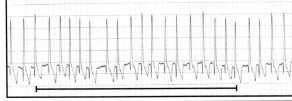

Lead II trace showing atrial fibrillation. The bar shows a 6-second interval.

The dog was closely monitored. It would be expected that he should be more relaxed, with a reduction in respiratory rate and effort, within an hour. Furosemide was continued intravenously to effect, with concurrent monitoring of renal parameters and electrolytes once or twice daily. The aim of diuresis was to improve respiratory parameters without causing excessive electrolyte depletion and azotaemia. Clinical parameters such as heart rate, respiratory rate, demeanour, appetite, water intake and urine output were monitored hourly initially, but this frequency may decrease with improvement. Further tests were postponed until the dog was more stable (in this case the following day).

Thoracic radiography and echocardiography showed findings consistent with DCM, resulting in congestive heart failure, pulmonary oedema and atrial fibrillation.

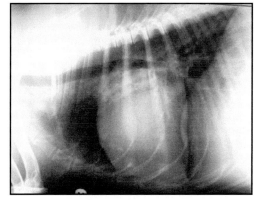

Lateral thoracic radiograph showing a generalized enlargement of the cardiac silhouette. The caudal vena cava is elevated and the lobar vessels are enlarged. The trachea is elevated by the enlarged cardiac silhouette and the lung fields show a predominantly interstitial pattern particularly prominent in the perihilar region.

Medical treatment was modified by adding an ACE inhibitor, pimobendan, oral furosemide, spironolactone and digoxin. Digoxin has a long half-life and therefore requires several days to take full effect; heart rate should then be well controlled, with mean 24-hour heart rate <110 beats per minute (measured using a Holter monitor). If tachycardia persists, diltiazem or a beta-adrenoceptor antagonist may be used in addition to the digoxin. Some Dobermanns have frequent and complex ventricular ectopy, and digoxin may be contraindicated in these cases.

At the time of admission to the hospital, a discussion was initiated with the owners about whether or not to resuscitate the dog if he had a further crisis and whether those attempts should be restricted to closed chest resuscitation.

Acute/chronic pain management

The presence of pain in cardiac patients is uncertain. Pain associated with ischaemia and narrowed blood vessels does not appear to be present in veterinary patients, although secondary muscular pain in the thorax due to the dypsnoea is a possibility in this case. Care should be taken not to confuse the signs of dullness and exercise intolerance with the side effects of any pain medication used. One would also need to be sure of the outcome measures for treating pain, such as reduction of anxiety associated with pain.

Non-steroidal anti-inflammatory drugs (NSAIDs) may be contraindicated if appetite and/or cardiac output and subsequent renal perfusion are poor.

Fear, stress, conflict concerns

Anxiety due to the dyspnoea may result in a positive feedback cycle, with anxiety leading to further dyspnoea. The best option in this case is to hospitalize the dog and give him opiates as an anxiolytic. During recovery and long-term management, events or contexts known previously to cause the dog anxiety should be identified and avoided. There is evidence that the use of touch reduces blood pressure and releases a variety of mood-enhancing neurotransmitters; the use of gentle commands may interrupt panic (see Chapters 4 and 8).

Nutritional requirements

Calorie requirements
The most important consideration in the dietary management of cardiomyopathy is 'calorie mismatch'. Dogs with DCM are often thin (cardiac cachexia) and maintenance of bodyweight in heart failure is associated with longer survival time (see Chapter 5). The most important consideration in this dog is therefore to maintain food intake. Dietary modifications in cases of advanced cardiac disease must take into consideration the potential benefits *versus* the possibility of the patient's not accepting the new diet. Dietary changes should be considered only when he is no longer in overt cardiac failure.

Sodium restriction?
Nutritional modulation of chronic cardiac disease has traditionally centred on restriction of sodium. However, excessive sodium restriction leads to two major problems: reduced palatability of the diet; and early and exaggerated activation of the renin–angiotensin–aldosterone system, which is counterproductive, as this contributes to the progression of disease in CHF. Therefore, recommendations for animals with advanced or symptomatic cardiac disease have shifted to *avoidance of excessive sodium intake* (>100 mg sodium per 100 kcal of food).

There is some debate about the benefit of further sodium restriction in advanced or refractory CHF. Recommendations for reducing sodium to 50–80 mg sodium per 100 kcal in patients with moderate heart failure (ISACHC stage 2 heart disease) and to <50 mg sodium per 100 kcal in patients with severe or refractory CHF are quoted in the literature. To achieve this usually requires the feeding of prescription diets designed for patients with cardiac disease. In cases where a commercial diet that has the desired sodium content and that the dog will accept cannot be found, formulation of a complete and balanced homemade diet suitable for patients with cardiac failure could be considered. Clients also need to be counselled about acceptable treats and ways of administering medications without the use of high-salt foods such as cheeses, condiments or luncheon meats. Tablets may be wrapped inside soft sweets (NB not chocolate) or, if the dog is being fed tinned prescription diet, small amounts of that food.

Nutraceuticals

Omega-3 polyunsaturated fatty acid supplementation in patients with advanced heart disease has been associated with some positive results, including: reduction in circulating inflammatory cytokines; better preservation of lean muscle mass; and improvement of appetite. Although an optimal dose has not been determined, daily doses of 40 mg/kg of eicosapentaenoic acid (EPA) and 25 mg/kg of docosahexaenoic acid (DHA) have been recommended.

DCM in certain breeds, such as American Cocker Spaniels, Newfoundlands and occasional Golden Retrievers, has been reported to respond favourably to taurine and/or L-carnitine supplementation (Kittleson *et al.,* 1997; Backus *et al.,* 2003; Bélanger *et al.,* 2005), although not all dogs with DCM will show improvement with such supplementation. Studies have suggested that Dobermanns have neither taurine deficiency-related DCM nor a positive response to dietary supplementation.

Physiotherapy

There may be some benefit to performing stroking massage on this dog – a calming technique that helps to relieve stress and anxiety. Involvement of the owners in this process may also help ease *their* anxiety.

Once acute cardiac failure has been controlled medically, a gentle cardiac rehabilitation programme may be of benefit. A staged programme, closely monitoring dyspnoea, can improve exercise tolerance and quality of life. Cardiac rehabilitation programmes in human patients include pre-exercise assessment, warm-ups, aerobic conditioning, cool-downs and ongoing monitoring. There is limited evidence of the benefits of such programmes in canine patients but they may be beneficial to offset physical deconditioning, especially if started at an early stage in the disease. Any programme should be designed and monitored by the veterinary surgeon.

Hydrotherapy

Hydrotherapy is not specifically indicated for this patient.

Acupuncture

Theoretically, lung and heart function could be affected by segmental acupuncture at thoracic paraspinal points, although this is unlikely to be used in practice. Secondary muscular pain in muscles overlying the thorax and neck may be effectively treated by local needling, with care not to needle in the interspaces. Needling over the cranial aspect of the sternum may be useful for both specific effects (segmental for the lung) and non-specific effects (e.g. anxiety). Acupuncture should only be used as an adjunct to the management of CHF and never as an alternative to medication.

Other nursing and supportive care

Resuscitation
Resuscitation equipment should be available. Cardiopulmonary–cerebral resuscitation (CCPR) may be required. The practice team must be aware of the extent of efforts to be made in resuscitating this patient (see above) and a sign put on the notes and kennels accordingly.

Monitoring
Frequent patient reassessment will help assess response and guide further treatments. Respiratory and heart rates, blood pressure and urine output should be recorded – initially at least every 15 minutes and then less frequently as the heart failure becomes controlled. Continuous ECG monitoring may be required.

Analysis of body condition score (BCS) is of particular importance in animals with oedema/ascites because, whilst they may weigh within the normal range (due to increased fluid retention), their body fat and muscle mass is likely to be markedly reduced.

Oxygen supplementation

To reduce stress to the patient, hands-free methods should be considered. Nasal oxygen is preferable; other possibilities are an oxygen cage, or holding an oxygen mask slightly away from the patient's muzzle. Whilst the patient is in overt cardiac failure, consideration should be given to reducing dyspnoea, e.g. positioning the dog in sternal recumbency with positioning aids or rolled-up towels either side (see Chapter 17).

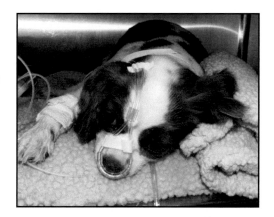

Nasal oxygen supplementation. (Courtesy of Yvonne McGrotty)

Comfort and stress avoidance

Dogs with acute heart failure have no reserve capacity, i.e. they cannot increase cardiac output to cope with increased demand, so stress should be avoided. Strict cage rest is essential. Normal body temperature must be maintained and the environment kept sufficiently warm.

Water

Fresh water should be freely available for the patient to drink. Very dyspnoeic patients may find it impossible to drink, so careful intravenous fluid therapy may be necessary. The patient on diuretic therapy will also need increased opportunity for urination via frequent short walks to the grass. If the patient is too ill for this, he may require bladder catheterization to prevent urine scalding.

Feeding

This patient is a 'fussy' eater and this, combined with cachexia and anorexia, means that he may require some encouragement to eat.

Owner advice and homecare recommendations

Feeding

Dietary management (see above) should be discussed and the owner educated on how to encourage the dog to eat:

- Feed small meals frequently
- Add moist food if the dog is eating a primarily dry food
- Warm the food to body temperature
- Add flavour enhancers (low-sodium)
- Add some chicken or other palatable foodstuff
- Add fish oil (high in omega-3 fatty acids).

The owner should be advised not to administer medication in high-salt foods (see above).

Monitoring

The owner should be informed on what is normal respiratory rate and rhythm and asked to monitor them regularly whilst the pet is asleep or at rest. A persistent increase in resting heart and respiratory rate is often an early sign of worsening heart failure. The owners should be made aware of the signs of heart failure: ascites, pulmonary oedema, syncope, exercise intolerance.

Relaxation

The owner should ideally dedicate some time each day to sitting with their pet, stroking and talking to him, helping to provide a calm and relaxing environment.

The owner can help to provide a calm relaxing environment. (Courtesy of Stephen Torrington)

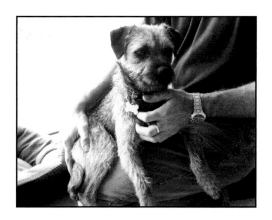

Exercise

Once CHF signs are controlled, gentle exercise can be introduced but should be well within the capabilities of the animal. Excessive exercise and walking outside in hot weather should be avoided.

Prognosis

The owner should be warned of the poor medium- to long-term prognosis for this patient and the possibility that he might die suddenly and unexpectedly due to an arrhythmia. The owners may be comforted to some extent by the assurance that little could be done in this circumstance, even by a trained professional.

References

Backus RC, Cohen G, Pion PD *et al.* (2003) Taurine deficiency in Newfoundlands fed commercially available complete and balanced diets. *Journal of the American Veterinary Medical Association* **223**, 1130–1136

Bélanger MC, Ouellet M, Queney G and Moreau M (2005) Taurine-deficient dilated cardiomyopathy in a family of golden retrievers. *Journal of the American Animal Hospital Association* **41**, 284–291

Kittleson MD, Keene B, Pion PD and Loyer CG (1997) Results of the multicenter spaniel trial (MUST): taurine- and carnitine-responsive dilated cardiomyopathy in American cocker spaniels with decreased plasma taurine concentration. *Journal of Veterinary Internal Medicine* **11**, 204–211

Case 16.2
Chronic heart failure in a dog

A 10-year-old neutered male Cavalier King Charles Spaniel was presented with a worsening cough of 4 months' duration and progressive exercise intolerance over the last week, when the owner had also noticed abdominal distension. The dog was currently being treated for stifle degenerative joint disease using NSAIDs. His BCS was 6/9.

The dog coughed regularly throughout the consultation and the cough was exacerbated by pinching the trachea. His heart rate was 150 beats per minute, with a regular rhythm. Femoral pulses were weak but no pulse deficit was detected. Mucous membranes were pale and capillary refill time was 2–3 seconds. On auscultation there was a grade 4/6 systolic murmur but no gallop sound or adventitious lung sounds were detected. There was a palpable abdominal fluid thrill. Serum biochemistry showed moderate azotaemia.

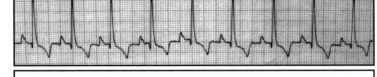

Lead II trace showing sinus tachycardia (170 beats per minute) and wide notched P waves, suggestive of left atrial enlargement.

An ECG showed signs suggestive of left atrial enlargement.

Radiographs showed signs suggestive of cardiogenic pulmonary oedema. There was a generalized loss of abdominal contrast consistent with ascites.

The cardiac silhouette is enlarged and the shape is suggestive of predominantly left-sided enlargement. There is also elevation of the trachea. The enlarged left atrium is causing compression and elevation of the mainstem bronchi. The lobar vessels are enlarged and there is a mild increase in perihilar interstitial markings, suggestive of cardiogenic pulmonary oedema.

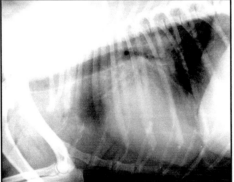
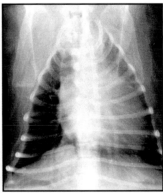

On echocardiography the atrioventricular valve cusps appeared thickened and irregular. There was moderate mitral valve regurgitation and the left atrium was enlarged. There was mild tricuspid valve regurgitation with a velocity <2 m/s and therefore not supportive of a diagnosis of pulmonary hypertension. Contractility was adequate and there was normal velocity flow in both the aorta and pulmonary artery. These findings were consistent with a diagnosis of atrioventricular valve disease resulting in CHF.

Agreed medical/surgical management

This condition is amenable to medical treatment with diuretics (e.g. furosemide, spironolactone), ACE inhibitors and pimobendan. In view of the pre-existing azotaemia, the dose of diuretics would normally be reduced. However, gastrointestinal absorption of drugs is likely to be suboptimal because the right-sided CHF will have reduced intestinal perfusion. The ascites should not be drained unless absolutely necessary, as this represents a significant protein loss to the dog.

The dog can be treated medically on an outpatient basis, with regular monitoring of renal parameters. The aims of treatment are: to control clinical signs such as coughing; to ensure that body condition is maintained; and to reduce the dose of diuretics to the lowest effective dose.

Acute/chronic pain management

The presence of pain in canine cardiac patients is uncertain (see Case 16.1).

Ongoing treatment of this dog's concurrent osteoarthritis will require an alternative to NSAIDs as the latter should not be used concurrently with ACE inhibitors which potentiate renal toxicity. The dog's azotaemia would also be a contraindication to the use of NSAIDs. Paracetamol ± codeine could be considered. Tramadol might be used as an alternative analgesic, although it does not have anti-inflammatory properties. Care should be taken not to confuse any potential side effects of tramadol (dysphoria and dullness) with a deterioration in the cardiac condition. Multimodal analgesia may mean that the dose of each individual medication can be reduced to mitigate problems. If osteoarthritis has resulted in hyperalgesia and/or allodynia, then gabapentin and/or amantadine may be considered, although gabapentin is contraindicated in human patients with advanced renal disease. The drug is partially processed through the liver in dogs (so it should not have a detrimental effect on the kidneys), but given the uncertainty about its pharmacokinetics in dogs and cats, it should still be used with care.

The use of warmth, massage, cold therapy and electrotherapy can be helpful to control pain as long as there is no local circulatory insufficiency. Additional treatments provided by the veterinary physiotherapist can also be valuable in this regard (see below).

Fear, stress, conflict concerns

Owners should be instructed not to 'force' the dog to go out on walks if he is reluctant, but rather to use enrichment inside the house and in the garden until any pain and exercise intolerance is improved. Alternatively, taking him out in the car may maintain his interest.

Significant chronic pain associated with the osteoarthritis may increase fearfulness and anxiety. Signs of sound sensitivity, anxiety around young bouncy dogs, withdrawal from the family or becoming more 'clingy' may indicate that pain is having a significant impact. As long as pain is also being addressed directly (see above), pheromone therapy and/or alpha-casozepine may be helpful in moderating anxiety associated with pain, although this is not a proven effect (see Chapter 4).

Nutritional requirements

Calorie requirements
Calorie mismatch is the most common problem in CHF. Cavalier King Charles Spaniels with mitral valve disease often have concurrent obesity and there is a clinical benefit in these cases of a careful weight loss programme (see Chapter 6). Weight management would also benefit this patient in reducing the pain associated with his osteoarthritis. However, once CHF has developed, as in this case, the dog is likely to begin to lose lean bodyweight because of cardiac cachexia; ensuring sufficient protein and calorie intake then becomes most important.

Sodium restriction
Changes to diet could be considered once the dog is out of fulminant CHF. Nutritional modulation of chronic cardiac disease has traditionally centred on restriction of sodium. However, excessive sodium restriction leads to the problems outlined in Case 16.1, and recommendations for the amount of dietary sodium to give are as detailed for that Case. Clients also need to be counselled about acceptable treats and ways of administering medications without the use of high-salt foods such as cheeses, condiments or luncheon meats.

Nutraceuticals
Omega-3 polyunsaturated fatty acid supplementation has been associated with some positive results in patients with advanced heart disease, including reduction in circulating inflammatory cytokines, better preservation of lean muscle mass and improvement in appetite. Furthermore, omega-3 fatty acids may also help decrease the inflammation associated with osteoarthritis in this case. Although an optimal dose has not

been determined, daily doses of 40 mg/kg of eicosapentaenoic acid (EPA) and 25 mg/kg of docosahexaenoic acid (DHA) have been recommended. The use of other nutraceuticals for osteoarthritis, such as glucosamine and chondroitin sulphate, have yielded mixed results in improving clinical signs. Although these agents have a very wide margin of safety, the use of additional medications in a dog already requiring various cardiac medications may compromise client compliance.

Physiotherapy

Exercise in heart failure
Gentle exercise is beneficial in CHF once the acute phase has been treated successfully. A gradually increasing walking programme would be helpful. A staged programme, closely monitoring respiratory rate and avoiding dyspnoea, can improve exercise tolerance and quality of life.

Osteoarthritis
In respect of the stifle DJD, the use of heat, massage, passive movements and stretches can be beneficial in improving comfort and mobility (especially in the mornings and prior to exercise). The use of cold therapy after walks is also useful to control pain and any localized inflammation/swelling caused through exercise, although such effects after exercise would indicate that the exercise was excessive. An appropriate low-impact exercise programme could be provided to the owners (see Case 14.8). All exercises (including walking) should be paced (within the tolerance of the patient) yet provided regularly (little and often) and this approach should be continued throughout the dog's life. This approach would also satisfy the requirements of the heart condition.

Hydrotherapy

Hydrotherapy is not indicated for this case unless medical management dramatically improves the clinical signs. It may help to improve the pain and restricted range of motion caused by DJD, but there is risk of collapse during swimming (the exertion required during these sessions should not be underestimated) which should therefore be avoided. An underwater treadmill may be less strenuous for the patient and therefore possible in this case, but the risks from the heart disease should be carefully weighed up against any possible benefits.

Acupuncture

The main indication for acupuncture in this patient is in the treatment of the pain of osteoarthritis. There is good evidence for the use of acupuncture in the treatment of pain of osteoarthritis of the human knee. Local needling around the stifle (ST36, BL40, SP9, SP10) and in secondary muscle pain in the hip (gluteals and lower back) represents segmental acupuncture.

Other nursing and supportive care

Considerations for comfort, stress reduction, feeding and monitoring are as for Case 16.1. Food intake should be monitored and care taken to avoid food aversion, e.g. he should not be force-fed. Water should be provided *ad libitum*.

Geriatric care
Because this patient is 10 years old and has DJD, thought should be given to the requirements of an aged patient. Plenty of padded bedding should be provided. Opportunities should be given for the dog to stretch his limbs, or physiotherapy performed to keep them mobile. In addition, it may also be necessary to turn him regularly to avoid atelectasis and resultant pneumonia and decubitus ulcer formation. Positioning him in sternal recumbency using positioning aids or rolled-up towels either side can also minimize hypostatic congestion. Small details, such as an increased opportunity for urination, are important for patients on diuretics, and can make all the difference to patient comfort. Exercise should be kept to a minimum (short distance walks requiring minimal effort only).

Owner advice and homecare recommendations

For considerations concerning dogs with osteoarthritis, see Case 14.8. If there are children in the household, they should be instructed to treat their pet with care. As this is an elderly dog prone to joint pain, there is an increased chance that he will be less tolerant of overenthusiastic handling. Dedicating time to sitting with the pet, stroking and talking to him, will help provide a calm and relaxing environment.

Exercise

The owners should be provided with an appropriate exercise programme designed specifically to cater for the dog's joint and cardiac needs, and an explanation should be given regarding the pacing of all activities.

Feeding

Owners should be educated as to the reasons for avoiding a high salt intake; suitable diets and treats (e.g. baked potato skins, proprietary low-salt snacks, fruit and vegetables) should be discussed. Methods of administering medication without disguising them in high-salt foods should be suggested (see Case 16.1).

Follow-up and monitoring

The owner should be advised to bring the dog back for frequent check-ups to monitor for signs of disease or deterioration. They should be warned that a persistent increase in resting heart and respiratory rate is often an early sign of worsening heart failure.

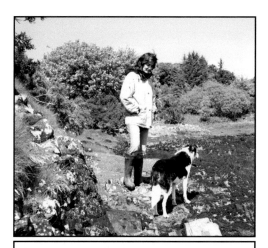

Sometimes just visiting new places to stand and watch, or gently explore, is enough stimulation for older or infirm dogs. (Courtesy of Samantha Lindley)

Case 16.3
Pericardial effusion in a dog

A 10-year-old entire male Golden Retriever was presented for investigation of ascites and exercise intolerance of 7 days' duration. He had concurrent moderate to severe degenerative joint disease, currently managed with NSAIDs. His BCS was 6/9. The dog was unpredictably aggressive in the hospital.

Heart rate was 120 beats per minute with a regular rhythm. Femoral pulses were weak but no deficit was detected. His mucous membranes were pale and capillary refill time was 2 seconds. On auscultation heart sounds were quiet; no murmur, gallop sound or adventitious lung sounds were detected. There was a palpable abdominal fluid thrill. Haematology, serum biochemistry and urinalysis were unremarkable.

An ECG showed low-voltage QRS complexes and electrical alternans. Radiographs showed enlargement of the cardiac silhouette and a generalized loss of abdominal contrast consistent with ascites but no evidence of a pleural effusion. Echocardiography showed signs consistent with a pericardial effusion resulting in cardiac tamponade. Careful inspection of the heart base and right atrial areas revealed no obvious intrapericardial mass.

ECG traces from leads I, II and III show low-voltage QRS complexes and also electrical alternans, a regular fluctuation in R wave amplitude.

Thoracic radiographs showing generalized enlargement of the cardiac silhouette, resulting in a globoid shape with a sharp outline.

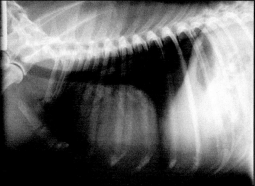

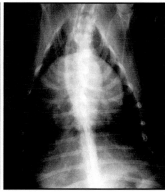

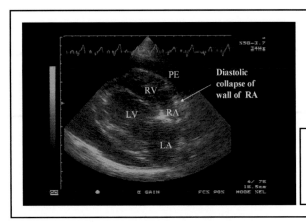

PE
RV
LV
RA
LA
Diastolic collapse of wall of RA

There is an echogenic space within the pericardium and diastolic collapse of the right atrium.

Agreed medical/surgical management

Prior to drainage of the pericardial effusion an intravenous catheter was placed to allow rapid administration of emergency drugs. Oxygen was provided by mask throughout the procedure and continuous ECG monitoring was also in place as the drainage catheter had the potential to provoke ventricular arrhythmias.

Percutaneous pericardiocentesis was performed under sedation, using a sterile urinary catheter guided ultrasonically into the pericardial space through a 14G intravenous catheter. Ultrasonography after the procedure showed complete drainage and resolution of the cardiac tamponade.

After the procedure the dog was made comfortable in a kennel whilst recovering from sedation. There is often a profound and rapid diuresis after pericardiocentesis and therefore the dog was taken outside regularly to allow him to urinate.

Echocardiography was repeated the following day to ensure that there was no early recurrence of the

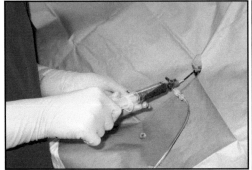

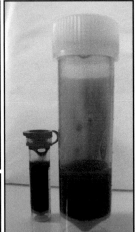

Percutaneous pericardiocentesis produced 800 ml of non-clotting serosanguineous fluid. Samples were sent for fluid analysis, including cytology and culture.

effusion. The intravenous catheter was then removed prior to discharge.

Although no intrapericardial mass was identified and no abnormal cells were detected on cytology, neoplasia such as mesothelioma could not be excluded, as reactive mesothelial cells resemble neoplastic cells and some intrapericardial neoplasms do not exfoliate cells readily. In this case the effusion recurred every 2–3 months and was treated by repeated percutaneous pericardiocentesis; an alternative approach would be to consider a partial pericardectomy.

Acute/chronic pain management

This dog should undergo a thorough examination for sources of pain (e.g. musculoskeletal, visceral, dental) as a possible cause of his unpredictable aggression. As he has osteoarthritis, in the absence of anything else obvious, he should have that pain addressed with NSAIDs at the standard dose for at least a month. Care should be taken using tramadol; there is a possibility that tramadol may make aggressive episodes worse in some individuals, although the link between worsening aggression and the mechanism of this is uncertain and there are insufficient data to avoid its usage where pain and suffering indicate it. If there is evidence of continued suffering in spite of the NSAIDs or evidence of central sensitization, then gabapentin and/or amantadine may be an additional or alternative option to tramadol, alongside the NSAIDs. If side effects develop with NSAIDS (e.g. gastrointestinal or renal), paracetamol ± codeine, prednoleucotropin or acupuncture should be considered. The use of heat, massage, cold therapy and electrotherapy can also be helpful (see Case 14.8).

Fear, stress, conflict concerns

This dog should have a full behavioural work-up to identify, if possible, the cause of his unpredictable aggression. Genuinely unpredictable aggression is usually indicative of a clinical cause (including brain disease). So called 'rage' in this breed has been variously linked with epilepsy and/or dietary sensitivity, but there are no convincing data to prove these connections (though it is difficult to collect reliable data or set up studies to test hypotheses convincingly).

Nutritional requirements

Protein loss

This dog should be fed an adequate amount of high-quality dietary protein because intermittent drainage of the pericardium will result in significant intermittent protein loss from the body, which needs to be replaced. This is particularly important in an older dog, such as this one, because dogs have proportionately less lean body mass and more fat mass as they age. Long-term feeding of a protein-restricted 'senior' diet may therefore not be appropriate in this case.

Neoplasia

If the dog does have pericardial neoplasia as a cause of his effusion, there may be benefit in feeding a high-fat diet (see Chapter 15).

Nutraceuticals

The dog may benefit from supplementation of omega-3 fatty acids and glucosamine for the degenerative joint disease (see Case 14.8).

There may also be a role for supplementation with omega-3 fatty acids to reduce his aggression. Although there is currently no evidence that this helps in aggressive dogs, there *is* some limited evidence in humans (Appleton *et al.,* 2008). In addition, a recent study showed that aggressive dogs have low plasma omega-3 fatty acid levels when compared to non-aggressive controls (Re *et al.,* 2008).

Dietary sensitivity

An exclusion diet (see Case 22.2) may be indicated at an appropriate stage of treatment to rule in or out dietary intolerance as a cause of unpredictable aggression. Such an approach must be carefully weighed alongside the nutritional considerations of his medical condition, especially given that the current evidence for this approach is inconclusive.

Physiotherapy

There is no specific indication for exercise in relation to pericardial effusion, but consideration of exercise should be made in relation to the dog's degenerative joint disease (see Case 14.8). If evidence of neoplasia should become apparent, the use of certain physiotherapy modalities would need reconsideration, as neoplasia is a contraindication to many of them.

Hydrotherapy

Hydrotherapy may be helpful as part of a programme to improve this patient's fitness and allow support of his joints whilst exercising. It is to be expected that this patient will be normal between recurrences of the pericardial effusion and therefore hydrotherapy poses no especial risks, although treadmill exercise underwater will be less strenuous and may be preferred to swimming.

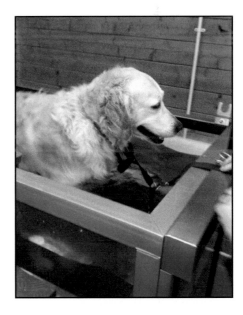

An underwater treadmill may be more suitable than swimming. (Courtesy of Samantha Lindley)

Acupuncture

Acupuncture is indicated here for the treatment of osteoarthritis. It is not an alternative to NSAIDs, but may be as effective as tramadol and other analgesics in reducing pain and central sensitization in combination with NSAIDs and is useful in treating muscle pain secondary to the pain of OA and postural shifts. Local needling in the areas of pain is indicated with recourse to electroacupuncture if the response to treatment is poor.

Monitoring

The patient should be monitored carefully before, during and after drainage, paying particular attention to respiratory and heart rate, pulse volume and heart rhythm. He should also be monitored carefully for arrhythmias, both during drainage of the pericardium and for several hours afterwards, when atrial fibrillation may occur due to re-expansion of the collapsed atria.

Oxygen should be administered if the dog shows signs of tachypnoea or of haemodynamic instability.

Fluid therapy

Animals with pericardial effusion have poor venous return and blood pressure, so intravenous fluids may be necessary in the short term to aid venous return and thus cardiac output. The aim is to drain the pericardial effusion as soon as possible to remove tamponade and thus restore blood pressure, but short-term fluids while this is achieved may be beneficial. However, care should be taken not to increase central venous pressure so much with the fluids that pulmonary oedema ensues. Profound diuresis after drainage will warrant frequent trips outside to allow urination. Weighing the dog every 12 hours after drainage will allow an estimation of the rate of loss of ascitic fluid.

Postoperative care

The pericardiocentesis site should be kept clean and monitored closely for signs of infection.

As the patient is elderly and has degenerative joint disease he may need gentle physiotherapy to help keep his joints mobile. It may also be necessary to turn him regularly to avoid atelectasis and resultant pneumonia.

Owner advice and homecare recommendations

See Case 14.8 for considerations in respect of degenerative joint disease.

Signs of recurrence

The owner should be informed that pericardial effusion may recur at any stage and should be advised of the signs to look for which might indicate recurrence and cardiac tamponade:

- Weakness, lethargy
- Ascites
- Exercise intolerance
- Weak pulse
- Pallor
- Dyspnoea – usually related to pain
- Collapse – exacerbated by exertion
- Cough – in the initial period
- Vomiting and/or diarrhoea.

They should be encouraged to contact the veterinary surgery immediately if any of these occur.

Behavioural considerations

This patient's aggression is described as unpredictable, but if there are patterns to when it occurs, e.g. during close handling, then some physiotherapy or play may need to be altered or avoided. If the behaviour is genuinely very unpredictable, there is no advice to give owners as to how to avoid it. The cause must be found. However, the aggression should be addressed as part of the overall evaluation of this patient and the severity of it will guide advice and treatment priorities.

References

Appleton KM, Rogers PJ and Ness AR (2008) Is there a role for *n*-3 long-chain polyunsaturated fatty acids in the regulation of mood and behaviour? A review of the evidence to date from epidemiological studies, clinical studies and intervention trials. *Nutrition Research Reviews* **21** (1), 13–41

Re S, Zanoletti M and Emanuele E (2008) Aggressive dogs are characterized by low omega-3 polyunsaturated fatty acid status. *Veterinary Research Communications* **32**, 225–230

Case 16.4
Aortic thromboembolism in a cat

A 10-year-old male neutered DSH cat was presented with sudden-onset unilateral left hindlimb paralysis. The cat had been on treatment for congestive heart failure (CHF) secondary to idiopathic hypertrophic cardiomyopathy (HCM) for 6 months.

On clinical examination the left hindlimb was cold, the muscles stiff and the nailbeds cyanotic. The left femoral pulse was absent. The cat was tachycardic (heart rate 200 beats per minute with a regular rhythm) and had a systolic heart murmur.

Clinical findings were supportive of a provisional diagnosis of aortic thromboembolism disease secondary to HCM.

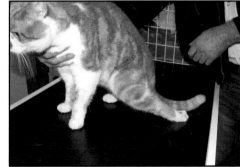

A typical presentation with sudden-onset unilateral left hindlimb paralysis. (Courtesy of Simon Swift)

Agreed medical/surgical management

The cat was given analgesia (see below). His current treatment for CHF (furosemide and an ACE inhibitor) was continued, with regular monitoring of renal parameters and electrolytes.

There are no prospective placebo-controlled trials yet published in the field of management of thromboembolism in cats and therefore each case has to be managed on an individual basis, prioritizing pain control and regular reassessment of limb function. Thrombolytic drugs such as tissue plasminogen activator could be considered but, as there is a significant risk of life-threatening complications (50% mortality in some studies) secondary to reperfusion syndrome, their use cannot be recommended at this time.

Drugs such as heparin or low-molecular-weight heparin (LMWH) can be used to prevent enlargement of the existing clot. Heparin therapy is easier to monitor (using activated partial thromboplastin time, APTT), as LMWH treatment requires an assay for anti-factor Xa antibody, which is not readily available. The advantage of LMWH, however, is that generally the volume required for injection is smaller, resulting in less patient discomfort. Whilst warfarin therapy is theoretically possible, the risk of fatal complications as a result of uncontrolled haemorrhage, and the need for frequent monitoring, make this approach inadvisable, particularly in cats that go outdoors and in multi-cat households. Aspirin and clopidogrel are anti-platelet drugs that have also received some attention for use in the prevention of further clot formation; there is currently little evidence proving their benefit and the results of ongoing studies will help to clarify this area.

It is important to set firm treatment goals, so as to avoid prolonging suffering in a patient with a poor prognosis; thrombosis is likely to recur within 6 months in the majority of cats with underlying heart disease. Euthanasia is indicated if the cat fails to respond to therapy and pain is uncontrollable.

Acute/chronic pain management

Acute pain
This is very important in this condition. Opioids should be used initially for acute pain management. Epidural morphine may be useful (see *BSAVA Manual of Canine and Feline Anaesthesia and Analgesia*). Aspirin, if given as an anticoagulant, may also provide some analgesia. Euthanasia should be seriously considered if pain cannot be adequately controlled.

Once the cat has recovered from the acute pain of the first few days, analgesia with oral transmucosal buprenorphine (see Chapter 3) may be helpful.

Chronic pain
If the cat is recovering but still unable to use his hindlimbs, he could strain his back and forelimb muscles by using them to move about. Secondary muscle pain should therefore be considered as an additional source of pain and discomfort for this patient. If aspirin is still being used, this may help. Acupuncture is often well tolerated and may be better indicated for muscle pain, although there is no currently no clinical evidence for this in animals. NSAIDs, in the form of meloxicam, may otherwise be helpful, but caution must be exercised with

NSAIDs since this patient is also receiving ACE inhibitors. Careful physical examination of the cat will determine whether he is suffering secondary muscle pain, bearing in mind that behavioural measures of suffering will be harder to assess.

Fear, stress, conflict concerns

At the veterinary clinic

- Assess how the cat perceives human attention; where cats are poorly socialized or wary of people, interactions may increase anxiety.
- If the cat is well socialized, reward and reinforce any positive experiences and associations with the veterinary practice and its team. Use positive touch (stroking and rubbing around the chin, grooming with a massaging groomer, gentle stroking of the chest) to encourage him to relax.
- Take time with the patient to help him relax before any intervention. This is particularly important if he is anxious about being handled.
- The use of pheromone therapy may be beneficial, especially if the cat is going to be in a cage.
- Minimize exposure to potential stressors, such as dogs and other cats, noises and strong odours.
- Use the space in the cage to provide a hiding area (a cardboard box will do with a blanket or soft bedding, or a towel can be hung up).
- Use minimal restraint during procedures where possible.

At home
Once the cat is at home, enhancing his core territory or environment will help him feel better (help him cope with his discomfort more easily). It is also necessary to make some adjustments so that an inactive and unwell patient can exploit the improvements in the environment:

- **Food.** Increase the number of feeding stations. The cat must also be able to reach food easily; if he has previously fed at a height he may not feel like jumping, so adjust the position of the food, whilst making sure this does not make him anxious about it being available to competitors (e.g. the pet dog or a possible intruding cat if the food is placed near the cat flap).
- **Water.** Cats generally prefer their water about a room's distance away from their food in a clear, wide bowl.
- **Access inside and out.** Cats normally have more than one access point into and out of their core territory (usually the house). Consider providing an additional access point, or ensure that he can use the existing access points (they are not too high or too difficult to negotiate when he feels unwell and uncomfortable). If the cat cannot resume going outside for some time, then this will need to be considered in his general management as a source of potential frustration and anxiety.
- **Mobility.** If the cat is moving around by pulling himself along by his forequarters, removing rugs and mats will help his progress through the house.
- **Scratching posts.** Are these easily accessible and appropriate? A horizontal scratch post can be provided, so that the cat can still reach it if he does not feel up to climbing.
- **Hiding areas.** Provide multiple safe and comfortable hiding areas at different levels, or make sure that there is a 'step' system to allow the cat to reach his old favourite places.
- **Beds.** Provision of new beds, such as radiator beds, may improve the comfort and wellbeing of the patient.
- **Play.** Modify games to very short bursts of gentle play, but continue to try to gently stimulate the cat.
- **Petting.** Use of gentle touch, stroking and grooming in ways that the patient will tolerate and enjoy will not only improve the patient's feelings of wellbeing but will also give the owner a sense of participating in their pet's treatment and nursing.

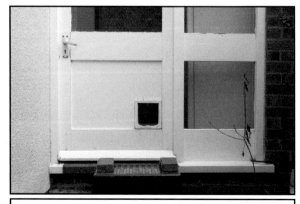

A step may be needed to maintain ease of access to the cat flap. (© Irene Rochlitz)

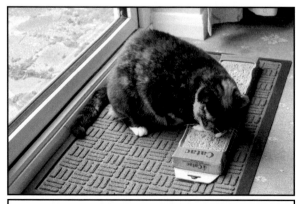

A horizontal scratching post may be useful for a cat with limited mobility. (© Irene Rochlitz)

Nutritional requirements

Patients with acute thromboembolisms are not usually amenable to nutritional modulation, at least initially. Resolution of the thromboembolus, or at least the pain associated with it, is usually necessary before the patient will accept food voluntarily. Although the priority will centre on simply finding a diet accepted by the patient, there should be some effort in identifying a palatable diet that is not high in sodium content. If the cat survives beyond the first day, daily food intake should be monitored carefully to ensure that he is eating to fulfil his resting energy requirement (RER; see Chapter 5). If he fails to do this, early consideration should be given to placing a feeding tube (preferably naso-oesophageal as this does not require an anaesthetic for placement). Cats that remain anorexic for a prolonged period with concurrent disease have a high risk of developing hepatic lipidosis, even if they were not obese to start with.

In the longer term, if the cat survives, supplementation of the diet with omega-3 fatty acids (such as fish oil) might be considered to reduce the risk of recurrent thromboemboli. There is evidence of the beneficial anti-thrombotic action of fish oil in human cardiac patients, though evidence for efficacy in cats with HCM is lacking.

Nutraceuticals
Low plasma vitamin B12 concentrations have been found in cats with aortic thromboembolism associated with cardiomyopathy (McMichael *et al.*, 2000), so there is a rationale for supplementing vitamin B12 in this patient. However, the effects of this on the pathogenesis of aortic thromboembolism have not been evaluated.

Physiotherapy

To counteract the muscle-wasting effects of the sudden-onset bilateral hindlimb paralysis, this cat should receive regular (three times daily) physiotherapy to maintain joint and muscle range, muscle strength, balance and proprioception, and joint stability. The success of this physiotherapy will be very dependent on his willingness to be handled and guided to perform certain activities. Massage, passive movements (including functional gait patterning – bicycling), assisted standing (using physio rolls or harnesses) and assisted walking (using harnesses) should all be included. Veterinary physiotherapists would also be able to perform joint mobilizations (including compressions) to maintain range and simulate weightbearing stresses during the non-mobilization period.

Hydrotherapy

Hydrotherapy is not specifically indicated for this patient.

Acupuncture

Acupuncture may provide additional pain relief if the cat is sensitive enough to the treatment (i.e. a good responder, bearing in mind that not every individual responds to acupuncture in the same way), but electroacupuncture may be necessary to give potent enough analgesia for such a painful condition. A sensible approach would be to needle over the lower back and sacrum.

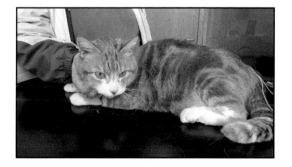

Electroacupuncture may be helpful for analgesia. (Courtesy of Samantha Lindley)

Other nursing and supportive care

WARNING
Indwelling venous catheters should NEVER be placed into veins of legs devitalized by occlusive emboli.

Cage rest and monitoring
Cage rest is required in a comfortable, warm environment. Affected animals may be hypothermic; however, excessive external warming should be avoided as this may result in peripheral vasodilation and shunting of blood and warmth away from vital organs.

The cat should be monitored for signs of pain:

- Vocalizing
- Unable to settle
- Rolling around
- Panting or open-mouth breathing.

Oxygen supplementation may be required (see Chapter 17).

Handling
Care must be taken when handling or restraining the cat as his limbs are likely to be sore to the touch, particularly in the early stages.

Dealing with limited mobility
Assisting the cat into a standing position for short periods during the day will help prevent pressure sores and urine scalding. If he has unilateral or bilateral hindlimb paresis, he will be unable to move around easily. Absorbent bedding or an incontinence pad should be provided and the cat monitored regularly for signs of skin sloughing and to prevent urine scalding. Placement of a urinary catheter should be considered early on in the course of treatment.

Without proximal control (trunk, hip and scapular muscles), limb movement is often difficult and uncoordinated. Transition from lateral recumbency into a sternal position may not be possible and the patient may require assistance to maintain this position.

Self-mutilation of distal limbs is commonly exhibited during convalescence and is characterized by excessive licking or chewing of the toes or lateral hock. Application of an Elizabethan collar, loose-fitting bandage, stockinette or other barrier is usually effective. If the limbs become traumatized, they should be bandaged.

Food and water
Water and food bowls should be placed within easy reach of the patient (but not too near to the litter tray if one is provided). As the cat is likely to be anorexic, he may need to be encouraged to eat using the following measures:

- Feed small meals frequently
- Hand-feed
- Add moist food if the cat is eating a primarily dry food
- Provide fresh food
- Warm the food to body temperature
- Add some chicken, fish or other palatable foodstuff
- Add fish oil (high in omega-3 fatty acids).

Rehabilitation
Inpatient rehabilitation, including gentle passive movement of affected limb(s), should commence once the signs of pain and discomfort have reduced or ceased. Lack of motivation and fatigue can often be responsible for slow progress of patients with aortic thromboembolism. Therefore, lots of fuss and encouragement should be given to the cat, in addition to using food and the owners as motivating factors. As time progresses, the amount of assistance should be varied in order to improve strength and balance.

Owner advice and homecare recommendations

Home environment
Attempts should be made to optimize the core territory and reduce the cat's general stress levels and insecurity after recovery and hospitalization (see 'Fear, stress', above). Until the cat is fully ambulatory, he may require a low-sided litter tray, and the owner's assistance may be needed to help him with balance and coordination. More gentle games may be required if the cat wants to play, and he should be discouraged from climbing.

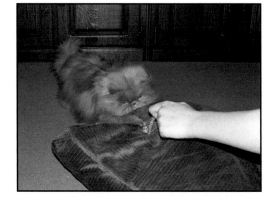

Gentle games are suitable while the cat's mobility is limited.
(© Samantha Elmhurst)

Self-mutilation

Self-mutilation of distal limbs is commonly exhibited during convalescence and is characterized by excessive licking or chewing of the toes or lateral hock. It is crucial that the owner is able to prevent this by applying an Elizabethan collar, loose-fitting bandage, stockinette or similar. If the limbs becomes traumatized, the cat should be brought back into the surgery to have bandages applied.

Follow-up and prognosis

The owner may require help and advice in managing the underlying heart failure. About half of all cats with heart disease fail to get their medication because giving tablets is difficult; strategies include the use of a pill popper. Monitoring the cat's respiratory rate is also important.

The owner should be made aware of the poor prognosis and likelihood of recurrence of thromboembolism, and of the signs to look out for:

- Acute-onset paralysis and pain (most common)
- Lameness or a gait abnormality
- Tachypnoea or respiratory distress
- Vocalization and anxiety.

References

McMichael MA, Freeman LM, Selhub J *et al.* (2000) Plasma homocysteine, B vitamins, and amino acid concentrations in cats with cardiomyopathy and arterial thromboembolism. *Journal of Veterinary Internal Medicine* **14**, 507–512

Case 16.5
Patent ductus arteriosus in a puppy

A 6-month-old entire female Border Collie puppy was presented with a continuous murmur loudest at the left cranial heart base.

Investigation involving haematology, serum biochemistry, electrocardiography, thoracic radiography and echocardiography was performed and results were consistent with a patent ductus arteriosus (PDA) which had not yet resulted in congestive heart failure (CHF).

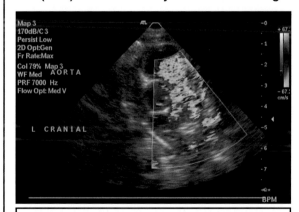

Colour Doppler image (left parasternal view) from a dog with a PDA, showing turbulent flow in the main pulmonary artery. (Courtesy of Diagnostic Imaging Department, Queen's Veterinary School Hospital, University of Cambridge)

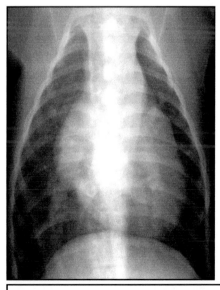

This DV radiograph shows three bulges – seen at 11–1, 1–2 and 2–3 o'clock – representing an enlarged aortic arch, pulmonary artery and left auricular appendage, respectively. A hypervascular lung pattern is also present. (Courtesy of Diagnostic Imaging Department, Queen's Veterinary School Hospital, University of Cambridge)

Agreed medical/surgical management

Treatment options, including surgical ligation or placement of an occlusion device, were discussed. Due to financial constraints, the owner chose to have the ductus ligated surgically.

A left lateral thoracotomy was performed, the ductus identified and carefully ligated. The thoracotomy was closed routinely and a chest drain placed. Once the puppy was returned to the kennel she was monitored continuously by a nurse until the chest drain was removed. The drain was suctioned hourly until it yielded minimal air or fluid (usually 6–8 hours); provided the dog is breathing normally, the drain can then be removed.

Echocardiography was performed 24 hours postoperatively and confirmed minimal residual flow through the ductus. During the period of hospitalization, the patient was monitored for signs of dyspnoea and infection, in addition to routine postoperative checks (see Chapter 12). Provided there are no wound complications, pain is well controlled, and the dog is mobile and eating/drinking voluntarily, she should be discharged within 2–3 days.

Acute/chronic pain management

Perioperative

Acute pain management around the time of surgery requires a multimodal approach: bupivacaine could be instilled into the chest and combined with parenteral methadone and NSAIDs. Epidural morphine given preoperatively can also be useful. Alternatively, an intercostal block with bupivacaine can be used preoperatively (or at the time of surgery), but care should be taken with doses if intrapleural bupivacaine is also given postoperatively (see Chapter 2). Whilst full mu opioids are very effective for pain control, they can suppress appetite (see below).

Postoperatively the dog can be sent home with NSAIDs, with the addition of tramadol or paracetamol + codeine, and assessed for signs of continuing pain.

Fear, stress, conflict concerns

It is particularly important to ensure that clinical signs prior to surgery and changes in interaction during recovery have not overly influenced this dog's socialization experiences and opportunity to learn normal social behaviour. The patient may have had limited interaction with other dogs, for example, or been restricted in her exposure to different environments due to her owner's concern about the heart disease. It is important to investigate any signs of fear or anxiety about exposure to new events, or problems associated with social interaction, and ensure appropriate behavioural advice to remedy these as soon as possible. In some cases where owners are concerned about health problems they may inadvertently reinforce undesired behaviours in their dog, so any signs of learned patterns of attention-seeking behaviour should also be identified and appropriate advice sought. As this is a young Collie, she may also have a high drive for exercise and need for mental stimulation as she recovers. Mentally stimulating games and training techniques can be used to maintain her interest during recovery.

Nutritional requirements

Growing dogs have specific nutritional requirements, such as higher protein and calcium needs, and these are best met by using complete and balanced diets designed for growth in dogs. Whilst it is uncommon for such patients to have problems with food intake postoperatively, there may be individuals where this does become a problem. Possible reasons for this include incomplete control of pain and the effects of analgesic agents on appetite and gastrointestinal function. Whilst full mu opioids are very effective for pain control they could suppress appetite. If the patient fails to eat sufficiently to meet its energy requirements (at least RER) by the second day postoperatively, there should be consideration of changing the type of analgesia. It would be very unusual to require a feeding tube in a case such as this puppy.

Physiotherapy

On the day of operation, whilst the patient is still drowsy, full-range passive shoulder movements should be performed to prevent muscle shortening and adhesions from the thoracotomy. Once awake, adequate analgesia will be necessary to allow physiotherapy input, which should be carried out three times daily.

Positioning is important in the early stages to encourage chest expansion and drainage of secretions (operated side uppermost) (see Chapter 17). From this position, the patient should be positioned with quarter turns to prone and supine, to allow the anterior and posterior chest walls to have unrestricted movement. Deep breathing should be encouraged (to re-expand the collapsed lung) via early mobilization, once it is practical to do so, 2–3 times a day.

Walks should be quickly increased in distance and passive movements continued to maintain joint range of all limbs, especially the shoulder on the operated side. Once the dog is moving well, exercises to encourage shoulder movement should be provided (including hydrotherapy, see below), as should exercises to encourage good posture and gait. These should be continued by the owners upon discharge.

Hydrotherapy

Once the drains have been removed, and all wounds are sealed, hydrotherapy can be started slowly and sensibly progressed. Hydrotherapy can be valuable to improve the dog's overall fitness, but may be particularly valuable in the early stages to ensure adequate shoulder movement and encourage chest expansion.

Acupuncture

Acupuncture is not indicated unless there is continuing postoperative pain.

Other nursing and supportive care

Postoperative care
Full details of postoperative care are given in Chapter 12, but the following should be considered specifically:

- Close monitoring for complications such as haemorrhage or pneumothorax
- Preventing hypothermia
- If possible, ensure that the puppy's bladder is empty before she comes round from the anaesthesia. Once recovered, she should be taken outside frequently to urinate.

Care of the thoracostomy tube
The thoracostomy tube should be capped when suction is not being used: the end of the tube should be folded over and secured with a gate clamp. The drain should be secured against the animal using a light bandage to prevent its being dislodged. Failure to do either of these can result in pneumothorax. The stoma around the tube should be kept clean.

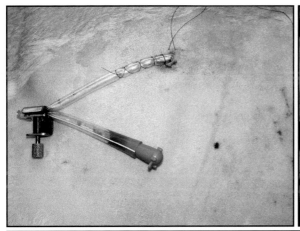 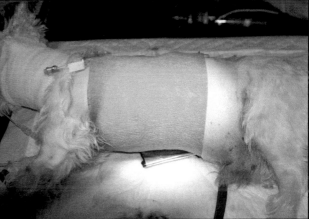

The thoracostomy tube is capped and secured and a light bandage applied. (Courtesy of Stephen Baines)

Wound management
The surgical wound must be kept clean and dry and monitored for signs of inflammation and infection. An Elizabethan collar should be applied (see Chapter 12 for more details on wound care).

Owner advice and homecare recommendations

Rest and exercise
To reduce the risk of seroma formation at the ventral extremity of the wound, the puppy should be rested with lead exercise gradually resumed over the first 4 weeks. She is likely to have a high drive for exercise and need for mental stimulation as she recovers; mentally stimulating games and training techniques should be used to maintain her interest during recovery.

Case 16.5 Patent ductus arteriosus in a puppy

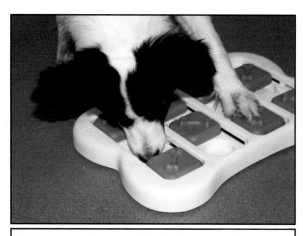

Toys with small treats hidden inside can provide useful mental stimulation with relatively little physical effort. (© Helen Zulch)

Follow-up

The owner should watch for signs of complications, such as exercise intolerance, cough and dyspnoea.

The owner should be instructed to keep the incision site clean and dry. The puppy should be prevented from licking at or chewing at the stitches. If necessary, an Elizabethan collar can be used. This is especially important if she is to be left alone. The wound will be checked 7 days postoperatively and auscultation repeated to confirm that the diastolic component of the murmur is absent.

Echocardiography is also repeated 6 months postoperatively. In this case, it showed normal cardiac chamber dimensions, resolution of the mitral regurgitation and no residual flow though the ductus.

Breeding restrictions

The owners should be advised that PDA is considered a heritable disease. Therefore, dogs in whom PDA has been diagnosed, with or without surgical correction, should not be used for breeding.

17

Patients with respiratory disease

Edited by Melissa Java and Lesley King

Introduction

Although often chronic in nature, respiratory disease commonly presents, in an emergency setting, as an acute exacerbation of disease. Patients in respiratory distress require immediate attention and therapy. These patients often present a challenge to the clinician, who has limited time to perform a physical examination and make a rapid assessment. All interventions must be carried out with minimal stress to, and manipulation of, the patient, because decreased gas transfer due to an inability to assume postural adaptations to hypoxia, accompanied by increased oxygen consumption caused by struggling, may combine to cause rapid desaturation and decompensation of the patient.

Emergency approach to acute respiratory distress

The general emergency approach to a dog or cat with acute respiratory distress includes minimizing stress, administration of oxygen, and careful treatment with anxiolytics or sedatives. As a general rule, oral drugs should be avoided in distressed respiratory patients because of the risks of aspiration associated with pill administration and questionable drug absorption from a hypoxic gastrointestinal tract. For animals with lower airway disease, bronchodilators are often also used. The beta-2 adrenergic agonist terbutaline can be given subcutaneously or intramuscularly, which makes it a convenient and effective bronchodilator for use in lower airway disease (particularly feline asthma) in the emergency setting. Phosphodiesterase inhibitors such as theophylline or aminophylline are usually administered orally, and therefore are usually not used in the emergency setting. Aminophylline, however, is available as an injectable form and can be given intravenously if it is diluted and given slowly. Glucocorticoids such as dexamethasone sodium phosphate are effective and inexpensive for parenteral use in the emergency setting. Inhaled aerosolized drugs may also be used in emergencies if the distressed patient tolerates their administration, but because of questionable drug distribution, they should not be used as a substitute for parenteral drugs in this setting. If the patient is too unstable for an intravenous catheter, these medications may be given intramuscularly.

If possible, the animal with upper airway disease should be positioned in sternal recumbency with the head and neck extended and the mouth open with the tongue pulled forward to facilitate the least resistance to air flow. Short-acting glucocorticoids may be given to treat inflammation and oedema/swelling, but may complicate a later diagnosis of neoplasia. If the animal is hyperthermic, active cooling should be performed. Animals with a mild to moderate degree of upper airway obstruction can be managed medically but have a risk of acute decompensation if they become stressed or overheated. Increased efforts to breathe associated with exercise or thermoregulation can worsen the degree of collapse of the upper airway, creating a vicious circle that can precipitate a dangerous crisis. Medical management of mildly affected animals with upper airway obstruction includes weight loss, exercise restriction, use of a harness rather than a neck collar, providing a cool environment, sedation as needed, and occasional use of corticosteroids. Any concurrent cardiac or endocrine disease should be addressed. Antitussives and bronchodilators may be added if required, and antibiotics based on culture and sensitivity results may also be indicated if secondary/concurrent bacterial infections or pneumonia are present. Antiviral and immunomodulatory drugs, accompanied by nutritional support, may be considered in cats with viral disease. However, most upper airway obstructive disease is progressive, therefore corrective surgery is often indicated for definitive treatment.

Intubation is indicated if the patient cannot be stabilized within a reasonable period of time. The function and patency of the upper airway should be assessed at this time. If intubation is not possible because of upper airway obstruction then an emergency tracheostomy should be performed. Thoracic and neck radiographs should be performed to evaluate for evidence of neoplasia and pulmonary parenchymal disease including aspiration pneumonia and non-cardiogenic pulmonary oedema. If the patient is intubated and there is evidence of pulmonary parenchymal disease or possible pneumonia, a sample should be obtained for airway cytology and bacterial culture and sensitivity testing. Empirical parenteral broad-spectrum antibiotics should be started while awaiting results.

If pleural space disease is strongly suspected on physical examination, immediate thoracocentesis should be performed as oxygen is being administered. Radiographs should be delayed until after the patient has been stabilized by therapeutic thoracocentesis. If a pneumothorax is thought to be present, then a dorsal thoracocentesis should be performed; whereas, if fluid is present then thoracocentesis should be performed ventrally. Ultrasonography may provide confirmation of pleural fluid and may be helpful as guidance for needle placement, but is not essential. Patients are often too distressed to resist the procedure; however, sedation may be required in certain patients. Fluid cytology should be performed, and aerobic and anaerobic culture and sensitivities should also be performed if there is suspicion of an infectious cause. A chest tube should be placed under general anaesthesia if negative pressure cannot be obtained, or if the patient requires multiple thoracocenteses.

Patients with pyothorax may require intravenous fluid resuscitation if they are in septic shock. Primary treatment may include medical management with chest tubes, long-term broad-spectrum antibiotics, and analgesia. Thoracotomy may be necessary if medical management fails, if there is indication of thoracic or pulmonary lesion(s), or if *Actinomyces* sp. has been isolated from the pleural fluid.

Oxygen therapy

Regardless of the underlying cause, oxygen supplementation is the first priority for any patient in respiratory distress. Oxygen can be provided by a number of different methods; the method chosen should provide adequate oxygen without causing further stress to the patient.

- Flow-by or facemask oxygen can be effective for the sedated or neurologically impaired patient; however, the majority of conscious animals do not tolerate the presence of a facemask long term.
- Flow-by oxygen is very useful for providing oxygen during short procedures, such as thoracocentesis or intravenous catheter placement.
- Nasal oxygen requires the placement of either nasal prongs or nasal cannulae (unilateral or bilateral) and is a very effective method for large dogs that are not panting or open-mouth breathing. Some dogs may paw at the cannulae and may therefore require an Elizabethan collar.
- An oxygen cage or incubator is another very effective method of oxygen supplementation. Most commercial oxygen cages monitor and display the inspired oxygen concentration and regulate the humidity and temperature. Disadvantages of this method include rapid loss of oxygen when the door is open, potential overheating of larger animals, and difficulty in accessing patients rapidly.

Venous access

Ideally, the next priority for any animal that is having difficulty breathing is to place an intravenous catheter in a peripheral vein. Clinical judgement must be used to determine whether catheter placement might cause undue stress, in which case efforts to stabilize the patient may take precedence. However, early establishment of vascular access can greatly facilitate crisis management if the patient decompensates, allows the administration of intravenous drugs for treatment of the problem, and permits blood samples to be obtained.

Further investigations

If the patient is in significant respiratory distress, radiography should be delayed until after stabilization. Sedatives and analgesics should be administered very cautiously, as drug-induced decreases in central respiratory drive may result in respiratory depression that could precipitate respiratory arrest. Drug doses should be minimized and clinicians should be organized and prepared to intubate any respiratory patient that has been sedated.

Based on the history and signalment, an initial brief physical examination, and observation of the pattern of respiration, the clinician is usually able to categorize the type of respiratory disease based on its location within the respiratory system. Specific therapeutic options and the long-term care of the stabilized patient will then depend on the underlying cause.

References and further reading

Brown D and Gregory S (2005) Brachycephalic airway disease. In: *BSAVA Manual of Canine and Feline Head, Neck and Thoracic Surgery*, ed. DJ Brockman and DE Holt, pp.73–83. BSAVA Publications, Gloucester

Demetriou JL, Foale RD, Ladlow J *et al.* (2002) Canine and feline pyothorax: a retrospective study of 50 cases in the UK and Ireland. *Journal of Small Animal Practice* **43**, 388–394

Hedlund CS (2002) Surgery of the upper respiratory system. In: *Small Animal Surgery*, ed.T Fossum, pp.620–628. Mosby, St. Louis

Holden D and Drobatz K (2005) Emergency management of respiratory distress. In: *BSAVA Manual of Canine and Feline Head, Neck and Thoracic Surgery*, ed. DJ Brockman and DE Holt, pp.73–83. BSAVA Publications, Gloucester

Johnson MS and Martin MWS (2007) Successful medical treatment of 15 dogs with pyothorax. *Journal of Small Animal Practice* **48**, 12–16

King LG and Boag A (2007) *BSAVA Manual of Canine and Feline Emergency and Critical Care, 2nd edn.* BSAVA Publications, Gloucester

Luis Fuentes V, Johnson L and Dennis S (2010) *BSAVA Manual of Canine and Feline Cardiorespiratory Medicine, 2nd edn.* BSAVA Publications, Gloucester

MacPhail CM (2007) Medical and surgical management of pyothorax. *Veterinary Clinics of North America: Small Animal Practice* **37**, 975–988

Payne JD, Mehler SJ and Weisse C (2006) Tracheal collapse. *Compendium on Continuing Education for the Practicing Veterinarian* **28**, 373–382

Rooney MB and Monnet E (2002) Medical and surgical treatment of pyothorax in dogs: 26 cases (1991-2001). *Journal of the American Veterinary Medical Association* **221**, 86–92

Waddell LS, Brady CA and Drobatz KJ (2002) Risk factors, prognostic indicators, and outcome of pyothorax in cats: 80 cases (1986-1999). *Journal of the American Veterinary Medical Association* **221**, 819–824

Clinical case studies

A variety of case scenarios in dogs and cats will now be presented to illustrate the considerations to be made and the options available within a specific clinical setting. Information relating to the rehabilitation and palliation of each condition has been contributed to each case by the authors in the first part of this Manual, plus notes on nursing and homecare from Rachel Lumbis RVN. The reader should refer back to the appropriate chapters for further details. Photographs used to illustrate the principles and techniques within the cases do not necessarily feature the original patient.

Case 17.1
Asthma in a cat

A 3-year-old castrated male Siamese cat had recently been diagnosed with feline asthma and was being medicated with an oral corticosteroid and bronchodilator. On examination he was breathing normally. The owners reported that they were having difficulty medicating him. He was an indoor-only cat and the only pet in a two-bedroom apartment. He was overweight (BCS 7/9) and had a dry, unkempt coat.

Blood tests, urinalysis and/or radiography were considered to rule out concurrent disease contributing to the poor hair coat.

Agreed medical/surgical management

Stress to this patient must be minimized by handling him sensitively. Oxygen should be provided if necessary during acute bouts. Short-acting parenteral glucocorticosteroids and bronchodilators should be used for immediate management of emergency crises, while oral corticosteroids and bronchodilators are usually used for long-term management. For better long-term compliance, inhaled corticosteroids or bronchodilators should be considered. It may also be necessary to consider repository subcutaneous corticosteroid therapy administered monthly.

Environmental issues in the apartment that might trigger asthma attacks should be addressed; these include dust, smoking, cat litter and air fresheners. Weight loss was advised.

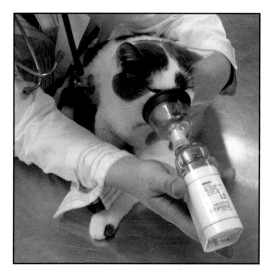

Use of a nebulizer to deliver an aerosol of salbutamol to a cat. (Reproduced from *BSAVA Manual of Canine and Feline Cardiorespiratory Medicine, 2nd edition*)

Acute/chronic pain management

Pain is unlikely to be an issue in this case but an open mind should always be kept in this regard. Secondary muscular pain in the thoracic and even abdominal muscles may be identified, and acupuncture could be indicated if these were considered to be significant and/or if acupuncture were being considered as part of the treatment (see below). It is sometimes possible for cats to develop pneumothorax, or even rib fractures, during severe asthma attacks, and in that event pain management will be necessary.

Fear, stress, conflict concerns

Care needs to be taken with altering the cat's environment suddenly (even if it is for the better), especially changing the cat litter. This may trigger toileting problems and increased stress for the patient (and owner). Change should be done relatively gradually and should consist of providing the cat with choices so that he can demonstrate his preference. A change in feeding regime may be helpful, with the cat working for his food (see below).

Nutritional requirements

Weight management

The predominant nutritional consideration in this cat is weight loss. The excess weight is a major consideration, since obese subjects have reduced respiratory function. Thus, the clinical signs are likely to have been exacerbated by the degree of adiposity. Further, since glucocorticoids may be used during management, this could lead to further weight gain if food intake is not properly regulated. It may be worth performing preliminary laboratory analyses to ensure that the cat is clinically well and that there is no evidence of another significant disease. Whilst weight loss is clearly beneficial, this should only be started when the cat is medically stable because sick cats have an increased risk of hepatic lipidosis if they are dieted too enthusiastically.

Given that there are no drugs authorized for weight loss in cats **(the weight loss drugs for dogs should not be used in cats)**, a conventional weight management regime would be recommended, involving appropriate dietary management and lifestyle alterations (see Chapter 6). Just before starting the weight management regime, the cat should be weighed and his body condition score assessed (see Chapter 6). This will enable the degree of excess weight to be estimated, and a target bodyweight set. A purpose-formulated diet, designed for feeding during weight management, can be commenced (see Chapter 6 for details on how to set target weights). The cat should be meal-fed; *ad libitum* feeding is usually inappropriate, especially for neutered cats as they do not regulate their intake well to match calorie needs.

If the diet is changed, **it is vital to ensure that the cat does not become anorexic.** Overweight cats that go off their food are at increased risk of developing potentially fatal hepatic lipidosis, so adequate food intake must be maintained – even if it means giving up on a weight loss diet which the cat finds unpalatable.

It would also be beneficial to increase activity levels, since this will improve fitness and burn calories. However, the level of activity must be carefully tailored to the abilities of the patient, and must not exacerbate clinical signs. Short periods of gentle activity would be recommended initially, and levels should only be increased when fitness has improved and it is safe to do so. Rather than vigorous play sessions, it may be sensible to increase activity in other ways. One approach would be to distribute (kibbled) food over a wide area to encourage movement.

If the clinical condition is more stable, weight loss has started and the cat is fitter, it may be possible to start introducing play sessions, as for a normal feline weight management regime (Chapter 6). Only one or two sessions of 2–3 minutes may be a sensible starting point.

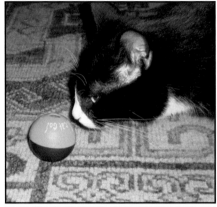

The cat should return to the clinic every 2 weeks initially, so that progress with weight loss can be monitored. The same set of electronic weigh scales should be used when weighing him, so that any changes are known to be due to genuine changes in weight rather than inaccuracies between scales. Most cats will lose between 0.5 and 1.0% of starting bodyweight per week. Dietary caloric intake may need to be modified if weight loss slows.

Once the cat has reached his target weight, a maintenance regime should be instigated. The transition should be made gradually; for example, the cat should continue to be weighed every 2 weeks, whilst his energy intake is increased incrementally by 10% at a time. Once weight has stabilized, the interval between weight checks can be gradually extended (monthly, 3-monthly, 6-monthly) but they should not be stopped altogether.

If dried food is being fed, a feeding toy can be used to increase activity at meal times. (Courtesy of Hilary Orpet)

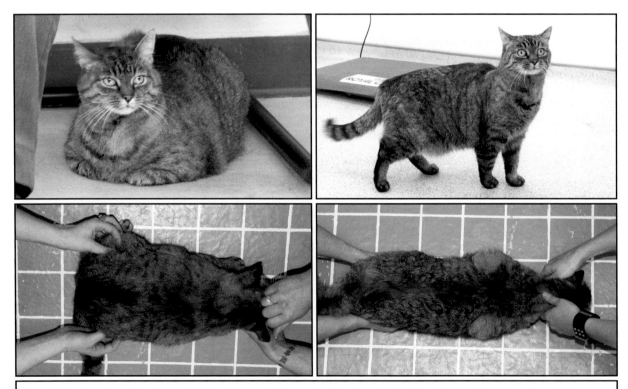

A weight management regime can be very successful in cats. (Courtesy of The Royal Canin Weight Management Clinic, University of Liverpool)

Nutraceuticals

The use of omega-3 fatty acids as adjunctive therapy for human adults and children with asthma has been associated with some success, especially when combined with antioxidants. This approach has not resulted in any measurable improvement in cats with asthma, although further evaluation is necessary before excluding this form of therapy.

Physiotherapy

The main physiotherapy input would be in respect of exercise, to improve exercise tolerance and help with weight loss. A slowly progressive exercise programme encouraging small periods of controlled play would be the preferred approach, which can be increased in time and complexity with ability.

> **WARNING**
> Manual techniques used on the chest may increase bronchospasm, so would not be recommended.

Hydrotherapy

Hydrotherapy is not indicated for this patient.

Acupuncture

There is much experimental work on the effects of acupuncture on the immune system of mice and rabbits, and some data from clinical studies in human patients. Although the experimental data look impressive, the effect in practice seems to be either relatively small or confined to a subpopulation of very sensitive acupuncture 'responders'. There are anecdotal reports of dramatic reduction in pruritus with atopy, for example, whilst the majority of atopic animals do not appear to respond at all in terms of their atopy, although they may respond to the analgesic effects of acupuncture.

Cats appear to be generally good acupuncture responders and, although there is no evidence of effect for feline asthma, it may be worth discussing the option with the owner. It must be made clear that this is not a substitute for specific medication, weight loss or environmental changes but rather is an adjunctive treatment.

> **WARNING**
> Safety considerations include consideration of immune status if corticosteroid doses have been prolonged or high (risk of infection), and avoidance of needling between the ribs on to pleura because of the risk of causing pneumothorax, especially when there is pre-existing lung pathology.

Other nursing and supportive care

Handling the cat in the clinic

Any physical examination should be performed rapidly and carefully, while avoiding stressing the cat, paying particular attention to his breathing pattern, auscultatory abnormalities, pulses and mucous membrane colour and perfusion. If he is very dyspnoeic on admission, it may be best to give him some immediate intravenous steroid treatment and a bronchodilator, and put him somewhere calm and quiet – with oxygen therapy – to calm down for some time before attempting full examination or other investigations.

- If the cat is acutely dyspnoeic and needs oxygen, an oxygen cage is usually the least stressful method. Another option is an Elizabethan collar with plastic wrap over the top to contain oxygen; however, many cats find this method stressful and do not tolerate it well.
- If the patient is in acute respiratory distress, ways to reduce any dyspnoea/orthopnoea should be considered, e.g. positioning the cat in sternal recumbency with positioning aids or rolled up towels either side.
- Venous access is vital in patients with compromised respiratory function, so a peripheral intravenous catheter should be placed and maintained.
- The provision of a vaporizer or nebulizer to humidify the air may help the cat to breathe more easily.
- Regularly monitor and record vital signs.

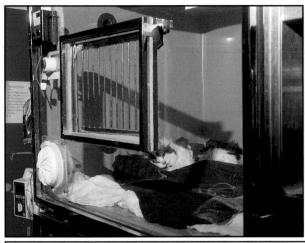 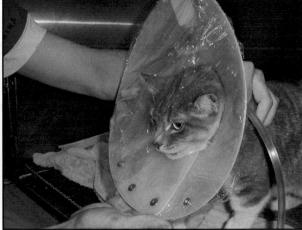

Alternative methods of oxygen supplementation for a dyspneoic cat.

Feeding

If the cat is anorexic and not interested in feeding, *he should not be force-fed*. This would cause stress, could result in a food aversion, and carries the risk of aspiration in a dyspnoeic animal. It is best to wait until the acute dyspnoeic episode is over and then to attempt to hand-feed small amounts of highly palatable fresh food such as tuna or chicken.

Owner advice and homecare recommendations

Management at home

Once a diagnosis is confirmed and a management plan has been drawn up, it is worthwhile remembering that most respiratory patients do much better in their own homes. As stress can trigger and exacerbate symptoms, the more that can be managed at home, the better for the cat.

A marked improvement in the cat's wellbeing can often be achieved by reducing its exposure to airway irritants and removing potential triggers such as household aerosols, cat litter dust and cigarette smoke. The owner should consider excluding the cat from their bedroom (to reduce exposure to human dander and house mites), although this must be weighed up against the potential stress that this may cause. Sudden changes in environmental temperature should be avoided. The home environment should be as stress-free as possible and the cat should be provided with an area within the apartment to which it can escape for peace and quiet.

Grooming the cat and putting aside some time to sit and fuss over him can help to promote relaxation, assuming he enjoys such contact.

Home monitoring

The owner should be advised of normal respiratory, heart and pulse rates and rhythms; regular monitoring while the cat is asleep or at rest is recommended.

An asthmatic cat will squat, with its shoulders hunched up and neck extended. A persistent increase in resting heart and respiratory rates, together with long periods of coughing, are often an early sign of an asthma attack. **Attacks can be mild or severe and it is vital that the owner seeks veterinary advice if they suspect that their cat is unwell.**

Medication

There are many treatment options for asthma available to complement standard pharmaceutical medications. These options include nebulizers, aerosol chambers and acupuncture (see above).

If the owners decide to try inhaled medication for the cat, the vet or nurse will need to demonstrate the technique to the owners.

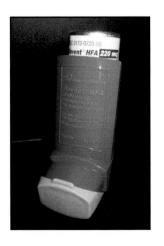

Standard metered dose inhaler for corticosteroid administration. (Courtesy of Lynelle Johnson; reproduced from *BSAVA Manual of Canine and Feline Cardiorespiratory Medicine, 2nd edition*)

Weight loss programme

The owners should be assisted in implementing the weight loss programme and advised on how to encourage the cat to exercise.

Case 17.2
Haemothorax in a dog

A 4-year-old female spayed Cocker Spaniel cross in ideal body condition was presented in a dyspnoeic and collapsed state. Clinical examination confirmed dyspnoea and muffled heart sounds, with reduced resonance on thoracic percussion. Mucous membranes were pale and peripheral pulses weak. The owner reported no known trauma or toxin ingestion, but mentioned that the dog 'eats everything off the streets'.

Ultrasonography confirmed pleural fluid. Aspiration cytology confirmed haemothorax. One-stage prothrombin time (OSPT) was markedly prolonged, and activated partial thromboplastin time (APTT) was also prolonged. A presumptive diagnosis of anticoagulant toxicity was made on the basis of these findings and the subsequent response to vitamin K therapy.

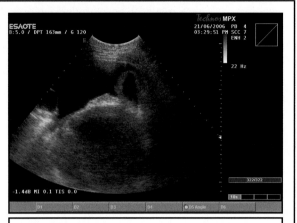

Ultrasound image showing anechoic fluid accumulating in the pleural space. (Courtesy of Frances Barr)

Agreed medical/surgical management

The dog was given oxygen therapy and thoracocentesis was performed, with concurrent intravenous volume resuscitation. A fresh whole blood transfusion was commenced, to replace clotting factors and red cells. (Alternatively, packed red blood cells and fresh frozen plasma could be used if available.)

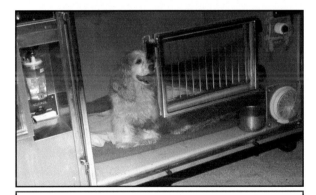

In emergencies involving dyspnoeic animals, oxygen can be supplemented using an oxygen cage.

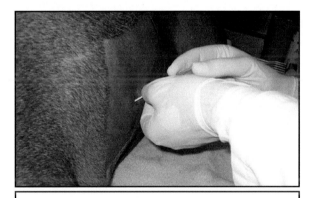

Thoracocentesis needle being placed in a dog. (Courtesy of Lynelle Johnson)

Subcutaneous vitamin K1 (2.5 mg/kg q12h) was given in the hospital, followed by oral vitamin K1 (2.5 mg/kg q12h) for 4 weeks; OSPT was then rechecked 48–72 hours after finishing the course. (For a *known* first-generation anticoagulant (warfarin) toxicity, 1 mg/kg orally q24h vitamin K1 should be instituted for 10–14 days, and OSPT rechecked 48–72 hours after finishing the course.) Vitamin K1 therapy should only be permanently stopped if OSPT is normal 48–72 hours after a course of therapy.

Acute/chronic pain management

The haemothorax in this patient may well be causing her pain and will contribute to her depressed state. Opiates can be considered: any concern about their respiratory depressant effects is counteracted by the fact that relief of any pain will improve ventilation by increasing chest excursion. Pethidine would be a good choice initially, because of its short duration of action, until the haemothorax has been drained. After that, methadone or buprenorphine would be good choices, depending on pain scoring: if pain is moderate, buprenorphine would be suitable.

Fear, stress, conflict concerns

The reasons for the dog's scavenging behaviour should be explored in the long term, to determine whether it is behavioural or clinical in origin. It may be that the behaviour has been inadvertently rewarded in the past, or she may be genuinely hungry and attempting to satisfy her appetite, or she may have a genuine pica as a result of an underlying problem such as gastrointestinal disease. However, it is likely that management with a muzzle is the most practical measure in the short term.

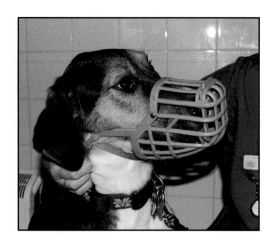

A basket muzzle, fitted here by the veterinary nurse, can help prevent a dog from eating inappropriate items while out on a walk. (Courtesy of Rachel Lumbis and Catherine Kendall)

Nutritional requirements

Feeding in the hospital

WARNING
The dog should not be fed while she is dyspnoeic (because of the risk of aspiration pneumonia) or while receiving a blood transfusion (because of the risk of vomiting during the transfusion).

After the initial 24 hours' stabilization, it is important to ensure that this patient eats while in the hospital. Her calorie requirements should be calculated (see Chapter 5). If she does not eat at least 85% of her calorie requirements for 3 days after hospitalization, consideration should be given to some form of assisted feeding. In this case, as feeding is likely only to be needed short term, a naso-oesophageal or oesophagostomy tube would be ideal; the naso-oesophageal route might be preferable as general anaesthesia is not required. However, it is important to ensure that blood clotting times are normal before the tube is placed, to avoid the risk of severe epistaxis (the extent of which may go unnoticed as the blood may be swallowed). Oesophagostomy tube placement is also *not* recommended in a patient with severe coagulopathy that has resulted in haemothorax – even after administration of fresh frozen plasma and vitamin K; these cases pose a risk, especially in dogs, where the procedure is not as straightforward as it is in cats). Before subjecting this patient to an oesophagostomy tube, clotting times must be completely normal. See Chapter 5 for details on tube placement and feeding.

Diet
There is no special advice about diet for this patient. After the initial injections of vitamin K1, she could be maintained longer term on oral vitamin K1, provided that efficacy is checked frequently by assessing clotting times. Absorption of oral vitamin K1 is increased 4–5 times if given with wet food of a high fat content.

Physiotherapy

As soon as the dog's condition is stable, gentle exercise should be introduced to encourage deep breathing to prevent any restriction of chest movement due to pleural thickening. This will also help reverse any atelectasis associated with the haemothorax, by increasing tidal volume and reversing small airway collapse, and therefore may also decrease the need for oxygen therapy.

WARNING
Vigorous exercise should be avoided whilst clotting is deranged.

Hydrotherapy

Hydrotherapy is not indicated for this patient.

Acupuncture

Acupuncture is not indicated for this patient.

Other nursing and supportive care

Care on admission

While the patient is in acute respiratory distress, ways to reduce any dyspnoea/orthopnoea should be considered, e.g. positioning her in sternal recumbency with positioning aids/rolled up towels on either side. Stressing, handling and restraining the dog should be minimized.

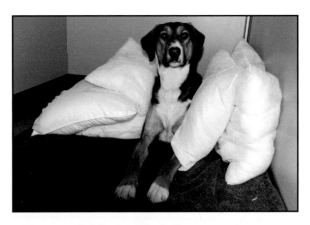

> Positioning in sternal recumbency with support on either side would be suitable for a dyspnoeic dog. (Courtesy of Rachel Lumbis and Catherine Kendall)

The dog should be given oxygen until the pleural fluid has been drained. Quiet dogs will often tolerate an intranasal oxygen tube well; this is the most efficient means of supplementing oxygen once coagulation times have been normalized. It is important that the oxygen is humidified by passing it through a humidifier bottle first. Failing this, an oxygen cage or Elizabethan collar with cling film could be used (as in Case 17.1).

WARNING
Nasal oxygen cannulae should be avoided while the coagulopathy is present, because they may induce haemorrhage from the vascular mucosa of the turbinates.

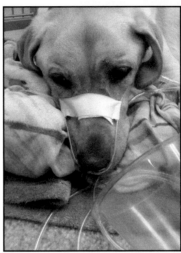
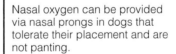

Nasal oxygen can be provided via nasal prongs in dogs that tolerate their placement and are not panting.

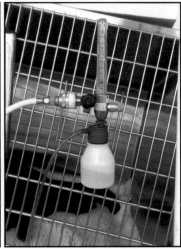

It is important that the oxygen is humidified by passing it through a humidifier bottle first. (Courtesy of Penny Watson)

Comfort and monitoring

Comfort and reassurance should be provided to the patient, along with a warm quiet environment. Opportunities for trauma must be avoided until the coagulopathy is under control (e.g. avoid letting her bash into kennel doors, etc.). The patient should be continually monitored for further signs of haemorrhage.

She should be taken outside, and gentle exercise introduced, once she is stable. This will also help to stop her becoming understimulated once she feels well.

Owner advice and homecare recommendations

Monitoring

Owners should be advised to look carefully for any signs of bleeding or recurrence of dyspnoea while the dog is still on vitamin K therapy. The owner should be requested to bring the dog back to recheck blood clotting 48–72 hours after completion of vitamin K1 therapy. If the initial course does not normalize clotting, vitamin K1 therapy will be reinstituted for a further week. Return for a further OSPT will be necessary 48–72 hours after completion of therapy.

Exercise

The owners should be advised to give the dog gentle exercise (see above) once her condition is stable. The amount of exercise should be within the capabilities of the animal.

Avoiding scavenging

The owners should be encouraged to acclimatize the dog to wearing a comfortable, basket-type muzzle whenever she has the opportunity to scavenge.

Case 17.3
Chronic bronchitis in a dog

An 8-year-old male castrated Bichon Frisé in ideal body condition was presented for re-evaluation of a chronic cough. He had previously been diagnosed with chronic bronchitis. He was breathing with a normal rhythm but had bilateral crackles. The owner reported that the dog coughed daily. The dog had also previously been diagnosed with diabetes mellitus, which had been stabilized, patellar luxation, and had moderate to severe periodontal disease.

Thoracic radiographs were taken to rule out other causes of coughing and crackles, such as tracheal collapse, heart disease, neoplasia and pneumonia. Blood samples were taken in order to perform a complete work-up and rule out other concurrent disease in this older diabetic dog. Airway sample cytology and culture were performed to evaluate the type of inflammation (neutrophilic/eosinophillic) and to rule out bacterial infection; the results showed a mild neutrophilic infiltrate. A sample of faeces was submitted for a Baermann test for lungworms; this was negative.

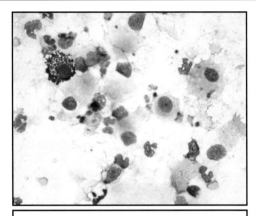

BAL sample showing a mixed inflammatory profile dominated by neutrophils and macrophages. (Courtesy of Brendan Corcoran. Reproduced from *BSAVA Manual of Canine and Feline Cardiorespiratory Medicine, 2nd edn*)

Agreed medical/surgical management

The dog was currently being medicated for his diabetes with Lente insulin (given twice a day) and an NSAID for chronic bilateral luxating patellae (grade III/IV).

Therapy for chronic bronchitis starts with bronchodilators (theophylline or terbutaline, orally). If coughing does not improve, corticosteroids will probably be required, but systemic corticosteroids will adversely affect the management of the diabetes by making the patient unpredictably insulin-resistant, and also cannot be given concurrently with the NSAIDs. Inhaled fluticasone is an option because this will provide local drug levels in the airways without systemic absorption. If inhaled anti-inflammatories are ineffective, NSAIDs should be stopped and oral glucocorticoids begun.

Glucose/ketones should be monitored, the teeth brushed, and dental extractions with cleaning considered. Surgical management of the luxating patellae had been discussed previously but, in view of the concurrent problems, conservative treatment had been decided upon as the pragmatic choice.

Acute/chronic pain management

Chronic pain
The main chronic pain issue to be dealt with in this patient is that from the luxating patellae and the periodontal disease. The patellar problem is likely to lead to lumbar pain because of the shift of weight from the hindlimbs to the lumbar muscles.

Chronic coughing is also likely to give rise to secondary muscle pain from the intercostal and other thoracic muscles, as well as exacerbating any concurrent muscle strain in, for example, the lumbar or abdominal muscles. The patient should be assessed to determine as far as possible how much his patellar problem is affecting him, and treatment devised accordingly.

The dog is already receiving NSAIDs. Acupuncture (see below) may be useful to avoid further additional medication. Tramadol, at the lowest starting dose since little is known about its action in sick dogs, may help to reduce suffering. Paracetamol, with codeine or alone, may be a useful adjunct if other NSAIDs are contraindicated, since it can be given alongside corticosteroids. Glucosamine and chondroitin supplementation seem to have analgesic effects in some individuals (see Nutrition) but should not be considered as sufficient analgesia alone. Pentosan polysulphate injections given once weekly for 4 weeks to assess effects, and thereafter as indicated, may also be useful; although the datasheet for Cartrophen recommends that it *not* be given concurrently with NSAIDs.

Fear, stress, conflict concerns

If the coughing causes pain or the bouts are prolonged, then anxiety is likely to be a factor and such a stressor may affect both the diabetes and the bronchitis. Continuing pain from the mouth and patellar problems will also be a source of conflict and anxiety as in any chronic pain condition. Recognizing and controlling the pain and cough are therefore most important.

If the owner recognizes signs of anxiety associated with the coughing bouts, teaching them a relaxation technique to use with the dog can be useful. Restriction of exercise should also be considered as a possible stressor, and alternative sources of mental stimulation provided, such as changed feeding regimes and mentally stimulating games such as hide and seek (see Chapter 4).

Nutritional requirements

Diet

The dog is already likely to be on a suitable diabetic diet. Any balanced diet fed in the same amounts every day could be used; on twice-daily insulin the dog should have half of his calorie requirements split into two meals a day and given at the same time as the insulin injections. The prescription diets for diabetic dogs have increased fibre content (usually mixed fermentable and non-fermentable) and also reduced caloric density compared with normal maintenance diets. These are suitable unless the dog is underweight, in which case a diet of normal caloric density should be chosen.

Bichon Frisés, like other terrier-type dogs, may develop diabetes mellitus secondary to chronic pancreatitis; if this is suspected as the underlying cause, a low-fat diet designed for intestinal disease (normal caloric density) or a low-fat maintenance diet may be chosen.

If the dog gains weight while on steroid therapy, reducing the amount of food fed or changing to a calorie-restricted diabetic diet might be considered, together with appropriate adjustments of the dose of insulin to balance the changes in food intake and steroid dose. On the other hand, if the dental disease reduces the dog's appetite and food intake, this change to a low-calorie diet would be inappropriate. Overall, then, this dog's calorie intake and choice of diet should be tailored to the individual circumstances. There are no particular recommendations for diet for his respiratory disease.

Nutraceuticals

Omega-3 fatty acid supplementation has been used in chronic respiratory conditions, such as asthma, in human patients. No data are available regarding its use in dogs with chronic bronchitis, although it is thought that supplementation could reduce the degree of chronic inflammation. Further research is warranted before any recommendation can be made. Omega-3 fatty acids have also been suggested to reduce joint inflammation in osteoarthritis (see Chapter 14).

Chromium picolinate was previously thought to increase insulin sensitivity; therefore, dietary supplementation of this micronutrient was considered potentially beneficial for diabetics. Results for improvement in diabetic management have not been positive, however, and this is no longer thought to be an important component of therapy.

Physiotherapy

Chronic bronchitis

It would be useful to determine when the dog coughs the most. It is likely that this will be in the mornings, after sleeping, and during or after exercise. If there is a pattern to his coughing, then treatment should be carried out around these times, e.g. first thing in the morning (directly after waking), before exercise and before bedtime.

Regular short sessions of chest physiotherapy and postural drainage (see Case 17.5) to clear retained sputum would be beneficial. The preferred positions for treatment would be alternate-side lying, standing and sitting, with double-handed percussion (coupage) carried out in each position for 2 minutes followed by six expiratory vibrations (see Chapter 9). This protocol should be carried out a minimum of four times a day. The dog may not cough at the time of treatment but may well cough 15–20 minutes afterwards (this is normal in babies who also cannot 'deep breathe' to command).

Exercise will also encourage deep breathing and sputum clearance, but will need to be tailored to the dog's ability (i.e. in respect of his luxating patellae). Regular exercise has also been found to control blood sugar levels in humans with diabetes mellitus and, in the long term, to lead to reductions in their required medications. Regulating the amount of exercise to the same amount each day (as much as possible) would also be important to this dog's diabetic stability.

Patellar luxation

There are several issues concerning the luxating patellae that need consideration. These are primarily to do with pain relief and associated musculoskeletal problems (e.g. muscle wastage, loss of joint range, alteration in dynamic muscular support to the stifles, reduction in balance and proprioception). See Case 14.6 for recommendations.

Secondary muscle and joint pain

The other issue that should be considered is in respect of secondary muscle and joint pain resulting from persistent coughing and compensatory postures. Once these have been identified as an issue, appropriate physiotherapy treatments may include joint mobilizations, soft tissue treatments (e.g. massage, myofascial release, acupressure) and electrotherapy modalities, including therapeutic laser therapy (see Chapter 9).

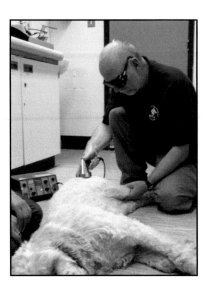

Laser therapy of the gluteal muscles. (Courtesy of Brian Sharp)

Hydrotherapy

Although hydrotherapy might help to improve the luxating patellae by improving muscle mass and strength, the physical effort of swimming will exacerbate the patient's cough and cause deterioration in this and his other medical conditions.

Acupuncture

The main indication for acupuncture is as an analgesic for the luxating patellae (see Case 14.6), especially if NSAIDs become contraindicated (e.g. if glucocorticoids are used for the bronchitis). However, in the course of examination, other sources of secondary muscle pain, partly due to postural changes (lumbar epaxial muscles especially) and partly due to coughing if the bouts are severe, should be identified as possible sources of continuing pain: muscles over the thorax, abdomen and even in the neck (especially lower neck and cranial trapezius muscles) can be strained secondary to coughing.

Most of the causes of chronic bronchitis are not likely to be amenable to acupuncture treatment, although it is possible that a small number of individuals with an allergic component to their disease may be sufficiently sensitive to the therapy that a response may be seen. However, acupuncture is not an alternative to conventional and specific therapy in this condition, neither is there any evidence that it is directly anti-inflammatory.

> **WARNING**
> - Avoid direct needling into the stifle joints and needling between the ribs on to pleura and lung.
> - Prolonged and high doses of glucocorticoids would mean that the use of acupuncture carries a relative caution (risk of infection) if the animal is severely immunosuppressed.
> - Acupuncture has been reported, anecdotally in humans, to alter the requirement for insulin temporarily, so it is recommended that glucose levels are checked in the 24 hours following acupuncture rather than assumed to be stable for the usually well controlled diabetic.

Other nursing and supportive care

- If the dog is hospitalized, he should be in a quiet stress-free environment, away from barking dogs and other unwelcome stressors.
- The provision of a vaporizer or nebulizer to humidify the air may help the dog to breathe more easily.

Diabetic routine in hospital

The dog should be kept to as near normal routine as possible to avoid diabetic complications. This includes feeding him the same food as at home in the same quantities and administering insulin at the same time of day. Food intake must be monitored carefully and alterations made to insulin given as necessary. For example, if food is withheld for sedation or general anaesthesia, usually half of the usual insulin dose is given and blood glucose monitored carefully while the dog is fasted and during anaesthesia. Blood glucose may need to be monitored frequently in any hospitalized diabetic patient (up to every 2, 4, 6 or 12 hours depending on circumstances). This is particularly important because the stress of hospitalization, procedures and concurrent diseases are all likely to affect glucose levels, even in previously well regulated diabetics.

Owner advice and homecare recommendations

Chronic bronchitis

Establishment of excellent client communications is critical so that client expectations are realistic and they adhere to the therapeutic regime. Owners should be advised that canine chronic bronchitis is a common, progressive airway disorder. Its signs can be greatly improved, but the disease is not curable. If the owner is currently using a lead when taking the dog out, it might be worth considering the use of a non-pulling harness or headcollar instead. The owners should also avoid, as much as is possible, exposing their dog to environmental stressors including house dust, vapours, chemical fumes, cigarette smoke, pollution, dust and grains. Inhalation of humidified air via a vaporizer or commercial humidifier/nebulizer, or placing the animal in a hot steamy bathroom, may liquefy secretions, hydrate the airways and reduce the dog's cough. The owners should be instructed in chest coupage (see above). If an inhaler is to be used (see Case 17.1), the owners should receive careful instruction and demonstration on how to use it.

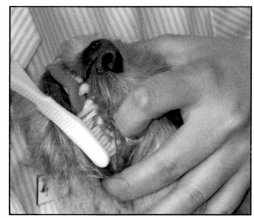

Dog wearing an Easy Walk® harness. (Courtesy of Premier Pet Products)

Particular care should be taken to explain the potential effects of various medications (e.g. steroids) on the control of the dog's diabetes mellitus. If the owner monitors blood glucose concentrations at home, they may be able to adjust for this themselves, with advice from the practice.

The owners should also be advised to keep the patient's weight stable. This is important for all its concurrent conditions (bronchitis, diabetes mellitus and luxating patellae).

Exercise
The owner should be provided with an appropriate exercise programme designed specifically to cater for the dog's needs, and an explanation should be given regarding the pacing of all activities. It is particularly important, in view of the diabetes, to keep the amount of daily exercise as constant as possible.

Dental prophylaxis
Routine dental prophylaxis may help maintain a healthy oral flora. The owners should be instructed on how to brush their dog's teeth effectively and a practical demonstration given. The owner should be encouraged to repeat this technique whilst in the practice, first on a model and then on their pet.

The dog is held across the muzzle. Brushing should be started at the back of the mouth and worked forwards. The bristles of the toothbrush are angled toward the gingival margin. (Reproduced from *BSAVA Manual of Canine and Feline Advanced Veterinary Nursing, 2nd edn*)

Case 17.4
Brachycephalic airway obstruction syndrome in a dog

A 2-year-old spayed female Pug was presented with severe stertor due to presumptive brachycephalic syndrome. The dog was obese (BCS 8/9) and very anxious. The owner had financial limitations.

Agreed medical/surgical management

The first requirement is for sedation to decrease the dog's anxiety and modify respiratory drive, thereby decreasing airway obstruction. Parenteral acepromazine is most effective, with the addition of butorphanol if necessary.

If the patient is hyperthermic, she should be cooled using water, ice and/or a fan, until rectal temperature is <39°C. Intravenous fluid therapy is required if she is dehydrated or hypovolaemic.

Oxygen therapy using flow-by, a face mask or oxygen cage may be necessary. If the patient is sedated enough, she may be positioned in sternal recumbency with her head and neck extended, her mouth open and tongue pulled forward.

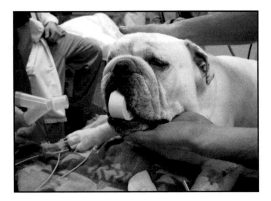

Flow-by oxygen being delivered to a brachycephalic dog. The patient's head is being held with the neck extended and the mouth propped open.

If there is no response to oxygen therapy, tracheostomy and airway examination should follow. Thoracic radiographs should be considered to rule out concurrent pneumonia.

Ideally, surgery to trim the overlong soft palate, stenotic nares and everted saccules should be carried out (see *BSAVA Manual of Canine and Feline Head, Neck and Thoracic Surgery*).

Acute/chronic pain management

Perioperative
Steroids may be given perioperatively to reduce the swelling in the airway; if steroids are used, NSAIDs are contraindicated. In this patient it would be best to avoid opioids, unless absolutely necessary, because of their respiratory depressive effects; if essential, it would be preferable to use shorter-acting drugs such as pethidine or butorphanol. Butorphanol may have the added advantage of preventing cough (so reducing cough-induced swelling). A topical local anaesthetic at the surgical site(s) immediately after surgery should be considered.

Chronic pain
Chronically, there may be secondary muscle pain in the muscles of the neck due to postural changes to ease breathing and the subsequent anxiety associated with breathing difficulties. Acupuncture (see below) is arguably the most useful treatment if these are identified, although massage (see Physiotherapy) may also be helpful.

Fear, stress, conflict concerns

If the patient is anxious because she cannot breathe, short-term sedation is indicated (see above) but, in the longer term, teaching the animal to relax on command may be useful (see Chapter 4). Rhythmical rubbing of the sternum to ease anxiety when the owner notices the patient is particularly anxious or breathless may be useful, both specifically to the patient but also to the owner. If the patient is also temperamentally anxious, i.e. anxious whether she is dyspnoeic or not, then this is likely to contribute to the problem. It may be helpful to explore changes to the environment, owner attitude and, possibly, the use of pheromone therapy and/or alpha-casozepine, although efficacy of either in this situation is unclear (see Chapter 4).

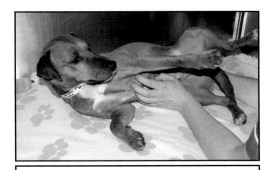

Veterinary nurse demonstrating rhythmical sternal rubbing to ease anxiety. (Courtesy of Rachel Lumbis and Catherine Kendall)

Nutritional requirements

Feeding in the hospital
For the first 24 hours, the dog's fluid and electrolyte requirements should be considered and supplied intravenously if she is too dyspnoeic to drink. Thereafter (from day 2), if the dog remains too dyspnoeic to be able to eat, consideration should be given to some form of tube feeding. Although this dog is obese, any weight loss in these circumstances of stress would be predominantly of lean body mass (see Chapter 5). A naso-oesophageal tube is not ideal in the light of all the airway problems and the fact that the nares are likely to be narrow. Oesophagostomy tube placement would also be very difficult in an obese pug – the thick neck would make this procedure almost impossible to do. If tube feeding proves necessary, a PEG tube (see Chapter 5) could be placed; if the dog is having an anaesthetic for airway examination and surgery, careful consideration should be given to whether she needs a PEG tube before the surgery, as that would be the ideal time to place it. The dog can be fed all or part of her daily calorie requirements via the tube, depending on the need (i.e. on whether she is eating any food independently). Details of calculating the amount to feed and introducing tube

feeding are described in Chapter 5. Total parenteral nutrition (TPN) or partial parenteral nutrition (PPN) are other options to provide nutrition in an animal that is dyspnoeic and anorexic in the hospital (see Chapter 5).

Long-term dietary management: weight loss

In the long term, the main aim in this dog will be weight loss, as the obesity and associated increase in peripharyngeal fat are likely to be contributing to her problems. Depending upon the timeframe between the current illness and the start of the weight management regime, it may be worth performing haematology and clinical biochemistry profiles to determine that the dog has no evidence of concurrent disease.

Options for weight management include drug therapy (e.g. dirlotapide or mitratipide), or a conventional strategy involving dietary caloric restriction. For both options increasing physical activity would be of benefit. Prior to starting the weight management regime, the dog should be weighed and body condition score assessed (see Chapter 6). This will enable the degree of excess weight to be estimated, and a target bodyweight set.

If dietary management is employed, a purpose-formulated diet, designed for feeding during weight management, should then be selected. The best diets are supplemented in protein, so that loss of lean tissue mass is minimized. It would be preferable to choose a diet that is high in fibre, since this may help to improve satiety and minimize negative behavioural manifestations from hunger. The amount of diet fed should be calculated based upon feeding a proportion (typically 50–65%) of maintenance energy requirements at target weight (not current bodyweight) (see Chapter 6). The owner should be instructed to weigh the daily food ration (rather than using a measuring cup) and feed the diet in a number (3–4) of small meals rather than as a single meal. Owners should be discouraged from feeding any additional food (e.g. tit-bits, treats) since these will slow progress with weight loss. If the owners wish to give rewards to their dog, a portion of the daily ration (e.g. dry kibbled foods) should be reserved for use in this way. Most dogs will lose between 0.5 and 1.5% of starting bodyweight per week. If the rate of weight loss is too fast, an increase in the dietary ration can be considered (typically 5%); conversely, where weight loss slows, and there is no other explanation (e.g. no change in exercise plan, no evidence of deviations from the diet), a reduction in dietary energy intake (again typically 5%) should be considered.

In addition to dietary management, the owners should be encouraged to put in place a daily exercise plan, tailored to their dog's abilities. Given the respiratory problems, the level and type of activity should be within the patient's capabilities; controlled exercise would likely be best, using a harness rather than a collar. If/when the dog improves (i.e. loses weight and becomes fitter) it may be possible to instigate some short play sessions. However, these should be low-intensity and of short duration, and not frenetic, since this may exacerbate clinical signs of respiratory compromise.

The dog should return to the clinic on a 2-weekly basis, initially, so that progress with weight loss can be monitored. The same set of electronic weigh scales should be used when weighing the dog, so that any changes are known to be due to genuine changes in weight rather than inaccuracies between scales. Once the dog has reached target weight, a maintenance regime should be instigated. The transition should be made gradually, e.g. the dog should continue to be weighed every 2 weeks, whilst the energy intake is increased

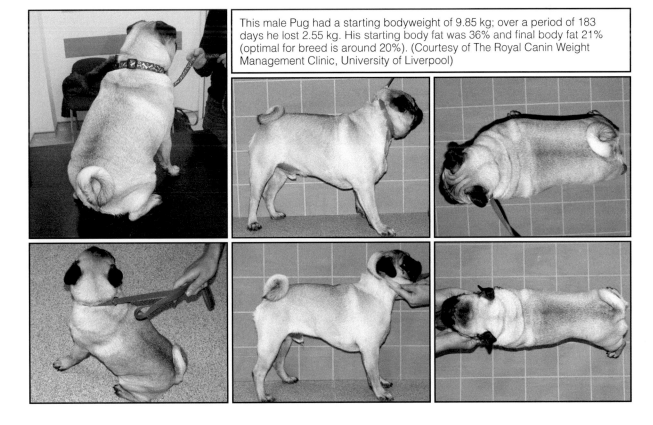

This male Pug had a starting bodyweight of 9.85 kg; over a period of 183 days he lost 2.55 kg. His starting body fat was 36% and final body fat 21% (optimal for breed is around 20%). (Courtesy of The Royal Canin Weight Management Clinic, University of Liverpool)

incrementally by 10% at a time. Once weight has stabilized, the interval between weight checks can be gradually extended (monthly, 3-monthly, 6-monthly) but they should not be stopped altogether.

Physiotherapy

Physiotherapy is not specifically indicated for this dog's main problem, but would have a useful input in the longer term in respect of exercise and increasing exercise tolerance. Input from a veterinary physiotherapist to work with the owner in developing an appropriately progressive exercise programme (so that all this dog's physical needs are addressed) would be the most effective way forward.

If neck or shoulder muscles are sore secondary to overuse in coughing, then the use of warmth and massage could prove beneficial. Gentle, calm techniques (such as stroking, kneading and picking-up) will help relax muscles and may also help to calm the dog. These are easy techniques to teach the owner so he/she can be involved in the treatment process and continue them at home (especially as there are financial limitations and the owner may not be able to afford treatments such as acupuncture).

Hydrotherapy

Hydrotherapy is not indicated for this patient.

Acupuncture

If secondary muscle pain is found on examination (likely to be in the muscles of the neck, but also possibly the pectorals and shoulder girdle muscles depending on the extent of physical exertion and posture change required to breathe), acupuncture can be used to target this directly. There may be some transient, but potent, anxiolytic and sedation effects. However, given the owner's financial limitations in this particular case, it is likely that the medication will be a cheaper option than acupuncture, with more predictable results.

Other nursing and supportive care

Reducing dyspnoea in the hospital
If the patient is in respiratory distress, dyspnoea/orthopnoea should be reduced as much as possible (see above). The dog should be kept in a cool environment if she is hyperthermic, and comfort and reassurance provided. Overheating is very common in these dogs, so body temperature needs measuring frequently and measures taken urgently to lower body temperature if it increases (see above). Venous access is vital in patients with compromised respiratory function; therefore, a peripheral intravenous catheter should be placed and maintained.

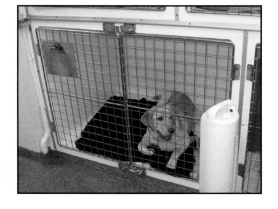

A fan can be used to keep a dog cool while caged in the clinic. (Courtesy of Liz Mullineaux)

Monitoring
Vital signs should be monitored and recorded regularly. Because of the narrowing of the dog's airways and the extra tissue in the pharynx, brachycephalic animals are at greater risk of airway blockage while under anaesthesia. During the postoperative period, the dog must be observed continuously until she is completely recovered from anaesthesia. Subsequently, close observation for dyspnoea and airway obstruction resulting from postoperative inflammation, oedema or haemorrhage is necessary.

Feeding
For several days following surgery, the dog must be observed while eating to ensure that aspiration does not occur. If a PEG tube is placed, the dog must be fitted with an Elizabethan collar to prevent premature removal of the feeding tube, although she should be closely monitored to ensure that this does not distress her unduly. The feeding tube must be flushed with 5–10 ml of water after each feed to minimize clogging (see Chapter 5).

Education about BAOS

It can be difficult to communicate to owners that their pet's congenital conformation is a risk factor for serious, even fatal, respiratory distress. However, the owner must be educated so that they are aware of the risk factors that may trigger a serious episode. Lifelong avoidance of all risk factors as much as possible is necessary.

The owners should be instructed not to force their dog to exercise and, especially, to limit exertion in high ambient temperatures to the absolute minimum. Increased panting can also cause swelling and narrowing of the airway, resulting in collapse or syncope. It is also important that they prevent the dog from becoming overexcited, as this can lead to collapse due to a lack of oxygen.

The owner should be advised about their pet's prognosis. Animals that have signs of upper airway obstruction and do not have surgery will often adjust their behaviour, reducing their activity. They may then survive for several years but will not be able to have a normal life. If additional factors are introduced, these animals usually will decompensate and become severely obstructed. Animals that have surgery to resect the obstructing soft tissue usually will improve but will never be normal.

Owners should be advised about the signs and identification of severe respiratory distress. Abnormal respiratory sounds (stertor, stridor, wheezing), abnormal posture (orthopnoea, head and neck extended, elbows abducted, sternal recumbency), abnormal mucous membrane colour (cyanosis), tachypnoea, weakness and exhaustion, altered respiratory effort (shallow and rapid, or laboured and forceful, or absent), and vigorous resistance to restraint are the typical signs present in animals with respiratory distress.

Weight loss

It is important to assist the owners in implementing a realistic and achievable weight loss programme for their dog (see above). They should be encouraged by stressing how much difference it will make to the dog's ability to breathe. Advice should be given on how to encourage the dog to exercise, e.g. toys and creative games to mentally stimulate her, such as seeking and finding food bowls containing some of her daily ration.

Exercise

The owners should be provided with an appropriate exercise programme designed specifically to cater for the dog's needs, and an explanation should be given regarding the pacing of all activities. The owner can also be taught simple massage techniques to help relax muscles and keep the dog calm.

Case 17.5
Tracheal collapse in a dog

A 7-year-old female spayed Maltese Terrier in ideal body condition was presented in orthopnoea, with significant upper airway noise. She was currently being treated with hydrocodone (antitussive), prednisolone and theophylline for tracheal collapse but was not responding to medical management.

Following emergency stabilization (see below) thoracic radiographs were obtained to rule out concurrent disease such as aspiration pneumonia. An endotracheal wash was obtained for culture and sensitivity testing.

Emergency treatment

As soon as the dog was admitted, oxygen therapy was commenced. She was sedated with parenteral acepromazine (butorphanol may be added if needed). She was positioned in sternal recumbency with her head and neck extended, her mouth open and her tongue pulled forward. The dog's rectal temperature was taken and she was cooled using cold water and a fan until her temperature was <39°C. Parenteral corticosteroids were administered to decrease airway oedema/inflammation.

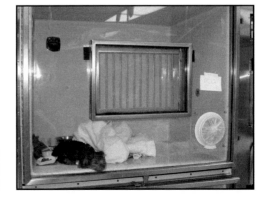

An oxygen cage is a very effective means of providing oxygen for small patients.

If there is no response to these measures, and airway obstruction due to the collapsing trachea continues, general anaesthesia should be induced, the dog intubated and positive pressure ventilation initiated as required.

Antibacterial agents should be commenced if airway culture is positive.

Medical and surgical options

Every effort should be made to manage the tracheal collapse with medical management. In addition to antitussives, this would include: exercise restriction; decreasing any anxiety/ stress (with possible need for sedatives/anxiolytics); weight management; and treatment of any concurrent pulmonary and/ or cardiac disease. Neck leads should be avoided and a harness used instead.

However, if there is ongoing airway obstruction, surgery should be considered. Controversy exists over the most effective treatment for tracheal collapse, i.e. surgical implantation of extratracheal prostheses *versus* intraluminal stent placement (Moritz *et al.*, 2004; Sun *et al.*, 2008). Both procedures show comparable survival rates. Established guidelines for intraluminal stent placement include: dogs who would not benefit from surgery (older dogs, obese dogs, or dogs with intrathoracic/mainstem bronchial collapse) and dogs who are not considered good anaesthetic/surgical candidates (underlying significant heart disease). Intraluminal tracheal stent placement offers the benefits of a minimally invasive procedure and shorter anaesthesia and recovery times. Antitussives are sometimes indicated while the trachea is healing, as excessive coughing can break the repair down.

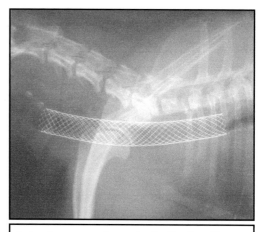

Lateral survey radiograph of a Toy Poodle following placement of an intraluminal self-expanding stent for collapse of the cervical and thoracic inlet portions of the trachea. (Reproduced from *BSAVA Manual of Canine and Feline Head, Neck and Thoracic Surgery*)

Acute/chronic pain management

Perioperative

If tracheal stent surgery is performed, steroids will have been given perioperatively to reduce the swelling in the airway, so NSAIDs are contraindicated. In this patient it would be best to avoid opioids unless absolutely necessary because of their respiratory depressive effects. If opiates are essential, then shorter acting drugs like pethidine or butorphanol would be preferable. Butorphanol may have the added advantage of preventing cough (so reducing cough-induced swelling). Topical local anaesthesia is not necessary for dogs that have had intraluminal stent placement.

Chronic pain

Chronic dyspnoea is likely to give rise to secondary muscle pain from the intercostals and other thoracic muscles; cranial trapezius may also be painful because of the tendency of this patient to extend its neck. This pain will increase anxiety and may further restrict breathing. The safest option for treatment here may to be use acupuncture (see below) but paracetamol added to the current treatment may also be helpful. Other NSAIDs are contraindicated in this patient because of the use of prednisolone. If the patient is sensitive to the effects of opiates, a combination of codeine and tramadol would be better avoided.

Fear, stress, conflict concerns

These may be significant depending on the degree of dyspnoea, the dog's temperament and response to veterinary intervention and hospitalization. Discussion with the owners of her likely response will be helpful in devising nursing care and in recognizing the signs of an abnormally severe response to her situation. See Cases 17.3 and 17.4 and Chapter 4 for management of anxiety.

Nutritional requirements

Feeding in the hospital

It is very likely that this dog will be unable to eat or drink sufficiently for the first few days due to the extent of her respiratory problems. For the first 24 hours, her fluid and electrolyte requirements should be supplied intravenously. Thereafter (from day 2), if she remains too dyspnoeic to be able to eat and drink, intravenous fluids should be continued and consideration given to some form of tube feeding. Neither a naso-oesophageal nor an oesophagostomy tube is ideal in the light of all the airway problems and increased potential for aspiration. A gastrostomy (PEG) tube would be preferable; if the dog is anaesthetized for airway examination and surgery, this would be a good time to place a feeding tube. The dog can be fed either all or part of her daily calorie requirements via the tube depending on need (i.e. whether she is eating any food independently). Details of calculating amount to feed and how to introduce tube feeding are given in Chapter 5. Total or partial parenteral nutrition are other options for nutritional support of an animal that is dyspnoeic (see Chapter 5).

Physiotherapy

If aspiration pneumonia is diagnosed and sputum retention is an issue, the dog should be positioned in the appropriate postural drainage position, with the affected segment uppermost and expiratory vibrations applied (see Chapter 9). It is recommended this is carried out 2–3 times daily (minimum). Head-down positioning should be avoided in dyspnoeic animals because it might worsen respiratory distress, and percussion should not be applied whilst the dog is dyspnoeic as it can cause breath-holding. If the dog is intubated and tracheal collapse is not below the end of the endotracheal tube, tracheal suction is also advised after postural drainage and vibrations to clear secretions. To achieve optimum V/Q matching, alternate-side lying is recommended whilst the patient is intubated, and side lying (good lung down) when the patient is extubated. If there is no aspiration, no physiotherapy is indicated.

Hydrotherapy

Hydrotherapy is not indicated for this patient.

Acupuncture

Not applicable, unless to treat secondary muscular pain.

Other nursing and supportive care

- If the patient is in respiratory distress, ways to reduce any dyspnoea/orthopnoea should be considered, e.g. positioning and oxygen therapy (see Case 17.2).
- Venous access is vital in patients with compromised respiratory function, therefore a peripheral intravenous catheter should be placed and maintained. Regular monitoring and recording of vital signs is essential.
- A stress-free environment and strict rest should be imposed.
- Body temperature should be monitored frequently and the dog cooled if necessary (see above).

Postoperative care
Following surgery, the patient should be monitored closely for signs of complications:

- Laryngeal paralysis
- Swelling of the airway
- Necrosis of the trachea
- Pneumonia
- Infection of the surgical site.

Following surgery, the dog must be fitted with an Elizabethan collar to prevent interference with the surgical site. This is also indicated if surgery has not been performed but the dog has intravenous catheters and feeding tubes *in situ*.

Feeding and tube care
If the patient has a PEG tube, feeding and tube care will be required as detailed in Chapter 5.

Owner advice and homecare recommendations

Feeding and weight management
Diet is critical and the owner must prevent the dog from becoming obese.

Follow-up and prognosis
The owners should be advised that wheezing, breathing with an expiratory effort, exercise intolerance, cyanosis and even syncope may be noted. Coughing may occur at any time during the day but is common following exertion (exercise intolerance), at night (nocturnal coughing) as secretions accumulate, or when the trachea is

irritated – for instance with 'lead pulling'. Exercise should be restricted for a period of around 4 months following surgical repair and a harness should be used instead of a collar. Over-exciting or stressful situations should be avoided or sedation given as needed if such situations are anticipated.

The owners should be made aware that tracheal collapse can be a progressive disease, and treatment with a tracheal stent is a *salvage* procedure, not a cure. Complications of stent placement include stent migration, stent fractures, granulation tissue formation, coughing, and infectious tracheitis. Therefore, regular routine follow-up radiography and/or fluoroscopy will be necessary to assess the overall integrity of the stent.

References

Moritz A, Schneider M and Bauer N (2004) Management of advanced tracheal collapse in dogs using intraluminal self-expanding biliary wall stents. *Journal of Veterinary Internal Medicine* **18**, 31–34

Sun F, Uson J, Ezquerra J *et al.* (2008) Endotracheal stenting therapy in dogs with tracheal collapse. *The Veterinary Journal* 175, 186–193

18

Patients with urogenital disease

Edited by Clive Elwood

Introduction

Diseases of the urogenital system can lead to problems with fluid balance, metabolic derangements, pain/discomfort, infection, dysuria, incontinence (with the potential for urine scalding) and inhibition of voiding behaviour. Appetite may be significantly affected and specific nutritional therapies may be appropriate. Understanding these derangements is important in determining care plans that allow owners to manage their pets' conditions at home whilst maximizing quality of life.

Fluid and electrolyte balance

Diseases that reduce the ability of the kidneys to concentrate urine (e.g. end-stage chronic kidney disease (also called chronic renal failure), chronic pyelonephritis, pyometra) are associated with an increased obligatory fluid loss. As a consequence, patients are more prone to dehydration and complications such as pre-renal renal failure, which can lead to a spiralling deterioration. Ensuring effective fluid throughput is, therefore, essential. In the acute stage of management, intravenous fluid therapy is usually most appropriate, but this is not suitable for management in the home. Fluid balance should be carefully monitored because, as well as an obligatory fluid loss, renal failure is associated with an inability to dilute urine beyond the isosthenuric range and, therefore, excretion of excess fluid. This must be recognized and taken into account when determining rates of fluid administration. In some circumstances it is appropriate to measure 'ins and outs', which requires urinary catheterization and a closed collection system. Close monitoring of bodyweight, tissue hydration and respiratory rate is important. Oedema (of the lungs or body) is more likely when there is accompanying hypoproteinaemia (e.g. in patients with protein-losing nephropathy) and/or poor vascular integrity, and also in small dogs and cats where accidental fluid overload occurs more easily, especially if some form of drip pump is not available. Fluid supplementation is also a key consideration in the management of feline lower urinary tract disease (FLUTD) and urolithiasis, as it reduces the concentration of calculogenic mineral.

Environmental inhibitions from kennelling mean that the patient may be more likely to be self-supportive at home and that some management strategies may have more chance of success. Fluid intake can, sometimes, be increased by offering food that has been liquidized to a slurry with added water. Dry diets are often less suitable for patients with urogenital problems because of the lack of accompanying water. In some circumstances, fluid can be administered enterally using assisted feeding techniques such as oesophagostomy and gastrostomy tubes (see Chapter 5). Fluid administered within 'food' must be taken into account when calculating total fluid needs. An alternative technique is the administration of fluids subcutaneously, by owners, to cats with chronic kidney disease (CKD). This is considered an acceptable technique by the Feline Advisory Bureau and has strong advocacy in some quarters. More details can be found at www.fabvets.org.

Renal failure is often accompanied by a diminished ability to excrete acid from the renal tubules and, accordingly, a metabolic acidosis. Acidic intravenous fluids (such as 0.9% sodium chloride, pH 5.0–5.5) are not, therefore, optimal and lactated Ringer's solution (pH 8.0) is generally more appropriate.

Hypokalaemia can be a significant problem, and has been a concern in the treatment of cats in the past, although newer renal support diets seem to have largely addressed this problem. Hypokalaemia should be actively addressed either during fluid therapy or through oral potassium supplementation, since it is detrimental to gastrointestinal function and appetite as well as causing significant muscle weakness and increasing the risk of fatal arrhythmias. Hypomagnesaemia is also a potentially significant metabolic derangement in renal disease and can potentially lead to cardiac arrhythmias, refractory hypokalaemia, hypocalcaemia and muscle weakness/hyperactivity (Khanna *et al.*,1998; Kimmel *et al.*, 2000).

Nutritional requirements

Nutritional support is considered an important facet of CKD management. Key elements are:

- Maintenance of calorie consumption
- Avoidance of excess amino acid turnover by minimizing catabolism of body protein and matching intake of protein to needs (as much as possible)
- Provision of essential nutrients whilst limiting potential uraemic toxins (e.g. phosphate)
- Ideally, an ability to 'fix' uraemic toxins within the bowel.

In practice, this means a protein/phosphate-restricted diet, and there is evidence that these 'renal' diets may slow the inevitable decline in renal function (Plotnick, 2007). See Chapter 5 and the case studies that follow for more details.

In animals with uraemia or other systemic effects of urinary tract disease, appetite is often diminished. This can produce conflict between the 'ideal' nutritional profile and what the patient will actually eat. This conflict may be overcome by using assisted feeding techniques and, potentially, appetite stimulants, but the desire to feed an 'ideal' diet should not override considerations of quality of life and practicability. In some circumstances it is better to feed a less-than-ideal diet for the sake of providing protein and calories, accepting that this may not be optimal for specific disease management. Budgetary and other practical considerations must also be taken into account, including the owner's home demands and their capacity to provide varying levels of support. In some cases a carefully formulated homemade diet, made with the help of a veterinary nutritionist, may offer a practical compromise solution.

Urinary tract diseases other than CKD, e.g. urolithiasis, may have specific nutritional requirements (see Chapter 5 and the cases that follow for more details). When embarking on dietary management strategies, the clinician must follow specific guidelines, because some of the therapeutic diets can have a very restricted nutritional profile and are not considered suitable for long-term management. Supplementation of standard diets may be necessary in specific cases, e.g. oral potassium supplementation for hypokalaemia. The benefits of more generic supplementation, such as with B vitamins, are unproven.

Anaemia

Chronic anaemia may limit quality of life in CKD in both dogs and cats. It is predominantly a result of a deficiency of erythropoietin (EPO). Recombinant human EPO is considered an acceptable treatment but requires additional supportive care, such as iron supplementation and close monitoring of haematological parameters. More recently, the EPO analogue darbepoeitin has become available and may offer a viable alternative.

Hypertension

Renal disease (CKD, glomerular disease) can be accompanied by clinically significant hypertension, leading to potentially life-ending complications such as retinal detachment and intracerebral haemorrhage. Control of blood pressure is, therefore, important. Current recommendations are given by the International Renal Interest Society (IRIS) and can be found at www.iris-kidney.com (see also *BSAVA Manual of Canine and Feline Nephrology and Urology*.) When giving anti-hypertensive treatment, particular consideration should be given to: side effects (e.g. weakness, lethargy, reduced appetite) that could have a significant impact on overall quality of life; fluid and nutritional balance; and assessment of the disease progression.

Management of severe uraemia/azotaemia

Management of acute and chronic azotaemia/uraemia can be achieved by peritoneal dialysis, haemodialysis or renal transplantation, but there are substantial practical and ethical difficulties with these treatments.

- Peritoneal dialysis is used, rarely, for temporary relief of azotaemia in acute renal failure (ARF) where recovery is possible, but practical difficulties, such as catheter maintenance, make it difficult to maintain for long periods.
- Haemodialysis is, theoretically, more practical for longer term use but requires substantial investment in expertise and equipment and is, currently, not readily available in the UK. Even in the USA, its use is limited to a small number of centres and then it is not typically used for chronic management.
- Renal transplantation in cats, which is generally accepted as an option in the USA, has been the subject of much ethical debate in the UK. The Royal College of Veterinary Surgeons has issued 'Guidelines for Renal Transplantation in Cats' (Annex p, 'RCVS Guide to Professional Conduct', www.rcvs.org.uk), which limits the procedure to specialist centres that fulfil specific criteria of care. To date, even those centres that could meet the requirements have not chosen to pursue this therapy.

Infection

Secondary infection is a serious complication of many urinary tract diseases, including CKD, obstructive diseases, urolithiasis and neoplasia. Predisposing factors include: dilution of urine; provision of privileged sites (e.g. uroliths); loss of mucosal integrity; altered urine chemistry; and failure of normal anatomical barriers. In addition, many interventions, such as urinary catheterization, increase the risk of infection by disturbing normal anatomical barriers and by providing a privileged site for bacterial multiplication. Most infections (70–75%) are with Gram-negative organisms such as *Escherichia coli*, *Proteus*, *Klebsiella*, *Pseudomonas* and *Enterobacter*, whilst 25–30% are with Gram-positive organisms such as *Staphylococcus*, *Streptococcus* and *Enterococcus*. Whenever possible, antibiotic selection should be based upon urine culture and sensitivity testing. If culture is not possible, and there is still evidence of infection, broad-spectrum options with good urinary tract penetration, such as amoxicillin/clavulanate (or just amoxicillin or ampicillin if the infection is confined to the lower urinary tract, since high urine concentration overcomes resistance in coagulase-positive *Staphylococcus*), fluoroquinolones and trimethoprim/sulphadiazine should be considered. In an entire male dog, it is important to use a drug with prostate penetrance for any urinary tract infection.

Antibiotic usage is considered to be a risk factor for the development of resistant infections, by promoting preferential selection of resistant strains in the gastrointestinal tract that can then ascend the urinary tract from the perianal skin area. This is particularly relevant when considering management of catheters, where it is better practice to avoid antibiotics whilst the patient is being catheterized. Secondary infections with sensitive organisms are then easier to treat with standard antibiotics once interventions cease.

Occasionally there is a need to use antibiotics to manage recurrent urinary tract infections, e.g. in chronic pyelonephritis. In these circumstances prolonged uninterrupted antibiotic usage is likely to induce bacterial resistance. Strategies such as intermittent dosing regimes (e.g. week on/week off), pulse dosing (e.g. once daily at night to allow retention of antibiotic in the urine overnight) and rotation of antibiotic class may be considered. *Escherichia coli,* in particular, can develop resistance during treatment, so it is wise to repeat culture and sensitivity testing after a few weeks of treatment and to change antibiotics as necessary. In rare circumstances, asymptomatic infection that is difficult or impossible to clear with antibiotics may be better managed without them.

Systemic infection (including acute pyelonephritis) is a serious potential complication of urinary tract infection. It is important, therefore, to warn owners managing pets with urinary disease to seek veterinary attention if there is malaise or signs of fever. Such signs should be considered potentially serious by the veterinary team and addressed in a timely fashion. A positive urine culture may indicate the likely infecting organism and antibiotic sensitivity pattern. It is important to note that many cases of pyelonephritis can be clinically mild in dogs and cats, particularly if there is concurrent disease, such as hyperadrenocorticism, suppressing clinical signs.

Protein-losing nephropathy

Chronic management of PLN can be difficult. Dietary management is discussed in Chapter 5 and in applicable cases below. Angiotensin converting enzyme (ACE) inhibitors can reduce urinary protein loss, particularly in glomerulonephritis, and thereby reduce hypoalbuminaemia and consequent oedema. Severe oedema may need careful nursing to prevent the development of decubital ulcers. PLN is a major predisposition to hypercoagulability and thromboembolism, and this should be considered in management. Optimal strategies for anticoagulation have not been determined, but options include heparin or low-molecular-weight heparins (with or without parenteral plasma) and platelet inhibitors such as clopidogrel or aspirin (although aspirin should be used cautiously because of potential renal and gastrointestinal side effects).

Lower urinary tract obstruction

Acute obstruction to urine flow is a life-threatening emergency because of consequences such as acidosis and hyperkalaemia. It is also, typically, very painful. Protocols for management are well described in the *BSAVA Manual of Canine and Feline Emergency and Critical Care.* Acute obstruction is a potential complication of chronic disease and any failure to pass urine should be considered significant.

Chronic partial obstruction to urine flow can have a major impact on quality of life and long-term health. As well as the pain of increased bladder pressure and the distress of urgency, urinary retention can lead to problems such as urinary tract infection and/or urolithiasis due to urine stagnation. Excessive stretching of the bladder wall, which can lead to loss of detrusor tone and an inability to void, can be long lasting but can respond to aggressive management with long-term bypass of the obstruction (e.g. by cystotomy tube).

Ureteral obstruction

Obstruction of ureters by uroliths or neoplasia, with consequent ureteric spasm, hydroureter and hydronephrosis, is painful. Management strategies may involve encouraging uroliths to pass, using fluids and diuretics, in which case attention must be given to analgesia and fluid balance. Unresolved unilateral obstruction may be manageable by stenting, nephrectomy or neo-ureterocystotomy, but bilateral partial obstruction is more difficult to manage because of concerns about loss of renal function and ureteric stenosis subsequent to surgery (Kyles *et al.,* 2005).

Analgesia

Diseases of the urinary tract can be associated with significant pain and morbidity. As well as obvious pain associated with conditions such as ureterolithiasis, attention must be given to the pain and distress of more common conditions such as cystitis, which can have a significant impact on quality of life. Spasmolytics such as propantheline bromide may be beneficial for the hypercontractile bladder. Because of effects on renal blood flow, non-steroidal anti-inflammatory drugs (NSAIDs) are often contraindicated, so alternative management such as tramadol, amitriptyline and/or gabapentin and/or amantadine (NB avoid using amitriptyline and tramadol together) should be considered (see Chapter 3). However, it should be noted that none of these drugs can be used with impunity when either hepatic or renal function is impaired. Whilst not toxic to either organ, the rate of elimination and/or detoxification is likely to be reduced in the face of dysfunction, so caution and a consideration of lower dose rates would be sensible. As with all painful conditions, an assessment of the degree of suffering the patient is experiencing is essential before one can make the kind of risk/benefit analysis that will help to guide the owner. It should also be remembered that pain is a stressor and is likely to contribute adversely to the progress of the concurrent disease as well as to the overall wellbeing of the patient.

Nursing care

Good nursing practice is the key to the avoidance of complications and maintenance of quality of life in patients with urinary tract disease. Increased urine production, reduced bladder volumes and increased stimulation of urination are all potential reasons for patients to need more frequent opportunities to urinate. In some patients, e.g. cats and highly behaviourally inhibited dogs, great care should be given to adjusting the litter or environment to facilitate voiding during hospitalization. In animals where voluntary urination is not possible, early recognition and sterile catheterization may be necessary to avoid complications such as detrusor muscle failure.

Incontinence may lead to soiling of the coat and chemical dermatitis. As well as strategies to maintain low bladder volumes, anticipation of needs and frequent close monitoring of the perineal area for soiling are important. Protection of the skin with petroleum jelly can be helpful to prevent scalding. If there is urine contamination, rapid cleaning followed by drying and protection is appropriate. Temporary use of nappies to soak up urine or, as appropriate, closed system indwelling urethral catheters or cystostomy tubes may be necessary.

The aim is always to return patients to care in the home as soon as is practical. Good communication with owners about specific care needs, and discussion of what is actually achievable in specific circumstances, should enhance compliance and improve the patient's quality of life.

References and further reading

Elliott J and Grauer GF (2007) *BSAVA Manual of Canine and Feline Nephrology and Urology, 2nd edn.* BSAVA Publications, Gloucester

Khanna C, Lund EM, Raffe M and Armstrong PJ (1998) Hypomagnesemia in 188 dogs: a hospital population-based prevalence study. *Journal of Veterinary Internal Medicine* **12**, 304–309

Kimmel SE, Waddell LS and Michel KE (2000) Hypomagnesemia and hypocalcemia associated with protein-losing enteropathy in Yorkshire terriers: five cases (1992–1998). *Journal of the American Veterinary Medical Association* **217**, 703–706

Kyles AE, Hardie EM, Wooden BG *et al.* (2005) Management and outcome of cats with ureteral calculi: 153 cases (1984–2002). *Journal of the American Veterinary Medical Association* **226**, 937–944

Plotnick A (2007) Feline chronic renal failure: long-term medical management. *Compendium on Continuing Education for the Practicing Veterinarian* **29**, 342–350

Clinical case studies

A variety of case scenarios in dogs and cats will now be presented to illustrate the considerations to be made and the options available within a specific clinical setting. Information relating to the rehabilitation and palliation of each condition has been contributed to each case by the authors in the first part of this Manual, plus notes on nursing and homecare from Rachel Lumbis RVN. The reader should refer back to the appropriate chapters for further details. Photographs used to illustrate the principles and techniques within the cases do not necessarily feature the original patient.

Case 18.1
Chronic kidney disease in a cat

A 13-year-old female DSH cat was presented with acute-onset disorientation due to bilateral retinal detachment. She was 10% dehydrated, depressed and in poor body condition (BCS 3/9). She had lost weight over the last few months and had a reduced appetite but was drinking more than usual.

Investigations confirmed hypertension and chronic kidney disease (CKD) with moderate azotaemia (including hyperphosphataemia) and a mild anaemia. Urine protein:creatinine ratio (UPC) was 0.2. There was no evidence of a urinary tract infection.

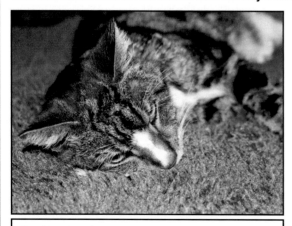

Cat with renal failure and hypertension.

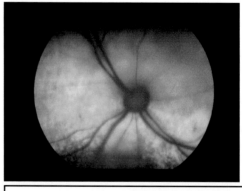

Retina from a cat with hypertension, showing areas of detachment dorsal and ventral to the optic nerve head. (Courtesy of David Gould)

Agreed medical/surgical management

Intravenous fluid and electrolyte therapy was instituted to correct dehydration and maintain hydration status and serum electrolytes. The potential for deficient water excretion and overhydration should be recognized and, once fully hydrated, inputs matched to needs. Hypokalaemia is a potential risk and potassium should be supplemented according to serum concentrations, initially by the addition of potassium chloride in fluids and then with oral potassium supplements as necessary. Hyperphosphataemia should be treated with oral phosphate binders (e.g. chitosan/calcium phosphate).

Associated renal secondary hyperparathyroidism may need further treatment with, for example, calcitonin, although the benefit of this is unproven in cats and dietary therapy is usually adequate (see below).

Anti-hypertensives were prescribed (amlodipine is the most appropriate). An ACE inhibitor is probably of no benefit because of the cat's low UPC and because ACE inhibitors are less effective at reducing blood pressure in cats than in dogs.

The anaemia was not sufficiently severe to impact on quality of life; should it become so, treatment with recombinant human erythropoietin or darbepoeitin could be considered.

Acute/chronic pain management

This patient may well have pain in the form of what human patients would call ' a headache', but treatment for the hypertension should resolve this. There should be no pain associated with the retinal detachment.

This cat had secondary renal hyperparathyroidism and some degree of bone resorption. This is reported to give significant pain in human patients and it should therefore be assumed that there is the possibility of a similar degree of suffering in cats. Treatment of the hyperparathyroidism should attenuate this to some degree, but the patient should be assessed for bone pain whilst being examined. Oral transmucosal buprenorphine (see Chapter 3) may be useful if skeletal pain is suspected.

Fear, stress, conflict concerns

This patient, as well as feeling ill, will be frightened and distressed because of the sudden blindness.

Reducing stress in the veterinary clinic

- Reward and reinforce any positive experiences and associations with the veterinary practice and its team. Use positive touch (stroking and rubbing around the chin – although the approach will need to be gentle and gradual, given the blindness – grooming with a massaging groomer, and gentle stroking of the chest) to release mood neurotransmitters, drop the blood pressure and encourage bonding. Such techniques will obviously only be useful in cats that enjoy handling and touch.
- Take time with the patient to help her relax before any intervention.
- Pheromone therapy may be useful, but should not replace identification of specific stressors, and appropriate behaviour therapy and pain relief.
- Minimize exposure to potential stressors such as dogs and other cats, noises and strong odours.
- Even though the cat cannot see, there may well be a strong desire to feel that she is hiding in or behind something. Use the space in the cage to provide a hiding area (a cardboard box will do with a blanket or bed).
- Use minimal restraint during procedures where possible.
- Continuity of scent stimuli helps cats to adapt to the clinic environment. Rather than removing all bedding each day, put extra beds or blankets in the pen and only remove some at each daily clean, so that some remain carrying the cat's scent.

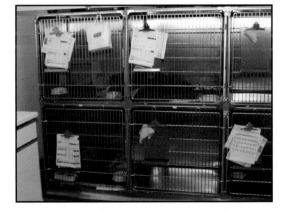

> Cats are best kennelled away from dogs and out of each other's line of sight.

Minimizing stress at home

The cat is miserable and feeling unwell. The owner should understand that the cat may not want handling, and that handling and approach should be careful. When she gets home there will need to be considerations of her ability to get about the house and access her resources, i.e. food, water, litter tray, hiding places, and the company of her owners if she is an affectionate cat. Moderation of the cat's core territory should consider the following.

- **Food.** Increase the number of feeding stations. The cat must also be able to reach food easily; if she has previously fed at a height she may not feel like jumping, so adjust the position of the food, whilst making sure this does not make her anxious about it being available to competitors (e.g. the pet dog or a possible intruding cat if the food is placed near the cat flap).
- **Water.** Cats generally prefer their water about a room's distance away from their food in a clear, wide bowl.
- **Access inside and out.** Cats normally have more than one access point into and out of their core territory (usually the house). Consider providing an additional access point, or ensure that she can use the existing access points (they are not too high or too difficult to negotiate when she feels unwell and uncomfortable).
- **Scratching posts.** Are these easily accessible and appropriate? A horizontal scratch post can be provided, so that the cat can still reach it if she does not feel up to climbing.
- **Hiding areas.** Provide multiple safe and comfortable hiding areas at different levels, or make sure that there is a 'step' system to allow the cat to reach her old favourite places.
- **Beds.** Provision of new beds, such as radiator beds, may improve the comfort and wellbeing of the patient.
- **Play.** Modify games to very short bursts of gentle play, but continue to try to gently stimulate the cat.
- **Petting.** Use of gentle touch, stroking and grooming in ways that the patient will tolerate and enjoy will not only improve the patient's feelings of wellbeing but will also give the owner a sense of participating in their pet's treatment and nursing.

Nutritional requirements

Encouraging food intake in the hospital

Cats in the middle of uraemic crises are often inappetent, and introduction of new therapeutic diets at this stage is difficult. The most important consideration in the short term is that the cat is encouraged to eat *something*. Transition to a renal diet is best attempted only when she is feeling better. Correction of her hydration status and blood pressure may improve her appetite and food intake. If she is nauseous or vomiting because of the uraemia, an anti-emetic might help her appetite. There is a temptation to use appetite stimulants in a case such as this. However, there is little evidence that these agents are effective at restoring appetite in cats with kidney disease and some are contraindicated in renal failure (see Chapter 5). Other methods of encouragement should be tried (see Nursing care, below). It is very important to keep a daily record of calorie intake; if the cat eats less than her resting energy requirement (RER; see Chapter 5) for more than 2–3 days, some form of tube feeding should be instituted. A naso-oesophageal or oesophagostomy tube would be indicated and would also allow administration of medication and fluid requirements while the cat is in the hospital (see Chapter 5 for more details).

Long-term feeding

Once the cat is stable and eating, it is important to try to move her over to long-term feeding of a phosphate-restricted renal diet. There is evidence that these diets significantly reduce renal secondary hyper-parathyroidism and increase the life expectancy of cats with CKD; in fact, they are the most effective treatment (see Chapter 5). Therefore, it is worth trying a number of different manufacturers' renal diets and also a variety of dried and moist foods before giving up. Some renal diets are sodium-restricted and some are not. It would be logical to believe that this cat should have sodium restriction to help control her hypertension. However, there is no evidence that sodium restriction lowers blood pressure in cats and there is some suggestion that it may be detrimental in some cases (see Chapter 5). Therefore, although it is wise to *avoid high-sodium tit-bits*, use of a low-sodium diet *per se* may not be helpful.

Nutraceuticals

Omega-3 fatty acids have been shown to have beneficial effects in renal disease in dogs (at least experimentally) through improving glomerular filtration rate and perfusion of the kidney. Fish oils (high in omega-3 fatty acids) may also attenuate inflammation, help preserve lean body mass and improve appetite (see Chapter 7). Supplementation with fish oil might therefore be advised for this patient. However, clinical studies demonstrating definite benefit of fish oil supplementation in naturally occurring CKD in cats have not been carried out.

Physiotherapy

Physiotherapy is not indicated for this patent.

Hydrotherapy

Hydrotherapy is not specifically indicated for this patient.

Acupuncture

There is good evidence from human studies that acupuncture is helpful in post-chemotherapeutic and postoperative nausea and vomiting (see Chapter 11); therefore, it is at least possible that it may also be helpful in the nausea caused by CKD. The mechanism of action is unknown, but if the cat is being seen regularly at the clinic and if she is not distressed by these visits then it would be worth trying some acupuncture to see whether her appetite and demeanour improve. The acupuncture points chosen could be general and easily accessible points; ST36 may be helpful if tolerated. **Safety considerations would be primarily immunosuppression and the risk of introducing infection with needling.** Absolute leucopenia would contraindicate acupuncture, but that is not to say that acupuncture must be avoided where immunosuppression is only a possibility. A neutrophil count should be used as a guide, although it should be borne in mind that uraemia impairs neutrophil function, even in the face of a normal count.

Other nursing and supportive care

- Vital signs, fluid input (oral and intravenous) and output, and blood pressure should be measured and recorded regularly.
- Intravenous fluid therapy should be maintained but access to water should also be provided.

Feeding
It is important to monitor daily calorie intake and insure that the cat eats to meet her RER. She should be encouraged to eat by trying the following strategies:

- Providing fresh, palatable food
- Adding moist food if the cat is usually fed a primarily dry food
- Warming the food to body temperature
- Adding some chicken or other palatable foodstuff
- Adding strongly smelling foods (e.g. pilchards or fish oil)
- Trying her favourite foods from home
- Feeding small meals frequently
- Hand-feeding
- Stroking the cat or providing privacy while eating.

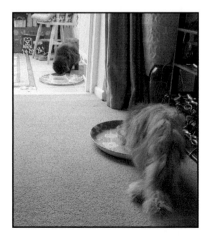

> Feeding from different positions or surfaces may encourage eating.

If she is not interested in eating, large amounts of food should not be left in the cage.

Care of feeding tube
If a feeding tube has been placed, this should be monitored carefully as the majority of complications involve tube occlusion or localized irritation at the tube exit site. Feeding and tube care are detailed in Chapter 5.

Comfort and care
Because of her poor vision, when cleaning out the patient's kennel, it is useful to try to maintain the same cage layout to avoid distress and confusion.

Owner advice and homecare recommendations

Eating and drinking
It is important to stress to the owner that the cat must always have free access to water. The owner should be advised to contact the surgery immediately if any concurrent illness stops the cat drinking. Advice should also be given on the use of the diet and why it is important: in this case, the dietary treatment is being used like a drug. The owner should be advised to monitor the cat's fluid intake and output, her appetite and her general quality of life.

> Cats generally prefer their water in a wide bowl and at a distance from their food. (© Samantha Elmhurst)

Litter trays

As the cat is polyuric, more litter trays may need to be provided if the owner is out for long periods. Soiled litter should be removed and topped up with a fresh supply. It is important that the cat's litter tray is cleaned regularly but complete cleaning out of the litter tray should only be done once a week, to maintain some continuity of environmental odour.

Accommodating to a blind cat

The owner will need advice about how to help a blind cat accommodate to its environment at home (see Fear, stress, conflict above).

Case 18.2
Chronic pyelonephritis in a dog

A 10-year-old neutered male Maltese Terrier was presented with intermittent pollakiuria, urinary tenesmus and haematuria, caused by recurrent urinary tract infections. Hair loss, abdominal enlargement and a pendulous prepuce were apparent. He had lost some muscle mass, although he was still bright and eating. He was less inclined to exercise than he had been.

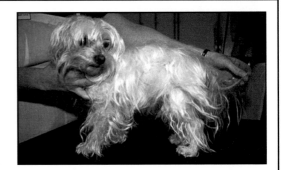

Maltese Terrier with hyperadrenocorticism and pyelonephritis.

Contrast radiography and abdominal ultrasonography showed bilaterally enlarged, plump adrenal glands and a slightly hyperechoic liver parenchyma. There were also dilated renal pelvises and ureters. Blood tests showed high alkaline phosphatase and there was a lack of cortisol suppression on a low-dose dexamethasone suppression test. Renal function was normal but the urine contained blood, protein and white cell casts.

A diagnosis was made of bilateral pyelonephritis with underlying hyperadrenocorticism.

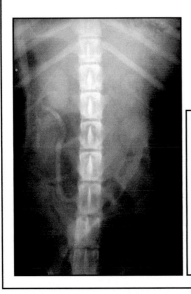

Intravenous urography showing a distorted renal outline, dilated renal pelvises and dilated ureters in a dog with pyelonephritis. Air bubbles, arising from the concurrent pneumocystogram, have entered the ureters.

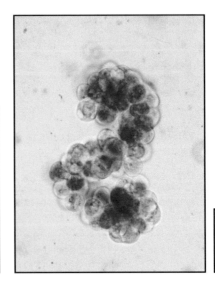

White cell casts in a urine sample.

Agreed medical/surgical management

The pyelonephritis was treated with a prolonged (6 weeks) course of an appropriate antibiotic, selected according to urinary culture of a sterile cystocentesed urine sample. In the long term, the dog might need ongoing intermittent or sustained antibiotic therapy, as indicated by response and monitoring of urine cultures.

The hyperadrenocorticism was managed with trilostane.

Chronic pain

The sources of chronic pain for this patient are: kidney pain; potential secondary muscle pain in the thoracolumbar longissimus and deeper paraspinal muscles, as well as abdominal muscles (see Chapters 3 and 11); and, potentially, bladder and urethral pain. Additionally, he may well have secondary lumbar and hip girdle pain from frequent squatting and straining; muscle weakness secondary to hyperadrenocorticism will increase the potential for muscle strain and pain. In addition, as this dog's hyperadrenocorticism is treated effectively, the pain associated with any underlying chronic degenerative joint disease would be unmasked.

As kidney function is normal, NSAIDs would be the first choice but only once the hyperadrenocorticism is under control (otherwise this will be the equivalent of concurrent use of NSAIDs and steroids, which will greatly increase the risk of gastrointestinal ulceration). However, there may be significant suffering on pain assessment, in which case tramadol, or paracetemol ± codeine, would be appropriate additions. If the bladder pain is uncontrolled and/or there is evidence of significant sensitization to pain, the addition of gabapentin or amitriptyline may be helpful (NB do not use amitriptyline with tramadol); as both gabapentin and amitriptyline require normal renal function for elimination, dosage should be considered in the light of biochemical analysis. Acupuncture may be a helpful adjunct (see below).

Fear, stress, conflict concerns

Pain and discomfort are always a source of stress and conflict, but specific treatment of the condition and management of pain should be sufficient in this patient.

Nutritional requirements

Dietary advice

There are no specific dietary modulations that have been identified to aid in the management of canine pyelonephritis. It should be stressed that this dog is suffering from an inflammatory disease and also has some loss of muscle mass, so *feeding a protein-restricted renal diet would be contraindicated*, unless he had sustained irreversible permanent CKD as a result of the pyelonephritis. As in any other inflammatory disease, adequate daily intake of a high-quality digestible diet is recommended. The dog's dietary intake should be monitored to ensure he is eating his daily energy requirements – although in a dog with hyperadrenocorticism, inappetence would be very unlikely, even in the presence of concurrent pyelonephritis.

Nutraceuticals

Cranberry juice capsules might be beneficial in helping to control this dog's urinary tract infection. There is some evidence that cranberry juice protects against infectious cystitis in humans (Jepson and Craig, 2008), although evidence of their effectiveness in dogs is currently only anecdotal.

Physiotherapy

This dog may benefit from a slowly progressive exercise programme as his condition improves, to help restore muscle and improve overall function (see Chapter 9). If treatment of the hyperadrenocorticism unmasks symptoms of an underlying degenerative joint disease, physiotherapy would also be helpful for that (see Chapter 14).

Hydrotherapy

As this dog is still bright, short sessions of gentle hydrotherapy may be beneficial to help improve his body condition and build up muscle mass. This will be much more effective than land-based exercise at building muscle and condition, as long as times are kept short to start with (considering his age and condition) and increased slowly, and provided he doesn't find the water stressful.

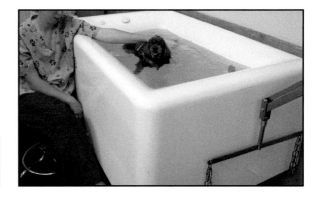

This small dog is undergoing gentle hydrotherapy in a small tub. If using a full-sized hydrotherapy pool, a person should be in the water with the dog. (© Janet Van Dyke)

Acupuncture

As an adjunctive source of analgesia for renal and muscle pain, acupuncture may well be helpful. The targets for needling would be trigger points (see Chapters 11 and 3) in the longissimus and abdominal muscles and paraspinal needling into multifidus from thoracolumbar to lumbosacral junction bilaterally and over the sacrum. **The main safety consideration would be significant immunosuppression; this increases the risk of introducing infection by needling.** If underlying degenerative joint disease has been unmasked, acupuncture can also be used to treat the pain of this condition (see Chapter 14).

Other nursing and supportive care

- While the patient is in the hospital, his fluid input, urine production and hydration status, and food intake should be checked frequently.
- This patient has an infection and is immunosupressed. Any downturn in status (reduced appetite, demeanour, fluid intake) should be carefully assessed because septic complications are possible without associated fever and overt inflammatory responses.

Urination

Frequent opportunities for urination should be afforded, as both the pyelonephritis and hyperadrenocorticism will lead to polyuria. If the dog has muscle weakness and significant polyuria, there is a risk of urination in the kennel and consequent urine scalding. This should be prevented as much as possible by frequent changes of bedding, walks outside, and bathing and drying him carefully if he becomes contaminated with urine.

Monitoring hyperadrenocorticism treatment

A small number of dogs have an adverse reaction to trilostane, sometimes resulting in acute-onset *hypo*adrenocorticism. Therefore, the dog should be carefully monitored, both in the kennels and at home, for any unusual behaviour: particularly, sudden-onset depression, vomiting, or a sudden reduction in eating or drinking. If these occur: the trilostane should be stopped pending further investigations; blood samples should be checked for electrolytes (sodium and potassium) and pre- and post-stimulation cortisol concentrations; and the dog should be put on intravenous fluids and, if in doubt, given a bolus of intravenous dexamethasone.

Owner advice and homecare recommendations

- It is important that the owner is aware that the dog has two problems, which are inter-related.
- The owner must be advised to complete the full course of antibiotics, regardless of whether or not the dog appears better.
- The owners should be informed that the dog's muscle strength will gradually improve as the hyperadrenocorticism is successfully treated and that they should be able to increase his exercise gradually.
- The polydipsia and polyuria should resolve quite quickly, but until they do, the owners will need to make allowance for the dog's frequent needs to urinate, e.g. by providing a dog flap or getting up in the night to let him out.

Informing the owners about hyperadrenocorticism

It should be explained that therapy for hyperadrenocorticism (Cushing's disease) is usually effective but is also usually lifelong. It is also important to explain to the owners that a small number of cases are due to macroadenomas in the pituitary gland and that these may eventually cause neurological signs. The possibility of side effects from the trilostane should be explained and advice given as to the signs to look out for (see above). Owners should be advised to ring the veterinary clinic immediately if they are worried.

Follow-up

Unresolved chronic pyelonephritis may lead to chronic kidney disease; it is important that the owners are aware of the importance of follow-up visits to check urine cultures and the effectiveness of treatment, particularly since dogs with kidney infections often show minimal clinical signs.

References

Jepson RG and Craig JC (2008) Cranberries for preventing urinary tract infections. *Cochrane Database Systematic Reviews* CD001321

Case 18.3
Protein-losing nephropathy in a dog

A 3-year-old male neutered Bernese Mountain Dog in ideal body condition was presented with ascites and peripheral oedema. He was quiet, had a diminished appetite and some developing decubital ulcers from excessive recumbency.

Investigations confirmed hypoalbuminaemia and protein-losing nephropathy (PLN) with a urine protein:creatinine ratio (UPC) of 5. There was an associated moderate azotaemia. Systolic blood pressure was moderately elevated.

No underlying predisposing cause was identified, despite extensive investigations. The main differential diagnoses were amyloidosis and glomerulonephritis. Kidney biopsy was not considered wise in view of the azotaemia and also the fact that the result would not change therapy or prognosis. It was decided to treat the patient as having suspected glomerulonephritis, given that there is no proven treatment for amyloidosis.

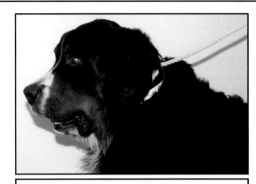

Bernese Mountain Dog presented with peripheral oedema. Decubital ulcers were apparent on close inspection.

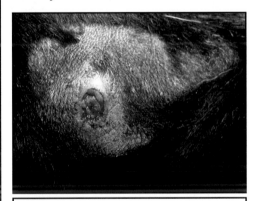

Decubital ulcer arising from recumbency and oedema. (Courtesy of Jonathan Bray)

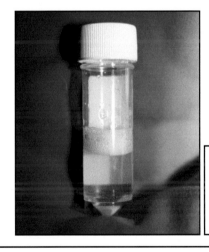

A frothy head on a shaken urine sample is an indicator of significant proteinuria.

Agreed medical/surgical management

The dog was given judicious intravenous fluid therapy to treat the azotaemia and to ensure that no pre-renal component developed. An angiotensin converting enzyme (ACE) inhibitor was then added, together with dietary and fish oil therapy (see below) to try and reduce glomerular protein loss. The dog's response to treatment was carefully monitored with regular re-checks to assess blood pressure, degree of azotemia and UPC. There was a particular concern to make sure that azotaemia did not increase significantly while on ACE inhibitor therapy.

Acute/chronic pain management

Chronic pain
The oedema may be painful, depending on the extent. The dog should be handled especially considerately and pain relief may be required. Since NSAIDs are contraindicated by the renal disease, paracetamol + codeine may be used short term until the oedema has improved.

Management of decubital sores (see below) will decrease any associated discomfort.

No concerns were specifically identified, but given the dog's quiet temperament he may be inclined to withdraw, which will make distinguishing signs of progressing disease difficult. Whilst the dog should be allowed sufficient time and space to rest during his illness, he should also be encouraged to spend time with the family and other people if he is sociable, be given gentle exercise in the garden, and have time spent with him grooming and touching him. Gentle play should be attempted if he can be encouraged to join in. In this case, such gentle activities may help prevent his decubital ulcers from getting worse.

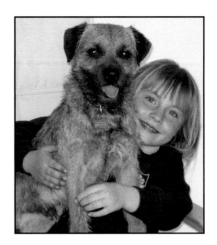

Dogs with a quiet temperament will benefit from gentle interaction with family members. (Courtesy of Stephen Torrington)

Nutritional requirements

Feeding in the hospital
The medium- to long-term aim in this dog is to move him on to a moderately protein-restricted and phosphate-restricted renal diet (see below). However, while he is inappetent in the hospital he may refuse any change of diet or clinical diet, and the immediate aim should be to encourage him to eat and fulfil his RER. This may involve tempting him with palatable foods. Temporary naso-oesophageal or oesophagostomy tube feeding (see Chapter 5) might be considered if needed to maintain energy and protein intake and prevent a further drop in plasma protein concentration.

Long-term feeding
Dietary therapy in the long term would revolve around the use of a protein- and phosphate-restricted renal diet. This is not only indicated in chronic kidney disease in dogs (where it increases the life expectancy) but is also, rather counter-intuitively, specifically indicated for glomerular disease where moderate protein restriction may actually increase blood albumin concentration by reducing glomerular damage and thus protein loss (see Chapter 5). The effectiveness of this strategy has been clearly demonstrated in glomerulonephritis in human patients and also in familial glomerular disease in dogs. The degree of protein restriction may not need to be severe to result in significant benefits. The major challenge in this case may be identifying a palatable diet that is protein-restricted. In some cases, formulation of a balanced homemade diet with the aid of a veterinary nutritionist may be necessary to improve food intake.

If the dog were not already azotaemic but just had proteinuria, it would have been worth instigating a trial treatment with a carefully designed novel protein diet, to rule out food hypersensitivity as an underlying cause of glomerulonephritis. To date, dietary hypersensitivity as a cause of glomerulonephritis has only been reported in Soft-coated Wheaten Terriers with protein-losing nephropathy and enteropathy (Vaden *et al.*, 2000) but it has been suggested as an unrecognized cause of IgA-associated glomerulonephritis in humans (Pouria and Barratt, 2008) and may also occur in some other dogs. Response to the diet should be monitored by measuring serum albumin and UPC, and the food changed to a traditional protein-restricted diet if there has been no measurable improvement after 4–8 weeks. **However, in this dog, the presence of significant azotaemia would make use of a renal diet, as soon as possible, preferable to a hypoallergenic dietary trial.**

Nutraceuticals
The addition of omega-3 fatty acids in the form of fish oil could also be beneficial in this dog. These have been shown experimentally to improve glomerular function and reduce glomerular inflammation in dogs.

Physiotherapy

In this case, peripheral oedema is best managed by a combination of effleurage massage (see Chapter 9) and exercise. Cold compression can be helpful in many cases when the oedema is caused through injury or surgery to a specific body area that can then be treated to limit the oedema, but is generally less effective when the oedema is more widespread due to hypoproteinaemia as it is in this case. Encouragement to exercise is a useful way of reducing oedema and simple walking is adequate.

Laser therapy of the wounds could be considered. However, evidence for the wound-healing properties of low-level laser therapy is controversial, and several systematic reviews of both human and animal studies have concluded that there is no firm evidence for its use, although the methodology of most of the studies was found to be poor. The use of laser on infected areas is also controversial; so, on balance, its use in this case would be best avoided.

Hydrotherapy

Generally speaking, the presence of open wounds is a contraindication to hydrotherapy, so the decubital ulcers will restrict its use in this patient.

In other patients, hydrostatic pressure (see Chapter 10) may help to reduce peripheral limb oedema if the patient is stood in water up to the shoulder, either in a pool on the ramp or in an underwater treadmill.

Acupuncture

Treatment of azotaemia-associated nausea

There is good evidence from human studies that acupuncture is helpful in post-chemotherapeutic and postoperative nausea and vomiting (see Chapter 11). It is possible, therefore, that it will also help with any nausea associated with azotaemia, which is also centrally mediated. The mechanism of action is unknown, but if the dog is feeling nauseous due to azotaemia, is being seen regularly at the clinic and is not distressed by these visits then it would be worth trying some acupuncture to see if his appetite and demeanour improved. The points chosen could be general and easily accessible points; ST36 may be helpful if tolerated. **Safety considerations would be primarily immunosuppression and the risk of introducing infection with needling, particularly as neutrophil function can be reduced in azotaemia.**

Treatment of decubital ulcers

Decubital ulcers sometimes appear to respond well to local needling; the needles should be applied in healthy skin as close as possible to the edge of the sore, about 2.5 cm apart. The clinical (human) and experimental (rats) evidence for the use of acupuncture in wound healing is good, although there is currently no evidence beyond anecdotal of its efficacy in dogs.

Other nursing and supportive care

The patient is dull and depressed. Time should be set aside to sit with him and give him some one-to-one attention. The owner should be encouraged to visit but the dog's reaction must be monitored carefully to ensure that he does not become distressed when the owner leaves.

Monitoring

- Whilst the patient is in the hospital, vital signs and fluid input (oral and intravenous) and output should be monitored and recorded.
- UPC, blood pressure, degree of azotaemia and electrolytes should be monitored closely after initiating therapy to assess the success of fluid and drug therapy and allow appropriate adjustments to be made.
- Daily measurement of bodyweight will give a good idea of the resolution or build-up of oedema because any short-term changes in weight will be due to fluid movements.

Urination

The patient should be given frequent opportunities to go outside to urinate, as he will be polyuric. He should be monitored carefully for any evidence of urine scalding; this dog may urinate in the kennel because he is depressed and polyuric. Any urine-contaminated bedding must be changed quickly and urine-contaminated fur washed and carefully dried. If frequent urine contamination becomes a real problem and threatens to significantly worsen the skin sores, it may be preferable to place an indwelling urinary catheter in the short term until he is more mobile. However, if this is done, it is vital to be as sterile as possible and to use a closed system to minimize the risk of urinary tract infections.

Placement of an indwelling urinary catheter can minimize the risk of urine scalding in a recumbent patient.

Decubital ulcers

Patient comfort should be maintained: the dog should have soft deep bedding and, if recumbent, be turned frequently (at least every 4 hours) to prevent further decubital ulcer formation. The bony prominences (e.g. elbows and ischial wings) are most likely to suffer from developing sores; these areas should, therefore, be padded using foam. The area around the sores should be clipped and cleaned with a mild antiseptic, then dried thoroughly and an appropriate cream or protective barrier film applied to the sores. Contamination and patient interference with the wounds should be avoided.

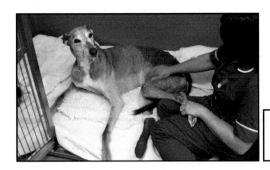

Soft bedding and physiotherapy can help reduce decubital ulcers.

Feeding

The patient should be encouraged to eat, as inadequate food intake will lead to negative nitrogen balance and will exacerbate the hypoproteinaemia. Methods of encouragement include: feeding small meals frequently; providing fresh, palatable food; hand-feeding; warming the food to body temperature; adding some chicken or other palatable foodstuff (preferably not high in salt). Large amounts of food should not be left in the kennel if the dog is not interested in eating. Force-feeding should be avoided as it can create food aversion.

Owner advice and homecare recommendations

Eating and drinking

Advice should be provided on the purpose of the diet.

It is essential that the owners understand that unlimited access to fresh water is vital for this dog. They should ring the surgery immediately if this is ever prevented (e.g. if the dog is vomiting and stops drinking).

Exercise and opportunities to urinate

The owners should be advised concerning gentle exercise. They will also need to make allowance for the dog's frequent needs to urinate, e.g. by getting up in the night to let him out.

Follow-up and prognosis

The owners should be advised that although the long-term prognosis is guarded because of the development of azotaemia, the drug and dietary treatment should increase the dog's life expectancy – as well as quality of life – by preserving remaining renal function as much as possible. They need to be aware of the signs to look out for that might indicate worsening renal function and/or a reduction in blood albumin concentration, e.g. anorexia, vomiting, increased polyuria/polydipsia, increased ascites. It is worth showing them how to measure the dog's girth with a tape measure so that they can assess any increase in ascites more objectively.

References

Pouria S and Barratt J (2008) Secondary IgA nephropathy. *Seminars in Nephrology* **28**, 27–37

Vaden SL, Hammerberg B, Davenport DJ *et al.* (2000) Food hypersensitivity reactions in Soft Coated Wheaten Terriers with protein-losing enteropathy or protein-losing nephropathy or both: gastroscopic food sensitivity testing, dietary provocation, and fecal immunoglobulin. *Journal of Veterinary Internal Medicine* **14**, 60–67

Case 18.4
Bladder transitional cell carcinoma in a dog

A 7-year-old female neutered Border Collie was presented with dysuria and haematuria. Urine could be passed with effort but there was some enlargement of the bladder. The dog was otherwise bright and alert, in good condition and eating, drinking and exercising normally.

Blood samples were taken for biochemical and haematology screens; results were unremarkable, showing no evidence of renal or hepatic dysfunction. Contrast radiography and ultrasonography revealed a mass at the bladder neck that involved the proximal ureter. A suction catheter biopsy confirmed transitional cell carcinoma (TCC).

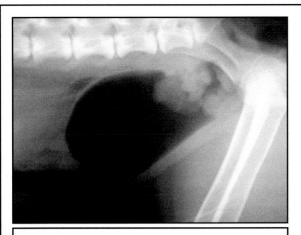

Pneumocystogram demonstrating masses in the trigone of the bladder.

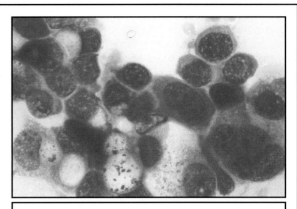

Cytological specimen showing transitional cell carcinoma cells. May–Grünwald–Giemsa; original magnification X1000. (Courtesy of Roger Powell, PTDS Laboratory Services)

Agreed medical/surgical management

A COX-2 inhibitor was used to palliate the tumour. Other chemotherapeutics (e.g. mitoxatrone) were considered but declined by the owner.

Monitoring of urine passage and temporary catheterization relief may be necessary pending response to drug treatment. If the dog becomes completely obstructed, a percutaneous cystotomy tube can be placed to bypass the urethra and avoid bladder overstretch, but this should only be a temporary measure as it carries a risk of ascending infection. Placement of an expanding urethral stent could also be considered as a means of relieving obstruction.

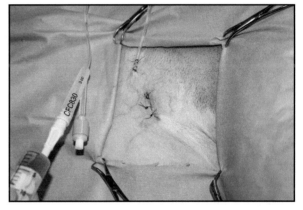

Surgical placement of a cystostomy tube. (Courtesy of Jonathan Bray)

Acute/chronic pain management

COX-2 inhibitors such as meloxicam should have an impact on pain and discomfort associated with the tumour. Tramadol, or paracetamol + codeine, may be helpful and can be used in addition to the NSAID if the patient starts to show signs of suffering. The dog should be monitored carefully for any side effects associated with long-term use of the COX-2 inhibitor, particularly gastrointestinal signs. Epidural analgesics may be helpful if she continues to have intermittent bad days.

Chronic pain
If signs of a chronic pain state develop, the use of amitriptyline, amantadine or gabapentin may be helpful (see Chapter 3).

Fear, stress, conflict concerns

Pain and discomfort are always a source of some stress and conflict and the dog should be monitored for changes in her normal behaviour that would indicate that she is suffering (see Chapters 3 and 4).

Nutritional requirements

This dog has a good appetite and no evidence of renal compromise, so there are no special dietary considerations and she can remain on her normal diet.

Potential dietary influences on development of TCC in dogs

It is possible that certain dietary ingredients either predispose to, or protect against, TCC in susceptible dogs, as is the case in people. This is not surprising, since diet influences urine composition. In one study in Scottish Terriers (which are known to be at increased risk of TCC), a diet high in green leafy or yellow–orange vegetables appeared to prevent or slow the development of TCC of the bladder (Raghavan et al., 2005) but it is not known whether feeding these vegetables AFTER the tumour has developed and in other breeds of dog would have any effect on tumour progression.

Obesity may also increase the effect of other risk factors for TCC in dogs (Glickman et al., 1989) but this is not relevant in this case as the patient is not obese.

Nutraceuticals

Other nutritional supplements such as antioxidants and omega-3 fatty acids have been proposed for other forms of canine cancer, but there are no studies supporting their use in bladder TCC.

Physiotherapy

Physiotherapy is not indicated for this patient.

Hydrotherapy

Hydrotherapy is not specifically indicated for this patient.

Acupuncture

Acupuncture is not indicated for this patient unless she is not obtaining adequate pain relief from conventional analgesics or there is a contraindication or adverse response to their use. There is no evidence that the use of acupuncture will have any effect (one way or the other) on the tumour itself and it will have limited effects on bladder function whilst a pathological lesion is present. If the owner elects to try conventional chemotherapy after all, there may be some value in using acupuncture to treat chemotherapy-related side effects (see Chapter 15).

Other nursing and supportive care

Comfort and pain recognition

If the patient is hospitalized, she should be observed for signs of pain and depression. A pain scoring system could be used to ensure a standardized approach to monitoring and pain management (see Chapter 3).

Monitoring urination

The bladder should be palpated at least twice a day, and after walks, to ensure that there is not a large residual volume of urine remaining which would increase the risk of secondary urinary tract infection and detrusor muscle over-stretch. The dog must not be left for long periods of time without bladder assessment. If there is persistent residual urine, then manual expression, intermittent catheterization, temporary tube cystostomy or urethral stenting may be indicated.

Cystostomy tubes

If a cystostomy tube has been placed it needs careful management. Complications are fairly common and include: recurrent and, eventually, antibiotic-resistant lower urinary tract infections followed by pyelonephritis; urine leakage; and subcutaneous peristomal leakage and infection. The tube should be kept capped and emptied regularly in a sterile manner. The dog should NOT be placed on prophylactic antibiosis as this increases the risk of superinfection with a resistant organism. Instead, the urine collected should be regularly tested with a dipstick and intermittent urine cultures and any infection developing should be treated with appropriate antibiotics, chosen on the basis of sensitivity testing.

Owner advice and homecare recommendations

Urination

The owners will need to monitor the dog carefully to ensure she urinates regularly and passes a good stream. If possible, they should be taught to palpate the bladder in the caudal abdomen for any residual urine afterwards (many owners can become quite proficient at this with practice). It is important to contact the surgery if the dog has a significant residual urine volume or if she becomes unable to pass urine.

If the dog is discharged with a cystostomy tube, the owner will need to empty the bladder at least three times a day to avoid stagnation of urine. Information on how to do this and on care of the catheter must be given, preferably in writing. Tube dislodgement is a serious complication: if the tube dislodges, the owner must contact the surgery *immediately*.

The owner should also monitor the urine carefully for any signs of urinary tract infection. It may be worthwhile asking them to bring regular urine samples into the practice for assessment for white cells cytologically (the presence of blood on a dipstick will not help identify urinary tract infections as the tumour is also likely to bleed).

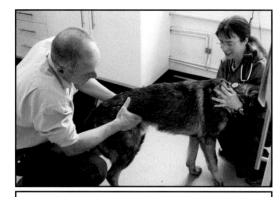

Teaching an owner to palpate a dog's bladder for subsequent assessment of voiding function at home.

Assessing pain

The owners need to know the signs of pain to look out for: depression is one sign, but irritability, anxiety and other changes in behaviour may be observed (Chapter 3 and 4). If appropriate, the owner can be shown how to use a pain scoring system to ensure a standardized approach. They must contact the practice if they are concerned that the dog is in pain.

Prognosis

It should be explained carefully and sensitively, but clearly, to the owners that the prognosis is poor and that they should consider euthanasia of the dog if urination becomes impossible or her pain becomes intractable. It should be noted that a tube cystostomy or urethral stent is a *temporary* solution.

References

Glickman LT, Schofer FS, McKee LJ, Reif JS and Goldschmidt MH (1989) Epidemiologic study of insecticide exposures, obesity, and risk of bladder cancer in household dogs. *Journal of Toxicology and Environmental Health* **28**, 407–414

Raghavan M, Knapp DW, Bonney PL, Dawson MH and Glickman LT (2005) Evaluation of the effect of dietary vegetable consumption on reducing risk of transitional cell carcinoma of the urinary bladder in Scottish Terriers. *Journal of the American Veterinary Medical Association* **227**, 94–100

Case 18.5
Urethral sphincter mechanism incompetence in a dog

A 4-year-old female neutered Dobermann was presented with a history of incontinence. She was unaware of the incontinence and left puddles after lying down. She was slightly obese (BCS 7/9) and was a family dog.

Investigations confirmed a caudally displaced bladder neck and no other reasons for incontinence other than urethral sphincter mechanism incompetence (USMI). A full medical work-up including blood screens failed to identify any underlying condition which might predispose to or exacerbate the USMI in this dog.

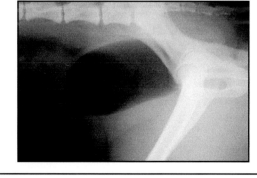

Caudal displacement and dorsal bulging of the bladder neck on a pneumocystogram is typical of USMI.

Agreed medical/surgical management

Medical control of the USMI was gained using a combination of phenylpropanolamine and estriol, together with initial antibiotics for a secondary urinary tract infection. Surgery was not considered necessary at this point, but could be considered in the future if medical management fails.

Acute/chronic pain management

This is not a painful condition.

Fear, stress, conflict concerns

It must be made clear to the owners that the dog should not be punished for 'accidents'. Training her to urinate on command may maximize the efficiency of the available opportunities to urinate, although it is possible that she may have acquired some aversion to urinating in front of the owners if they have made an issue of her urinating inappropriately in the hope that this would limit 'accidents'. Some enquiries into the dog's attitude about urinating in the garden/cryptically/in front of the owners should make the situation clearer.

Nutritional requirements

Weight management

The obesity in this patient is likely to be exacerbating her incontinence, and so a weight management regime is required. As weight loss progresses, the requirement for pharmaceuticals may decline; even small amounts of weight loss can produce benefits, although the effect is likely to be greatest if/when a lean body condition (BCS 4/9) is reached.

Details of weight loss regimes are given in Chapter 6. In this case, it would be feasible to use either a conventional weight management regime or drug therapy (e.g. dirlotapide or mitratapide). In addition, the owners should be encouraged to instigate a daily exercise plan, tailored to their dog's abilities.

The dog should return to the clinic on a 2-weekly basis initially, so that progress with weight loss can be monitored. The same set of electronic weigh scales should be used every time so that any changes are known to be due to genuine changes in weight rather than inaccuracies between scales. Most dogs will lose between 0.5 and 1.5% of starting bodyweight per week.

Once the dog has reached her target weight, a maintenance regime should be instigated. The transition should be made gradually: the dog should continue to be weighed every 2 weeks while energy intake is increased incrementally by 10% at a time. Once weight has stabilized, the interval between weight checks can be gradually extended (e.g. monthly, 3-monthly, 6-monthly). It is vital that weight checks are not stopped altogether because weight management helps to control clinical signs with USMI, rather than curing the disease outright. Therefore, if weight rebound occurs, so will the clinical signs. The preference would be to ensure that the dog remains in optimal (even lean e.g. BCS 4/9) body condition throughout life.

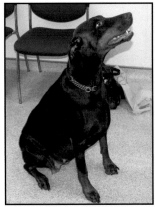
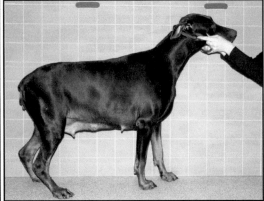
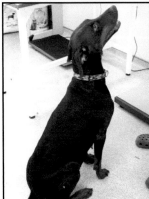
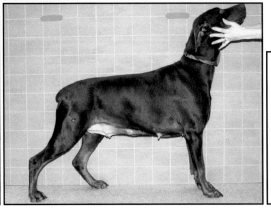

A Dobermann before **(top)** and after a weight management programme. Starting bodyweight was 50 kg and she lost 4.5 kg (19%) slowly but steadily over 468 days. Her body fat content decreased in that time from 46% to 32%, so all weight lost was adipose tissue. (Courtesy of The Royal Canin Weight Management Clinic, University of Liverpool)

Physiotherapy

Physiotherapy is not indicated for this patient.

Hydrotherapy

Hydrotherapy may theoretically help with weight loss, because during the session metabolic requirements are increased, but this is probably over-emphasized as a benefit of hydrotherapy where dogs are usually swum or treadmill walked a maximum of twice a week. The urinary incontinence in this dog would also lead to a requirement for increased monitoring and cleaning of the pool or tank.

Acupuncture

Acupuncture is often reported anecdotally to be useful in incontinence in the bitch, but there is no mechanism to suggest why it should have an impact on a caudally placed bladder. In SL's experience those incontinent canine patients (both male and female) who respond to acupuncture have associated lumbar pain and are not responding convincingly to the medications described above. Acupuncture would thus not be recommended in this patient.

Other nursing and supportive care

- The use of barrier creams until the dog becomes continent may help to prevent urine scalding.
- Clipping and cleaning the perineal region to help prevent urine scalding may be useful, although it is more important in long-haired dogs.
- Incontinence pads will increase the patient's comfort and wick away excess moisture.
- The patient should be offered frequent opportunities to urinate.

Owner advice and homecare recommendations

Education about the condition
Breed and gender could be predisposing factors in this dog but it is important also to stress that the dog's concurrent obesity will exacerbate the condition. This should give the owner motivation to persevere with the weight loss programme. The owner should also be informed that these dogs are at increased risk of urinary tract infection when incontinent.

Urination
The owner should be advised to allow the dog frequent opportunities to urinate, including last thing at night to try to prevent overnight incontinence. As discussed above, they should not chastise the dog for incontinence but might consider training her to urinate to order, so that they can ensure her bladder is empty last thing at night. The dog should not be left for long periods without access to outdoors. For example: if the owners are out at work for long periods in the day, could they ask a neighbour to let the dog out for them?

The owner should be advised about some of the clinical signs that they may observe if the incontinence recurs:

- Patches of urine where she has been lying
- Excessive licking of the vulva
- Evidence of bladder infections
- Infection and smell around the vulva
- Leakage of urine when she barks.

They should contact the surgery if any of these occur. Careful observation by the owner for recurrence of signs usually reveals when the dose needs to be increased and this should be carried out in consultation with the veterinary surgery.

Drug side effects
Phenylpropanolamine can cause hyperexcitability, irritability, panting or anorexia. Oestrogens can potentially cause bone marrow suppression. Owners observing any side effects should be advised to stop the drugs immediately and contact their veterinary surgeon for further advice.

Case 18.6
'Idiopathic' cystitis in a cat

A 3-year-old neutered female Oriental cat was presented with recurrent bouts of pollakiuria, urinary tenesmus and haematuria. She was of nervous disposition and was kept as an indoor cat in a household with two other cats. She was fed a dry diet *ad libitum* with the other cats, and was in ideal body condition.

A bladder biopsy indicated interstitial cystitis. No other diseases were identified on a full medical work-up.

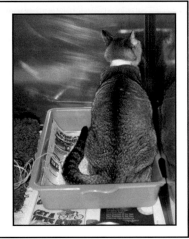

Oriental cat demonstrating urinary tenesmus. The patient is receiving intravenous fluids.

Agreed medical/surgical management

The main therapeutic strategies for this cat will revolve around reducing stress and increasing water intake in food (see below). If these do not work alone, a tricyclic antidepressant such as amitriptyline (5–12.5 mg per cat q24h) or clomipramine could be considered. There is some evidence that amitriptyline can work in cystitis by modifying neurogenic inflammatory responses (Chew *et al.,* 1998), though one study questioned its efficacy and noted that there may also be a rebound worsening of clinical signs when the drug is stopped (Kruger *et al.,* 2003). Amitriptyline is bitter and difficult to administer. A liquid form is available but is fruit-flavoured, which is also unacceptable to many cats. It is contraindicated in impaired renal and hepatic function and should be used with extreme caution in animals with dysrhythmias.

It should be stressed that feline interstitial cystitis is *not* caused by bacterial infection. The true efficacy of different treatment strategies can be difficult to assess in individual cases because the disease is self-limiting but recurrent.

Acute/chronic pain management

Interstitial cystitis can be a painful condition and NSAIDs can be helpful during acute episodes, preferably meloxicam since it is authorized for long-term use in the cat. If amitriptyline is used concurrently with meloxicam, renal function should be checked regularly since amitriptyline requires competent renal function for elimination.

Fear, stress, conflict concerns

There is good evidence that idiopathic and interstitial cystitis are diseases of a susceptible individual cat put into a 'provocative' environment, and that stress is a trigger. It is therefore important to try to identify and address any stressors in the cat's environment, such as bullying by other cats, the arrival of a new baby, moving house, etc. There is some evidence to suggest that modification of the cat's core territory (see Case 18.1) can be helpful in reducing the severity and frequency of bouts of cystitis (Buffington *et al.,* 2006), by allowing the cat to cope more effectively with its stressors. Pheromone therapy may also be helpful and – although there is no clear evidence – there are increasing anecdotal reports of the apparently successful use of alpha-casozepine. Specific behavioural problems will need to be assessed on an individual basis and treated appropriately (see *BSAVA Manual of Canine and Feline Behavioural Medicine*).

Nutritional requirements

Moist food
In addition to reducing stress, the only other treatment shown to be effective in placebo-controlled trials of cats with idiopathic cystitis was feeding a moist (as opposed to a dry) lower urinary tract clinical diet (Markwell *et al.,* 1999). It was suggested that the most important aspect of the diet was the increased water content, since it is

known that cats fed dried food generally produce more concentrated urine than cats fed canned food and this is likely to be a risk factor for idiopathic cystitis. Since this patient was being fed on dried food, the initial strategy should therefore be to try to move her on to a moist diet. It may be that the *type* of diet is less important than the addition of water, so it may not be necessary in this case to move the cat on to a specific lower urinary tract diet – but this hypothesis has not yet been tested in placebo-controlled trials. Monitoring serial urinalysis in order to track urine specific gravity may provide information for further adjustment, such as adding water to wet food.

Some cats (only a small percentage) have a taste/texture preference for dried food. If that is the case in this cat, then it would be wise at least to feed a dried diet marketed for lower urinary tract disease, since these diets also try to encourage increased water intake by other means (e.g. reduced residue decreasing faecal water loss, increased salt content). However, it would also be important to try to increase water intake in other ways (e.g. using water fountains to encourage drinking). Again, monitoring serial urine specific gravities would help assess the success of this strategy.

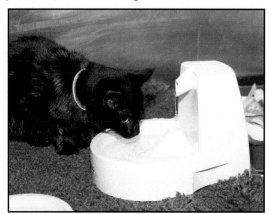

Some cats prefer to drink from free-flowing water, like this drinking fountain.

Nutraceuticals

The use of nutraceuticals for the treatment of cats with idiopathic or interstitial cystitis has not been associated with particular success. A randomized blinded placebo-controlled trial did not reveal a positive response to glycosaminoglycan supplementation (see Chapter 7 for more details).

Physiotherapy

Physiotherapy is not indicated for this patient.

Hydrotherapy

Hydrotherapy is not specifically indicated for this patient.

Acupuncture

Acupuncture has been reported anecdotally to be useful in cases of interstitial cystitis. The mechanisms are likely to be: augmentation of central pain processing to assist in 'winding down' the painful and sensitive bladder; pain relief during attacks; mild anxiolysis; and pain relief for any secondary lumbar muscular pain. If the patient becomes very distressed at being presented to the clinic, caution and careful assessment of the risk and benefits are required; the stress of a visit to the clinic might precipitate an episode, over-riding any benefit of the acupuncture. House visits would not usually be a good alternative, as bringing the whole procedure to the cat's core territory may prove a greater – and potentially more damaging – stressor than visiting the clinic. Local treatment of any obvious painful areas in the lumbar muscles should be combined with segmental needling of lumbar and sacral multifidus muscles (see Chapter 11).

Other nursing and supportive care

Limiting stress in the hospital

The time this cat spends in the hospital should be limited: the visit to the clinic may be stressful in itself; and returning to a multi-cat household after an absence could precipitate difficulties between the cats.

If the cat is kept in for work-up, measures should be taken to reduce stress such as:

- Trying to confine her to a cat-only ward (see Case 18.1)
- Maintaining a quiet, peaceful environment
- Using pheromone therapy in the ward (although there is no specific evidence for its use in this situation)
- Spending time with the cat – grooming and hand-feeding (assuming she enjoys human contact)
- Using techniques requiring minimal restraint.

It may also help to ask the owner about the cat's normal behaviour and environment, and to:

* Use the same litter as is used at home
* Provide a bed or box for the cat to hide in
* Feed the same diet as fed at home, whilst taking into account the requirements of increased water intake (see above).

It is worth remembering these strategies whenever the cat comes into the clinic in future for repeat visits or routine visits such as vaccinations. It would be best if these visits did not trigger a recurrence of the cystitis. The provision of a 'cat only' waiting room, or screened off part of the waiting room, might help reduce stress on these routine visits.

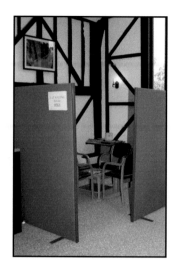

A screened off area of the waiting room, specially for cats, can help reduce their stress.

Drinking and urination
Free access to water should be provided and moist food fed (see above). Urine samples can be collected as required for analysis: the use of specially designed cat litter can help in this.

Owner advice and homecare recommendations

Follow-up and prognosis
Owners should receive extensive advice about minimizing stress and about dietary management. It is important to emphasize that idiopathic and interstitial cystitis are not infectious conditions and are not life-threatening, but *will* recur. Clinical signs usually become less severe and frequent with time. Owners should be advised to monitor for signs of recurrence but only to contact the surgery if these become more severe, frequent or prolonged than usual.

References

Buffington CA, Westropp JL, Chew DJ and Bolus RR (2006) Clinical evaluation of multimodal environmental modification (MEMO) in the management of cats with idiopathic cystitis. *Journal of Feline Medicine and Surgery* **8**, 261–268

Chew DJ, Buffington CA, Kendall MS, DiBartola SP and Woodworth BE (1998) Amitriptyline treatment for severe recurrent idiopathic cystitis in cats. *Journal of the American Veterinary Medical Association* **213**, 1282–1286

Kruger JM, Conway TS, Kaneene JB *et al.* (2003) Randomized controlled trial of the efficacy of short-term amitriptyline administration for treatment of acute, nonobstructive, idiopathic lower urinary tract disease in cats. *Journal of the American Veterinary Medical Association* **222**, 749–758

Markwell PJ, Buffington CA, Chew DJ *et al.* (1999) Clinical evaluation of commercially available urinary acidification diets in the management of idiopathic cystitis in cats. *Journal of the American Veterinary Medical Association* **214**, 361–365

Case 18.7
Acute urinary obstruction in a cat

A 3-year-old male neutered DSH cat was presented with acute urinary obstruction. The owner reported that the cat had been straining to urinate non-productively for 24 hours. He was an indoor-only cat, fed on dry food *ad libitum* and was in ideal body condition.

On clinical examination, the cat had a full, tense bladder that could not be expressed manually. There was evidence that he had been licking his penis and had caused local trauma. The cat was distressed and in pain.

Blood samples revealed azotaemia with hyperkalaemia and acidosis, and confirmed post-renal renal failure.

Agreed medical/surgical management

An intravenous catheter was placed. ECG monitoring was instigated for arrhythmias that might be caused by the hyperkalaemia. Life-threatening electrolyte/acid–base disturbances should be treated immediately with dextrose ± insulin or calcium gluconate (see *BSAVA Manual of Canine and Feline Emergency and Critical Care*).

Catheterization was attempted, under careful sedation, to unblock the urethra. If this proves unsuccessful, emergency cystocentesis can be carried out, taking care to empty the bladder as much as possible to reduce the risk of rupture, followed by repeat catheterization. A temporary cystostomy and/or emergency perineal urethrostomy (see *BSAVA Manual of Canine and Feline Abdominal Surgery*) is indicated if it proves impossible to clear the urethra. The patient should be monitored for haematuria and urethral spasm. Post-obstructive diuresis may require increased fluid rates and may result in hypokalaemia, so hydration status, renal function and electrolytes should be monitored. The degree of permanent renal dysfunction (if any) can be assessed after the cat has recovered by re-checking the serum creatinine and urine specific gravity.

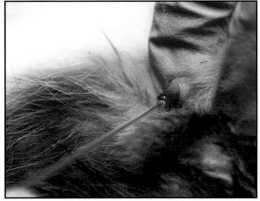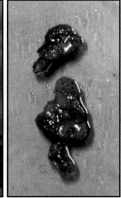

Using a urethral catheter to unblock a cat with a urethral obstruction. This mucoid/struvite plug is approximately 2–3 mm wide and 2 cm long.

Acute/chronic pain management

Perioperative
Partial mu agonists (e.g. buprenorphine) should be suitable for perioperative analgesia in this case. NSAIDs should be avoided in patients with azotaemia. Diazepam, by virtue of its central muscle relaxant properties, may help to reduce discomfort arising from urethral muscle spasms and can be used alongside the buprenorphine.

Chronic pain
Chronic pain management should not be required unless the cat develops chronic non-obstructive FLUTD, in which case chronic pain management should be administered as per Case 18.6.

Fear, stress, conflict concerns

Apart from age, breed, sex and dietary factors, the risk factors for struvite uroliths in cats are poorly understood. Unlike in humans and dogs, struvite uroliths do not appear to be infection-induced in cats. The risk factors for the formation of mucoid plugs are even less well understood. Stress has *not* been recognized to date as a risk factor for obstructive FLUTD, although stress *is* implicated as a risk factor for oxalate urolith formation in humans, and is proposed to act via effects on the hypothalamic/pituitary axis and ADH production. It is possible, therefore, that stress might play a role in the condition in cats; consideration should be given to the cat's home environment (see Case 18.1).

Nutritional requirements

Diet in the hospital
In the first 24 hours the most important consideration is resolution of the cat's electrolyte abnormalities and therefore feeding is not so important. Thereafter, the cat should be fed on a moist diet, because a reduction in urine specific gravity is helpful in any form of cystitis and in reducing the risk of struvite calculi (see below). However, it is unwise to feed an acidifying diet (i.e. a diet manufactured specifically for treatment of struvite calculi in cats) for several days after the relief of the obstruction, because obstructed cats will also have a metabolic acidosis (due to reduce renal acid excretion), which will take a few days to resolve.

Long-term diet
As in Case 18.6, the most important consideration is to feed the cat a moist diet long term to increase water intake. This may suffice if the patient has previously been fed on a dry diet.

Various other dietary strategies have been suggested to reduce the recurrence of struvite calculi in cats. These include: acidifying the urine; reducing dietary magnesium; and reduced relative supersaturation with struvite. Urinary acidifiers can be added to normal food, but it is important to monitor urine pH to assess efficacy. Some of the dietary manipulations that reduce the risk of struvite formation may, conversely, increase the risk of oxalate formation; if possible, the diet should be designed to reduce the risk of both.

There are no known dietary (or other) manipulations which reduce the risk of mucoid plugs in cats.

Diet if there is permanent renal damage

If follow-up blood samples show that the cat has developed permanent renal dysfunction as a result of post-renal failure, he should preferentially be moved on to a manufactured low-phosphate renal diet (rather than a lower urinary tract diet) if possible, as this will significantly increase life expectancy (see Chapter 5 and Case 18.1).

Nutraceuticals

Glycosaminoglycan supplementation might be considered for this patient, although there is no evidence for a beneficial effect in cats with obstructive FLUTD (see Chapter 7).

Physiotherapy

Physiotherapy is not indicated for this patient.

Hydrotherapy

Hydrotherapy is not specifically indicated for this patient.

Acupuncture

Acupuncture has been reported, anecdotally, to cause sufficient relaxation of the urethra to ease catheterization in some patients. Needling should be segmental and concentrated over the sacrum, whilst the cat is sedated for catheterization. Acupuncture may also provide mild adjunctive anxiolysis and sedation.

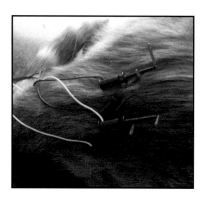

Needling over the sacrum (electroacupuncture in this example) has been reported to be useful when attempting to unblock an obstructed urethra. (Courtesy of Samantha Lindley)

Other nursing and supportive care

Monitoring

- While the cat has serious hyperkalaemia and the ECG indicates life-threatening changes, continuous monitoring is needed to guide treatment and evaluate the response. A pain condition scoring system can be used.
- Once the acute condition has been managed, and the cat relieved of its obstruction, vital signs and fluid input (oral and intravenous) and output should be monitored.
- Following removal of the urinary obstruction, intravenous fluid therapy and regular monitoring of electrolytes should be maintained until post-obstructive diuresis ceases.
- Urine production should be recorded daily and the patient watched for signs of dysuria/haematuria. The bladder should be palpated at least twice a day, and after each urination, to assess for any residual urine that may prompt a need for manual expression, catheterization or anti-inflammatory therapy.

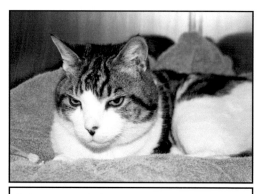

Following relief of the acute urinary obstruction, the cat is receiving intravenous fluids.

Patient comfort and stress relief

Warmth, comfort and a clean environment (including keeping the litter tray clean) should be provided. In-hospital stress should be reduced as much as possible (see Case 18.6).

Owner advice and homecare recommendations

Diet and water intake

The owners should be advised of the importance of keeping to the prescribed diet and, especially, of the need to encourage increased water intake.

Follow-up and prognosis

The owners should be warned to look out for signs of recurrence of either stones or obstruction and to contact the surgery if they recur. The main problem with urolithiasis is the risk of obstruction. This can be life-threatening, especially in male cats, so the owner must contact the veterinary surgery immediately if the cat is straining unproductively to urinate. It is possible for owners to confuse this with constipation, so this should also be discussed.

If the cat has had a perineal urethrostomy, it will be at increased risk of urinary tract infections and the owner should also be advised to monitor for signs of these, such as urinary frequency, urgency and straining, bloody urine and malaise (as a result of fever and systemic responses).

Case 18.8
Urolithiasis in a dog

A 5-year-old neutered male Miniature Schnauzer in normal body condition was presented with an acute onset of abdominal pain. Clinical examination revealed that the pain was perirenal and there was palpable unilateral renomegaly.

Investigations confirmed unilateral hydronephrosis and hydroureter due to obstruction with a radiopaque, probably oxalate, urolith. The dog was not azotaemic. Blood samples taken prior to commencing intravenous fluid therapy showed normal total and ionized calcium concentrations and no other evidence of an underlying cause (normocalcaemic calciuria). Urinalysis showed the presence of oxalate crystalluria.

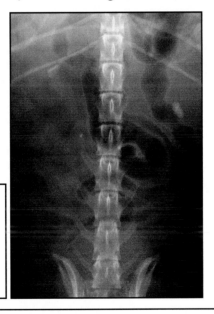

This plain abdominal radiograph shows bilateral radiopaque nephroliths and a radiopaque object on the right, between the kidney and the bladder, suspected to be a ureterolith.

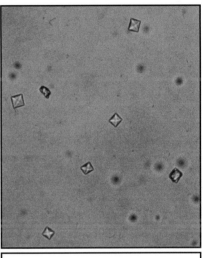

Calcium oxalate crystalluria, consistent with oxalate urolithiasis.

Agreed medical/surgical management

The dog was managed with saline diuresis and pain relief (see below) for 24–48 hours. If this fails to displace the stone(s), surgical management is indicated (either a unilateral ureteronephrectomy after confirmation of normal function in the contralateral kidney with an intravenous urogram or placement of ureteral stents to bypass the blockage).

Acute/chronic pain management

Acute pain

The pain associated with ureteric calculi should not be underestimated. Acute pain management should include a full mu agonist opioid (methadone or morphine). Although the patient is not azotaemic, NSAIDs should be avoided until potential obstruction is relieved. If opioids are insufficient to control the pain, dexmedetomidine (CRI at 0.5–1 mg/kg/h) should be considered.

Chronic pain

Chronic pain should not be an issue in this patient, although in human patients such painful conditions have been reported to produce secondary somatic pain (i.e. in the body wall) which then continues long after the condition is surgically or medically resolved. If this is present, one would expect the patient to be re-presented with similar signs (i.e. abdominal pain) but no renomegaly or urolith. In such patients, searching for myofascial pain in the thoracolumbar segments may be useful, treating any found with acupuncture (see below).

Fear, stress, conflict concerns

There are no specific concerns in this patient. However, stress is implicated as a risk factor for oxalate urolith formation in humans, where it is proposed to act via effects on the hypothalamic/pituitary axis and ADH production. It is possible, therefore, that stress might play a role in the condition in this dog, so it might be worth discussing this with the owners and reducing any obviously exciting and stressful conditions.

Nutritional requirements

Diet in the hospital
The most important consideration while the dog is in the hospital is that he eats, rather than giving him a specific diet. Therefore it is best in the short term to offer him a palatable diet – preferably similar to his usual food, and moist rather than dried (see below) – and to consider moving him on to a prescription diet later, once he is stabilized. The pain associated with the calculi, and the effects of the opiates, will be likely to make him anorexic but he should eat readily after the stones have been removed. If this is not the case, and he fails to meet his RER after successful treatment, temporary tube feeding with an oesophagostomy or naso-oesophageal tube might be considered.

Long-term dietary management
The dietary recommendations for calcium oxalate urolithiasis keep changing and it is important to note that diets are *never* calculolytic for this type of stone (i.e. they cannot dissolve them) but simply aim to prevent recurrence. They predominantly do this by trying to reduce the supersaturation of urine with oxalate, by promoting inhibitors and reducing promoters. Even so, there is a high recurrence rate, particularly in breeds like this one, which is at high risk of oxalate urolithiasis for as yet poorly understood reasons.

The most important, and consistent, consideration is that water intake is increased. A study has shown that Miniature Schnauzers fed on dried food produced more concentrated urine than when fed on canned food (i.e. they failed to increase their water intake to make up for the reduced water in the food), whereas Labrador Retrievers produced urine of the same specific gravity regardless of the diet fed (Stevenson *et al.*, 2003).

The long-term use of a diet formulated for prevention of oxalate stones should be considered in this case (preferably the canned form). However, many of these diets are protein-restricted but have increased fat levels.

WARNING
It is essential to check that this Miniature Schnauzer is neither hyperlipidaemic nor prone to pancreatitis *before* prescribing such a diet. Such diets can lead to recurrence of (potentially fatal) bouts of pancreatitis. In dogs with hyperlipidaemia or pancreatitis, feeding a highly digestible diet with good moisture content, and even adding extra water to the food, is the best compromise.

Weight management
This dog is in normal body condition, so weight loss is not a consideration. However, obesity has been identified as a risk factor in calcium oxalate urolithiasis in dogs (Lekcharoensuk *et al.*, 2000); where a dog with the condition is overweight a weight management programme (see Chapter 6) would be wise.

Physiotherapy

Physiotherapy is not indicated for this patient.

Hydrotherapy

Hydrotherapy is not specifically indicated for this patient.

Acupuncture

Acupuncture is not indicated for this patient unless he is re-presented with similar signs (no renomegaly/urolith) as described in 'Chronic pain', above. Searching for the relevant myofascial trigger point would then be theoretically (based on observations in human patients) useful. Treating the pain associated with the initial condition is likely to require strong electroacupuncture, but the situations in practice when this would be practical or superior to opiate use would be few and far between.

Monitoring

The saline fluid therapy requires careful monitoring and the dog's urine output also needs monitoring during the initial presurgical period: both to ensure there is a good output (i.e. no complete blockage) and also to note whether any stones are passed.

Food intake should be recorded and pain assessed.

Urination

During the diuresis, the dog should be taken outside frequently to pass urine. It is usual to turn off the drip but leave it attached and carry the bag out attached to the dog. Measures should be taken to ensure that he does not become urine-scalded while on diuresis; soiled bedding must be changed frequently, and any urine-stained fur and skin washed and carefully dried.

Owner advice and homecare recommendations

Water and urination

Free access to water is essential at all times and the dog must be given plenty of chances to urinate to prevent the presence of urine in the bladder for long periods.

Follow-up and prognosis

The owners should be advised that urolith removal does not alter the factors responsible for their formation, and that recurrence is very likely. This will help to minimize any sense of failure when the uroliths recur. This should be balanced against the need to motivate the owners to, at least, slow recurrence by trying to adhere to dietary manipulations. The owner should watch for any evidence of dysuria or haematuria and bring the dog back to the veterinary surgery when these occur.

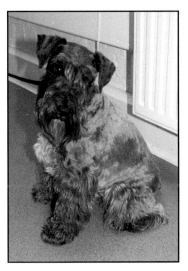

> Miniature Schnauzers are predisposed to oxalate urolithiasis. Owners should be advised that recurrence is likely.

References

Lekcharoensuk C, Lulich JP, Osborne CA *et al.* (2000) Patient and environmental factors associated with calcium oxalate urolithiasis in dogs. *Journal of the American Veterinary Medical Association* **217**, 515–519

Stevenson AE, Hynds WK and Markwell PJ (2003) Effect of dietary moisture and sodium content on urine composition and calcium oxalate relative supersaturation in healthy miniature schnauzers and labrador retrievers. *Research in Veterinary Science* **74**, 145–151

Case 18.9
Prostatitis in a dog

A 9-year-old male entire crossbred dog was presented with acute-onset abdominal pain and fever. There were signs of early septic shock and the dog was markedly depressed.

Physical examination revealed a swollen, painful prostate gland. Prostatic imaging and sampling, and urinalysis, confirmed acute bacterial prostatitis and an associated urinary tract infection.

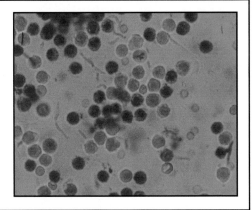

> White blood cells and bacterial rod forms in a urine sample.

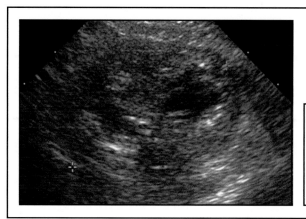

Ultrasonographic appearance of the prostate from a dog with acute prostatitis. The gland is enlarged (4.1 cm) and of a mixed, irregular echogenicity. Some hypoechoic (probably fluid-filled) spaces are apparent.

Agreed medical/surgical management

Intravenous fluid therapy and antibiotics were administered. Ampicillin (broad-spectrum) was given initially, as this would penetrate the inflamed prostate gland but not the uninflamed blood–prostate barrier. Following culture and sensitivity testing, oral therapy with a more specific antibiotic with good prostatic penetrance was given. Analgesia was provided (see below). Chronic management includes advising prophylactic castration to prevent recurrences. (See *BSAVA Manual of Canine and Feline Reproduction and Neonatology* for more details on management of prostatic disease.)

Acute/chronic pain management

Acute pain

Opioids may be useful in the transition from acute pain around the time of treatment to longer lasting pain. Morphine is better avoided because there is concern (possibly unfounded) about urethral sphincter spasm. Pethidine is too short-acting and would entail regular painful injections. Therefore, methadone may be the best choice of opioid here. Failure to control pain adequately with opioids should prompt use of additional drugs; lidocaine and/or ketamine CRI may be very useful. Epidural local anaesthetics should be avoided if there are early signs of septic shock (it could worsen the hypotension), but epidural morphine can be useful and is safe in early septic shock because it is unlikely to cause further vasodilation.

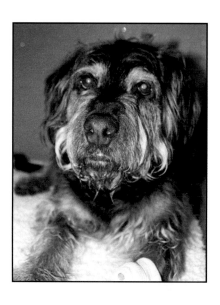

A swollen, painful prostate gland in this patient was associated with acute-onset abdominal pain and fever.

Chronic pain

If chronic pain remains after acute intervention, NSAIDs would be the first choice of analgesic, followed by the addition of tramadol or paracetamol + codeine if the dog is still depressed and suffering.

Fear, stress, conflict concerns

Pain and discomfort always produce stress and conflict, but these should resolve as the condition is treated. Castration can cause problems for the occasional dog who may find that it is hard to communicate with other male dogs, and there are anecdotal reports of loss of confidence/anxiety states after castration. This is not a reason not to perform the surgery, but the possibility of behavioural changes after castration should be included in the list of possible side effects explained to the owner.

Nutritional requirements

Feeding in the hospital

It is important that the dog eats during the acute phase of treatment. Depending on the severity of abdominal sepsis, there may be an increase in protein requirements (e.g. if there is peritonitis) so feeding of a diet formulated for critical care might be ideal. However, the dog may be unwilling to eat because of the pain and opiate analgesia. His daily energy intake should be carefully monitored; if this fails to meet at least 50% of his RER for 3 days, some form of assisted feeding should be instituted, such as an oesophagostomy or naso-oesophageal tube (see Chapter 5).

Long-term diet
If the dog is to be castrated, the owner should be warned that in most cases energy requirements will decrease after neutering, and so food intake will probably have to be reduced to maintain stable bodyweight.

Physiotherapy

Physiotherapy is not indicated for this patient.

Hydrotherapy

Hydrotherapy is not specifically indicated for this patient.

Acupuncture

Acupuncture is not specifically indicated for this patient.

Other nursing and supportive care

Monitoring
Intravenous fluid therapy requires careful monitoring. The dog should also have access to water *ad libitum*. Food intake should also be monitored. A pain scoring system will help a consistent approach to pain assessment.

Urination and defecation
Urine production and hydration status should be checked frequently. Sometimes dogs with acute prostatitis will be unable to urinate because of urethral spasm and it is important to recognize and treat this quickly to prevent detrusor muscle over-stretch. The patient requires frequent opportunities for urination and defecation. Constipation due to pain and/or physical obstruction is possible, and the addition of stool softeners (e.g. lactulose) could be considered. Urine samples may be required for assessment of case progression.

Deterioration
The patient should be observed for signs of clinical deterioration, such as fever, dehydration, septicaemia or endotoxaemia.

Postoperative care
An Elizabethan collar may be required to prevent the dog interfering with the surgical wound. See Chapter 12 for a full discussion of postoperative care.

Owner advice and homecare recommendations

The owners should be advised to complete the full course of antibiotics prescribed, regardless of whether or not the dog appears better.

Follow-up
Owners should be advised how often to return the dog to the clinic for reassessment and urine culture.

They should monitor the dog for any signs of dysuria, haematuria or urethral obstruction, and contact the surgery immediately if any of these happen. It is important to emphasize the risk of permanent detrusor over-stretch and persistent bladder atony, resulting in an inability to urinate, if obstruction is not treated quickly.

19

Patients with gastrointestinal, liver or pancreatic disease

Edited by Penny Watson

Introduction

Diseases of the gastrointestinal tract, liver and pancreas in dogs and cats can occur separately or concurrently. The most important considerations for supportive care in all of these diseases are: fluid and electrolyte balance; nutrition; and, particularly for pancreatic disease, analgesia. There are also particular nursing, homecare and infection control considerations for the dog or cat with vomiting and diarrhoea.

Fluid and electrolyte balance

Vomiting and/or diarrhoea rapidly result in dehydration and electrolyte and acid–base imbalances, particularly if there is a concurrently reduced, or absent, oral intake of fluids and food.

The most profound imbalances occur with gastric and upper intestinal losses. Disease that is confined to the colon is unlikely to result in significant electrolyte or acid–base imbalance. All but the most mildly affected dog or cat with vomiting, small intestinal diarrhoea, pancreatitis or acute liver disease will require intravenous fluids and electrolytes. Mildly affected animals, without clinically detectable dehydration and which are still drinking, could be treated with oral fluid and electrolyte replacement. The aim of supportive care is to restore lost fluids and reverse dehydration and electrolyte imbalances within the first 12–24 hours of therapy; thereafter, nutritional therapy should be considered.

If the patient remains clinically dehydrated after 24 hours of intravenous fluids, a careful re-evaluation of the fluid rate should be made, as it is likely that this is inadequate. It is easy to underestimate the fluid deficit and required fluid rate, particularly in large breed dogs. More details on fluid therapy can be found in the BSAVA Manual of Canine and Feline Emergency and Critical Care.

Vomiting and diarrhoea from any cause can result in a variety of acid–base and electrolyte disorders. In one study of upper intestinal foreign bodies in dogs, the most common of these were hypochloraemia, hypokalaemia and metabolic alkalosis, regardless of the site of obstruction (gastric or jejunal). It is a mistake to assume that pure gastric vomiting will result in alkalosis whilst intestinal disease will result in acidosis: in fact, the acid–base disturbances resulting from vomiting and diarrhoea are unpredictable and can only be addressed by individual measurement (Boag et al., 2005). Acid–base

disorders do not always need specific treatment: often they will normalize provided the kidneys are functional and the animal is given sufficient fluid therapy. Nevertheless, in a few cases (e.g. severe metabolic acidosis in a dog with acute pancreatitis and concurrent diabetic ketoacidosis), intervention will be required. More details on treatment of acid–base disturbances are found in the BSAVA Manual of Canine and Feline Emergency and Critical Care.

Hypokalaemia is a significant and common finding in both dogs and cats with gastrointestinal disease, but especially in cats and small-breed dogs, and particularly in pancreatitis. Cats with gastrointestinal disease are very susceptible to hypokalaemia; not only is there reduced intake of potassium and the loss associated with vomiting, but cats are particularly susceptible to the increased renal loss associated with diuresis. Marked hypokalaemia is life-threatening and even mild to moderate hypokalaemia will reduce gastrointestinal motility and so delay recovery from the primary disease. Standard crystalloid solutions, including lactated Ringer's, do not contain sufficient potassium to replace needs and ongoing losses. It is therefore essential in all dogs and cats with significant vomiting and diarrhoea to measure serum potassium concentrations and supplement fluids as necessary, preferably according to a sliding scale (Figure 19.1).

Blood potassium concentration (mmol/l)	Potassium to add to fluids (mmol/l)
3.5–5.5	20
3.0–3.4	30
2.5–2.9	40
2.0–2.4	60
<2.0	80

19.1 Potassium supplementation requirements. Note that lactated Ringer's (Hartmann's) solution already contains 5 mmol/l potassium. Addition of >20 mmol/l of potassium to intravenous fluids requires the availability of potassium measurement on site and well controlled fluid infusion rates: preferably an infusion pump. The infusion rate of potassium should not be increased above 0.5 mmol/kg/h.

Protein, blood and glucose loss

Some gastrointestinal diseases are associated with significant hypoproteinaemia. This needs to be addressed, usually by dietary means, but also in some cases by intravenous infusion of plasma or albumin. Diseases associated with hypoproteinaemia include chronic liver disease (where there is reduced hepatic production of albumin and globulins (except gamma-globulins)) and protein-losing enteropathies: lymphangiectasia; severe small intestinal inflammatory bowel disease; and small intestinal and gastric neoplasia, particularly lymphoma.

Hypoproteinaemia predisposes to thromboembolic disease and some animals with liver and/or pancreatic disease (particularly acute disease) are prone to diffuse intravascular coagulation. In these circumstances, a plasma infusion, with or without heparin therapy, might be considered, although its use and efficacy in preventing or treating thromboembolic disease in small animals is controversial.

Low blood glucose concentration can be a significant and life-threatening complication in gastrointestinal disease, particularly in small-breed dogs with liver disease or pancreatitis. It is therefore important to measure blood glucose and address any deficiencies urgently. Hypoglycaemia can contribute to the encephalopathy seen in liver disease and will result in irreversible brain damage if not addressed.

Hyperglycaemia is a relatively common finding in dogs and particularly cats with acute pancreatitis and/or hepatic lipidosis. It may be transient and reversible or it may result in diabetes mellitus. The presence of concurrent ketoacidosis in dogs or cats implies diabetes and the need to instigate insulin therapy. In the absence of ketoacidosis, the hyperglycaemia may be reversible and the clinician is left to decide whether simply to monitor blood glucose concentration while instituting other treatment, or whether also to treat judiciously with soluble insulin; there is some evidence that controlling the hyperglycaemia associated with critical illness is associated with a better outcome.

Some dogs and cats with severe inflammatory bowel disease, gastrointestinal neoplasia or liver disease may suffer from microcytic anaemia. In liver disease, this is due predominantly to iron chelation by hepatocytes, although there may be concurrent gastrointestinal blood loss due to portal hypertension. In intestinal disease, anaemia is associated with chronic blood loss into the gut and therefore a true iron deficiency. With small intestine or gastric bleeding, there may be overt malaena; faeces may appear normal in colour if blood loss is low grade and prolonged, but there will still be significant anaemia (Ristic and Stidworthy, 2002). In these cases, serious consideration should be given to administration of a blood transfusion, particularly if surgery is considered for biopsy and placement of feeding tubes. Animals with iron deficiency are unable to replace even modest blood losses associated with surgery.

Nutrition

Adequate and appropriate nutrition is essential for, and central to, the treatment of diseases of the liver, pancreas and gastrointestinal tract (see Chapter 5 and the cases below). The gastrointestinal tract, pancreas and liver are central to the digestion, absorption and metabolism of dietary components, so changes in the diet will have profound effects on the diseases and healing of these organs. It is no longer acceptable or appropriate to starve animals with gastrointestinal, pancreatic or liver disease, except in the very short term (up to 3 days) in acute disease. Even then, recent work in puppies with parvovirus has suggested that early feeding (within the first 12 hours) results in faster recovery (Mohr et al., 2003) and evidence in human medicine suggests early feeding also improves outcome in severe acute pancreatitis (Meier and Beglinger, 2006) so the 'knee-jerk' reaction of starving any animal that is vomiting should be reconsidered carefully in every case.

Many animals with gastrointestinal disease will need some form of assisted feeding because nausea and postprandial pain will reduce or abolish voluntary intake. Even in the face of ongoing vomiting, tube feeding can hasten recovery as at least some of the food reaches the intestinal tract and provides nutrition for enterocytes (Mohr et al., 2003). The concurrent use of antiemetics should increase the amount of food absorbed. If the animal is undergoing laparotomy for investigation or treatment, or indeed being given a general anaesthetic for any reason, it is important to consider whether a feeding tube should be placed at the time of surgery. In cats undergoing intestinal biopsy for investigation of gastrointestinal disease, tube placement is almost always required, and similarly for many dogs. It is better to place a feeding tube that is subsequently not used than not to place one and be faced with an anorexic animal after surgery that needs another anaesthetic for tube placement.

Analgesia

The clinician should not underestimate the need for analgesia in patients with gastrointestinal disease, particularly in acute or chronic pancreatitis but also in gastrointestinal motility disorders and biliary tract disease. Acute and chronic pancreatitis are associated with very significant pain. As with other diseases, cats with pancreatitis are inclined to withdraw and do very little in response to pain, and this gives rise either to the idea that they are 'hiding' it or that they are not actually in pain. However, cats with pancreatitis certainly do suffer pain, just as dogs and human patients do, and it needs addressing.

There can be some difficulty in finding a suitable analgesic in gastrointestinal disease, particularly because of the propensity for non-steroidal anti-inflammatory drugs (NSAIDs) to contribute to gastrointestinal ulceration and to renal compromise in dehydrated animals. However, difficulty in finding a suitable analgesic is not a reason not to use one. Selection of appropriate analgesics is addressed in the case studies that follow and in Chapters 2 and 3.

In acute pancreatitis, there is documented evidence that intragastric feeding of a high-fat diet causes postprandial pain in humans; anecdotally, the same appears to be true in dogs, so even changing to a low-fat diet may reduce postprandial pain in canine pancreatitis. The effect of dietary fat in feline pancreatitis is unknown. Liver disease is associated with pain if the liver capsule becomes stretched (such as in feline hepatic lipidosis) or inflamed, or if there is biliary tract disease or obstruction, as pain receptors in the liver are predominantly located in the capsule and biliary tract but not in the hepatic parenchyma.

Nursing and infection control

The most important considerations when nursing patients with gastrointestinal disease are: feeding; frequent cleaning of vomitus and diarrhoea from the cage and patient; and controlling the spread of infection. Animals with acute pancreatitis or severe gastrointestinal disease or hepatic encephalopathy will be nursed in intensive care, with all the implications this carries for care of the patient, feeding tubes and therapeutic and monitoring equipment.

Many gastrointestinal diseases are infectious to other inpatients and some can be transmitted to people. This is made worse because organisms spread in the faeces will be liberally distributed around the hospital by an animal with diarrhoea. Agents such as canine parvovirus and feline coronavirus are highly infectious to other animals within the hospital; therefore, isolation facilities with very careful control measures are required to limit their spread. Other infections, such as salmonellosis, campylobacterosis or cryptosporidiosis, are infectious to nursing staff and owners, as well as to other animals. Careful cleaning of the environment, personal hygiene and education of the owners are vital to prevent zoonotic infection. Contact with immunosuppressed animals (e.g. inpatients on chemotherapy) or people should be completely avoided until the infection is eliminated.

Homecare

Homecare of the animal with gastrointestinal disease has its own challenges. Owners (and animals in their home environment) may not be very good at keeping to prescribed diets. In addition, canine diarrhoea is a major concern to owners that should not be underestimated, particularly if the urgency associated with colonic involvement means that the owner is frequently woken at night or is often clearing up diarrhoea from the kitchen floor. In these circumstances, rapid resolution of the diarrhoea becomes a priority.

References and further reading

Boag AK, Coe RJ, Martinez TA and Hughes D (2005) Acid-base and electrolyte abnormalities in dogs with gastrointestinal foreign bodies. *Journal of Veterinary Internal Medicine* **19**, 816–821

Hall EJ, Simpson JW and Williams DA (2005) *BSAVA Manual of Canine and Feline Gastroenterology, 2nd edn.* BSAVA Publications, Gloucester

Meier RF and Beglinger C (2006) Nutrition in pancreatic diseases. *Best Practice in Research: Clinical Gastroenterology* **20**, 507–529

Mohr AJ, Leisewitz AL, Jacobson LS *et al.* (2003) Effect of early enteral nutrition on intestinal permeability, intestinal protein loss, and outcome in dogs with severe parvoviral enteritis. *Journal of Veterinary Internal Medicine* **17**, 791–798

Ristic JM and Stidworthy MF (2002) Two cases of severe iron-deficiency anaemia due to inflammatory bowel disease in the dog. *Journal of Small Animal Practice* **43**, 80–83

Clinical case studies

A variety of case scenarios in dogs and cats will now be presented to illustrate the considerations to be made and the options available within a specific clinical setting. Information relating to the rehabilitation and palliation of each condition has been contributed to each case by the authors in the first part of this Manual, plus notes on nursing and homecare from Rachel Lumbis RVN. The reader should refer back to the appropriate chapters for further details. Photographs used to illustrate the principles and techniques within the cases do not necessarily feature the original patient.

Case 19.1
Acute parvovirus infection in a puppy

An 8-week-old entire female Rottweiler puppy was presented with acute haemorrhagic gastroenteritis. The pup had been bought a week ago and the owner was already very fond of her. There were no other dogs in the household.

On clinical examination, the puppy was 5–10% dehydrated and very hunched up, suggesting pain. She also had haemorrhagic diarrhoea. A faecal ELISA test confirmed parvovirus (CPV-2) infection.

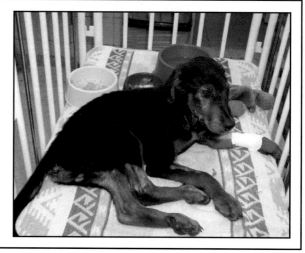

Puppy with parvovirus infection. Following analgesia she is comfortable but she is very cachexic and in clear need of nutrition. (Courtesy of Johan Schoeman)

Agreed medical/surgical management

The puppy was admitted and barrier-nursed in isolation (see later).

Blood and urine samples were collected just prior to commencing intravenous fluid therapy with twice-maintenance rates of lactated Ringer's solution, supplemented as necessary with replacement potassium (based on serum levels measured in pretreatment blood sample; see Figure 19.1 in the Introduction to this chapter). In a puppy, it is very important to make sure this infusion rate is NOT exceeded, as it is very easy to over-infuse small animals. Urine output should be monitored because renal shutdown is a serious complication (and will reinforce the care needed not to over-infuse the puppy). It is also important to ensure that the dehydration is being adequately addressed, i.e. has been reversed within about 12 hours, because it is also easy to *under*-infuse puppies. If the puppy is too collapsed and dehydrated to allow placement of an intravenous fluid line, intramedullary infusion of fluids is an acceptable alternative. Whichever route is used, an infusion pump is recommended to allow careful control of infusion rates and avoid mistakes.

It is important to check the patient's blood glucose on admission, and frequently thereafter, as hypoglycaemia is not uncommon in puppies with parvovirus; any hypoglycaemia needs addressing urgently by adding 2.5% or 5% dextrose to the intravenous fluids.

If the puppy is very hypoalbuminaemic, a plasma transfusion may be given. A colloid could be used instead, but plasma from a vaccinated dog has the added advantage of antibodies, which may help the puppy.

A CBC showed marked neutropenia. Intravenous antibiotics are indicated to protect against septicaemia of gut origin. This is likely to occur because of the severe intestinal wall damage combined with neutropenia. A combination of fluoroquinolones and amoxicillin might be chosen in an adult dog, but in a young large-breed dog fluoroquinolones are contraindicated because of their detrimental effect on cartilage. In this case, the animal should be given intravenous amoxicillin only, until fully rehydrated; treatment with intravenous gentamicin can then be considered, taking care to dose correctly and in full knowledge of the potential for nephrotoxicity.

Antiemetics may be used: maropitant is a good choice and is authorized in the UK. If this does not work, ondansetron can be used.

It is important wherever possible to use an infusion pump when rehydrating small puppies to prevent over- or under-infusion of fluids. Urine output should be monitored.

Recombinant feline interferon-omega treatment could also be used. Although by no means essential, this has been shown to reduce mortality in both challenge and field trials of canine parvovirus infection (Martin *et al.*, 2002; de Marin *et al.*, 2003).

Early feeding is also important (see below).

Once the dog has recovered from the initial acute phase, antiparasitic (e.g. anti-*Giardia*) treatment can be considered. Pups with heavy parasite burdens appear predisposed to more severe parvoviral infections.

Acute/chronic pain management

Parvoviral haemorrhagic gastroenteritis can be a very painful condition, so serious consideration should be given to analgesia. There is very little information about the use of analgesics in young animals, and even less about their use in those with underlying serious disease, so great care should be taken in the choice of analgesic in this case. **NSAIDs are contraindicated in view of the patient's age and condition.**

Opioids are likely to form the mainstay of analgesic treatment. Pethidine (meperidine) is potentially useful because of its spasmolytic properties, but it cannot be given intravenously and the frequent intramuscular injections that would be needed would be uncomfortable for the puppy. Partial agonists may provide inferior analgesia to a pure mu agonist.

A fentanyl constant rate infusion (CRI) or application of a fentanyl patch should be considered, while bearing in mind that it takes 24 hours for analgesia to be achieved by this route and there is a danger of removal by the puppy. Further work in canine paediatric patients is needed before lidocaine CRI can be recommended, although potentially it may have other beneficial effects as a prokinetic and anti-inflammatory/antioxidant.

Fear, stress, conflict concerns

Eight weeks is a particularly vulnerable age for puppies, and pain and disease will compound the stress that she is under. As well as medical help and acute pain management, she should get as much company and attention as is compatible with care and hygiene precautions. Assuming she survives, it will be important to counsel the owners as to her socialization and early experiences, since she will have not only lost valuable time in becoming familiar with normal surroundings, but there is also a danger that negative associations will already have been made because of pain and distress at such a young age.

While the puppy is sick, it is natural for the owners to give her their attention as soon as she makes a noise or seeks reassurance. This is understandable, and necessary during an acute phase of illness. However, the owner should be given advice about controlling attention when she recovers, to prevent her becoming very dependent or developing attention-seeking behaviours.

Nutritional requirements

Feeding in the hospital

Traditional nutritional management of puppies with parvoviral enteritis has typically entailed waiting until gastrointestinal signs resolved before attempting to feed. More recently, a clinical trial has demonstrated that early enteral nutrition achieved via naso-oesophageal feeding is well tolerated in such cases. This resulted in a renewed interest in pursuing nutritional support, even in cases where animals have significant gastrointestinal disease. Mohr *et al.* (2003) performed a randomized study in 30 dogs with parvovirus infection (15 in each group) which were all 8–24 weeks old. The trial compared the outcomes of *either* feeding *nil per os* until 12 hours after the vomiting stopped (mean 50 hours from admission) *or* giving early enteral nutrition by naso-oesophageal tube from 12 hours or less from admission. The enteral nutrition was combined with the use of antiemetics but, despite this, a proportion of the food fed was vomited back. Nevertheless, the early fed group had faster resolution of vomiting and diarrhoea, greater weight gain, reduced catabolism, and evidence of improved gastrointestinal barrier function (i.e. reduced permeability).

So, early feeding is advised in cases of parvovirus infection. It is likely that some sort of assisted (i.e. tube- or syringe-) feeding will be necessary in most cases, as these animals are usually very inappetent. Naso-oesophageal tubes would be most appropriate in the majority of cases.

The puppy was fed via a naso-oesophageal tube.
(Courtesy of Johan Schoeman)

The composition of the diet may not be as important as the ability to administer it via feeding tubes. Therefore, diets designed for convalescence are usually recommended for such cases (Mohr *et al.* used a canine convalescence diet in their study). Meeting full energy requirements may not be possible in such cases, but even small amounts of enteral nutrition may confer benefits by improving intestinal barrier function, speeding gut wall healing and reducing bacterial translocation into the circulation (see Chapter 5). Infrequent episodes of vomiting may not necessarily preclude continuing with enteral support; only in circumstances where the degree of vomiting may compromise the dog's intravascular fluid volume should discontinuation of feeding be considered. An alternative is *microenteral* nutrition, where small amounts of food are administered continuously using a syringe pump. Partial parenteral nutrition might also be considered if the puppy is not keeping down very many calories (see Chapter 5).

Antiemetics will also be necessary in most cases (see above).

Nutraceuticals

It would be rational to believe that oral supplementation of glutamine might be indicated in this case, since glutamine is a preferred energy source for enterocytes and also for the gut immune system (see Chapter 7). However, there is no published evidence to date supporting the supplementation of glutamine specifically in gastrointestinal disease in dogs.

A number of studies have looked at the effects of antioxidants, such as vitamin E and lutein, on the immune status of healthy dogs; some studies suggest that some antioxidants enhance immunity. Panda *et al.* (2009) showed evidence of oxidative stress in red cells of dogs with parvovirus infection, but there are no studies on the use of antioxidants in clinical parvovirus infection in dogs.

There might also be a theoretical rationale for the addition of probiotics to the diet of dogs after recovery from the acute phase of parvovirus infection, to encourage restoration of normal gut flora. There is some evidence for the efficacy of probiotics in acute viral enteritis in children, but the effect is confined to certain strains of probiotic bacteria (Vandenplas *et al.*, 2007). There is currently no evidence for the efficacy of probiotics in viral diarrhoea in dogs.

Feeding at home after discharge
See Homecare, below.

Physiotherapy

Physiotherapy is not indicated for this patient.

Hydrotherapy

Hydrotherapy is not specifically indicated for this patient.

Acupuncture

Not applicable, unless the pain is not being controlled in any other way.

Other nursing and supportive care

Infection control
The puppy will need careful barrier nursing to prevent infection of other outpatients and inpatients, and also to prevent personnel who are nursing the dog from transmitting the virus out into the external environment and to their pets at home. If isolation facilities and barrier nursing (see below) are not possible in the practice, serious consideration should be given to transferring the puppy to a facility that can achieve effective infection control. Infected puppies will only shed large amounts of virus for about 4–5 days from the onset of clinical signs. However, the virus will survive in the environment for months to years, provided it is not exposed to sun or effective disinfectants. The environment should be cleaned with a suitable disinfectant: many disinfectants and detergents do not kill parvovirus.

Essentials of barrier nursing

- The kennel should be isolated away from the main ward. It should be in its own unit, with separate handwashing facilities and its own equipment and cleaning tools.
- Thermometers, stethoscopes and other monitoring equipment should also be separate and kept within the isolation ward. Of particular note here are pens: these can easily 'walk' out of the isolation ward and transfer infection; they should remain within the ward.
- As far as possible, nominate just one person to nurse the dog and try to minimize their contact with other animals in the practice (particularly those that are young or immunosuppressed).
- Staff should only enter the ward wearing protective clothing, including gloves and boots, and should dip their feet in a viricidal bath on the way in and out of the ward. They should routinely disinfect their hands on the way in and out of the ward. Consideration should be given to showering before re-entering the normal ward, or returning home to any vulnerable pets.

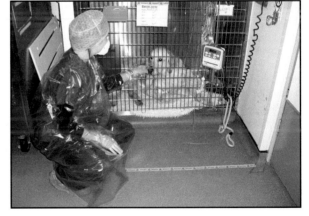

A patient receiving barrier nursing care. (Reproduced from *BSAVA Manual of Canine and Feline Advanced Veterinary Nursing, 2nd edn*)

Monitoring and comfort
A clean and comfortable environment should be provided, including warmth and absorbent disposable bedding. Vital signs should be monitored and the puppy watched for signs of pain.

Episodes of vomiting and diarrhoea must be recorded, to allow effective fluid replacement and also to allow monitoring of the effectiveness of antiemetic treatment. If the patient becomes soiled with vomitus or diarrhoea, she should be bathed immediately and then dried with an absorbent towel. The application of barrier cream to the hindquarters following episodes of diarrhoea should be considered to prevent scalding.

Fluids and food
It is important to check regularly that the intravenous fluids are running and that the rate is correct and electrolytes (particularly potassium) are supplemented appropriately.

If a feeding tube has been placed, this should be monitored carefully as the majority of complications involve tube occlusion or localized irritation at the tube exit site. The puppy may need to be fitted with an Elizabethan collar to prevent premature removal of the feeding tube. The feeding tube should be flushed with 5–10 ml of water after each feed to minimize clogging

Owner advice and homecare recommendations

Feeding and advice on weight gain

Parvovirus infection results in severe damage to the intestinal wall, which takes months to heal in puppies that survive the acute episode. In some cases, gut function never returns to normal and the dog is a permanent 'poor doer'. It is important to warn the owner carefully about this. This puppy will require a large amount of energy to grow, especially as she is of a large breed. Her body will prioritize protein and calories for growth against weight gain (filling out) and the owner should therefore expect her to look thin until she is at least 6 months old. Initially, it would be wise to discharge the puppy on a highly digestible prescription diet designed for intestinal disease, which should be fed little and often. However, if possible, she should be weaned slowly on to a large-breed growth diet more appropriate to her long-term needs. Regular endoparasite control is wise.

Monitoring clinical signs

The owner should be advised that it is normal for the puppy's stools to be a little loose at first. If diarrhoea persists or vomiting occurs, the owner should be encouraged to contact their veterinary surgeon. Following any episodes of loose stools or diarrhoea, the puppy's hindquarters should be bathed.

It is not uncommon for puppies recovering from parvoviral disease to develop an intussusception, so any acute worsening of clinical signs should be taken seriously and the puppy re-presented to the veterinary surgeon.

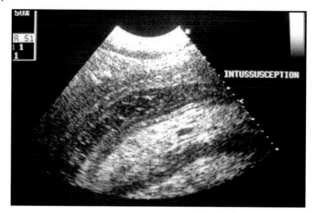

Ultrasound scan of an intussusception in a dog. (Courtesy of Diagnostic Imaging Department, Queen's Veterinary School Hospital, University of Cambridge)

Infection control and vaccination advice

It is important to check the vaccination status of other in-contact dogs and discuss future vaccination of this puppy. There are no other dogs in this household, but owners of other dogs that visit or that the puppy meets should be warned about the infection risk. Although she will only shed virus for 4–5 days from the onset of clinical signs, the virus shed into the environment before she was hospitalized can remain viable for months to years, and it is important to explain this to the owner. The environment (inside and outside the house) should be disinfected as much as possible. Household bleach (sodium hypochlorite) is effective against canine parvovirus; it should be diluted 1:32 with water and left in contact with surfaces for 10 minutes to be effective. Steam cleaning of surfaces that cannot be bleached may also be effective.

Maternal antibodies can interfere with the effect of vaccine and can result in a window of risk for infection in young puppies. Rottweilers are also recognized to have increased susceptibility to canine parvovirus and some of the newer subtypes of CPV-2 may be partly resistant to vaccination. If the puppy has sustained an infection in spite of vaccination, it would be appropriate to contact the vaccine manufacturer and to fill in a yellow 'lack of efficacy' form for the Veterinary Medicines Directorate. Immunity after natural infection like this is strong and prolonged – maybe even lifelong – so this puppy will probably not need parvovirus vaccinations in future.

References

de Marin K, Maynard L, Eun HM and Lebreux B (2003) Treatment of canine parvoviral enteritis with interferon-omega in a placebo-controlled field trial. *Veterinary Record* **152**, 105–108

Martin V, Najbar W, Gueguen S *et al.* (2002) Treatment of canine parvoviral enteritis with interferon-omega in a placebo-controlled challenge trial. *Veterinary Microbiology* **89**, 115–127

Mohr AJ, Leisewitz AL, Jacobson LS *et al.* (2003). Effect of early enteral nutrition on intestinal permeability, intestinal protein loss, and outcome in dogs with severe parvoviral enteritis. *Journal of Veterinary Internal Medicine* **17**, 791–798

Panda D, Patra RC, Nandi S and Swarup D (2009) Oxidative stress indices in gastroenteritis in dogs with canine parvoviral infection. *Research in Veterinary Science* **86**, 36–42

Vandenplas Y, Salvatore S, Vieira M, Devreker T and Hauser B (2007) Probiotics in infectious diarrhoea in children: are they indicated? *European Journal of Pediatrics* **166**, 1211–1218

Case 19.2
Inflammatory bowel disease in a dog

A 2-year-old entire female West Highland White Terrier was presented with chronic intermittent vomiting and small intestinal diarrhoea. The patient's clinical signs are made much worse by stress, such as fireworks and visits to the vet, suggesting a superimposed 'irritable bowel' component to the problem. After stress, she exhibits signs of abdominal pain (stretching, moaning, borborygmi) followed by explosive diarrhoea for 24 hours. She is a slightly thin, rather excitable dog with over-attached owners (a young married couple with no children) who become very anxious when she has a bad episode. The episodes are becoming worse with each subsequent stressful event.

Faecal samples showed no pathogens or parasites, and there were only partial responses to treatment with fenbendazole (to rule out giardiasis), an exclusion diet (to rule out food intolerance) and metronidazole (to rule out antibiotic-responsive diarrhoea). Inflammatory bowel disease (IBD) was diagnosed on the basis of endoscopic duodenal biopsy samples.

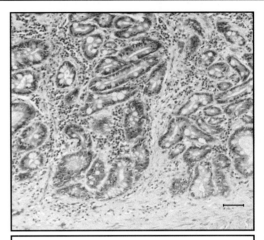

Section of duodenum from a dog with inflammatory bowel disease, showing a moderate increase in numbers of lymphocytes in the lamina propria. H&E; bar = 50 µm.

Agreed medical/surgical management

The dog was managed medically long term with continuation of the hypoallergenic diet and attempts to control stressful events. IBD can be a difficult disease to control and often requires multimodal treatment to reduce: intestinal inflammation; the immune response; and environmental triggers such as small intestinal bacteria, food antigens or stress.

In addition to long-term dietary treatment, she may need long-term or intermittent prednisolone and/or metronidazole. The prednisolone should be titrated to the lowest effective dose, preferably every other day, to minimize iatrogenic hyperadrenocorticism. An alternative might be to try ciclosporin, which is effective in some cases of IBD. Control of stress will be an important component of this dog's treatment.

Acute/chronic pain management

Low-dose amitriptyline may be helpful in controlling the pain of IBD; it may also regulate sleep and act as an anxiolytic. A suggested starting dose, to minimize side effects, would be 0.5 mg/kg orally q12h. It should be noted, however, that that this dose will not have an antidepressant effect (i.e. dealing with stress and anxiety as a phenomenon separate from the medical condition). Amitriptyline requires competent renal and hepatic function for clearance, so a biochemical blood screen is advised prior to commencing treatment; the drug should be used with caution in cases of cardiac arrhythmia. Amitriptyline may cause transient gastrointestinal signs and could potentially cause adverse behavioural changes, although this is not common.

Tramadol may also be helpful in this condition, but amitriptyline and tramadol should *not* be used together (possibility of serotonin syndrome; see Chapter 3).

Fear, stress, conflict concerns

Addressing the dog's nervous behaviour
This dog requires a behavioural assessment and possible referral to a behaviourist to determine the cause of her excitable and nervous behaviour. Physical signs resulting from stress often occur as a result of dogs being in a situation of *chronic* stress, with additional sources of *acute* stress that precipitate bouts of disease. The relationship between the dog and her owners may need to be addressed, as a common source of chronic anxiety is where owners are inconsistent in their responses to their dog (i.e. showing different responses to the same behaviour by the dog). This would need to be addressed by giving the owners a programme of advice,

where they respond consistently to their dog, ignoring undesired behaviours and rewarding desirable ones. In addition, the specific events that precipitate bouts of disease will need to be addressed, such as the fear of fireworks, with specific desensitization (to the vet visits and to noises) and counter-conditioning programmes (see *BSAVA Manual of Canine and Feline Behavioural Medicine*).

Addressing the over-attachment

Mutual over-attachment will require gentle weaning off the attention (in both directions) and the owners will need to stop showing sympathy when the dog looks anxious. Since ignoring such behaviour will be difficult for these owners, it will be more useful for them to be bright and jolly with her and to start training her to undertake alternative behaviours when she starts to look anxious. Relaxation therapy, pheromone (DAP spray, collar or diffuser) therapy and alpha-casozepine (see Chapter 4) would all be worth trying in this case, although there is no evidence of specific efficacy in IBD.

<h2 style="background:#888;color:#fff;display:inline-block;padding:2px 8px;">Nutritional requirements</h2>

Nutrition for IBD

Diet may have a significant role in controlling signs in dogs with IBD. However, there is a wide range of response, and diet alone is not effective in a great number of cases. This dog showed only a partial response with a hypoallergenic diet, showing that food intolerance was not the whole cause of its condition, although it is still possible that an inappropriate gut reaction to diet is one component. A diet trial to rule out food allergy should be carefully designed, using a single protein source. The protein should be identified as 'novel' on the basis of a full dietary history obtained from the owners, and all titbits should be avoided. Details of undertaking an effective dietary trial are given in Case 22.2.

Feeding a very digestible diet is also important in IBD, to reduce the work required from the compromised gut.

Nutrition for irritable bowel disease

Dietary composition can have a profound effect on gut motility (see Chapter 5), so some dietary manipulations might help control this dog's irritable bowel disease. Increasing non-fermentable fibre in the diet can help in some cases. Fermentable fibre may also be helpful because the production of short-chain fatty acids from gut fermentation (particularly butyrate) provides nutrition for colonocytes. Decreasing dietary fat might also help control the irritable bowel signs. Diets with different consistency (tinned, dried) have different transit times through the gastrointestinal tract (see Chapter 5), so manipulations of dietary consistency might also be tried.

<h2 style="background:#888;color:#fff;display:inline-block;padding:2px 8px;">Physiotherapy</h2>

There may be some benefit from performing stroking massage on this dog. This is a calming technique (see Chapter 9) that helps to relieve stress and anxiety. Involvement of the owners in this process provides them with some control over the situation and my help ease their anxiety.

<h2 style="background:#888;color:#fff;display:inline-block;padding:2px 8px;">Hydrotherapy</h2>

Hydrotherapy is not specifically indicated for this patient.

<h2 style="background:#888;color:#fff;display:inline-block;padding:2px 8px;">Acupuncture</h2>

Theoretically, acupuncture could have a positive effect on functional conditions such as 'irritable bowel' type problems, but the results of studies and one systematic review (Lim *et al.*, 2006) in humans are so far inconclusive. Irritable bowel syndrome is known to show a high placebo response to a number of interventions and that makes trial design difficult with an intervention such as acupuncture (see Chapter 8). One study did use the so-called 'placebo' (Streitberger) needle and was inconclusive (Schneider, 2006). Segmental acupuncture into multifidus muscles of the caudal thoracic and lumbar spine, and ventral points, would target the correct areas and may have a 'normalizing' effect on the gut. There may also be transient sedative and anxiolytic effects (see Chapter 11).

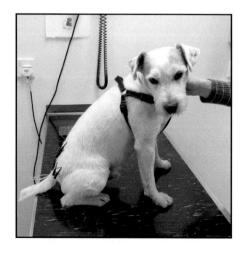

Acupuncture may have transient sedative and anxiolytic effects. (Courtesy of Samantha Lindley)

Other nursing and supportive care

Reducing stress

This dog was not hospitalized for the condition but will have repeated visits to the veterinary clinic, either for the IBD or for routine vaccinations, and these could be stressful. Measures should be taken to reduce this stress as much as possible. As part of a desensitization programme, the practice must become involved in helping the patient to make positive associations with visits to the practice – making a fuss of her, feeding her (but being careful to feed something appropriate for her condition) – and helping the owners not to rush the process by recognizing the early signs of anxiety that indicate that the programme is being pushed too far and too fast.

Feeding

It is important whenever the dog stays at the veterinary clinic that she receives her normal diet, since any sudden changes are very likely to upset her gut. It is important to discuss this with the owners; if necessary, they should leave some of her normal food with the practice if it is not normally in stock.

Owner advice and homecare recommendations

Working with the owners

The owners have an important role to play in the long-term management of this dog – both in controlling her IBD and in controlling her stress and irritable bowel. It is therefore important to have a good relationship between the owners and veterinary staff from the outset. The basic pathophysiology, treatment and prognosis of the diseases should be explained to the owners, along with potential uses and side effects of drugs used to treat them. The important role of the owners in helping with long-term control, working in partnership with the veterinary practice, must be stressed.

It is important to explain that both IBD and irritable bowel are lifelong diseases – they cannot be diagnosed, treated and then cured. The clinical signs can often be well controlled, so the owners should not be disheartened, but the disease is always present and signs can recur with various triggers. Using a common, well recognized human example to illustrate this can help; for example, asthma, where the disease is ever-present but acute attacks can be prevented by avoiding triggers.

The owners should be encouraged to discuss progress frequently with the practice: it helps if they can liaise predominantly with one veterinary surgeon (an 'advocate for the patient'), who has particular responsibility for the case and so knows the details whenever the owner contacts the practice (see Chapter 1).

The owners can help manage the dog particularly in the following ways:

- Long-term management of the IBD: with appropriate education and support, owners often become very good at titrating dietary and drug therapies optimally to control the dog's clinical signs
- Long-term management of the irritable bowel: the owners will have an important role in helping to reduce the dog's stress (see above). In addition, owners can be taught stroking massage to help relieve stress and anxiety in the dog and themselves.

Dietary management

It is important to explain any dietary manipulations carefully to the owners. In particular, if the dog is receiving a hypoallergenic diet, they need to understand the importance of strictly avoiding any other protein sources. It is also important to consider any other members of the family who may give tit-bits (e.g. young children) and also any neighbours.

References

Lim B, Manheimer E, Lao L *et al.* (2006) Acupuncture for treatment of irritable bowel syndrome. *Cochrane Database Systematic Reviews* CD005111
Schneider A, Enck P, Streitberger K *et al.* (2006) Acupuncture treatment in irritable bowel syndrome. *Gut* **55**, 649–654

Case 19.3
Acute severe pancreatitis in a dog

A 5-year-old neutered male Yorkshire Terrier was presented after protracted vomiting, in a collapsed and dehydrated state, with marked abdominal pain and some signs of systemic inflammatory response, after eating pork fat. The dog was normally fed a diet consisting solely of homemade food and table scraps, as he refused to eat manufactured petfood. He was in normal to slightly thin body condition and very nervous and attached to the owner, a retired elderly lady who spent all her time at home with him.

Acute severe pancreatitis was diagnosed on the basis of ultrasonographic appearance of the pancreas and raised pancreatic enzymes. A biochemistry screen showed azotaemia (likely prerenal), elevated liver enzymes and neutrophilia. The dog was given an 'organ score' of 2 or 3, which represents the number of organs apparently compromised in addition to the pancreas on admission (see *BSAVA Manual of Canine and Feline Clinical Pathology*). This suggested a rather poor prognosis and the dog was admitted to the intensive care unit.

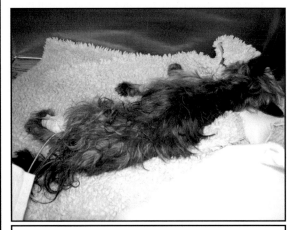

Yorkshire Terrier in the intensive care unit. An intravenous fluid line is in place plus a urinary catheter to allow monitoring of urine output.

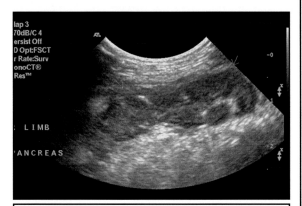

Ultrasonogram showing acute pancreatitis. Note the hypoechoic (black) pancreas surrounded by hyperechoic (white) mesentery. (Courtesy of Diagnostic Imaging Department, Queen's Veterinary School Hospital, University of Cambridge)

Agreed medical/surgical management

The dog was placed on intravenous fluids, and his blood glucose and potassium monitored frequently and supplemented as necessary. His urine output was monitored and was good once the fluid therapy had commenced. He was given analgesia as a priority (see below) and covered for secondary infections of gut origin with intravenous amoxicillin/clavulanate. Any vomiting was treated with an antiemetic (initially maropitant).

After 24 hours, once the dog was rehydrated, early consideration was given to feeding (see below). A plasma transfusion was also considered, to help replenish plasma α_1-antitrypsin and β_2-macroglobulin.

The dog recovered and was discharged after 7 days.

Acute/chronic pain management

Acute pain

Acute pancreatitis is associated with pain that can be severe. Treatment involves a staged approach of administering successively more potent analgesics, as is necessary. One important consideration in this case is that the drugs could not be given orally because of the dog's vomiting, so drugs that could be given systemically were needed.

Pain associated with pancreatitis is often refractory to opioids, and can be very difficult to treat. NSAIDs are usually contraindicated in pancreatitis because of the increased risk of gastrointestinal and renal toxicity. Other options are CRIs of lidocaine, ketamine and medetomidine, either alone or in combination. A combined CRI of morphine + lidocaine + ketamine (MLK) or a fentanyl CRI may also be used. Epidural morphine may be more effective than systemic opioids, and, because analgesia is likely to be necessary for several days, epidural catheterization would be better to allow longer-term treatment by this route.

There is some evidence in human patients to suggest that interpleural analgesia with local anaesthetics is effective in acute pancreatitis, but this has not been investigated in dogs.

Chronic pain

This appears to be an isolated attack of acute pancreatitis. However, it is possible that the dog has underlying chronic pancreatitis; if this is apparent, consideration should be given to long-term analgesia as necessary (see Case 19.4).

Fear, stress, conflict concerns

In the hospital environment

This patient will find not only his condition but also isolation from his owner and the hospital procedures stressful, especially as he starts to recover. As well as being detrimental to psychological welfare, there is increasing evidence that many disease processes can be exacerbated (or caused) by 'stress' (see Chapter 4). Discussion with the dog's owner will help discover what he likes in the way of attention, grooming, stroking (or not). Trial and error may reveal that he is happier in a quiet, dark kennel or with the ability to retreat into a box if

he feels overwhelmed by his surroundings, but this should not be assumed – the dog may be interested and stimulated by activity around it. The owner will be able to inform the practice staff of the dog's attitude to other dogs – if he is very fearful then he should be placed as far away from other dogs as possible, not allowed to meet them when he can eventually be walked out of his kennel, and kept in a high kennel out of the eyeline of other dogs. Pheromone therapy may be helpful in this situation.

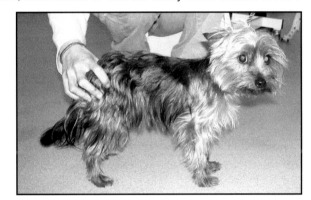

Hospital procedures can be stressful for an anxious dog.

Long-term treatment for 'stress'

Pancreatitis can be triggered by stress. Therefore, referral for behavioural assessment should be considered if there is a suggestion that this or previous episodes have been triggered or compounded by stress. The behavioural assessment will aim to determine the motivation for the nervousness and whether dependence on owner attention is important.

The source of the anxiety should be investigated, including finding out about the early socialization period. Often, high dependence on owners is a strategy for coping with perceived stressors – seeking attention is both reinforced by the owner and 'works' to help the dog cope with the stressor. This may be associated with separation-related behaviour (see *BSAVA Manual of Canine and Feline Behavioural Medicine*), the occurrence of which should be investigated in this dog. Identifying specific stressors is particularly important, as acute stress can precipitate bouts of disease, and addressing these may reduce recurrence.

The refusal to eat petfood may have arisen because its taste was associated with consequent pain. Where owners are anxious about their pet eating, they may also encourage 'fussiness' by immediately offering an alternative, more palatable food. Gentle weaning off the owner's attention should be considered, though it must be remembered that this may be a mutual over-dependence. Clomipramine and other tricyclic antidepressants should be avoided: TCAs have been reported to trigger pancreatitis in humans, and clomipramine has been reported to do this in one dog (Kook *et al.*, 2009).

Nutritional requirements

In the hospital

The traditional approach to the nutritional management of dogs with acute pancreatitis has centred on offering *nil per os* until vomiting and abdominal pain resolves, and offering a low-fat diet once the dog is eating voluntarily. However, this approach led to prolonged starvation of affected patients. Recent studies in human patients and canine models strongly support early feeding, preferably enterally, in severe acute pancreatitis – and the more severe the pancreatitis, the earlier the feeding should be. This is because food helps maintain gut wall integrity, reduces septic complications and speeds recovery (Meier and Beglinger, 2006). There is no evidence in support of the traditional view that feeding stimulates more inflammation by causing pancreatic enzyme release; indeed, there is some evidence to the contrary, i.e. that feeding reduces intrapancreatic enzyme release by encouraging normal release down the duct.

Every effort should be made to use the enteral route for nutritional support. Some patients may be managed with low-volume naso-oesophageal feeding using a low-fat liquid diet. If the dog is vomiting, the food should be combined with the use of antiemetics to try to reduce the amount brought back. Even in the face of some vomiting, enteral feeding can be worthwhile. This technique of tube feeding also affords the ability to aspirate stomach contents, thereby relieving stomach distension caused by fluid pooling in the stomach, which is a known cause of pain in human patients with acute pancreatitis.

Oesophageal and gastrostomy feeding tubes have been used in dogs with acute pancreatitis, with various degrees of success. This approach is reserved for dogs that tolerate enteral feeding without marked exacerbation of vomiting and abdominal pain. The diet used should be low in fat, as fat triggers more severe postprandial pain and may also trigger the pancreatitis itself. One practical approach to the institution of feeding in acute pancreatitis used by the author [PJW] is to start with baby rice mixed with water and then gradually move on to a low-fat diet over a few days.

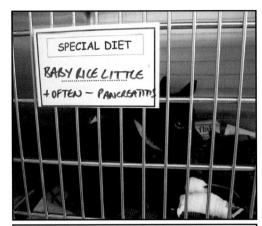

Baby rice mixed with water is a good initial diet to use orally in dogs with pancreatitis.

Dogs that require abdominal surgical exploration (e.g. because of pancreatic abscessation, biliary obstruction) may benefit from a jejunostomy feeding tube, which allows enteral nutrition to occur whilst bypassing the upper gastrointestinal tract. Jejunostomy feeding tubes require advanced surgical skills and also intensive care postoperatively, as jejunal feedings are usually done via continuous infusions of liquid diets, and animals must be closely monitored for complications.

An alternative 'middle way' would be to use a nasojejunostomy tube, which does not require surgery to be placed and yet allows feeding beyond the pancreas and the least stimulation of pancreatic secretions. This technique is commonly used in human patients, but has only recently been described in a small number of dogs and would require technical skills to implement.

In most animals, at least some of the daily calorie requirements can be given enterally. However, in those in which enteral nutrition cannot be implemented (i.e. those with intractable severe vomiting) or those in which only a small proportion of the calorie intake can be delivered enterally, parenteral nutritional support (see Chapter 5) should be considered. Formulation of total parenteral nutrition (TPN) is very difficult to accomplish in practice, and so these cases are usually managed at referral institutions. Commercial ready-made parenteral nutrition (PN) solutions (with or without lipids) are an alternative that could be implemented in general practice, provided the practice is equipped to deal with the special requirement for safe administration (e.g. aseptic placement of long-term catheters, infusion pumps, intensive care monitoring). Solutions providing partial parenteral nutrition (PPN) are easier to use in practice, and can be given via a peripheral vein, but only supply 50% or less of daily calorie requirements. Once vomiting subsides, efforts should be made to introduce enteral feeding as soon as possible (e.g. an animal could receive parenteral nutrition for only 3 days).

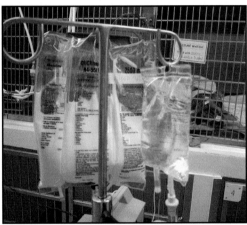

PPN solution in use in the intensive care unit. Such a solution can provide up to 50% of the calorie requirements intravenously for the patient.

Long-term feeding

It is advisable to feed this dog long term on a low-fat diet to reduce the risk of recurrence of the pancreatitis. The pork may, indeed, have been a trigger for the disease, and perhaps that is all he needs to avoid in the future. However, terriers are predisposed to acute pancreatitis, so avoiding potential future triggers seems wise. The diet should also be easily digestible. Commercial veterinary low-fat diets or low-fat over-the-counter diets are available. However, in a case such as this, where the dog refuses commercial diets, a low-fat homemade diet should be formulated. For short-term use (i.e. 2 weeks) the diet need not necessarily be complete and balanced. However, for long-term management, formulation of a complete and balanced low-fat homemade diet is advisable. This is best achieved through consultation with a veterinary nutritionist. The owner must also be carefully advised to avoid high-fat tit-bits and be made aware of what constitute high- and low-fat treats.

Nutraceuticals

There have been several studies evaluating the use of glutamine (both enterally and parenterally) in acute pancreatitis in human patients and in animal models. Whilst there have been some positive results (see Chapter 7), no trials have been done in naturally occurring pancreatitis in dogs or cats. There have also been some individual studies in humans of other specific supplements added to enteral nutrition in acute pancreatitis, including arginine, omega-3 fatty acids and probiotics, but studies are too few and too small to draw definite conclusions.

Physiotherapy

Physiotherapy is not specifically indicated for this patient, although the use of gentle massage may help with pain relief. If myofascial trigger points were identified (see Acupuncture, below) there would be some benefit in using trigger point therapy/acupressure treatment in preference to acupuncture, as this may be able to be provided by the owner following appropriate teaching.

Hydrotherapy

Hydrotherapy is not specifically indicated for this patient.

Acupuncture

A careful reduction of opiate medication may be possible if the patient responds well to acupuncture. Segmental acupuncture can be performed by needling from caudal thoracic to cranial lumbar segments – targeting multifidus muscles at these levels. Examination of the rectus abdominis muscles for myofascial trigger points (see Chapter 11) may yield a further target for treatment, along with points in the linea alba. Electroacupuncture may be necessary to effect sufficient analgesia.

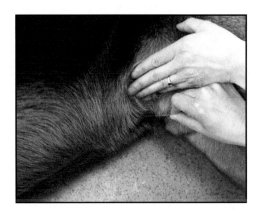

Needling the linea alba. (Courtesy of Samantha Lindley)

Other nursing and supportive care

Care in the ICU
While the dog is in the intensive care unit, he must be checked frequently (preferably at least hourly). The following should be monitored:

- Temperature, pulse rate and volume, and respiratory rate
- Pain score: preferably using an objective measure (see Chapter 2)
- Fluid rate and urine output
- Serum electrolytes (particularly potassium) and glucose
- Any signs of developing coagulopathy (e.g. petechiae).

The kennel must be kept clean of any vomit and a comfortable environment provided.

Feeding
If the dog is receiving *nil per os*, wiping his gums and mucous membranes with wet cotton wool may help him feel more comfortable.

If a feeding tube has been placed, this should be monitored carefully as the majority of complications involve tube occlusion (see Chapter 5). If microenteral or jejunostomy nutrition is indicated, food intake should be carefully monitored with the use of a fluid pump; a fresh bag and new solution should be provided every 12–24 hours to prevent bacterial or yeast growth.

On removal of the feeding tube, oral feeding can be gradually reintroduced over several days provided there is no recurrence of clinical signs. The diet should be minimally reliant on pancreatic enzymes for digestion and therefore low in fat and highly digestible (see above).

Owner advice and homecare recommendations

Avoiding recurrence
The owner should be advised that there is currently no specific 'cure' for pancreatitis and that episodes could recur, so the aim is to reduce triggers. These might include stress and high-fat diets.

- The owner should be instructed not to feed high-fat food, table-scraps or snacks.
- Suggest suitable low-fat treats that the owner can offer the dog, e.g. cooked potato, rice, pasta, small

amounts of cooked vegetables, cooked chicken *without the skin*. Things to AVOID include cheese, chicken skin and bacon.

- Reiterate the importance of reducing the dog's stress if this is triggering recurrences (see 'Fear, stress', above).

Recognizing repeat episodes

The owner should observe their pet for gastrointestinal signs (e.g. vomiting, diarrhoea) as well as cranial abdominal pain, apathy and anorexia. These signs may indicate the return of pancreatitis. The owner should be advised that pancreatitis can range from a mild, self-limiting disease to a severe and life-threatening condition and that they should contact the veterinary surgery if clinical signs persist for more than a few hours.

In the long term, a small number of dogs develop diabetes mellitus and exocrine pancreatic insufficiency as a result of chronic ongoing pancreatitis (see Case 19.4). If this dog has more than one episode of pancreatitis, it would be wise to warn his owner about these potential long-term possibilities, so that they are recognized if they occur.

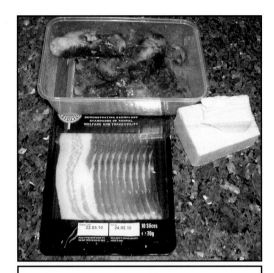

High-fat tit-bits such as sausages, bacon and cheese should be **avoided** in dogs predisposed to pancreatitis.

References

Kook PH, Kranjc A, Dennler M and Glaus TM (2009) Pancreatitis associated with clomipramine administration in a dog. *Journal of Small Animal Practice* **50**, 95–98

Meier RF and Beglinger C (2006) Nutrition in pancreatic diseases. *Best Practice in Research in Clinical Gastroenterology* **20**, 507–529

Case 19.4
Chronic pancreatitis in a dog

A 9-year-old neutered male Cocker Spaniel was presented with a history of short bouts of anorexia and vomiting, occurring about once a month and usually resolving without veterinary attention. The owners used supermarket own-brand tinned dogfood. The dog's appetite had recently increased and he produced poorly formed voluminous faeces. He was moderately overweight but was beginning to lose weight.

Blood test results were unremarkable, apart from elevated pancreatic specific lipase and repeatedly subnormal trypsin-like immunoreactivity, suggesting developing exocrine pancreatic insufficiency (EPI). Ultrasound examination showed a mass in the pancreas, and an exploratory laparotomy was therefore performed to obtain a biopsy sample to rule out neoplasia. Biopsy confirmed a diagnosis of relatively end-stage chronic pancreatitis.

The dog had also developed a mucopurulent conjunctivitis, which was diagnosed as keratoconjunctivitis sicca (KCS) on Schirmer tear testing.

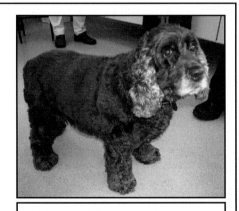

Cocker Spaniel with chronic pancreatitis.

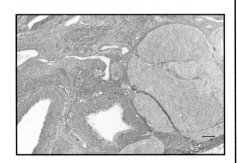

Section of pancreas showing chronic pancreatitis with marked fibrosis (stained red) surrounding sparse remaining acini. Sirrius red stain; bar = 100 μm.

The dog was placed on dietary management (see below). Pancreatic enzymes were added to each meal immediately before feeding.

Topical ciclosporin ointment was administered for the KCS. The owner was warned that diabetes mellitus might develop long term (see below).

If diarrhoea continued, a short course of metronidazole (10 mg/kg orally q12h) could be considered to control any secondary small intestinal bacterial overgrowth (common in EPI). A faecal culture and parasite examination would also be wise. It is also important to check serum cobalamin concentration and supplement parenterally if it is low.

Chronic pancreatitis in English Cocker Spaniels is believed to be an autoimmune duct-destructive disease. Therefore, steroid therapy might be indicated, although it would be more effective earlier in the course of the disease. It is important to monitor the dog's liver function carefully in the long term because, for currently unknown reasons, many Cocker Spaniels with chronic pancreatitis ultimately die of liver failure. Acute flare-ups of pancreatitis are treated symptomatically with analgesia (see below) and fluid therapy as necessary. Severe acute flare-ups are treated as in Case 19.3.

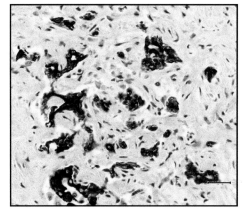

Section of pancreas from a Cocker Spaniel with chronic pancreatitis, stained immunohistochemically for cytokeratin, demonstrating duct destruction. Mouse anti-human AE1/AE2; bar = 30 μm.

Acute/chronic pain management

Chronic pancreatitis can be a very painful condition – not only during acute flare-ups but also in the long term.

Acute pain
Restricting dietary fat can have some impact on postprandial pain (see below). Supplementation of pancreatic enzymes in the food has been suggested as a method of pain control, although there is no real support for this in human or canine studies. However, in this dog, enzyme supplementation will be necessary clinically.

NSAIDs are best avoided as analgesics because of the risk of gastrointestinal ulceration and because some degree of prerenal azotaemia is common in pancreatitis. Paracetamol (± codeine) could be used for mild to moderate pancreatic pain, provided there was no evidence of liver dysfunction, and is the first drug suggested in human medicine for this condition. Tramadol could be tried if paracetamol does not work or is contraindicated, although initial vomiting/diarrhoea and dysphoria should be looked for. In at least one study in human patients (Wilder-Smith *et al.*, 1999), tramadol interfered significantly less with gastrointestinal function and was rated significantly more effective than morphine. Mild sedation from tramadol (see Chapter 3) may make assessment of this dog's condition difficult, since it may be misinterpreted as dullness due to the disease.

In more severe pain a short stint of opioids could be tried (not morphine because this would require oral dosing and bioavailability via this route is poor); pethidine is a good visceral analgesic, although short-acting; buprenorphine or methadone are alternatives. The use of opioids in pancreatitis, either acute or chronic, is no longer contraindicated since theoretical concerns about the sphincter of Oddi have been discounted. If opiates do improve the patient's wellbeing, one could try oral transmucosal buprenorphine (see Chapter 3). This is not much used in dogs as yet, and the drug is not as well absorbed as in cats, but some recent work has shown that it is absorbed so it may be worth trying. Doses of at least 30 micrograms/kg have been suggested, although this is often accompanied by excess salivation.

Analgesia in very painful acute flare-ups should be given as Case 19.3.

Chronic pain
If the dog's pain remains intractable, immunosuppressive doses of steroids might be considered since the condition is thought to be autoimmune in Cocker Spaniels, and effective suppression of the inflammation should reduce associated pain.

TENS (see Physiotherapy, below) and acupuncture (see below) may also provide pain relief.

The physiological changes associated with chronic pain are indistinguishable from those of chronic stress (since pain is a stressor) (see Chapter 3). Behaviourally, changes may include dullness, agitation, sound sensitivity, panting and trembling, and avoidance of previously accepted stimuli.

The dog may also have learnt that specific events predict a painful consequence, such as when owners pick him up or when he eats. As with any event perceived as aversive, he may have developed patterns of behaviour that successfully avoid the painful event. This may be running away when the owners approach, or showing aggression so that they do not continue to approach, or a capricious appetite (enjoying one type of food for one or two meals and then refusing to eat it). Where such responses have developed, they may continue even when pain has resolved, and may then require specific programmes of desensitization and counter-conditioning to resolve (see *BSAVA Manual of Canine and Feline Behavioural Medicine*).

Nutritional requirements

Type of diet
Dogs with chronic pancreatitis should be fed long term on a low-fat diet. High dietary fat concentrations are definitely associated with postprandial pain (and thus often sequential food aversions) and may also trigger acute recurrences of disease. Dietary fat restriction, together with analgesia, are the most important long-term management considerations in this case. Either a low-fat prescription diet formulated for gastrointestinal disease or an over-the-counter low-fat diet might be used. It is also important to advise the owner to avoid high-fat tit-bits. In many dogs with chronic pancreatitis, low-fat but high-fibre diets for weight loss are not well tolerated and can trigger abdominal pain and vomiting – probably due to gastrointestinal stretching by the fibre.

Weight management
Many dogs with chronic pancreatitis are overweight. Although the link between obesity and pancreatitis is unclear, it is wise to diet the overweight patients. A standard approach to weight management can be followed (see Chapter 6) but high-fibre weight-loss diets should be used with caution, and withdrawn if any adverse signs (e.g. postprandial pain) are noted.

Dogs developing end-stage pancreatitis, however, will develop EPI and begin to *lose* weight. They can usually be maintained well on a low-fat diet with enzyme supplementation and do not require a specific weight-loss diet or regime.

Nutraceuticals
In this patient the cause of the chronic pancreatitis is unlikely to be primary hypertriglyceridaemia. However, in those cases where it is, supplementation with concentrated omega-3 fatty acids could aid normalization of the serum lipid profile and lower the risk of recurrence of pancreatitis.

Physiotherapy

Ensuring this dog receives adequate paced activity (regular walks) will help weight control and maintain physical fitness, in addition to providing mental stimulation and distraction to influence chronic pain status positively. Through careful placement of electrodes, TENS (see Chapter 9) may provide effective pain relief through segmental innervation (see above).

Hydrotherapy

Hydrotherapy is not indicated for this patient.

Acupuncture

Acupuncture may be indicated for analgesia. Paraspinal needling of caudal thoracic and cranial lumbar segments will segmentally target the pancreas. Ventral points in cranial rectus abdominis and possibly linea alba (CV points) may give an additional effect if the patient will allow safe needling in this position. Electroacupuncture may be needed to provide sufficient analgesia (see Chapter 11).

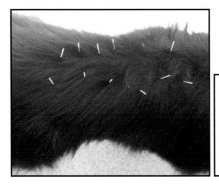

Paraspinal needling for pancreatitis pain. (Courtesy of Samantha Lindley)

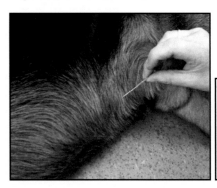

Needling the rectus abdominis muscle. (Courtesy of Samantha Lindley)

Other nursing and supportive care

Pain and condition scoring
Whenever the dog visits the surgery for assessments, his pain should be objectively scored as much as possible and recorded. This allows better monitoring of the efficacy of any dietary or analgesic treatments.

His weight should also be carefully monitored. He needs to lose weight, but is also developing EPI, which could cause him to lose *too much* weight. Careful records should also be kept of bodyweight and BCS.

Management of acute flare-ups
In-patient management of acute flare-ups of disease are as described in Case 19.3.

Owner advice and homecare recommendations

It is important to educate the owner about chronic pancreatitis and to warn them that this is a chronic, progressive disease which is usually controllable but not curable. It is rarely life-threatening (except in severe acute flare-ups) but tends to progress slowly to end stage, with the development of exocrine and endocrine insufficiency, e.g. diabetes mellitus. This dog already has EPI and the owner should be warned that he may develop diabetes in the near future. They should be warned of the signs to look out for (sudden-onset increased drinking and urinating) and to take the dog to the vet if these occur.

Pain
The potential pain associated with the condition should be explained and the owners encouraged to 'pain score' their pet to allow them to assess the efficacy of analgesics and dietary manipulations. Owners will often be more aware of how much pain the dog *was* in after the pain has been reduced with a low-fat diet and analgesia: he may for example be more playful and stop stretching after meals, indicating a significant reduction in postprandial pain that was previously not recognized.

Chronic pancreatitis is common in people and some owners may have personal or close family experience of the disease, showing great concern about the amount of pain their dog may be suffering, and sometimes even requesting euthanasia for that reason. These owners should be reassured that the dog's pain is being addressed and treated – in most cases very effectively.

Dietary advice
The owners should be given careful advice about long-term feeding of a low-fat diet (see above). In particular, if owners are looking to buy an 'over-the-counter' low-fat diet, they should be educated about reading petfood labels and working out the dietary fat concentration. As a rough guide, they should aim for a diet with <10% DM dietary fat. They should be shown how to convert fat concentration on a canned food label from total (moist matter) fat to dry matter (DM) fat to allow meaningful comparisons.

Percentage oil 'as fed' = Fat = x %

Total moisture content = y %

Then, fat content (dry matter) = $(x / 100 - y) \times 100$ %

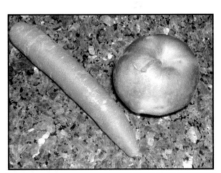

Carrots and apples can be used as low-fat tit-bits.

Alternatively, the veterinary surgeon could give suggestions of appropriate 'over-the-counter' low-fat tinned or dried foods that are known to them – to save the owner all the calculations.

Owners should be carefully advised about avoiding high-fat tit-bits and on what is, and isn't, a high-fat food. For example, owners often do not perceive cheese, chicken skin or meat gravy as being high in fat. It should be stressed that feeding these could trigger a potentially serious bout of disease.

Finally, in discussions of diets, it may help to identify and explain previous food aversions shown by the dog as a result of postprandial pain. It is not uncommon for dogs with chronic pancreatitis to have a very 'picky' appetite. The owners may feed more and more expensive (high-fat) foil-packed diets in an attempt to get the dog to eat, only to find the dog eats one meal of that diet and then refuses it. This often seems to be due to a food aversion as a result of postprandial pain, because such dogs will often willingly eat an apparently 'unappetizing' low-fat diet enthusiastically and repeatedly. Owners of these dogs often fear that their dog will not eat that 'cheap diet' – but they should be encouraged to at least try it as they may be pleasantly surprised.

References

Wilder-Smith CH, Hill L, Osler W and O'Keefe S (1999) Effect of tramadol and morphine on pain and gastrointestinal motor function in patients with chronic pancreatitis. *Digestive Disease Science* **44**, 1107–1116

Case 19.5
'Triaditis' in a cat

A 10-year-old neutered male DSH cat was presented with diabetes mellitus (DM) that was difficult to control.

The cat had 'triaditis' (pancreatitis + inflammatory bowel disease + chronic cholangitis), which had been diagnosed by pancreatic, liver and small intestinal biopsy 4 years earlier. He was managed with a short course of steroid therapy and had been on dietary management since then.

Diabetes was diagnosed 6 months ago and had been difficult to control because the cat intermittently went off his food, making the owner worry about how much insulin to give him. The cat was thin and losing weight. He was fed a variety of types and amounts of food to try to make him eat, but there was no consistent plan. The cat has access to outdoors and is a hunter. As he does not use a litter tray, the owner cannot monitor urine glucose concentrations.

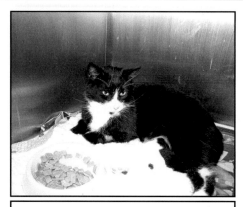

DSH cat with triaditis, refusing the food offered.

Agreed medical/surgical management

Stabilizing the diabetes mellitus

The cat will probably need hospitalizing for a few days to try to institute the best plan for stabilizing his DM and preventing further weight loss. A 24-hour glucose curve and fructosamine measurement will give some idea of the efficacy of the current dose of insulin. Biochemistry and haematology screens, a urine sample (preferably with culture of a cystocentesis sample) and abdominal ultrasonography will give baseline information about his current health status and any concurrent diseases that may be causing insulin resistance. The aim is to achieve a long-term 'stable' diabetic regime (as outlined below) and then adjust the regime on a temporary basis when the underlying diseases flare up.

A suitable diabetic regime which might be instituted for this patient consists of:

- Twice-daily subcutaneous Lente insulin, with the dose adjusted carefully to individual requirements
- Feeding the same amount of food every day (either meal-fed or *ad libitum*)
- Selecting and feeding an appropriate diet for a thin diabetic cat, with which both the owner and cat will be happy (see below)
- Ruling out and treating any concurrent diseases: not just the triaditis (see below) but also any urinary tract or other endocrine disease; in an older cat, ruling out hyperthyroidism and acromegaly are particularly important (see *BSAVA Manual of Canine and Feline Endocrinology*).

Specific considerations for diabetic management with triaditis

- Recurrent pancreatitis and cholangitis will certainly lead to periods of diabetic instability. These can be accepted as long as the cat is stable in between episodes. Acute flare-ups of the pancreas and liver diseases should be treated symptomatically, and insulin treatment adjusted temporarily as necessary (e.g. if the cat misses a meal, usually only a half dose of insulin is given).
- IBD is less likely than the pancreatitis or cholangitis to cause acute changes in insulin requirements, but is still a consideration: steroid treatment for the IBD is very debatable given the DM. It might be possible to manage this cat's IBD with diet alone. Failing that, an alternative drug such as chlorambucil might be considered. If steroids are used, the dose should be kept stable long term so that the insulin dose can be adjusted and also kept stable.
- This cat's weight loss and poor coat strongly suggest the development of exocrine pancreatic insufficiency (EPI) as a result of chronic pancreatitis. This could be confirmed by measuring serum feline trypsin-like immunoreactivity (TLI), although TLI may be in the normal range if it is concurrently being elevated by a bout of pancreatitis. Trial supplementation of the food with pancreatic enzymes might be worthwhile, even if TLI is normal. However, it should also be noted that insulin dose will probably have to be increased when enzymes are added to the food.
- Hyperthyroidism would be the other important differential for poor coat and weight loss.

Acute/chronic pain management

Analgesia for pancreatitis

This cat has confirmed chronic pancreatitis, which is known to be a very painful condition in people. Cats with even severe pain do not often display the signs that their owners or even the veterinary team expect. The response of most cats to pain is to 'do nothing' and withdraw, so it should be remembered that a quiet cat is not necessarily a happy cat and these patients MUST be given the benefit of the doubt that their pain is significant. Certainly, during episodes of anorexia, it is likely that the cat has significant epigastric pain.

NSAIDs are contraindicated because of the potential to cause gastrointestinal ulceration and also the high prevalence of prerenal azotaemia in pancreatitis. The most practical analgesic to use in this patient might be

oral transmucosal buprenorphine (20–30 micrograms/kg q8–12h) which can be dispensed for home use by the owner.

If the cat is hospitalized and in pain, the options are not straightforward: lidocaine CRI is likely to be contraindicated in cats because of toxicity and cardiovascular effects; ketamine CRI would be safe and may be worth trying, but there is no evidence of efficacy for visceral pain; dexmedetomidine CRI is likely to reduce splanchnic blood flow and is therefore also likely to be contraindicated. Opiates are thus the best option in the hospitalized cat.

Amitriptyline (5 mg at night) appears to be useful for visceral pain in cats, but can be difficult to administer because it is so bitter. It requires competent renal and hepatic function, so may be contraindicated if the cholangitis becomes obstructive.

TENS (see Physiotherapy, below) and acupuncture (see below) may also provide pain relief.

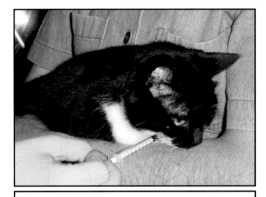

Administering oral transmucosal buprenorphine. (Courtesy of Polly Taylor)

Fear, stress, conflict concerns

Since exposure to stressors can precipitate bouts of IBD and also complicate diabetes control, it is important that this cat has as few stressors as possible in his life; as he has quite enough clinical stressors, he can do without any environmentally, or must at least be able to deal with them if they occur. Reducing stress is best achieved by making his life as predictable and controllable as possible. In other words, any changes in routine should be gradual, and any potential stressors identified and minimized. Optimizing core territory would be ideal; as the owner already has quite a lot to deal with in managing this cat, these measures could be introduced gradually and form part of the ongoing information given by the practice team to the client.

- **Food.** The cat must be able to reach food easily; if he has previously fed at a height he may not feel like jumping, so adjust the position of the food, whilst making sure this does not make him anxious about it being available to competitors (e.g. the pet dog or a possible intruding cat if the food is placed near the cat flap).
- **Water.** Cats generally prefer their water about a room's distance away from their food in a clear, wide bowl.
- **Access inside and out.** Cats normally have more than one access point into and out of their core territory (usually the house). Consider providing an additional access point, or ensure that he can use the existing access points (they are not too high or too difficult to negotiate when he feels unwell and uncomfortable).
- **Scratching posts.** Are these easily accessible and appropriate? A horizontal scratch post can be provided, so that the cat can still reach it if he does not feel up to climbing.

Nutritional requirements

Preventing hepatic lipidosis

Cats with concurrent diabetes mellitus and other liver diseases are at increased risk of developing hepatic lipidosis, even if they are thin to start with. For this reason, it is particularly important to ensure that this cat does not go off his food for more than 1 or 2 days whenever he has an episode of 'triaditis'. If attempted dietary changes to treat the condition result in anorexia, he should be rapidly put back on to a diet he accepts.

While the cat is in the hospital, his daily food intake should be carefully measured. If he fails to eat his resting energy requirement (RER; see Chapter 5) for more than 3 days, some form of tube feeding should be instituted. Appetite stimulants are unlikely to be effective, since anorexia is due to

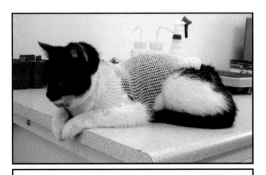

If there is prolonged anorexia and development of hepatic lipidosis, gastrostomy tube feeding would be appropriate. The feeding tube is covered with a body bandage.

gastrointestinal discomfort; furthermore, many are contraindicated in liver disease (see Chapter 5). In this case, naso-oesophageal or oesophagostomy tube feeding would be most appropriate, since the need for assisted feeding is likely to be temporary – while the inflammatory disease subsides. If the cat has a prolonged bout of anorexia and is developing hepatic lipidosis, some form of gastrostomy tube feeding would be necessary.

Choice of diet

In cases where the patient has a number of medical problems, many of which could respond to different nutritional approaches, it may be useful to prioritize the medical problems that could respond to dietary changes:

1. Diabetes mellitus
2. Liver disease
3. IBD and pancreatitis.

Dietary considerations for diabetes

Consistent and reliable food intake is a priority in all diabetic patients. This can be challenging to achieve in cats that have access to outdoors and that have a varying appetite and a varied diet. It would be preferable to identify one diet to be consumed by the cat reliably, rather than focusing on a particular diet profile or composition. The same measured amount of a manufactured diet should be fed every day. Meal feeding in time with insulin injections is less important in diabetic cats than in diabetic dogs because cats have constant gluconeogenesis, even in the postprandial phase, which smoothes out any postprandial glucose peaks. They can therefore be fed *ad libitum*, if this is preferred, provided that they consume the same TOTAL calorie intake daily.

Other considerations include manipulating protein content. In recent studies (e.g. Frank *et al.*, 2001) diets high in protein and low in carbohydrate have been demonstrated to reduce insulin requirements and even to revert some diabetic cats to a non-diabetic state. However, this manipulation is more effective in overweight diabetic cats (with presumed type II DM) than in thin diabetic cats, such as this case, with presumed insulin-deficient DM. High-protein diets are also quite palatable; this could increase reliable food intake and aid in preserving lean body mass.

Dietary considerations for the liver

High-protein diets are NOT contraindicated with this cat's liver disease. Protein restriction is only a consideration in parenchymal liver disease, where there is a significant effect on liver function. This cat has biliary tract disease, which typically does not affect liver function. The only consideration with biliary tract disease is to limit the fat content of the diet (as the associated biliary stasis may reduce fat emulsification).

Dietary considerations for IBD and pancreatitis

High protein could aggravate IBD, as the increase in protein antigens could further stimulate the immune response. If the nature of this cat's IBD is related to food intolerance, it would be possible to identify a novel protein source that could be used to control the IBD. The fact that this cat hunts would make this approach extremely difficult – the cat may be allergic to mice and may also eat the neighbour's cat's food!

Dietary fat is another potentially important factor. Although pancreatitis in cats is not usually related to dietary fat content, the suspicion of EPI may make fat assimilation an issue. However, dietary fat will probably not need restricting in this case because supplementation with pancreatic enzymes will improve digestion and fat absorption.

Manufactured or homemade diet?

It is almost always best to use a manufactured rather than a homemade diet, not only because of the strict nutrient requirements of cats (see Chapter 5) but also because it is very difficult to keep the calorie content of a homemade diet stable from day to day. In a few cases, it may be necessary to formulate a complete and balanced homemade diet, if the cat will not reliably eat a suitable manufactured diet. The homemade diet in this case would ideally fulfil the following requirements: high protein using a novel protein source; moderate to low fat content; and choosing ingredients that the cat would accept reliably. In order to formulate such a diet, a veterinary nutritionist should be consulted. Great care would need to be taken to avoid nutrient deficiencies and to ensure a consistent calorie content from day to day.

Vitamin requirements

It may be necessary to supplement fat-soluble vitamins in this case because the cat has three conditions which can cause fat maldigestion and thus reduce absorption of fat-soluble vitamins: cholangitis; chronic pancreatitis (and probable EPI); and IBD. Vitamin E can be supplemented safely without monitoring. Vitamin K should be supplemented if the cat has prolonged coagulation times. Vitamin D supplementation may be necessary if he has a measured low ionized calcium concentration.

Water-soluble B vitamins will also be lost in increased amounts in the polydipsia/polyuria associated with DM, and so should be supplemented. Serum vitamin B12 should be specifically measured in this patient: it is very likely to be low if he has EPI because in cats the pancreas is the only source of intrinsic factor required to absorb vitamin B12 in the ileum. If serum B12 is low, it should be supplemented by injection.

Nutraceuticals

Chromium picolinate was previously thought to increase insulin sensitivity; dietary supplementation of this micronutrient was therefore considered potentially beneficial for diabetics. Results for improvement in diabetic management have not been positive, however, and therefore this is no longer thought to be an important component of therapy.

Antioxidant supplementation could potentially be beneficial in liver diseases associated with biliary stasis, such as cholangitis, because refluxed bile is a potent oxidant toxin in the liver. In addition to vitamin E supplementation, there is a logical reason to supplement S-adenosylmethionine and silibilin in this patient, although there is a paucity of clinical studies documenting their use in cats with cholangitis.

Physiotherapy

Through careful placement of electrodes, TENS (see Chapter 9) may provide effective pain relief through segmental innervation, but this depends on the settings used and requires adequate compliance from the patient.

Hydrotherapy

Hydrotherapy is not specifically indicated for this patient.

Acupuncture

The pain of chronic pancreatitis may be alleviated by acupuncture (but see considerations below). Needling along caudal thoracic and cranial lumber segments into the multifidus muscles will segmentally target afferent nerves from the pancreas (see Chapter 11). Ventral points in the rectus abdominal muscle may complement the effect but may be difficult to treat practically. Care should be taken to avoid needling into the abdominal cavity if ventral points are used.

Acupuncture has been anecdotally reported to stimulate appetite in a variety of species, including the cat. However, if this cat's lack of appetite is due to gastrointestinal pain, as it is likely to be, encouraging him to eat may be less helpful. It has also been reported, anecdotally, that acupuncture can alter insulin requirements (in humans), so this might temporarily confuse the picture further (it is a transient effect).

Other nursing and supportive care

Monitoring and routine

While in the hospital, the cat's food intake and daily water intake should be carefully monitored and recorded. He should also be regularly assessed for pain.

The cat should have a consistent routine in the hospital of feeding and insulin treatment, which should mimic its home routine as much as possible. Stress should be avoided as much as possible, as this will affect both insulin requirements and blood glucose measurements.

Monitoring diabetic control

Blood for glucose curves should be taken with as little stress as possible as cats are very susceptible to stress hyperglycaemia, which would render a glucose curve uninterpretable. In a referral setting, it might be possible to measure continuous interstitial blood glucose concentration less stressfully (Ristic et al., 2005), but this requires expensive equipment. A more practical solution might be to get the cat used to ear-pricks for sampling. This also has the advantage that, if the cat tolerates it, it can be used for home monitoring as well (see below). If frequent venous blood samples are being taken for glucose measurement, care must be taken not to over-bleed the cat and significantly deplete its circulating fluid volume!

While the cat is in the hospital, urine glucose and ketone concentrations can also be monitored if the cat can be encouraged to use a litter tray with non-absorbable litter. This

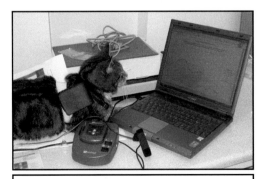

Continuous monitoring of interstitial blood glucose concentrations in a diabetic cat. (Courtesy of Michael Herrtage and Lucy Davison)

might be transferred to the home setting if the owner is willing, although this cat has not used a litter tray at home before so it may not start now.

Care of feeding tubes

If a feeding tube has been placed, this should be monitored carefully as the majority of complications involve tube occlusion. See Chapter 5 for details of feeding and tube care.

Owner advice and homecare recommendations

Diabetes management and control

The owners will need to be given detailed information and advice about management of this challenging case at home. The presence of complicating diseases which are likely to affect the cat's appetite and diabetic control in a rather unpredictable manner means that he is going to be more difficult to treat than the straightforward diabetic case, so the owners will need to be committed. Nevertheless, cases like this can do very well in the long term provided the owner and veterinary team are committed and can work together. It is helpful if one veterinary surgeon in the practice is responsible for most communications with the owner, as they will be up to speed with the cat's history and requirements.

The dietary and treatment advice outlined above should be carefully explained. In this case, the cat is already on insulin therapy so it is assumed that this has already been explained to the owner. However, in a newly diagnosed diabetic cat, it would also be important carefully to demonstrate correct storage, mixing, measuring and administration of insulin.

The amount of home-monitoring of this cat's diabetes that is possible or undertaken will depend on his temperament and the owner's and vet's preferences. Monitoring this cat with urine glucose measurements may not be practical, as he does not use a litter tray and goes outdoors. It is perfectly possible to home-monitor blood glucose concentrations in many cats using appropriate equipment. The owner should regularly contact the veterinary surgery with the results and should be advised not to alter insulin doses without veterinary advice. This is particularly important where diabetic instability is to be expected; too-frequent changes in insulin dose in response to temporary changes in requirements due to the underlying diseases are to be avoided. However, where an owner does not wish to monitor a cat at home, reasonable stability can be achieved with intermittent monitoring at the practice using blood fructosamine concentrations. Tight control of blood glucose is ideal, because cats have been shown to suffer from some degree of hyperglycaemia-induced islet cell damage.

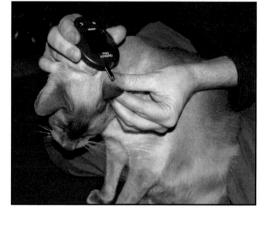

Blood glucose can be monitored at home relatively easily.
(Courtesy of Danièlle Gunn-Moore)

Feeding

- The owner should be given careful advice about feeding (see above).
- They should also be warned that the cat is very likely to go off his food occasionally because of the underlying cholangitis and pancreatitis but not to worry unduly about this.
- They should be advised not to worry if the cat misses one meal but otherwise appears bright.
  o They should still administer insulin, but half of the usual dose.
  o It is also wise to leave food down for the cat in case he becomes hypoglycaemic, as this should drive him to eat.
- If the cat misses more than one meal, or is unwell or vomiting, the owners should contact the veterinary surgery immediately.

References

Frank G, Anderson W, Pazak H *et al.* (2001) Use of a high-protein diet in the management of feline diabetes mellitus. *Veterinary Therapeutics* **2**, 238–246
Ristic JM, Herrtage ME, Walti-Lauger SM *et al.* (2005) Evaluation of a continuous glucose monitoring system in cats with diabetes mellitus. *Journal of Feline Medicine and Surgery* **7**, 153–162

Case 19.6
Chronic hepatitis in a dog

A 9-year-old spayed female Labrador Retriever was presented for investigation of gradual weight loss. She had previously been overweight.

Significantly elevated liver enzymes were found on a biochemical blood screen and the liver appeared rather small and diffusely hyperechoic on ultrasound examination. Coagulation times and platelet counts were normal. Liver biopsy confirmed chronic hepatitis of unknown aetiology. Staining for copper showed no evidence of copper storage disease.

The dog also had degenerative joint disease (DJD) in the hips and elbows; without adequate analgesia she refused to walk and became very stiff.

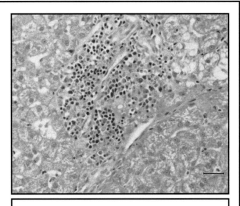

Liver section from a dog with chronic hepatitis, showing a multifocal lymphocytic infiltrate and some early fibrosis. H&E; bar = 30 μm.

Agreed medical/surgical management

Treatment for chronic hepatitis in dogs is challenging when the cause is unknown, and remains symptomatic. Some Labrador Retrievers suffer from a form of copper storage disease, and in these cases, copper chelation and a low-copper diet would be indicated. However, in this dog the cause is unknown. Some cases may be autoimmune. Others may be caused by infectious disease; there is a suspicion that an unidentified virus may cause at least some cases of idiopathic canine chronic hepatitis. It is therefore hard to know whether to use steroid therapy or not. In a patient such as this, with a lymphocytic infiltrate and only early fibrosis and no evidence yet of portal hypertension or ascites, a course of steroid therapy might be tried, with careful monitoring of clinical response and hepatocellular enzymes to assess response to treatment.

Other therapy is non-specific and supportive but nonetheless helpful: the dog should be fed a high-quality appropriate diet (see below); and therapy with antioxidants (see below) and ursodeoxycholic acid could be considered. Ursodeoxycholic acid may act synergistically with antioxidants but has some anti-inflammatory and antioxidant activity itself, which means that it may be indicated in any chronic hepatitis. However, there is very little firm evidence base for the efficacy of any treatments in canine chronic hepatitis.

The other major problem in this patient is finding an appropriate safe treatment for her degenerative joint disease in the face of liver disease (see below).

Acute/chronic pain management

Liver biopsy
Preoperative pethidine is useful for liver biopsy (especially if anaesthesia is not used, when it may reduce panting and improve the clarity of imaging). If analgesia is required postoperatively, buprenorphine would be appropriate.

Degenerative joint disease
This dog needs analgesia to maintain a good quality of life. NSAIDs should be avoided unless there is no alternative. Liver disease is a contraindication to their use and serious hepatotoxicity has been reported with some NSAIDs in dogs (MacPhail *et al.*, 1998). In the absence of NSAID use, tramadol will usually help with the affective (suffering) component of the pain. The patient should be monitored for dullness, dysphoria and vomiting. If hyperalgesia and/or allodynia are present (see Chapter 3), gabapentin may be considered daily in divided doses. Gabapentin is partially metabolized through the liver in dogs, so it may be better avoided in this patient. Continued weight loss should help the dog to cope with her joint problems and the owners should be given a target weight.

Nutraceuticals (see below) might also be used long term to help treat joint pain. Acupuncture (see below) would be indicated, and heat, massage, cold therapy and electrotherapy may also be valuable (see Physiotherapy, below).

If pain relief is not achieved by any other means, NSAIDs may still be worth considering as long as the owner is fully informed of the risks and whilst monitoring the patient very carefully.

Fear, stress, conflict concerns

Pain and anxiety are inextricably linked (see Chapter 3). Pain can also give rise to conflict and understimulation because the patient may want to exercise more than her condition allows (see Chapter 4). Finding alternative ways of delivering food can be helpful; for example, feeding the food ration in divided portions, with two at specific mealtimes as usual and then random delivery of food balls; using 'hide and seek' or finding dry food in a box of shredded paper (so long as the dog does not decide to eat the paper too); training exercises and fun games, which involve finding food. Such measures will also help to take her mind off her pain. Exercise should be moderate, frequent and interesting – meeting other people and dogs, if she enjoys that. Comfort in terms of her bed and travelling in the car should also be addressed (see Case 14.8).

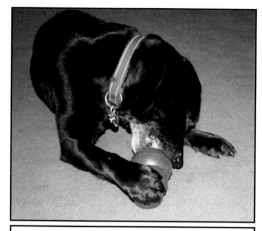

Hiding dried food in a toy can help increase stimulation in a dog with restricted exercise. (© Helen Zulch)

Nutritional requirements

Nutrition for chronic hepatitis

Nutritional modulation of chronic hepatitis entails consideration of several factors. Dogs with chronic hepatitis can be in a catabolic state, which may explain the recent weight loss noted in this patient. Energy density of the diet, as well as palatability, should be factored into the nutritional plan. The dog should be fed a digestible high-quality diet, little and often – the latter because it reduces the work required by the liver at each meal. A diet formulated for gastrointestinal or liver disease would be suitable, although care must be taken not to restrict protein unless necessary, because dogs with chronic hepatitis are at risk of going into negative nitrogen balance with protein restriction.

Another consideration includes whether the dog is demonstrating, or is at risk of developing, hepatic encephalopathy (HE). This case is unlikely to have acquired portosystemic shunts and HE yet, but may develop them later on. At that point, mild protein restriction might be considered, although the focus is moving away from this towards other means of controlling HE. Protein restriction is required only if signs of HE cannot be controlled with medical management (i.e. antibiotics, lactulose, feeding little and often). The reason to reserve protein restriction for cases where HE is present is because inappropriate or excessive protein restriction can exacerbate endogenous protein catabolism and worsen signs of HE. In addition, much of the ammonia in the portal blood comes from small intestinal enterocyte metabolism, which is unavoidable. Both the digestibility and source of protein may be important in the likelihood of precipitating an HE crisis. Animal-based proteins are typically highly digestible, but non-animal protein sources such as soya may be better tolerated in dogs with HE.

Dietary fibre may have a beneficial effect in dogs with chronic hepatitis. Zinc supplementation has also been recommended. Some Labrador Retrievers and other breeds have chronic hepatitis associated with copper build-up in the liver, and in these cases it is important to feed a copper-restricted diet. However, this is not necessary for this patient. More details on dietary management of liver disease are given in Chapter 5.

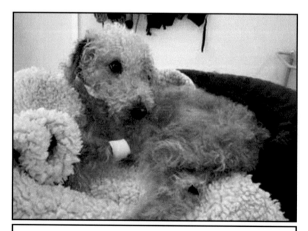

Copper storage disease is well known in Bedlington Terriers.

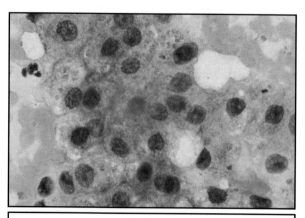

Copper granules are visible in the hepatocytes. Giemsa; original magnification x1000. (Courtesy of Elizabeth Villiers)

Nutraceuticals for liver disease

Several nutraceuticals are often used in canine chronic hepatitis. Veterinary studies have documented reduced hepatic glutathione concentrations in dogs and cats with liver disease, suggesting a possible role for glutathione precursors such as *S*-adenosylmethionine (Center *et al.*, 2002). Silymarin (family of active ingredients from milk thistle) is also often used and has been shown to be protective in acute *Amanita* mushroom toxicity in dogs (Vogel *et al.*, 1984). There is some evidence also for the efficacy of Vitamin E in chronic hepatitis (Twedt *et al.*, 2003).

Nutraceuticals for DJD

Nutraceutical agents proposed for joint disease include chrondroitin sulphate and glucosamine. However, there are limited data supporting their use (see Chapter 7). Other more recent strategies include the supplementation of omega-3 fatty acids, which may reduce joint inflammation and thus reduce requirements for non-steroidal therapy. Further work is required to confirm the benefits of omega-3 fatty acid supplementation in dogs with osteoarthritis. Nutraceuticals can either be supplemented separately or formulated within a diet designed for joint disease. In this case, because of the need to avoid NSAIDs, it would certainly be worth trying nutraceuticals as part of the programme of pain management for the joints.

Weight management

Usually, in an overweight dog, a careful weight-loss programme is an important part of controlling the pain associated with the DJD. However, in this patient, the liver disease itself is causing weight loss and so such a programme will not be necessary – or wise. An appropriate diet to support the liver takes priority.

Physiotherapy

The main physiotherapy involvement would be in respect of DJD in the hips and elbows. The use of heat, massage, passive movements and stretches can be beneficial in improving comfort and mobility (especially in the mornings and prior to exercise). The use of cold therapy after walks is also useful to control pain and any localized inflammation/swelling caused through exercise.

DJD is progressively detrimental to an animal's strength, joint and muscle range, balance, proprioception, joint stability and stamina. To counter these effects an appropriate exercise programme should be provided to the owners, which is low impact and addresses all of these elements. Hydrotherapy can be a particularly useful component of this programme (see below). All exercises (including walking) should be paced (within the tolerance of the patient) yet provided regularly (little and often), and this approach should be continued throughout the dog's life. All activities should be markedly reduced during 'flare-ups' of the DJD, and steadily returned to normal as the 'flare-up' subsides. If the DJD remains under control, the exercise programme should be gradually progressed.

Other interventions that can be beneficial for patients with DJD are those provided by the veterinary physiotherapist, and include joint mobilizations (to improve joint range and reduce pain), soft issue techniques (such as myofascial release and trigger pointing) and electrotherapy (TENS, laser) for pain relief, and NMES for weakened muscles (see Chapter 9).

Hydrotherapy

Hydrotherapy, using swimming or an underwater treadmill, may help with joint pain and mobility (see Chapter 11). Sessions should be short, as there is an underlying medical condition, possibly reduced cardiovascular fitness, and the dog is already stiff and refusing to walk. Someone will need to be in the pool to help and reassure the dog. The owners will need to be closely involved to give updates of progress in between each session to make sure it is helping. An underwater treadmill may be easier for the dog initially as it is less strenuous.

Acupuncture

Acupuncture is indicated in DJD (see Case 14.8). It is not, as far as is understood, anti-inflammatory but can be a potent analgesic, depending on the sensitivity of the patient to the stimulus. Local (segmental) needling appears to be most effective (see Chapter 11). Acupuncture must be used with caution if there are bleeding disorders or coagulopathies, especially in the closed fascial compartments of the lower limb (small risk of compartment syndrome).

Other nursing and supportive care

This dog will be hospitalized for a short time for the liver biopsy. Whatever sampling method is used (laparotomy, laparoscopy or ultrasound-guided biopsy), it is important to assess coagulation times and platelet counts *first*. If coagulation times are prolonged, vitamin K injections for 24 hours may help, or fresh frozen plasma may need to be given.

It is important to hospitalize the dog for 12–24 hours *after* the liver biopsy:

- Monitor closely for any signs of haemorrhage from the biopsy site
- Check the dog's pulse rate and volume, and mucous membrane colour at least hourly for 12 hours
- If there are signs of developing hypovolaemia, an emergency laparotomy may be required to stop the bleeding. This is unusual but occasionally occurs
- Monitoring PCV is *not* an effective way of looking for acute bleeding as, initially, the PCV does not change.

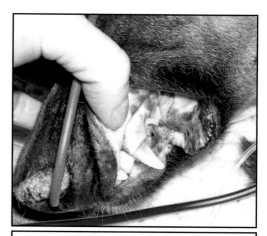

The sudden development of very pale mucous membranes should trigger an emergency laparotomy to stop bleeding from the biopsy site.

Owner advice and homecare recommendations

Advice on long-term management of dogs with DJD is detailed in Case 14.8.

Understanding and managing chronic hepatitis

The pathophysiology and prognosis of the chronic hepatitis should be carefully explained to the owner. Many people have some experience of either viral or alcoholic hepatitis in their own family and therefore it should be carefully explained that there is no evidence of human–dog transmission of a hepatitis virus. Owners should understand that in most cases the cause of the disease is not known and that it is therefore likely to progress to end-stage disease and cirrhosis; i.e. the dog is likely eventually to die of its disease (and there is no option for liver transplantation in dogs). However, in many dogs, this takes months to years and meanwhile, with careful management, they can maintain a good quality of life. The treatment and dietary advice given is designed to support the liver for as long as possible.

The owner should be advised of the signs they might see if the liver disease progresses, and to contact the surgery if any of these occur:

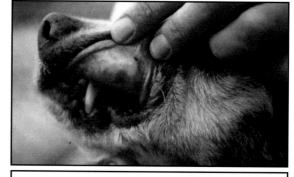

Jaundiced mucous membranes. (Courtesy of Michael Herrtage)

- Anorexia, vomiting or diarrhoea, sometimes with blood
- Abdominal swelling associated with ascites
- Jaundiced mucous membranes.

Follow-up and prognosis

Regular re-checks should be arranged, to assess both liver enzymes and the DJD. The owner should be encouraged to ring the practice if they are worried about the dog, and preferably to talk to the same members of the team each time who know her history.

References

Center SA, Warner KL and Erb HN (2002) Liver glutathione concentrations in dogs and cats with naturally occurring liver disease. *American Journal of Veterinary Research* **63**, 1187–1197

MacPhail CM, Lappin MR, Meyer DJ *et al.* (1998) Hepatocellular toxicosis associated with administration of carprofen in 21 dogs. *Journal of the American Veterinary Medical Association* **212**, 1895–1901

Twedt DC, Webb CB and Tetrick (2003) The effect of dietary vitamin E on the clinical laboratory and oxidant status of dogs with chronic hepatitis. *Journal of Veterinary Internal Medicine* **17**, 403 [abstract]

Vogel G, Tuchweber B, Trost W and Mengs U (1984) Protection by silibinin against *Amanita phalloides* intoxication in beagles. *Toxicology and Applied Pharmacology.* **73**, 355–362

20

Patients with oral or dental disease

Edited by Peter Southerden

Introduction

A wide range of problems affect the oral cavity, involving – either individually or in combination – the teeth, soft tissues and bone. Such problems include infections (e.g. periodontal disease, caries, osteomyelitis), trauma (fractures to teeth or bone, injury to soft tissues), neoplasia, congenital and developmental abnormalities (e.g. cleft palate, malocclusions) and a variety of immune-mediated and ulcerative conditions.

The problems that these create for the patient include:

- Pain:
  o This may be present all the time, or only when the patient tries to eat, swallow, engage in play and/or groom itself
  o Pain and odd sensations may lead to behavioural changes, including fear, aggression and bizarre behaviours such as backing away from familiar objects (not only the food bowl)
  o Pain and altered sensation may lead to self-mutilation through pawing or scratching at the face or through excessive rubbing
- Compromised nutrition:
  o The patient may pick out only those foods that it can eat easily, or which are appealing enough to overcome the anticipation of oral discomfort
  o Owners may feed more treats or tit-bits to tempt their pet
- Excessive salivation: this can potentially lead to lipfold dermatitis.

The problems for the owner include:

- Concern about pain, although pain is not always obvious
- Concern about the change in eating habits, with a consequent alteration in what they choose to feed their pet
- Concern about changes in behaviour that will often not be obviously related to mouth or teeth problems
- Concern about the smell from the pet's mouth
- Concern about saliva staining around the mouth and on the forelimbs.

The oral cavity

Specific factors relating to the anatomy, environment and function of the oral cavity have a direct impact on rehabilitation following surgery or disease and on palliative care. The anatomy of the oral cavity is complex. The relationship between hard and soft tissue is unique: the periodontium is a highly specialized structure responsible for maintaining teeth within maxillary and mandibular bone, and is vulnerable to the impact of the diverse bacterial population found in plaque. The mouth is an open ecosystem where bacteria are always present. Plaque bacteria exist in a biofilm within which they are more than 1000 times less sensitive to antimicrobials than are free-floating (planktonic) bacteria (Wolf, 2005). The healthy oral cavity is bathed in saliva; this is immunologically important, aids in mastication and maintains the integrity of the teeth.

The oral cavity has numerous functions:

- Oral competence is the ability to hold food and saliva in the mouth without drooling
- Chewing, swallowing and digestion:
  o The specialized lining of the mouth and the salivary glands provide lubrication that aids swallowing and the digestion of food
  o Chewing is also important for digestion
  o The oral cavity helps in swallowing, as the tongue and the mouth push the food towards the oesophagus
- Behaviour:
  o The ability to prehend and hold objects is important in working dogs and during play in pet dogs
  o Normal vocalization and social interaction is also, in part, dependent on a healthy oral cavity.

Surgical principles

Many conditions of the oral cavity can be treated specifically, often surgically. In these cases rehabilitation relies on excellent perioperative analgesia, a good surgical technique, and nursing skills to encourage a quick return to normal oral function.

Perioperative analgesia

Surgical manipulation of tissues within the oral cavity results in a greatly enhanced nociceptor response (peripheral sensitization and 'wind-up') to any additional perioperative stimulation (Beckman, 2006). Central sensitization may occur if this peripheral sensitization remains untreated. Pre-emptive analgesia in the immediate preoperative period avoids peripheral sensitization and limits subsequent wind-up (see

Chapters 2 and 3). The use of multimodal pain management, using a combination of opiates, non-steroidal anti-inflammatory drugs (NSAIDs), alpha-2 agonists and NMDA (*N*-methyl-D-aspartate) receptor antagonists, is appropriate for oral surgery. However, local and regional anaesthesia are more easily delivered to the oral cavity than to many other areas and are highly effective; they should therefore form a central part of the pain control strategy for oral surgical procedures.

Local anaesthetic techniques aim to produce complete analgesia in the target area by inhibiting transduction, transmission and modulation of stimuli along the nociceptive pathway. This may allow a lighter plane of anaesthesia to be achieved and a consequent reduction in the complications associated with general anaesthesia. Lidocaine has a rapid onset but a short duration of action (1–2 hours), whereas bupivacaine has a relatively slow onset of action but much longer duration (up to 8 hours). Combining the two agents can overcome their individual limitations, producing a rapid onset and an extended duration of effect. The longer duration of action of bupivacaine can contribute towards analgesia in the immediate postoperative period, when the patient may not be able to demonstrate the normal behavioural changes indicative of pain.

Self-traumatization of the tongue by chewing during the immediate postoperative period is a theoretical concern following a mandibular alveolar nerve block as this may anaesthetize the glossopharyngeal nerve that has a sensory function in the tongue. Such traumatization can be limited through careful observation and by allowing recovery in sternal recumbency, thus reducing deviation of the tongue to one side.

Technique and potential complications

Hypothermia during anaesthesia has a major impact on postoperative recovery and is a major concern during many dental surgical procedures, especially those involving the use of water-cooled high-speed dental burs, which expose patients to copious cold water oral lavage. The oral cavity is highly vascular and forms part of the thermoregulatory apparatus, hence the increased susceptibility to hypothermia after dental procedures. Complications of hypothermia can include hypoxaemia, hypovolaemia, coagulopathies, prolonged drug action and increased mortality (see Chapter 12). Prevention of hypothermia is critically important and attention should be paid to monitoring body temperature, maintaining room temperature, warming fluids and inhalant gases, forced air blankets, heat pads and keeping the patient as dry as possible.

Teeth are commonly involved in oral surgery; they may be the subject of extraction for specific dental problems, but they may also be involved in jaw fractures, tumour resection and other surgical procedures. It is important when performing an oral surgical procedure that teeth are not overlooked. They should not be damaged unnecessarily by pins or screws or when used as anchorage for acrylic and wire splints. In young cats and dogs, particular attention should be paid to unerupted permanent tooth buds, as trauma to them may affect eruption and normal jaw development.

Where pulp exposure has occurred (accidentally or iatrogenically) teeth must be treated endodontically or extracted. Untreated pulpitis due to pulp exposure is painful and will lead to pulpal necrosis, periapical inflammation and possibly osteomyelitis. Traumatically injured teeth where pulp exposure has not occurred should also be monitored, as pulpitis and its sequelae may result.

Poor tooth extraction technique can cause damage to blood vessels and nerves, resulting in haemorrhage and paraesthesia, and is thought to be one cause of feline orofacial pain syndrome. Ocular penetration is a recorded complication following extraction of the maxillary molar teeth in dogs. Root remnants should not be left *in situ* if there is evidence of periradicular infection, inflammation or endodontic disease. Even in cases where the root remnant appears healthy, its extraction is preferable; healthy root remnants should *only* be left in place if they can be monitored radiographically.

Normal or functional, pain-free occlusion should be the aim of all oral surgical procedures. The mouth should be able to close comfortably without teeth traumatizing soft tissue or each other. Regular checking of occlusion, especially during fracture repair, is important. This can be facilitated by intubation through a pharyngostomy incision.

Wound healing

In general, the oral cavity is an environment that is favourable for wound healing. It has an excellent blood supply. Oral wounds are bathed in saliva, which has antibacterial properties and provides an ideal moist environment. Oral wounds epithelialize faster and have lower levels of inflammatory infiltration than skin wounds (Ten Cate, 2003).

A detailed understanding of the use of various mucosal and mucoperiosteal flaps, their manipulation and the establishment of non-tension primary wound closure is vital for optimal postsurgical wound healing (see *BSAVA Manual of Canine and Feline Wound Management and Reconstruction*). Maintenance of the integrity and competence of the lips, cheeks, tongue and oral mucosa is essential for normal oral function.

Suture materials used in oral surgery should avoid or limit bacterial adhesion and proliferation. Absorbable monofilament sutures such as poliglecaprone 25 perform better than multifilament or non-resorbable materials. Sutures are usually placed in a single interrupted pattern and in a single layer; however, an additional submucosal layer of continuous poliglecaprone 25 or polydioxanone can be used if some tension is unavoidable.

Antibiosis

Bacteraemia can result from periodontal therapy, tooth extraction or surgical treatment of oral trauma (Gorrel, 2004). Prophylactic antibiotics are currently indicated in elderly, debilitated and immunocompromised patients and those with pre-existing cardiovascular or other systemic disease.

Antibiotics are not indicated as the first line of control for periodontal disease because of the wide variety of potential pathogens, the variable penetration into gingival crevicular fluid, and the greatly increased resistance to antibiotics of bacteria within biofilms. Professional periodontal therapy followed by mechanical plaque control is the treatment of choice. Antibiotics may be useful as an adjunct in the control of chronic periodontal disease where optimal treatment is impossible.

Chlorhexidine gluconate is the oral topical antibacterial of choice. It is available as a flushing solution, gel or toothpaste, at concentrations between 0.5 and 2%. It has been shown to prevent the normal progression of periodontal disease in dogs over several years (Hennet, 2002). It is also useful in controlling plaque bacteria in other chronic oral diseases, including chronic gingivostomatitis in cats, where it is important in the long-term management of refractory cases.

Pain management and palliative care

Palliation, with particular attention to pain relief and the return to or maintenance of normal inanition, is necessary for conditions that cannot be treated surgically, either for financial reasons or because they are not amenable or responsive to surgery. These would include: inflammatory conditions such as feline chronic gingivostomatitis, which does not improve after, or that is not amenable to, surgery; craniomandibular osteopathy; conditions where there is irreversible loss of structure and function (e.g. in neoplasia); or conditions that are not well enough understood (e.g. feline orofacial pain syndrome).

NSAIDs are the first-line treatment of choice in both dogs and cats, unless specifically contraindicated or where there is a specific requirement for corticosteroids (as in immune-mediated conditions). Where NSAIDs do not appear to control the pain, the addition of tramadol (with care in cats) with gabapentin, amantadine or amitriptyline can be helpful, although the clinician should always be clear as to the outcome measures they are expecting and add each medication in logical progression. For example, if the patient appears miserable and listless, assuming that there is no other organic cause for this, the addition of tramadol may be helpful. If there are clear signs of central sensitization (the animal will not tolerate even light touch of its face or gums, where previously it would accept this attention) and/or of neuropathic pain (e.g. sudden, paroxysmal attacks on its own face), then gabapentin, amitriptyline or amantadine may be better choices.

Chronic inflammation

Chronic inflammation is a feature of a number of oral conditions and is often associated with the host's immune response to plaque. Professional periodontal therapy, selective tooth extraction, mechanical plaque removal (tooth brushing) by the owner and use of topical oral chlorhexidine will often control inflammation. In some cases systemic antibiotics and NSAIDs may be useful.

Nutrition

Studies have shown that humans and animals that are nutritionally depleted have poorer recovery from surgery, decreased immune function, longer hospitalization, and increased risk of morbidity compared with well nourished patients (Han, 2004). Inappetence or dysphagia are common signs in patients with chronic oral disease or who have had oral surgery. Soft, palatable food is often better for patients with oral pain or who are recovering from surgery, combined with adequate analgesia, which is also essential. Patients that have undergone major surgical procedures, such as jaw fracture repair or tumour resection, are often best managed using a feeding tube such as a naso-oesophageal, oesophagostomy or gastrostomy tube (see Chapter 5).

In the immediate postoperative period a specialized recovery diet that combines high calorie density, high digestibility and palatability is useful. Once a patient has a normal appetite, this food can be replaced by a conventional soft diet until oral wounds have healed. This can take up to 2 weeks, depending on the cause and severity of the oral wound. Hard food and biscuits can gradually be reintroduced at this stage.

It is tempting for owners to encourage inappetent patients to eat with frequently offered highly palatable treats, such as biscuits and sweets. However, it is important to advise owners that high-sugar diets predispose to dental caries and should therefore be avoided.

References and further reading

Beckman BW (2006) Pathophysiology and management of surgical and chronic oral pain in dogs and cats. *Journal of Veterinary Dentistry* **23**, 50–60

Gorrel C (2004) *Veterinary Dentistry for the General Practitioner.* Elsevier, Oxford

Han E (2004) Esophageal and gastric feeding tubes in ICU patients. *Clinical Techniques in Small Animal Practice* **19**, 22–31

Heath S, Rusbridge C, Johnson N and Gunn-Moore D (2001) Orofacial pain syndrome in cats. *Veterinary Record* **149**, 660

Hennet P (2002) Effectiveness of a dental gel to reduce plaque in beagle dogs. *Journal of Veterinary Dentistry* **19**, 11–14

Lemke KA (2007) Pain management II: local and regional anaesthetic techniques. In: *BSAVA Manual of Canine and Feline Anaesthesia and Analgesia, 2nd edn,* ed. C Seymour and T Duke-Novakovski, pp. 104–114. BSAVA Publications, Gloucester

Reiter A (2007) Dental surgical procedures. In: *BSAVA Manual of Canine and Feline Dentistry, 3rd edn,* ed. C Tutt *et al.*, pp.178–195. BSAVA Publications, Gloucester

Ten Cate AR, Bartold PM, Squier AC and Nanci A (2003) Repair and regeneration of oral tissues. In: *Ten Cate's Oral Histology: Development, Structure and Function,* ed. A Nanci, pp. 397–416. Mosby, St Louis

Wolf HF (2005) *Color Atlas of Dental Medicine.* Thieme, Stuttgart

Clinical case studies

A variety of case scenarios in dogs and cats will now be presented to illustrate the considerations to be made and the options available within a specific clinical setting. Information relating to the rehabilitation and palliation of each condition has been contributed to each case by the authors in the first part of this Manual, plus notes on nursing and homecare from Rachel Lumbis RVN. The reader should refer back to the appropriate chapters for further details. Photographs used to illustrate the principles and techniques within the cases do not necessarily feature the original patient.

Case 20.1
Right mandibular fracture in a puppy

A 12-week-old female Chihuahua puppy was presented with a right mandibular fracture distal to the fourth deciduous premolar, caused by a bite from another dog. The puppy had a full set of deciduous teeth but none of her permanent teeth had erupted. The lower jaw had drifted to the right, causing a significant malocclusion. The puppy was reluctant to eat or to be syringe-fed because of pain from the fracture.

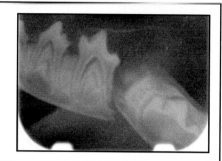

Radiography confirmed a fracture of the right mandible.

Agreed medical/surgical management

Conventional methods of fracture fixation, such as plates, pins or external fixators, were not appropriate in this case because of the puppy's size and the probability of iatrogenic damage to permanent tooth buds and adjacent neurovascular structures. (In cases where permanent dentition has erupted, interdental wiring and acrylic materials can be used to stabilize mandibular fractures, but this is more difficult in patients with deciduous dentition.) The case was managed using a tape muzzle to provide stability for the fracture and to hold the jaw in normal occlusion.

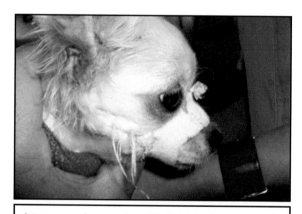

A tape muzzle was placed to hold the jaw in normal occlusion.

An oesophagostomy tube was placed and the puppy fed entirely through this for the first 7 days so that normal occlusion could be maintained, and to avoid inflicting pain by having to manipulate the fractured mandible whilst removing and replacing the tape muzzle.

Acute/chronic pain management

As with all pain assessments, a risk–benefit analysis must be made. It would be better in this patient to achieve effective perioperative analgesia with opioids and limit any problems with chronic pain as far as possible.

An opioid should be incorporated into the patient's premedication. In view of the puppy's age, pethidine (4 mg/kg i.m.) was used. At this age cardiac output may still be rate-dependent; therefore, using pethidine should help to prevent opioid-induced bradycardia during anaesthesia. The maximum duration of action of pethidine is about 2 hours, but by the time its effect would be waning, the mandibular nerve block should be effective. A mandibular nerve block, on the ipsilateral side to the fracture, was performed using bupivacaine 0.25% (see *BSAVA Manual of Canine and Feline Anaesthesia and Analgesia*). Great care should be exercised to avoid overdosage in such a small dog.

Opioids should be continued after the procedure, using methadone. There is less risk of bradycardia with methadone if the dog is not undergoing anaesthesia. The short duration of pethidine analgesia, and the fact that the injection stings, means it is less desirable for continuing long term as postoperative analgesia. Buprenorphine would be an alternative to methadone.

The puppy is likely to continue to be in pain after the procedure, or even after healing; a pain assessment will determine whether this is so (see Chapter 3). NSAIDs would be the treatment of choice. There appears to be some controversy about the dosing of NSAIDs in young animals; this patient, at 3 months, is not strictly paediatric (6 weeks and under) and it has been suggested (Mathews, 2008) that patients over 12 weeks require full dosing with analgesics to achieve sufficient pain relief. Using the lower end of the dose range without an initial loading dose (e.g. for carprofen and meloxicam), but checking that analgesia has been achieved, may be the sensible option.

A few days of transmucosal buprenorphine might help, although evidence in dogs suggests that doses need to be higher (30 micrograms/kg q8–12h) than in cats and may be associated with excessive salivation. If the patient becomes distressed on recovery, sedation may be provided with a low dose of acepromazine (0.005

mg/kg i.v.), repeated every 12 hours if necessary.

Tramadol would be indicated to reduce suffering, but the size of this patient would make administration more difficult. The drug can be dispensed in gel capsules but it is unlikely that she will take these if she is reluctant to eat. Tramadol is not only unauthorized for use in dogs but is also not recommended in human medicine for paediatric use, so extra caution should be used in animals under 3 months of age. Amitriptyline is a possibility for continuing pain and in the event of the development of a chronic pain state but, again, its effects on young animals have not been elucidated. Gabapentin is used in human paediatrics at reduced dosages, but this does not necessarily make it safe for the young animal.

Fear, stress, conflict concerns

This patient is a young dog that is in the process of learning about the world. The tendency for the owner will be to protect her and withdraw her from socialization and new experiences. Pain control (see above) is necessary to ensure that the puppy can continue to be introduced to the world without distress or making unpleasant associations. Pain, in itself, will make her more anxious; if experiences are associated with the pain, then these will be feared on each occasion they are encountered. Introduction to people is still possible, but they will need to be gentle and aware of the problems, avoiding the puppy's jaw area during interactions. Introduction to dogs should be limited to older calm dogs that can be approached cautiously by the puppy. Introduction to other experiences, such as household items, car travel, traffic, etc., should be undertaken with special caution, watching the puppy's reaction and ensuring that habituation and not sensitization is taking place (see Chapter 4).

Nutritional requirements

Dogs with severe oral trauma requiring significant surgical repair may need a feeding tube (see Chapter 5). As small toy breeds such as Chihuahuas are prone to the development of severe hypoglycaemia if there is poor food intake, establishing a means of providing adequate nutrition is strongly recommended. At the time of surgical repair, an oesophagostomy tube was placed to allow the puppy to be fed a diet to meet her growth requirements. A naso-oesophageal tube would be less ideal, as it is less easy to manage and more likely to be removed by the patient, meaning it can only be used for short-term feeding.

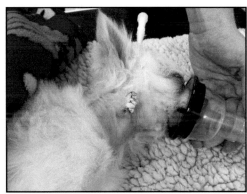 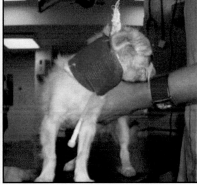

An oesophagostomy tube was placed under general anaesthesia. A bandage was applied to prevent self-trauma and to hold the tube in the correct position.

Diets typically used for tube feeding are energy-dense high-protein gruel-type diets. In this case, a moist growth (puppy) diet could be modified (liquidized with water) to enable its use in tube feeding. Daily calorie requirement should be calculated, feeds should be given little and often, and a record sheet kept of feeds and daily calorie intake (see Chapter 5). **Note that a 12-week-old puppy has an energy requirement approximately twice that of an adult dog, so the *calculated* RER should be doubled.** Tube feeding can be discontinued when the dog can eat voluntarily.

Physiotherapy

Gentle massage and application of warmth to the masseter and temporalis muscles (postoperatively and once pain is controlled) would theoretically be useful, but the size of the muscles in this patient would make such an approach challenging. Once adequate healing is confirmed and diet can progress from soft food, it would be beneficial to introduce increasingly more bulky and harder food to encourage progressive opening of the mouth and use of the jaw. Mixing the moist puppy diet with a dried puppy diet would therefore be helpful at this stage.

Hydrotherapy

Hydrotherapy is not indicated for this patient.

Acupuncture

Acupuncture may be helpful in providing adjunctive analgesia if it is tolerated by the puppy. Needling around the head (temporalis muscles and midline points such as GV17 and 20), Yintang and Taiyang (if tolerated) would be the most useful, although any points that may be strongly stimulated may help via a heterosegmental effect (descending inhibitory pain pathways; see Chapter 11).

Other nursing and supportive care

Monitoring

The puppy should be observed and monitored for signs of pain and discomfort. These signs would include:

- Depression
- Ptyalism
- Dysphagia
- Pawing at the mouth
- Reluctance or refusal to eat or drink, especially cold water.

Postoperative care

The puppy must be kept warm in the immediate postoperative period (note the fleecy bedding and blanket in the photo above). Hypothermia is a significant risk in such a small, young animal and will significantly delay anaesthetic recovery and increase risk if not addressed.

Accommodation

Ideally, the puppy should have access to a blanket, soft toy or other belongings from home to make her feel more secure. If she is hospitalized for a long period, it is useful for her to be able to see what is going on to prevent understimulation, but she will also need access to quiet. Young puppies are likely to be fearful and anxious, and will therefore benefit from frequent attention and close contact.

Medication

Care should be taken when administering any oral medications not to cause pain attempting to open the puppy's mouth. It may be preferable to give medications parenterally while the dog is hospitalized or to give liquid medications via the feeding tube to avoid opening the mouth at all.

Feeding

If a feeding tube has been placed, this should be monitored carefully, as the majority of complications involve tube occlusion or localized irritation at the tube exit site. Feeding and care of the tube are detailed in Chapter 5.

Once the tube has been removed, the puppy should be encouraged to eat and drink, and intake recorded. It is best not to force-feed, as this can lead to development of food aversion, especially where there is oral pain.

Owner advice and homecare recommendations

Chewing

The owner should be advised that for the immediate postsurgical period, it is important to prevent the puppy chewing on or biting any hard or solid structures. She should not catch stones or other hard substances, or play over-zealous games such as tug-of-war. Suitable, safe toys and chews can be recommended.

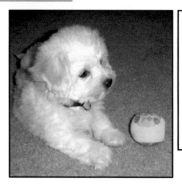

This puppy has been provided with a soft chew toy. (Courtesy of Gary M. Landsberg; reproduced from *BSAVA Manual of Canine and Feline Behavioural Medicine, 2nd edn*)

Monitoring

The owner should watch for signs of pain (see above) and for further signs of dental trauma:

- Abscessation, swelling or pain
- Teeth that are pink/purple often indicate bruising as a result of blood being released from vessels in the tooth pulp and haemoglobin passing into the dentine
- A grey or black tooth is almost certainly dead.

Follow-up

The owner must be advised when to return with the puppy for postoperative veterinary dental checks. This will provide an opportunity to conduct an examination of the oral cavity, as well as enquiring about the pet's health and wellbeing at home. On these visits, the owner should take the puppy to the nurse to be 'fussed over', put on the table and generally handled and rewarded, to get her used to coming into the surgery. Caution should be exercise regarding puppy parties, however, given the patient's size and possible continuing pain. Follow-up radiographs will be required to assess fracture healing and to confirm that deciduous teeth have been shed and permanent teeth have erupted normally.

Long-term tooth care

Once the fracture has healed and the veterinary surgeon has established that there is no continuing pain, the owner should be educated about how to introduce the puppy to having its teeth cleaned. Brushing techniques can be demonstrated on a model or 'demonstrator' dog. It is better if the dog becomes used to an oral hygiene programme at an early age:

1. Flavoured toothpaste should be placed on the brush and the puppy should be encouraged to lick the brush, with no attempt made to brush the teeth or restrain the puppy.
2. Once the puppy becomes comfortable with the process, the client can begin to touch the teeth gently.
3. Eventually, full brushing can take place.

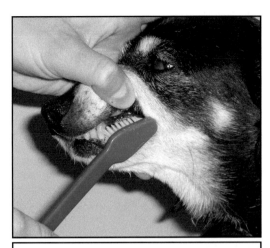

Brushing a dog's teeth can be demonstrated to owners so they can do this at home. (Courtesy of Rachel Lumbis)

References

Mathews KA (2008) Analgesia for pregnant and pediatric dogs and cats. *Veterinary Clinics of North America: Small Animal Practice* **38** (6), 1299–1301

Case 20.2
Chronic gingivostomatitis in a cat

A 10-year-old neutered male DSH cat was presented with lethargy, inappetence, signs of severe pain when trying to eat, and weight loss. Clinical examination revealed that he was in rather poor body condition, with marked gingivostomatitis.

The cat had mild to moderate build-up of calculus on his teeth. The inflammation was moderate to severe and affected primarily the gingiva associated with the maxillary premolars and molars and the mandibular molars, and non-gingival oral mucosa, especially in the region of the glossopalatine folds. There was moderate enlargement of the submandibular lymph nodes. Previous treatment had included routine scaling and polishing, intermittent antibiotics, and repeated injections of long-acting corticosteroids.

Blood samples were taken and showed normal T4 and no evidence of chronic renal failure. The cat was FeLV/FIV-negative but tested positive for feline calicivirus by virus isolation.

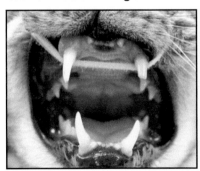

Severe inflammation affecting the gingival and oral mucosa lateral to the glossopalatine arch. (Courtesy of Lisa Milella)

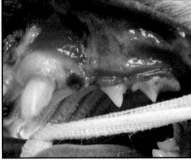

Inflammation extending to non-gingival oral mucosa above the left maxillary canine and premolars. (Courtesy of Lisa Milella)

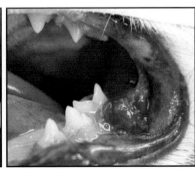

Inflammation and gingival hyperplasia distal and buccal to the left mandibular molar. (Courtesy of Lisa Milella)

Feline chronic gingivostomatitis (FCGS) is a syndrome characterized by persistent severe inflammation of the oral mucosa. A recent study suggested that FCGS has a prevalence of 0.7% in cats visiting first-opinion small animal veterinary practices (Healey *et al.*, 2007). Cats with FCGS present with signs of inappetence, lethargy and weight loss that are directly related to oral pain. Extraction of all premolars and molars, and sometimes also canines and incisors, is the treatment of choice. Preoperative radiographs are required to check for tooth resorption, retained roots and variations on normal dental anatomy; postoperative radiographs are important to confirm complete extraction of all tooth roots. FCGS will resolve in about 80% of cases treated in this way (Hennet, 1997).

Following full-mouth radiography, all teeth except the canines and incisors were extracted using an open (surgical) technique (see *BSAVA Manual of Canine and Feline Dentistry*). Mucoperiosteal flaps were sutured with 1 metric (5/0 USP) poliglecaprone using a simple interrupted pattern. Sutures were placed about 3 mm apart and the ends kept short in order to minimize postoperative plaque accumulation.

Refractory cases can often be successfully managed using a combination of topical chlorhexidine, systemic NSAIDs and systemic antibiotics (when required). Lyon (2005) demonstrated that, in cases where extraction of all the teeth was not desired, a combination of immunomodulation with ciclosporin, together with laser resection of proliferative tissue, produced a clinical improvement. Treatment with systemic or intralesional feline omega interferon has proved successful in some cases of refractory FCGS, though there are few peer-reviewed publications to support its use for treating FCGS (Southerden and Gorrel, 2007). Anecdotal evidence suggests that this treatment is less effective in cats that have not had extraction of at least all premolar and molar teeth.

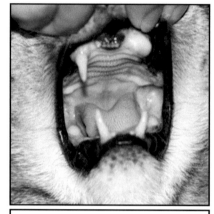

All premolars and molars have been extracted and the inflammation has resolved. (Courtesy of Lisa Milella)

Perioperative
Prior to surgery and postoperatively, oral transmucosal buprenorphine (see Chapter 3) may be a useful short-term measure. Tramadol (but see below for warnings concerning tramadol in cats) may be an effective alternative until meloxicam can be started, its delay being necessitated by the previous use of corticosteroids in this patient.

During surgery, mandibular/maxillary nerve blocks would be useful (see *BSAVA Manual of Anaesthesia and Analgesia*) but care should be taken not to exceed the toxic dose; cats are noted to be particularly susceptible. It is important to be aware that the patient may cause lingual trauma postoperatively before he recovers from the block because of a lack of sensation in the tongue, assuming he still has some teeth, if both mandibular nerves are blocked.

Long-term chronic pain
Chronic pain management is essential. The previous treatment with corticosteroids means that NSAIDs are contraindicated until the effects of the steroids have worn off but, where appropriate, meloxicam would be the first-line treatment of choice.

Tramadol can be used for analgesia in cats but seizures have been reported at the dosages used for the dog; 1–2 mg/kg could be used but owners should be warned of the possibility of seizure. This dosage is also difficult to deliver, though the drug can be dispensed into gel capsules. The drug is also very stable and so could be hidden in strongly smelling food, but this may still be detected and rejected.

Continuing severe pain would justify considering gabapentin or amitriptyline, both of which can be used concurrently with NSAIDs. Renal and hepatic function should be checked prior to treating with amitriptyline or gabapentin, as both are likely to require competent hepatic and renal function for clearance.

> **WARNING**
> * Amitriptyline should not be used with tramadol.
> * Amitriptyline should be used with extreme caution in patients with cardiac dysrhythmias.

The presence of chronic pain is a stressor. Additional stress in the clinic or at home will not help either the condition or the general wellbeing of the patient. There are two major considerations: treatment and handling at the veterinary clinic; and the patient's home environment.

Reducing stress in the veterinary clinic

- Reward and reinforce any positive experiences and associations with the veterinary practice and its team. Use positive touch, such as stroking and rubbing around the chin (unless mouth pain makes this painful in itself), grooming with a massaging groomer and gentle stroking of the chest, to release mood neurotransmitters, reduce blood pressure and encourage bonding. Such techniques will only be useful in cats that enjoy handling and touch.
- Take time with the patient to help him to relax before any intervention.
- Pheromone therapy may be useful, but should not replace identification of specific stressors, and appropriate behaviour therapy and pain relief.
- Minimize exposure to potential stressors, such as dogs and other cats, noises, and strong odours.

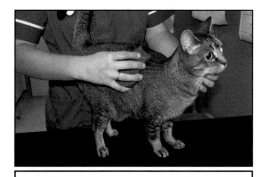

It may be beneficial to groom the cat gently, using a soft-bristled brush or a massaging groomer. (Courtesy of Rachel Lumbis and Catherine Kendall)

- Use the space in the cage to provide a hiding area (e.g. a cardboard box with a blanket or bed) and visual baffles (a towel over the cage door or hung to separate the cage) so the cat can *choose* to see and be seen or to hide.
- Use minimal restraint during procedures where possible.
- Continuity of scent stimuli helps cats to adapt to the clinic environment. Rather than removing all bedding each day, put extra beds or blankets in the pen and only remove some at each daily clean, so that some remain carrying the cat's scent.

Minimizing stress at home

The cat is feeling unwell. The owner should understand that he may not want to be handled, especially around the mouth, and that approach should therefore be careful. Enhancing the cat's core territory or environment will help him feel better (help him cope with the discomfort more easily), but it is also necessary to make some adjustments so that an inactive and unwell patient can still exploit the improvements in his environment.

- **Feeding.** This patient is inappetent and may need his appetite stimulating. Novel areas and food delivery may be helpful if an unpleasant association has been made with the routine feeding bowl/area. However, the usual bowls should not be removed; alternatives should be added elsewhere. Ensure the cat can easily reach the food (if he has previously fed at a height he may not feel like jumping), so adjust the position of the food, whilst making sure this does not make the cat anxious about it being available to competitors (the pet dog or a possible intruding cat if the food is placed near the cat flap, for example).
- **Water.** Cats generally prefer their water about a room's distance away from their food in a clear, wide bowl. It may be worthwhile putting down additional water bowls.
- **Access inside and out.** Cats would normally have more than one access in and out of their core territory (usually the house). Consider providing a second access point or ensure that the cat can use the existing access points, i.e. that they are not too high or too difficult to negotiate when the cat feels unwell and uncomfortable.
- **Scratching posts.** Are these easily accessible and appropriate for the patient? If the cat tends to scratch on horizontal surfaces, then a horizontal scratch post should be provided. If the post is an integral part of a piece of cat furniture then the patient should still be able to reach it if he does not feel up to climbing.
- **Hiding.** Provide multiple safe and comfortable hiding areas at different levels, or make sure that there is a 'step' system to allow the cat to reach its old favourite places.
- **Beds.** Provision of new beds such as radiator beds may improve comfort and wellbeing.
- **Play.** Modify games to very short bursts of gentle play, but continue to try to gently stimulate the cat.
- **Touch.** Use gentle touch, stroking and grooming in ways that the patient will enjoy to improve feelings of wellbeing and also to give the owner a sense of participating in their pet's treatment and nursing.

Nutritional requirements

Recording food intake

Cats with painful oral lesions such as stomatitis will often become inappetent. A careful record should be kept of the cat's calorie intake while he is hospitalized. If he eats significantly less than his resting energy requirement (RER; see Chapter 5), early consideration should be given to instituting nutritional support because this cat will be at risk of developing hepatic lipidosis secondary to anorexia, even if he is not overweight to start with.

Assisted feeding in hospital

Forced- or syringe-feeding could lead to the development of food aversion, which would be counterproductive. At the time of surgical repair, an oesophagostomy tube can be placed to allow the cat to be fed a diet that meets its nutritional requirements. An alternative would be a naso-oesophageal tube (see Chapter 5). A diet balanced for cats should be used, rather than a human tube-feeding diet, because cats have specific nutritional requirements. The cat should be fed his RER. Tube feeding can be discontinued when he eats voluntarily.

Encouragement to eat at home
Because of the chronicity of the gingivitis, this cat may need ongoing encouragement to eat sufficiently at home as well as in the hospital (see later).

Physiotherapy

- This cat may benefit from the application of warmth and gentle massage to the jaw muscles to help with pain and muscle relaxation, although this will be dependent on his tolerance to being handled around this area.
- Postoperatively, cold therapy can be applied (using cold flannels) for several days to help with pain relief and control of inflammation.
- After 3–5 days, warmth can again be applied.

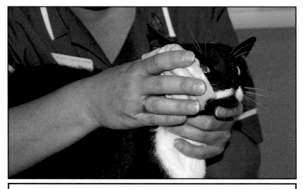

Warmth is best applied via warm flannels to the jaw area for approximately 10–15 minutes. (Courtesy of Rachel Lumbis and Catherine Kendall)

Hydrotherapy

Hydrotherapy is not indicated for this patient.

Acupuncture

Anecdotally, acupuncture has been used to treat the pain of chronic gingivostomatitis. There is currently no evidence that it has a direct anti-inflammatory effect, so no change in the appearance of the gums would be expected after treatment, but rather an improvement in the cat's demeanour and appetite. Acupuncture would ideally aim to target the head, and in this way, segmentally, the mouth. Needling should be performed in the midline, GV17 and GV20, plus Yintang and Taiyang, as well as the temporalis and masseters if tolerated.

Other nursing and supportive care

Monitoring
Hypothermia is a significant risk postoperatively. The cat should be kept warm during the recovery period, his temperature monitored, and action taken if his body temperature remains low. He should be observed and monitored for signs of pain and discomfort. These signs would include:

- Depression
- Ptyalism
- Dysphagia
- Pawing at the mouth
- Reluctance or refusal to eat or drink, especially cold water.

Feeding
If a feeding tube has been placed, this should be monitored carefully, as the majority of complications involve tube occlusion or localized irritation at the tube exit site. Feeding and care of the tube are detailed in Chapter 5.

Once the tube has been removed, the cat should be encouraged to eat and drink, and intake recorded. It is best not to force-feed, as this can lead to development of food aversion, especially where there is oral pain.

Grooming
It is likely that this cat will have ceased grooming himself due to the oral pain, particularly postoperatively. It may be beneficial to sit and gently groom him, using a soft-bristled brush or a massaging groomer. It would also be advisable to clean his eyes and nose, using warm damp cotton wool.

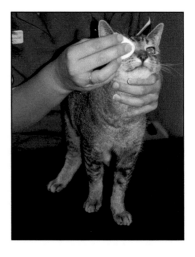

Cleaning the eyes with warm, damp cotton wool. (Courtesy of Rachel Lumbis and Catherine Kendall)

As well as the care considerations outlined above, grooming, in those cats that enjoy it, appears to be helpful in promoting relaxation and a decrease in anxiety. Simple methods of physiotherapy can be provided by owners several times daily (see above).

Grooming a cat that enjoys this will help the animal to relax and involve owners and their families in caregiving. (© Samantha Elmhurst)

Medications

Dosing this cat orally is going to be very difficult: giving medicines with food or as liquids should be considered. Regular visits to the veterinary surgery may be required if slow-release injections are used.

Diet and feeding

The owner should be asked to monitor the cat's food intake carefully and to contact the veterinary surgery quickly if he becomes inappetent. It is likely that the cat will prefer moist to dried food in the short to medium term as it is likely to be less painful to eat, but in the long term most cats will eat hard food if offered. If the cat is appetent, the use of strong-smelling soft food, such as pilchards, may help encourage food intake. Placement of food and water bowls should be considered (see above).

Oral hygiene

Twice-daily oral flushing with chlorhexidene will be helpful, if the cat will tolerate it. The owner should be informed that there may be some bloody saliva from the mouth and this can be carefully cleaned away using warm water.

Optimal homecare would include thorough tooth brushing of any remaining teeth. The owner should be instructed when to start this. A demonstration of how to restrain the cat and how to brush its teeth should also be provided, even if it involves the use of a model. However, one must be realistic about the fact that not all cats will tolerate this, and restraint will add to its stress and discomfort. Few cat owners are able or willing to perform dental homecare to a sufficient level to prevent plaque accumulation but its importance in plaque-sensitive FCGS cats should be emphasized.

Follow-up

The owner must be advised when to return for postoperative veterinary dental checks. This will provide an opportunity to conduct a full oral cavity examination, as well as to enquire about the pet's health and wellbeing at home. Active homecare and dental prophylaxis can also be discussed again.

References

Healey K, Dawson S, Burrow R *et al.* (2007) Prevalence of feline chronic gingivo-stomatitis in first opinion veterinary practice. *Journal of Feline Medicine and Surgery* **9**, 373–381

Hennet P (1997) Chronic gingivo-stomatitis in cats: longterm follow up of 30 cases treated by dental extractions. *Journal of Veterinary Dentistry* **14**, 15–21

Lyon KF (2005) Gingivostomatitis. *Veterinary Clinics of North America: Small Animal Practice* **35**, 891–911

Southerden P and Gorrel C (2007) Treatment of a case of refractory feline chronic gingivostomatitis with feline recombinant interferon omega. *Journal of Small Animal Practice* **48**, 104–106

21

Patients with ocular disease

Edited by David L. Williams

Introduction

In any patient with ocular injury or ill health, preserving vision and, perhaps even more importantly, reducing ocular pain must be the prime objectives. The veterinary practice has the opportunity to deal with patients in a holistic manner so that, even if appropriate treatment for the ocular condition is not immediately available, pain relief can be given and an appropriate environment arranged if the animal's sight is impaired, even as referral to a veterinary ophthalmologist is being arranged.

Ocular pain
Ocular surface irritation
The cornea is arguably the most highly innervated area of the body surface and it is therefore not surprising that trauma to the ocular surface produces trigeminal stimulation and pain. Indeed, what is perhaps surprising is the limited degree to which corneal ulcers, for example, produce blepharospasm, lacrimation and other obvious signs of pain in dogs and cats compared with human patients. Is it the case that companion animal species have lower levels of corneal innervation than people, or is it that the expression of such a painful stimulus is diminished in these animals? The latter seems more likely given that animals with a lack of corneal sensation (i.e. brachycephalic dog breeds such as the Pug and Pekingese, which have a reduced trigeminal nerve density in the superficial cornea) have a tendency to deep and potentially perforating ulcers, and the equivalent feline breeds (i.e. Persian, Burmese) have a tendency to develop corneal sequestrum (Blocker and Van Der Woerdt, 2001; Kafarnik et al., 2008). These particular animals also appear to have a reduced blink rate (although to date there are few firm data on normal blink rates across different breeds and species) and increased tear film evaporation, with a more rapid tear film break-up time, compared with other breeds of dogs and cats. It is therefore likely that the sensation of ocular surface irritation is important in provoking blinking and spreading of the tear film and in maintaining ocular surface health.

What then of animals with a pathologically reduced tear film in keratoconjunctivitis sicca (KCS)? Topical ciclosporin or tear replacement drops may be prescribed, but is there also the potential for ocular irritation in aqueous tear film deficiency? In a normal eye, ocular surface irritation from a noxious stimulus, be it physical or chemical, will provoke lacrimation, which will soothe the ocular surface and, it is hoped, remove the irritant focus. In KCS this opportunity is absent, and the animal will blink instead. However, in a dry eye, the more that blepharospasm occurs, the greater is the likelihood of trauma to the epithelial surface and also the likelihood of pain. This is known from studies of human patients with KCS (Nichols, 2006) but it is not known whether the same stimulus is experienced by dogs and cats. Some animals with KCS do exhibit increased blinking to the point of frank blepharospasm, but others do not. Two features of canine KCS may limit the extent of pain: a classic sign of the condition is a mucoid discharge, which serves to lubricate the otherwise dry ocular surface; secondly, personal observation suggests that dogs with dry eye have a reduced corneal sensation (as do human patients with the same condition).

An important feature of substantial ocular surface irritation is the reflex nervous stimulation through an antidromic trigeminal reflex arc, the so-called trigeminopupillary reflex, which causes profound miosis and a breakdown in the blood–aqueous barrier (Micieli et al., 1990). From a teleological perspective, this could be seen as the eye arming itself, as it were, against the possibility of a corneal penetration. Were such penetration to occur, fibrin within the aqueous would be available to clot and block fluid outflow through the perforation. The profound iridal sphincter constriction and ciliary body spasm themselves cause pain and the use of a cycloplegic drug, such as atropine, to paralyse the ciliary body is important for pain relief in such cases. Another method of reducing this irritation would be to combat the afferent rather than the efferent arm of the reflex. Topical NSAIDs can be effective in this, but the use of contact lenses should also be considered where there is profound irritation from exposure of a central corneal ulcer or from an irritant focus such as an ectopic cilium. A contact lens can provide relief from discomfort in the period before surgery to remove the offending noxious stimulus.

Appropriate medications for corneal and conjunctival pain include topical anaesthetics such as tetracaine or proxymetacaine. These can provide immediate analgesia but have deleterious effects on epithelial health and healing and so cannot be used long term. Systemic agents such as NSAIDs have some effect, but for severe pain, opiates such as methadone or tramadol can be useful. Recently, topical morphine at 0.5–1% has been reported as a potent ocular surface analgesic in dogs without deleterious effects on corneal epithelial migration or ulcer healing (Stiles *et al.*, 2003), although medication with this agent by such a route is not authorized for use in animals.

Inflammatory disease

In patients with uveitis, miosis and ciliary body spasm are key initiating factors in producing pain. Limited extrapolation from humans emphasizes the importance of cycloplegics (e.g. topical atropine) and the value of systemically administered pain relief through opiates – from tramadol, in relatively mild cases, to methadone in severe cases. Quite how useful NSAIDs are in these cases is unclear but, if opiates are not appropriate (e.g. in an animal being discharged home), systemic or topical NSAIDs should be considered to reduce pain and inflammation.

Glaucoma

Glaucoma is widely considered to be an extremely painful condition, at least in the acute phase. The ophthalmologist's prime aim, quite understandably, is to reduce intraocular pressure, and treatment with topical prostaglandin analogues or with intravenous mannitol infusions is usually successful in producing this rapidly. Pain relief is also important and it is unclear how many ophthalmologists and veterinary surgeons pay enough attention to pain relief in these situations, whether pressure reduction is successful or otherwise. More details of pain relief in glaucoma are given in the cases that follow.

Perioperative analgesia

For many years eyelid and corneal operations, as well as intraocular surgery, were performed without much consideration of pain relief apart from NSAIDs for a short period postoperatively. However, more emphasis is now being placed on intraoperative analgesia: nerve blocks in the lids during entropion surgery (Giuliano, 2006); retrobulbar injection for ocular surgery and enucleation (Accola *et al.*, 2006); and intracamerally (i.e. intraocular) in phacoemulsification (Gerding *et al.*, 2004).

Restoring and maintaining vision

One of the key aims of a veterinary ophthalmologist is to maintain vision where present, and restore it if compromised. There are no studies in the peer-reviewed literature that determine the quality of life for blind dogs and cats, though they often appear to cope well. The importance of vision relative to olfactory and auditory senses has been considered to be lower in animals, given their excellent senses of smell and hearing, than in people. However, in a recent study undertaken by the author it was demonstrated that sudden blindness caused by retinal detachment, sudden acquired retinal degeneration or glaucoma does have a profound effect on quality

of life in dogs (Williams and Jenkins, 2010) particularly in regard to their communication with other animals and their ability to exercise off the lead. Interestingly, from the same study, animals that had been blind for some time showed a somewhat improved quality of life over more recently visually deprived animals, presumably as they learned to cope better with their environment as the period of blindness increased.

Nevertheless, the primary aim of the veterinary surgeon should be to treat blindness, whether because of corneal obscuration in keratitis or trauma, lens opacification in cataracts, retinal detachment or degeneration, or optic neuropathy in glaucoma. The potential stress of surgery or repeated topical medication should be taken into consideration when attempting a cost–benefit analysis in such cases, but in most situations the decision will fall on the side of treating the animal rather than keeping the *status quo*, unless the animal is elderly with other concurrent health issues or financial constraints render treatment impossible for the owner. While our prime aim is the welfare of the animal itself, recommending a highly costly course of action to an owner unable to afford such an intervention may be unnecessary and could induce owner guilt. A comment that blind dogs and cats cope very well with their disability can resolve potential owner anguish.

Helping a blind cat or dog cope with its visual disturbance involves simple rules such as: not moving furniture around; using stair gates early in the onset of blindness; talking to animals more as they are approached; and getting down to the animal's level to experience potential difficulties it may have. Useful further reading on this is listed below.

References and further reading

Accola PJ, Bentley E, Smith LJ *et al.* (2006) Development of a retrobulbar injection technique for ocular surgery and analgesia in dogs. *Journal of the American Veterinary Medical Association* **229**, 220–225

Blocker T and Van Der Woerdt A (2001) A comparison of corneal sensitivity between brachycephalic and Domestic Short-haired cats. *Veterinary Ophthalmology* **4**, 127–130

Chester Z and Clark WT (1988) Coping with blindness: a survey of 50 blind dogs. *Veterinary Record* **123**, 668–671

Gerding PA Jr, Turner TL, Hamor RE and Schaeffer DJ (2004) Effects of intracameral injection of preservative-free lidocaine on the anterior segment of the eyes in dogs. *American Journal of Veterinary Research* **65**, 1325–1330

Giuliano E (2006) Regional anaesthesia as an adjunct to eyelid surgery. *Proceedings, British Association of Veterinary Ophthalmologists Congress* [available online at http://www.bravo.org.uk]

Kafarnik C, Fritsche J and Reese S (2008) Corneal innervation in mesocephalic and brachycephalic dogs and cats: assessment using *in vivo* confocal microscopy. *Veterinary Ophthalmology* **11**, 363–367

Micieli G, Tassorelli C, Viotti E *et al.* (1990) The trigeminal pupillary reflex as a model of vegetative-nociceptive interaction: physiological and clinical aspects. *Functional Neurology* **5**, 239–244

Mitchell N (2009) *Caring for the Blind Cat*. Lifelearn, Guelph

Nichols KK (2006) Patient-reported symptoms in dry dye disease. *Ocular Surface* **4**, 137–145

Stiles J, Honda CN, Krohne SG and Kazacos EA (2003) Effect of topical administration of 1% morphine sulfate solution on signs of pain and corneal wound healing in dogs. *American Journal of Veterinary Research* **64**, 813–818

Williams D and Jenkins C (2010) Quality of life assessments in blind and partially sighted dogs. *Scientific Proceedings, BSAVA Congress 2010: Veterinary Programme* p.438 [abstract]

Clinical case studies

A variety of case scenarios in dogs and cats will now be presented to illustrate the considerations to be made and the options available within a specific clinical setting. Information relating to the rehabilitation and palliation of each condition has been contributed to each case by the authors in the first part of this Manual, plus notes on nursing and homecare from Rachel Lumbis RVN. The reader should refer back to the appropriate chapters for further details. Photographs used to illustrate the principles and techniques within the cases do not necessarily feature the original patient.

Case 21.1
Corneal ulceration in a dog

A 10-year-old crossbreed bitch from a rehoming charity was presented with ocular pain, manifesting as constant narrowing of the palpebral fissure in both eyes. There was blepharitis bilaterally and both corneas demonstrated opacity and surface irregularity, with conjunctival hyperaemia. Closer investigation revealed a superficial epithelial abrasion across the entire cornea in both eyes, with concurrently constricted pupils.

Schirmer tear test results were 2 mm/min in each eye, confirming profound keratoconjunctivitis sicca (KCS). The intraocular pressure was 9 mmHg in each eye, showing that there was a degree of intraocular inflammation (probably as a reflex uveitis secondary to ocular surface pathology).

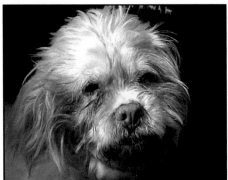 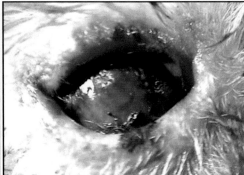

Bilateral corneal disease with dry eye.

Agreed medical/surgical management

Immediate amelioration of the ocular pain experienced by this patient is essential (see below).

The obvious medication to use in cases of dry eye is topical ciclosporin, although the proprietary preparation is expensive and this could be a problem given that this dog is from a rehoming shelter. Ciclosporin can be made up in corn oil at much less expense, although the cascade system prevents such use of generic preparations and supply of such a product not under the cascade system is a contravention of the Veterinary Medicines Regulations 2008 section IV subsection 27.2(a).

A carbomer-based tear replacement gel should also be applied.

Acute/chronic pain management

Much of the ocular pain from this condition probably arises from the iridal and ciliary body spasm occasioned by the uveitis. Topical atropine, given twice or three times daily, might be valuable to ameliorate these noxious intraocular inflammatory sequelae, although it has the disadvantage that further reduction in tear production may occur.

Longer-term pain relief with topical anaesthetic is not appropriate as this compromises healing of the corneal erosion. Topical ketorolac may be useful, but a small number of cases of corneal stromolysis with severe destructive stromal melting have been reported with this drug, so frequent evaluation of the eye is required. Unlike systemic NSAIDs, topical ketorolac can be used in the presence of systemic corticosteroids. There is some evidence that the topical use of morphine in 1% solution can provide analgesia without adverse effects on corneal healing.

The use of systemic corticosteroids should be avoided because they *may* have a deleterious effect on corneal epitheal healing and will also preclude the use of systemic NSAIDs to control the pain. Provided the dog has *not* received corticosteroids, systemic NSAIDs would be the first analgesic of choice. If these are ineffective (or contraindicated because of recent steroid use or side effects), tramadol may help to relieve suffering. If tramadol is not effective or causes unacceptable side effects, paracetamol ± codeine is an alternative (or addition in the absence of side effects).

Fear, stress, conflict concerns

This patient is in pain and is likely to be more anxious and reactive than usual. Approach to her head should be preceded by talking to her and by gentle touch. Owners and/or carers should bear in mind that the dog will need to be approached considerately. If the owner/carer reacts to her rubbing her eyes, she may learn to repeat the behaviour, so the owner should act pre-emptively and distract her. Interactions with other dogs should be kept to a minimum whilst she is recovering, unless the other dogs are well known to her and are calm on their approach. Although there is no evidence of specific efficacy in cases such as these, pheromone therapy may be helpful when the dog is kennelled at the practice and/or at the shelter (see Chapter 4).

Nutritional requirements

There are no specific nutritional requirements for this patient. Since oxidative stress plays an important part in the ocular surface pathology of KCS and ulcerative keratitis (Williams, 2008), optimal dietary antioxidant intake may be important.

Physiotherapy

Physiotherapy is not indicated for this patient.

Hydrotherapy

Hydrotherapy is not indicated for this patient.

Acupuncture

In theory, acupuncture could help to control the pain of corneal ulcers, but only as an adjunct to specific treatments, not as an alternative. It has been used in a variety of ophthalmic conditions in people but, as yet, there is no conclusive evidence of its effects. Segmental needling to the head – temporalis muscles, midline points (GV17, GV20), Yintang, Taiyang *if tolerated* – would be the logical choice, although if the patient is sensitive enough to the treatment any easily accessed points (e.g. SI11, GB30, ST36) may provide useful heterosegmental analgesia (see Chapter 11). The author [DLW] has preliminary unpublished data from dogs affected with KCS showing that acupuncture can be effective in increasing tear production as well as improving ocular comfort.

Other nursing and supportive care

Inpatient care and prevention of ocular trauma
Persistent vocalizing, coughing, barking or getting over-excited should be avoided during hospitalization. Time should be taken to sit with the anxious patient and provide reassurance. Careful monitoring for deterioration is required; infected ulcers can progress rapidly to melting ulcers. A dry eye lubricant should be used regularly (see above).

An Elizabethan collar should be fitted to prevent the dog from pawing her eyes and causing self-trauma. She should also be discouraged from rubbing her face on cage bars and other items.

Applying topical medication
- Before the application of topical medication, any ocular discharge should be gently removed; otherwise there may be reduced therapeutic effect. The nature and extent of the discharge should be recorded.
- When applying more than one topical medication, at least 6 minutes – preferably 10–15 minutes – should be left between applications; otherwise efficacy will be reduced.
- Drops must always be applied before ointments.
- If a mydriatic has been prescribed, the dog should *not* be taken outside immediately afterwards as she will be unable to constrict her pupil(s) and will therefore be uncomfortable and photophobic.

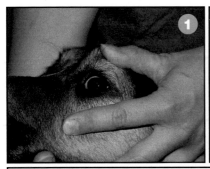 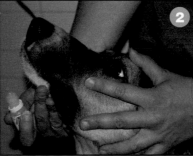 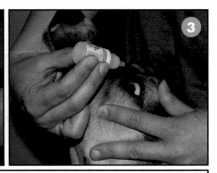

How to administer eyedrops to a dog. 1. Open the dog's upper and lower eyelids with one hand. 2. Tilt the dog's head back. 3. Apply one drop only on to the eye surface with the other hand. NB More than one drop increases reflex tearing, washing out medication and lowering its efficacy. (Courtesy of Rachel Lumbis and Catherine Kendall)

Owner advice and homecare recommendations

Prevention of trauma to the eye
The owner/carers should understand that it is vital that the dog does not interfere with healing or aggravate the injury. To this end, an Elizabethan collar or paw bandages should be fitted when the dog is left alone to prevent self-trauma. The dog should have only lead exercise until the ulcer has healed.

Monitoring for ocular pain
The owner should be warned about the signs of ocular pain:

* Self-trauma (rubbing of the eyes)
* Blepharospasm
* Photophobia.

Because of this patient's condition there will *not* be an increase in lacrimal flow to provide a further clue to the presence of ocular pain.
The owner should also be advised about the signs of infection:

* Purulent ocular discharge
* Redness
* Swelling.

The owner/carer should be advised to bring the dog straight back to the surgery if any of these are observed. They will also need to be advised how often they should bring her back to the surgery for routine re-checks in the absence of any complications.

Application of topical therapy
The owner should be shown how to apply topical ophthalmic medication. They will also need advice on applying multiple drugs (see above).

References

Williams, DL (2008) Oxidative stress and the eye. *Veterinary Clinics of North America: Small Animal Practice* **38**, 179–192

Case 21.2
Glaucoma in a dog

A 7-year-old male Bassett Hound was presented with a red, painful and apparently blind left eye. Intraocular pressure (IOP) in the left eye was 52 mmHg; the normally sighted right eye had an IOP of 22 mmHg (ideal upper limit 20 mmHg). Further investigations confirmed that the dog had glaucoma, an inherited condition in the breed.

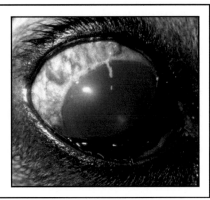

The glaucomatous eye on presentation, showing pupillary dilatation and episcleral engorgement.

Agreed medical/surgical management

Glaucoma may present acutely, as here, and is painful and blinding. In the past, immediate reduction in IOP was achieved using systemic hyperosmotic agents, such as glycerol by mouth or mannitol by intravenous infusion. Today, use of a topical prostaglandin analogue such as latanoprost is indicated. In many cases a reduction to normal IOP (<20 mmHg) occurs within 30 minutes of latanoprost administration, accompanied by intense miosis. Long-term control of the glaucoma using a carbonic anhydrase inhibitor such as dorzolamide is probably better than the continued miosis resulting from latanoprost administration, although the benefit of the prostaglandin analogue is that administration is once or twice daily while the carbonic anhydrase inhibitor needs to be given topically three or four times a day.

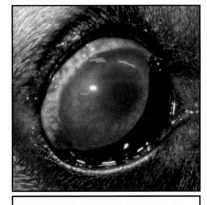

The eye 30 minutes after topical administration of latanoprost. There was miosis of the pupil and a reduction in IOP from 52 mmHg to 22 mmHg.

The other eye needs prophylactic medication with either a beta-blocker such as timoptol or a carbonic anhydrase inhibitor such as dorzolamide. Evidence shows that such medication of an as yet unaffected fellow eye delays the onset of glaucoma significantly, although it is still likely to occur in the other eye at some stage (Miller *et al.*, 2000).

Pain relief is generally provided by the reduction in IOP, although normalization of IOP is not guaranteed with anti-glaucoma medication.

A surgical approach – to reduce aqueous production or increase aqueous outflow – may be required, using a drainage implant or cyclodestructive treatment to obliterate the ciliary body that produces the aqueous. In severe cases enucleation or implantation of an intraocular prosthesis may be required. The latter procedure may bring with it ethical questions, since eviscerating the globe rather than enucleation is a technique for owner satisfaction rather than for the animal's benefit. Enucleation is the technique with fewer postoperative complications and preserving a blind eye is not in the animal's direct interests.

Acute/chronic pain management

Glaucoma can be a very painful condition – as painful in humans, it is said, as an acute intervertebral disc protrusion – so the pain should not be underestimated. However, the most effective pain relief will be achieved with prompt treatment of the condition (see above).

In the short term:

- Systemic NSAIDs may be helpful, although efficacy in glaucoma appears, anecdotally, to be lower than for ameliorating musculoskeletal or visceral pain
- Tramadol may also help to reduce suffering, though take care with vomiting and/or dysphoria
- Gabapentin may also be useful in painful glaucomatous eyes (Kavalieratos and Dimou, 2008)
- Opiates may be useful, but any that routinely cause vomiting, such as morphine, should be avoided, because vomiting will increase IOP.

Case 21.2 Glaucoma in a dog

The patient will need a gentle approach, being aware that approach from his left side may startle him and increase anxiety, or may even induce aggression, depending on his temperament and experience. The veterinary team and owners will need to bear this in mind when interacting with the patient, using their voices to alert him to their approach and gentle touch to help him accept handling around the painful eye.

Nutritional requirements

There are no specific nutritional considerations for this patient.

The patient should be approached gently from the non-blind side. (Courtesy of Rachel Lumbis and Catherine Kendall)

Physiotherapy

Physiotherapy is not indicated for this patient.

Hydrotherapy

Hydrotherapy is not indicated for this patient.

Acupuncture

In theory, acupuncture could have a role in pain relief in glaucoma but conventional treatment of the condition is the priority, with consideration of acupuncture only if the conventional treatment is unsuccessful or associated with unacceptable side effects. Studies on the use of acupuncture in human patients with glaucoma are inconclusive (Law and Li, 2007).

Other nursing and supportive care

Approach and handling
This needs to be gentle (see Fear, stress, conflict concerns, above).

Applying topical medication
See Case 21.1.

Owner advice and homecare recommendations

Administration of topical medication
Long-term administration of topical medication may be necessary. Application should be demonstrated to the owner.

Monitoring for recurrences or development in the other eye
The owner should be warned about the signs of ocular pain and advised to present the dog to the veterinary surgeon if these occur:

- Self-trauma (rubbing of the eyes)
- Blepharospasm
- Ocular redness and pupillary dilatation
- Epiphora
- Photophobia.

References

Kavalieratos CS and Dimou T (2008) Gabapentin therapy for painful, blind glaucomatous eye: case report. *Pain Medicine* **9**, 377–378

Law SK and Li T (2007) Acupuncture for glaucoma. *Cochrane Database Systematic Reviews* CD006030

Miller PE, Schmidt GM, Vainisi SJ, Swanson JF and Herrmann MK (2000) The efficacy of topical prophylactic antiglaucoma therapy in primary closed angle glaucoma in dogs: a multicenter clinical trial. *Journal of the American Animal Hospital Association* **36**, 431–438

22

Patients with dermatological disease

Edited by Hilary Jackson

Introduction

The effect of pain or discomfort induced by intractable pruritus on an animal's quality of life has not traditionally been addressed at length in veterinary dermatology texts, yet chronic skin disease undoubtedly has a significant impact on the health and well-being of both the pet and the family.

Skin innervation and the perception of pain and pruritus

Pain and itch are both elicited by noxious stimuli and are transmitted by unmyelinated C fibres and myelinated Aδ fibres. The sensations of pain and itch share many cutaneous mediators but are very distinctly separate sensory modalities. For example, itch is transmitted by a different subgroup of peripheral C fibres. As well as there being many cutaneous nerve receptors present in both the dermis and epidermis, there is increasing evidence that the cells of the epidermis, i.e. the keratinocytes, play an integral part in sensory perception. Once itching has started, the surrounding skin tends to be very sensitive to gentle, usually non-noxious, stimuli such as touch, and this can provoke further pruritus – a phenomenon known as allokinesis. Pruritus can also be exacerbated by dry skin (xerosis) or heat.

Pruritus in dogs

Assessment

Pruritus in the dog is typically manifested as scratching, licking, 'scooting' (rubbing the perineum along the ground), rubbing or head shaking. In order to assess the extent of the problem properly, it is essential to ask the owner if any of these activities have been observed.

Owner tolerance and family routine are important factors. If the owners are out all day at work and the dog sleeps overnight in a room that is distant from them, the severity of pruritus may be underestimated and it will be better tolerated than by an owner who is at home all day and lets the dog sleep in the bed or bedroom overnight. Additionally, dogs and owners will have different individual internal thresholds of tolerance to discomfort. All too familiar is the contrast between the owner who phones the clinic every time their dog scratches and the owner who presents a dog with lichenified, hyperpigmented and alopecic skin that apparently appeared only 'yesterday'.

Objective evaluation of both pet and owner by the attending veterinary surgeon is necessary to assess the severity of the disease correctly.

Numerical scales have been developed for research purposes to evaluate owner perception of pruritus and these are usually used in conjunction with a uniform assessment of clinical signs (CADESI = Canine Atopic Dermatitis Extent and Severity Index). These measures are becoming routinely employed in the evaluation of specific therapeutic interventions for canine atopic dermatitis. In clinical practice it is often useful to ask the owner to grade the degree of their pet's pruritus from 0 (none) to 10 (severe). If this is done at every visit, a more accurate assessment of any therapeutic or management intervention can be made.

The severity of pruritus can be assessed, in part, by examination of the skin. The presence of advanced excoriation and self-trauma is a clear indication of severe disease. However, some animals can be quite pruritic yet show only minor evidence on clinical examination; therefore, listening to the owner's description is an essential part of assessment. Close observation during the consultation is often helpful: a severely pruritic dog or cat will continue to scratch or lick in the clinic, whilst the more mildly affected animal will often be too distracted by the novel environment to demonstrate its pruritic state.

Management

The key to successful management is identification and management of the cause of the pruritus. In-depth discussion of the causes of pruritus and appropriate diagnostic techniques is beyond the scope of this chapter and the reader is referred to many of the excellent veterinary dermatology texts currently available, including the *BSAVA Manual of Canine and Feline Dermatology*.

The most common causes of pruritus in dogs are parasitic infestations, microbial infections and/or allergic skin diseases such as atopic dermatitis. Parasitic infestations should always be ruled out with appropriate tests such as skin scrapings and examination of coat brushings; in many cases, however, trial therapy with a parasiticide is the only effective means of excluding such a cause. Superficial infections with bacteria and/or *Malassezia* can be readily identified using skin surface cytology, and treatment of these infections often results in amelioration of pruritus.

Atopic dermatitis requires more in-depth investigation, and successful management relies on identification and control of the specific disease triggers. Although environmental allergens are commonly implicated, food allergens should also be considered in dogs with non-seasonal disease; a limited antigen diet, followed by provocation, is always recommended in these cases. Therapeutic interventions that have been shown to have efficacy for canine atopic dermatitis include calcineurin inhibitors (oral ciclosporin, topical tacrolimus) and glucocorticoids (oral or topical). Oral glucocorticoid doses should be tapered to the lowest dose administered every 48 hours that controls pruritus. There is less evidence for the efficacy of antihistamines, essential fatty acids and Chinese herbal supplements as monotherapeutic agents, although these treatments may be beneficial as steroid-sparing agents.

Allergen-specific immunotherapy is estimated to be effective in 60–70% of dogs with atopic dermatitis triggered by environmental allergens and is a good therapeutic option for a young dog because there are few long-term side effects of this treatment. However, the effects of this therapy are not clinically apparent until a few months into treatment and additional therapies are usually required to control pruritus during the initial stages.

Pruritus in cats

Assessment

Cats can be more difficult to assess than dogs. Pruritic skin diseases can manifest as self-induced alopecia induced by localized overgrooming and/or excoriations, often severe. The differential diagnosis for such conditions includes pain and psychological causes, as well as pruritus, although the evidence suggests that psychological causes are much less common than is often supposed. The licking or scratching that creates these lesions is usually performed in private, so cats are rarely presented to the veterinary surgeon as 'pruritic' but rather for investigation of the self-induced lesions. Many cats will become quite reclusive on account of their discomfort. Lethargy, inappetence and weight loss can also result from severe skin disease. The differential diagnosis for pruritus in cats includes parasitic infestation, microbial infections and allergic skin disease as the most common underlying aetiologies.

Management

Successful management of the allergic cat relies on identification and elimination of specific disease triggers. The role of parasites, especially fleas, should not be underestimated. Trial therapy with a parasiticide may be the only effective means of determining whether parasites such as fleas are involved, since the cat is likely to remove any evidence from the hair coat during grooming. Severely pruritic cats usually respond to short-term glucocorticoid therapy, although the effective dose is usually double that required in the dog.

Pain

The presence and degree of pain arising from dermatological conditions is often more difficult to assess than itch. Loss of appetite, weight loss and a lack of enthusiasm for walks or play are often present, but are not specific indicators of pain.

Dermatological pain is often associated with ulcerative conditions in which epidermal integrity has been compromised or where inflammation of the dermis or hypodermis is present. When epidermal integrity becomes compromised, bacteraemia, septicaemia, electrolyte and fluid loss may ensue and all contribute to the 'sick' patient. Erosive or ulcerative conditions affecting skin folds (intertrigous areas), footpads or mucosal surfaces in particular can cause distress and unwillingness to eat, to posture to urinate or defecate, or to ambulate. Dogs and cats with claw or footpad disease often present either with lameness or with an unwillingness to walk on hard or uneven surfaces.

Many of the severe ulcerative dermatological diseases arise from uncommon to rare autoimmune diseases. When, and only when, a definitive diagnosis has been made of autoimmune disease, high-dose glucocorticoid therapy, alone or in combination with other drugs, is required for long-term treatment. The immunosuppressive, anti-inflammatory and analgesic properties of glucorticoids are often highly beneficial to these patients, but alternative pharmacotherapy should be used to control pain until a definitive diagnosis has been made.

Many cases of otitis externa, with or without otitis media, can be extremely painful, and it is not uncommon for dogs to be presented for referral with a chronic disease history associated with unrecognized pain and discomfort. Clinical signs can be subtle and it is not until after successful treatment that the full impact of the previous discomfort may be realized. Affected dogs are often apparently 'head shy' and resent being touched around the ears. They can also present with aggression that is directed at their owners when topical medication of the ears is attempted.

For practical 'take home' pain relief, NSAIDs can be given as long as the patient is not taking glucocorticoids; tramadol or paracetamol + codeine are alternatives.

Chronic effects

The effect of chronic skin disease on the human–animal bond should not be underestimated, particularly when chronic pain is affecting the animal's normal behaviour, or where pruritus is affecting both the pet's and the owner's daily routine or causing sleep deprivation to both parties.

Further reading

Martin D and Martin A (2006) Pain management and anesthesia in veterinary dermatology. *Veterinary Clinics of North America: Small Animal Practice* **36**, 1–14

Mueller R and Jackson HA (2003) Atopy and adverse food reaction. In: *BSAVA Manual of Small Animal Dermatology, 2nd edn,* ed. AP Foster and CS Foil, pp.125–136. BSAVA Publications, Gloucester

Olivry T, Mueller RS and The International Task Force on Canine Atopic Dermatitis (2003) Evidence-based veterinary dermatology: a systematic review of the pharmacotherapy of canine atopic dermatitis. *Veterinary Dermatology* **14**, 121–146

Clinical case studies

A variety of case scenarios in dogs and cats will now be presented to illustrate the considerations to be made and the options available within a specific clinical setting. Information relating to the rehabilitation and palliation of each condition has been contributed to each case by the authors in the first part of this Manual, plus notes on nursing and homecare from Rachel Lumbis RVN. The reader should refer back to the appropriate chapters for further details. Photographs used to illustrate the principles and techniques within the cases do not necessarily feature the original patient.

Case 22.1
Chronic otitis externa in a dog

An 8-year-old female West Highland White Terrier had a history of chronic recurrent otitis externa. The first episode noted in the veterinary medical record was at one year of age. Since then there have been intermittent episodes, two or three per year, which have been treated symptomatically with various topical veterinary ear drops. Although her owners report that the problem generally settles down after the drops are applied for a few days, the dog never seems completely comfortable. Over the past few weeks she had become uninterested in walks or playing with her toys, and there is a bilateral malodorous otic discharge. Her owners have been applying an otic preparation, which was prescribed a few months ago, but this does not seem to help. She also licks her paws, axillae and groin.

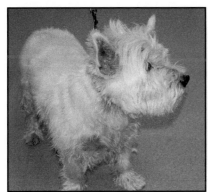 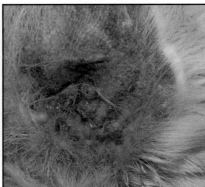

Severe chronic otitis externa. A purulent discharge can be clearly seen. (Courtesy of Peter Forsythe)

Physical evaluation revealed a bilateral purulent otic discharge, obscuring visualization of the ear canals and evaluation of the integrity of the tympanic membrane. The ear canals were painful on palpation and the right ear canal was thickened and lacked pliability. The external auditory orifices were narrowed by swollen tissue. The ventral and dorsal interdigital spaces were erythematous with patchy alopecia present.

Cytology of the otic discharge revealed numerous rod-shaped bacteria and degenerate neutrophils to be present bilaterally. Cytology from the interdigital spaces showed numerous *Malassezia* organisms. Swabs were taken for culture and sensitivity, and routine pre-anaesthetic blood work and urinalysis were undertaken.

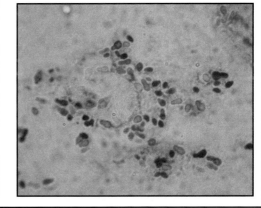

Malassezia organisms in a cytology smear. Diff-Quik; original magnification X100

Agreed medical/surgical management

Ear flushing under general anaesthesia is indicated, performed with irrigating saline. During the procedure it is important to establish the integrity or otherwise of the tympanic membranes, since rupture will predispose to otitis media. The degree of stenosis of the ear canals should be checked. A 7-day course of prednisolone prior to ear flushing may be appropriate to reduce inflammation and swelling of the ear canals.

Topical antimicrobial therapy for any ear infection is superior to systemic antibiotics. However, the ear canal must be clean and dry. In many cases it is necessary to repeat the flushing procedure during the course of treatment. Sequential examination with an otoscope accompanied by ear cytology should be used to monitor progress. Once the acute otitis has been addressed, future successful management relies on identification and control of the underlying atopic dermatitis (see Case 22.2).

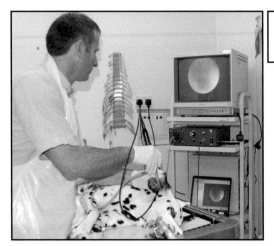

Performing video-otoscopy (VO) on an anaesthetized dog.

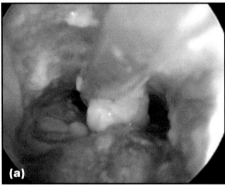 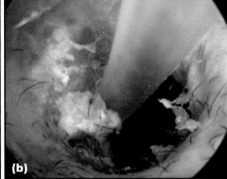

Flushing technique using a VO system. **(a)** Note the polypropylene catheter targeting tenacious debris. **(b)** The same ear canal after several cycles of flushing and suctioning. Reproduced from *BSAVA Manual of Canine and Feline Endoscopy and Endosurgery.*

Tissue calcification can occur with chronic otitis externa and this may lead to recurrent inflammatory episodes if it provokes a foreign body reaction. If otitis does not resolve, or is recurrent in the face of effective management of underlying disease, then the possibility of calcification should be considered. Persistence of middle ear disease associated with damage to the lining of the tympanic bulla is also a possibility. Effective assessment for these problems requires CT or MR imaging, these being more sensitive than radiography. Where significant tissue changes are present, surgical management of the ear disease is often the only option which will give sustained pain relief.

The *Malassezia* pododermatitis can be treated with topical washes or soaks in a shampoo containing miconazole. On occasion, adjunctive systemic treatment is also required using itraconazole or ketoconazole.

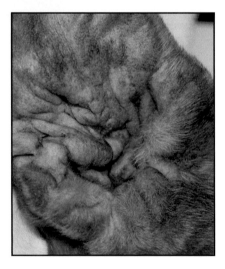

Chronic otitis externa results in hyperplasia of the affected tissue, stenosis of the ear canals and impaired conductive hearing.

Acute/chronic pain management

The pain and distress caused by otitis should not be underestimated.

Short-term glucocorticoids are helpful for their anti-inflammatory properties. They are usually continued for 7–10 days after the flushing procedure, to limit any exacerbation of inflammation caused by the procedure itself. Non-steroidal anti-inflammatory drugs (NSAIDs) are effective, but should only be used as an *alternative* to glucocorticoids, *not concurrently.*

For pre- and postoperative pain management, tramadol or paracetamol + codeine can be an effective adjunctive treatment. Tramadol capsules may need to be split or the drug dispensed into gel capsules to start this small patient off at a low dose (3 mg/kg q8–12h). The aim of tramadol is to reduce suffering by dissociating the animal from its pain, but it should be used *alongside* an anti-inflammatory agent where that is indicated, not instead of one. Tramadol or paracetamol ± codeine can be used concurrently with *either* glucocorticoids or NSAIDs.

Acupuncture may be helpful adjunctively (see below).

Pseudomonas ear infections are often associated with ulceration of the ear canal, pain and discharge, and many regularly used ear cleaners can 'sting'. Topical antimicrobial treatment promotes recovery; therefore, adjunctive pain relief can be withdrawn as the animal becomes more comfortable and inspection of the ear shows resolution of the otitis.

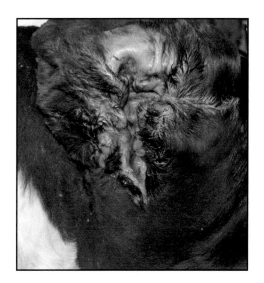

> Significant ulceration and discharge are associated with a pseudomonal ear infection. This patient had previously undergone lateral wall resection. (Courtesy of Peter Forsythe)

Fear, stress, conflict concerns

Chronic dermatological conditions, especially those involving pain, self-mutilation and/or pruritus, may predispose patients to appear tense, hypervigilant, anxious and/or snappy and 'grumpy'. Itch and pain are often perceived to be worse at night; therefore, rest and deep restorative sleep may be compromised. Sleep deprivation exacerbates pain. The use of pain relief at night, especially if it contains a component of central sedation, may be useful in minimizing this problem.

There are two main options for sedation of an anxious or agitated animal. The benzodiazepines diazepam and alprazolam can be used to effect, but one should beware of possible disinhibition of excitement/aggression. Acepromazine (ACP) combined with opioids can be a useful alternative to the benzodiazepines. Like these, ACP has a variable effect depending on the individual, but 0.01–0.03 mg/kg is recommended; the length of sedation following ACP is highly variable and may be prolonged so dosage frequency will need to be adjusted according to individual response. For additional sedation, butorphanol is preferable. If analgesia is required, as well as sedation, one of the mu receptor agonists is better. The choice depends upon the required duration: pethidine (meperidine) has the shortest duration at 30 minutes; methadone and morphine are longer lasting but beware of vomiting with morphine; buprenorphine is the longest lasting, using the lower dose for sick animals and higher doses for bouncy adults.

Such patients may have also developed learned fearful and/or aggressive behaviours as a result of having their feet and ears examined, bathed and treated. Simple techniques, such as warming the bottle of ear drops in the hand before applying, and drizzling the drops from the outside of the ear into the external meatus rather than pushing the nozzle into an inflamed and painful ear, may be helpful. Serious aversions would need to be treated by desensitization (see *BSAVA Manual of Canine and Feline Behavioural Medicine*), re-training the dog between bouts of otitis rather than during an acute flare-up. Short-term medicating by the practice nurse may be preferable to the dog's learning to be more fearful or aggressive of the procedure carried out by the owner. Further behavioural therapy may be helpful, but in the short term the ear treatment should not be made into an 'issue'. Ideally, these problems should be identified and dealt with prior to a crisis occurring.

Nutritional requirements

Food allergy/intolerance
A significant proportion of allergic skin diseases in dogs (including otitis) may be due, at least in part, to food allergy; thus, it is well worth ruling this out with a careful diet trial at some time during the work-up (see Case 22.2).

Essential fatty acids
Addition of extra essential fatty acids to the diet may help reduce inflammation and improve coat quality. Most of the commercially available limited antigen diets have an enhanced omega-3 and omega-6 essential fatty acid content, but the optimal ratio of omega-3 to omega-6 fatty acids for dogs with skin disease is currently unknown.

Physiotherapy

Physiotherapy is not indicated for this patient.

Hydrotherapy is not indicated for this patient.

> **WARNING**
> Ear disease can be made worse if water gets into the ear canal during swimming or hydrotherapy.

Acupuncture

As far as is currently understood, acupuncture does not have a direct anti-inflammatory effect, so should not be used as an alternative to anti-inflammatory agents. However, it may be used in combination with such agents to achieve two main effects: disease modification (long term); and analgesia for short-term pain relief.

Immune modulation
There appears to be a small population of atopic animals (and people) who respond dramatically well to acupuncture. This modulation of immune function is thought to be mediated via endorphins and to be similar to the effects of exercise. The acupuncture points are likely to be non-specific, but well tolerated limb points in muscle (LI11, SI11, ST36) are often used. Needling through areas of infected skin should be avoided.

Analgesia
Analgesia for the painful ear may be achieved via segmental needling in the temporal muscle and in healthy skin around the base of the ear. If this is not well tolerated by the dog, then the use of general points (GV14, GV17, ST36, LI11) may provide analgesia through heterosegmental and segmental effects (see Chapter 11). Sedation and a reduction in anxiety may be a useful side effect of treatment.

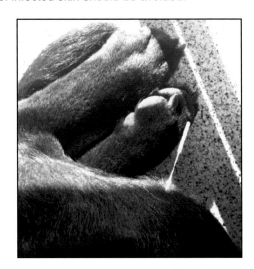

Acupuncture needle in ST 36.
(Courtesy of Samantha Lindley)

Other nursing and supportive care

Ear cleaning
The frequency of ear cleaning should be individualized according to the needs of the patient. Over-cleaning can lead to maceration of the epithelial lining and should be avoided.

Ear drops will not be effective if there is a lot of waxy debris or residual discharge within the ear canal. Before each application, the canal should be cleaned carefully using an appropriate ear cleaning solution. The patient should be allowed to shake its head and any residual cleaner should then be carefully wiped away. *Cotton buds are not recommended for routine cleaning by clients.*

Patient handling and restraint
Ear disease can be very painful, so it is important to restrain the dog well and carefully during ear treatments to avoid injury to staff and patient. Dogs that are in pain and showing signs of aggression may need to be muzzled. In some cases, the ear canal may be too swollen and painful for a complete treatment. Sedation for cleaning or a preliminary course of treatment may then be indicated. Unnecessary contact with the affected ear(s) should be avoided when restraining the patient for another reason or when stroking her.

Pain and self-trauma
The patient should be observed for signs of pain (depression, head shaking/rubbing, pawing at the ear). Self-trauma is a perpetuating factor in ear disease. The use of an Elizabethan collar or paw bandage(s) can help reduce further trauma, but the use of Elizabethan collars in ear disease should be avoided if possible as they increase local humidity and perpetuate infection.

Owner advice and homecare recommendations

Education about ear disease

The owner should be educated about the predisposing factors for otitis, including poor conformation of the ears and excessive swimming with the head under water. They should also be warned that otitis externa can impair conduction of sound to the tympanum, resulting in conductive deafness. This may be temporary if it is associated with discharge, but can become permanent if there are chronic tissue changes.

Medication and ear cleaning

The use of topical treatments should be explained to clients carefully.

- The owner should be shown how to clean the ears at home:
  - o The ear should be flooded with cleaner and then massaged for up to 5 minutes to allow penetration deep down into the ear
  - o The excess cleaner and debris should then be removed using cotton wool
  - o Cleaners are often required daily when treatment is initiated to remove excessive debris; however, the frequency of use should be reduced as the infection resolves to avoid maceration of the lining of the ear canal.

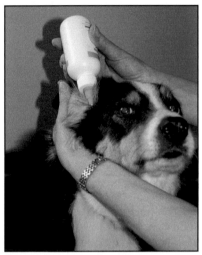

- Always demonstrate to owners the correct way to apply medication and topical therapy, to ensure that effective treatment is being given. As with any demonstration, it is often helpful to demonstrate first and then get the owner to repeat the procedure (on the other ear) to show that they are confident about what they have been shown.
- If the dog is not tolerant of the application of ear drops, the owner may require assistance, but it is worth mentioning that patience and gentle persuasion (treats) can often result in fractious or painful animals accepting the treatment.
- It is important to stress to the owner that nothing should be poked down the ear canal as this will be painful and could also cause further trauma.

Owners should be taught the correct way to give ear drops.

Case 22.2
Non-seasonal pruritus in a dog

A 4-year-old neutered male Labrador Retriever had a history of non-seasonal pruritus affecting his paws, ventral abdomen, limbs and face. He also had a history of recurrent otitis externa and superficial pyoderma. The pruritus had started when he was 18 months of age. Due to the non-seasonal nature of the pruritus, a differential diagnosis of atopic dermatitis triggered by food and/or environmental allergen(s) was considered, and a dietary trial was undertaken (see below).

Since being neutered the dog had had a tendency to gain weight. He also had hip dysplasia and had developed osteoarthritis, the discomfort of which was particularly evident in the winter months. He was medicated with meloxicam as needed to control pain.

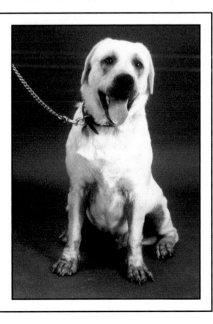

Labrador with atopic dermatitis. Note the self-induced alopecia, erythema and lichenification on his limbs, paws and ventral abdomen. (Reproduced from the *BSAVA Manual of Small Animal Dermatology, 2nd edn*)

Agreed medical/surgical management

In this particular dog it would be prudent to avoid systemic gluco-corticoids, given his tendency to gain weight and the concurrent treatment with meloxicam. Weekly bathing with a shampoo containing benzoyl peroxide may be helpful to prevent infections and remove allergen from the hair coat. Acute local flare-ups could be treated immediately with a topical hydrocortisone aceponate spray for 3–5 days. If pruritus is more sustained, he should be examined for physical and cytological evidence of secondary infections on the skin and in his ears. Appropriate antibacterial or antifungal treatment is often sufficient to restabilize an individual. Antihistamines and essential fatty acids (see below) may be of benefit if administered daily as a long-term treatment but are not effective in treating acute episodes.

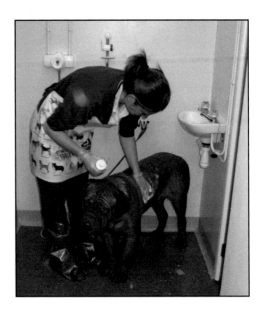

Medicated shampoo being applied to a pruritic dog. (Courtesy of Liz Mullineaux)

A 6-week limited antigen dietary trial should be carried out (see below). Following this, serum allergy testing and intradermal testing may be used to identify hypersensitivity to environmental allergens if allergen-specific immunotherapy is to be initiated. This mode of treatment is a safe long-term option but may take months to full effect, and adjunctive treatment is often required in the interim period.

Acute/chronic pain management

Itch or pain?

This dilemma is discussed in the introduction; in this atopic patient it is hoped that, having identified the cause of itch, it can be limited and managed by the treatment outlined.

The main consideration for pain management is likely to be where the patient self-mutilates or scratches or rubs to such an extent as to cause damage to, and pain from, the skin and underlying tissue. In the absence of glucocorticoid treatment, NSAIDs would be the first treatment of choice.

Chronic pain

Tramadol should help if the patient starts to show signs of struggling with his pain. If there is evidence of central sensitization (hyperalgesia and allodynia; see Chapter 3) then the addition of gabapentin or amantadine can be useful. However, human patients have reported itch as a potential side effect of gabapentin, particularly at higher doses, and this has also been reported anecdotally in one dog.

With regard to the osteoarthritis, NSAIDs should continue to be the mainstay of treatment for as long as this is appropriate and effective. Again, it is important to remember that NSAIDs should not be used concurrently with steroids. The addition of acupuncture (see below) may have benefits and should, on the basis of anecdotal reports, help in about 80% of cases of uncomplicated osteoarthritis in dogs. More details on analgesia in canine osteoarthritis are given in Case 14.8.

Fear, stress, conflict concerns

Prior to diagnosis the dog was very pruritic. This would manifest mainly at home and particularly during the evening. Additionally, he slept in his owners' bedroom and was routinely waking them up with his constant licking and scratching. As a consequence, both he and his owners were losing sleep, which was a source of stress for all concerned. Quality of life issues are a major concern for families with children affected by atopic dermatitis but this aspect is often overlooked in veterinary medicine. Frustration and stress can also arise from the chronic relapsing nature of poorly controlled disease and the financial and time commitments that burden the owners of severely affected dogs. The options for medical sedation of an anxious or agitated animal are discussed in Case 22.1, though these are short-term measures.

Punishment is inappropriate for licking/scratching behaviours, however annoying they may be to the owner. Punishment (either physical or verbal) will have one of three effects: reinforcement as an attention-seeking behaviour (confusing assessment of the effectiveness of the treatment); driving the patient to become cryptic in its behaviour (also confusing the assessment); or, if too effective in stopping the behaviour, causing other unwanted behaviours to manifest since the patient has a high drive to perform the scratching behaviour. Showing sympathy toward the dog may also reinforce the behaviour as an attention-seeking behaviour. The options for the owner are:

- **Ignoring the behaviour.** This is difficult if the dog is damaging himself; strategies such as collars or socks may be employed but are typically not very effective and can cause distress. They may also predispose to interdigital infections. Plastic claw covers may help limit the damage done by scratching, whilst allowing the patient to perform the desired behaviour and obtain some relief.
- **Distraction.** This is not appropriate at night if the owners are trying to sleep, but may help in the day or the evening. Play, a brief walk or visit to the garden, training exercises and/or relaxation techniques may be helpful, BUT it is vital that these are not seen as rewarding the scratching behaviour. Such techniques should be used when the worst of the scratching/licking is anticipated (i.e. pre-emptively before the behaviour starts). Once the behaviour has started, directing any attention towards the dog can reinforce the behaviour. In an emergency, the owner can do something that gains the dog's attention but without direct interaction. For example, the owner could run into another room or family members could start laughing in another part of the house, such that the dog stops scratching and seeks them out, but the behaviour is not directly reinforced.
- **Cooling.** At night it is helpful to keep the room in which the dog sleeps as cool as possible; a fan may help with this. Access to cool tiles, or even using chilled or dampened towels laid against the dog, may provide a distraction to soothe the itch. The use of sedating antihistamines prior to bedtime may also promote rest.

Clearly, NONE of these strategies is an alternative to diagnosis and treatment, but they may aid owner and patient whilst treatment is taking effect.

Nutritional requirements

Adverse reactions to food

A population of dogs with dermatological disease respond to dietary restriction and clinically relapse on challenge with food. It is not known at this time whether this is truly immunologically mediated (food allergy) or a non-immunological reaction (food intolerance). Thus the descriptive term 'adverse food reaction' is most appropriate. In a significant proportion of dogs with non-seasonal pruritus, their disease may be triggered, at least in part, by dietary components; thus, it is well worth ruling this out with a careful diet trial at some time during the work-up.

This involves taking a careful history of the complete diet, including treats and snacks. A diet containing a novel protein to which the patient has not been previously exposed can then be selected. This can be homemade or manufactured. Home-cooked diets usually require more effort on the part of the owner and compliance tends to be reduced when these are employed. An example of a suitable diet in many dogs is cooked fish and mashed potato. This can be safely fed for 3–4 weeks without supplementation, but lifelong use will require the advice of a veterinary nutritionist to ensure that the diet is balanced.

The diet should be fed for a significant amount of time to assess the full response: most dermatologists recommend 6–12 weeks, although some response is often apparent after 4 weeks. It is very important that the owner does not feed any tit-bits or snacks during this time. Owners often underestimate the significance of breaking the diet once; for example, one snack containing a protein that the dog is allergic to can set back the trial by weeks. Ensuring that neighbours and young children in the family do not give tit-bits is also important.

Another approach is to use hypoallergenic diets in which the protein and carbohydrate source may not be novel to the animal but the diet is hydrolysed so that all dietary antigens are reduced to molecular weights that are assumed to be too small to provoke an immune response. These diets are more expensive than novel protein diets and often less palatable. Failure to respond to one novel protein or hydrolysed diet trial may not rule out food allergy completely, as the individual response can be variable. A second dietary trial is sometimes required. If an animal does well on a home-cooked diet it is optimal to change to a similar commercially available diet for long-term feeding, as this will be nutritionally balanced. Occasionally, and for reasons not currently understood, some dogs only tolerate home-cooked food. If this is the case, then a veterinary nutritionist should be consulted regarding supplementation to balance the diet.

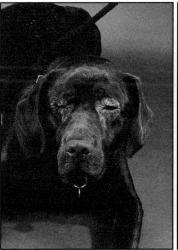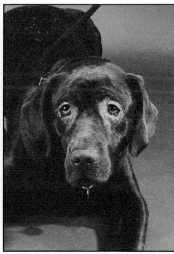

(Left) A 10-month-old female spayed Labrador Retriever with adverse food reaction. Clinical signs are facially orientated. (Right) The same dog after 4 weeks on a hypoallergenic diet trial. (Reproduced from *BSAVA Manual of Canine and Feline Dermatology, 2nd edn*)

A diagnosis of an adverse reaction to food can only be confirmed if the dog relapses after eating an offending food. This usually invokes a relapse of previously existing clinical signs within hours to days of introducing the food.

Supplements for skin health

There is evidence that dogs with atopic dermatitis triggered by environmental allergens have structural impairment of the epidermal barrier, the consequences of which might be enhanced transepidermal allergen penetration, increased transepidermal water loss and/or establishment of microbial infections. Ceramide-1 is an important component of the lipid barrier in the cornified layer of the epidermis. It contains α-linoleic acid; thus, supplementation with this omega-6 fatty acid has the potential to enhance skin barrier function.

Most commercially available limited-antigen diets have an enhanced omega-3 and omega-6 essential fatty acid content, though the optimal ratio of omega-3 to omega-6 fatty acids for dogs with atopic dermatitis is currently unknown. It is usually more cost-effective to feed one of the diets designed for dogs with atopic dermatitis than to supplement the regular diet with essential fatty acid capsules or liquid.

Supplements for joint health

See Chapters 7 and 14.

Weight management

This dog has the additional problem of a tendency to gain weight, which may be exacerbated by any steroid used for treatment of his dermatological disease. Any increase in bodyweight could have a negative impact on other medical problems, such as increasing the pain from hip dysplasia. Therefore, the initial priority with regard to weight management would be to ensure that he does not gain weight during the initial stages of therapy. Given that dietary change may be a key component of initial therapy for the pruritus, it would not be prudent to consider a purpose-formulated weight loss diet immediately. Instead, the priority should be to regulate intake closely on the diet chosen for dermatological disease. In this respect, the daily intake should be carefully calculated, with an aim of feeding at or just below (~80–90%) maintenance levels.

The owner should be instructed to weigh the food out precisely with kitchen scales, and it may be best to feed rations over a number of (e.g. 3–4) smaller meals. It is essential to avoid feeding tit-bits, not only to maximize the chances of success of the exclusion diet trial, but also to prevent unnecessary caloric intake. It should also be noted that supplementation with essential fatty acids, whilst potentially beneficial, will also increase caloric intake.

In addition, an exercise plan should be devised to maximize energy expenditure, whilst taking into account the orthopaedic concerns. Novel exercise techniques, such as hydrotherapy, may prove beneficial in stimulating activity and encouraging weight loss. The clinician should weigh the dog regularly and monitor progress, and ensure that weight is stable.

If, despite these preventive measures, the dog gains weight, it may be necessary to instigate a more formal weight management regime. If the dog does not respond to the food trial, a conventional programme with a purpose-formulated weight loss diet can be used. However, if skin signs respond positively to a single-source protein-source diet, it would be preferable to stay on that diet to avoid relapse. Since many exclusion diets are high in calories, achieving weight loss with such a food may prove challenging. For this, it may be preferable to ensure that a commercial exclusion diet is used, rather than a home-prepared recipe. Provided there are no specific contraindications, it may be worth considering drug therapy for weight loss (see Chapter 6).

Physiotherapy

See Cases 14.3 and 14.8 for physiotherapy for hip dysplasia and osteoarthritis, respectively.

Hydrotherapy

Hydrotherapy may also be useful for hip dysplasia (see Case 14.3) and for weight loss, especially where exercise is impeded by joint pain and obesity. **Hydrotherapy can be used safely in pruritic cases, as long as the skin problem has been controlled.** In cases where otitis externa is a risk, cotton wool should be placed in the ears before the session (and removed afterwards). Showers after hydrotherapy sessions, with or without any recommended shampoo, will help to remove any potential irritant from the chlorine in the pool water, which should be a minimal risk if the water chlorine concentrations are kept correct. Abnormal pH levels in the water may also cause irritation to skin.

Acupuncture

The most obvious indication is to help with the pain of the osteoarthritis (see Case 14.8).

A proportion of dogs (and humans) appear to be so sensitive to the effects of acupuncture that significant relief from atopic/allergic conditions is achieved (see Case 22.1: Immune modulation). This is an observed rather than a proven effect and probably applies to a relatively small percentage of the population. However, if the only alternative, having tried all other approaches, is lifelong glucocorticoids, or if the dog reacts adversely to any other treatment, then acupuncture could be offered. Weekly or twice-weekly treatment, including electroacupuncture if necessary, should be tried for at least 4–6 weeks. The acupuncture points are likely to be non-specific, but limb points such as ST36 and LI11 are commonly used from both a neurophysiological and a traditional perspective. The effect is hypothesized to be mediated by endorphins (see Chapter 11) and may modulate immune function in the same way as do optimum levels of exercise. Needling through infected areas of skin should be avoided. Discrete lesions can be treated if they are particularly troublesome; the technique involves needling in healthy skin close to the margin of the lesion. **Acupuncture is not an alternative to diagnosis and specific therapy where indicated.**

Other nursing and supportive care

Pain and self-trauma

The patient should be observed for signs of pain/itch (depression, scratching). The use of an Elizabethan collar or paw bandage(s) can help reduce self-trauma as a short-term measure, but Elizabethan collars should be avoided if there is ear disease. Clipping hair and removing dead skin and crusted material allows more successful topical treatment of the affected area. In some instances of severe skin damage, moist, antiseptic bandages may need to be applied. Affected area(s) should not be touched when restraining the patient or stroking him. Bathing affected dogs in cool water can be beneficial. *Do not use hot water because it can intensify itching.* The frequency of bathing should be restricted to only a few times a week, to avoid drying the skin out and increasing the itchiness. Emollients or humectants applied after bathing may limit this drying effect.

It is useful to keep the animal busy/occupied whilst in the hospital to distract him from the skin irritation. Toys can be used and/or try and situate him in a kennel where he can observe people coming and going.

Depending on the suspected cause of the pruritus, bedding should be selected carefully. Padded or stuffed bedding harbours dust mites. For patients with proven sensitivity to dust mites, it should be replaced with an easily washed towel or fleecy veterinary bedding. Coarse fibres may irritate already pruritic skin and could be replaced with something softer.

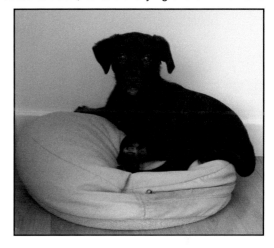

Padded beds can harbour dust mites.

Weight management

The nurse will have an important role to play in any weight loss programme. Regular re-checks for weighing, and for dietary and exercise advice, along with encouraging and motivating the owner, are all important parts of the weight loss programme (see Chapter 6).

Owner advice and homecare recommendations

Considerations for skin disease

The owner should be reminded that skin disease is often managed, not cured and, as a result, can be the cause of significant frustration. Support for the owner is therefore paramount and a patient, listening ear is likely to be appreciated.

The importance of carrying out treatment as directed must be stressed to owners, particularly the importance of sticking to the appropriate diet if food allergy is confirmed. The owners should also ensure that the dog has access to a comfortable bed, as well as to cool areas, to ease his itching.

Routine flea and tick prophylactics are to be recommended on all animals in the household, as bites from ectoparasites can exacerbate pruritus in animals with atopic dermatitis. Various sprays are available to control household dust mite populations but there is currently insufficient evidence to recommend these for use in the environment of dogs with dust mite hypersensitivity.

Considerations for osteoarthritis

- The owners should consider the surface on which he walks – trying to keep to grass or firm sand where possible rather than concrete. Non-slip rugs on laminate or tiled floors can be used to help movement around the house.

- A ramp may be useful to aid getting into and out of cars or to avoid steps.
- As dogs become more unsteady with arthritis they often hesitate going down steps. The use of a lead slipped around the dog's neck may give him extra confidence and the owner should encourage him also to use a wall (if available) against which to steady himself.
- This young dog is likely to enjoy play and exercise. Creative games such as hide and seek can be used to stimulate him mentally.

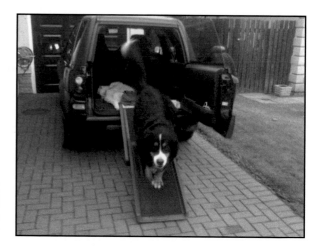

Ramps can help dogs with limited mobility get in and out of cars. (Courtesy of Samantha Lindley)

Index

Page numbers in *italics* indicate figures
For clinical use of drugs, see individual case studies

Index